Interpersonal Psychotherapy

Interpersonal Psychotherapy

A Global Reach

EDITED BY

MYRNA M. WEISSMAN

JENNIFER J. MOOTZ

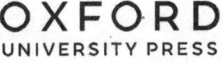
OXFORD
UNIVERSITY PRESS

OXFORD
UNIVERSITY PRESS

Oxford University Press is a department of the University of Oxford. It furthers
the University's objective of excellence in research, scholarship, and education
by publishing worldwide. Oxford is a registered trade mark of Oxford University
Press in the UK and certain other countries.

Published in the United States of America by Oxford University Press
198 Madison Avenue, New York, NY 10016, United States of America.

© Oxford University Press 2024

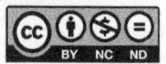
CIP data is on file at the Library of Congress

ISBN 978–0–19–765208–4

DOI: 10.1093/oso/9780197652084.001.0001

Printed by Marquis Book Printing, Canada

Human attachments are critical to well-being. Their severance through death, disputes, life changes, or their absence is associated with distress. This simple truth holds across different cultures and situations and is a reflection of our common humanity. IPT is one method in an evidence-based toolbox to repair these human fractures.

This book is dedicated to my late husband Gerald L. Klerman, whose early death in 1992 prevented him from seeing the endurance and global reach of his ideas. He would be pleased and not surprised as he truly believed in the common humanity of all people and their need for human attachments. Appreciation and affection to my husband Jim Frauenthal for supporting this effort all the way.
Myrna M. Weissman
2023

Dedicated to my beloved "attacharinos" Elia and Nora.
Jennifer J. Mootz
2023

CONTENTS

"Never let a good crisis go to waste." This is advice attributed to Winston Churchill and explains the context of our book.[1] It was largely written during the pandemic crisis, which decreased travel, extended the global reach, and increased mental health attention. The abrupt transition to telehealth and virtual platforms made communication possible. The deaths and disruptions of the virus exacerbated interpersonal problems of grief, disputes, life transitions, and loneliness, heightening mental health demand and requiring new ways of providing care. The pandemic was a fitting context for a book on global reach.

Interpersonal Psychotherapy: A Global Reach describes the rapidly expanding global dissemination of interpersonal psychotherapy (IPT), including the development of new training, technologies, and the use of IPT all over the world and in diverse populations. Many of the advances described occurred over the last 5 years; some accelerated during the pandemic. Many, if not most, of these developments are underreported in scientific journals, making this volume a resource for those looking to investigate and implement IPT in their own settings. For instance, the Finnish government has initiated widespread training of health workers in IPT. The World Health Organization, under the guidance of Mark Van Ommeren, endorsed IPT as an evidence-based intervention for depression and translated the group IPT manual into numerous languages. IPT has also been adapted as self-guided therapy. Task-shifted delivery of IPT has proliferated, and digitized versions of web-based and mobile applications have emerged. This book covers training considerations, especially for task-shifted or lay providers; use of technology; and the continuing evidence base of IPT. The book includes implementation in low- and middle-income countries (LMICs) and humanitarian settings that have limited funds for research and dissemination. Providing practical guidance and experience, global experts from different countries describe the implementation of IPT in their settings, sharing templates of training and adaptation. The book does not focus on the pandemic. Lessons learned from it— mental health impact, consequent implementation, training, and technological advances—are discussed. Our main goal is to provide practical information on the adaptation and use of IPT in different settings and in countries around the world. Chapters are practical, succinct, and clinically oriented.

This book is unique in several ways. It is written by the originator of IPT and includes descriptions of a recent modification of IPT, interpersonal counseling (IPC), which has been implemented by community health workers in LMICs. The techniques, strategies, and problem areas are identical in IPT and IPC. The IPT scripts have been simplified in IPC, and it is briefer. The co-author has experience in training and implementation of IPT in low-income settings globally and in the United States. She has led several initiatives to design new technology that can help support scalable solutions to increase access and reach of IPT. Both authors have real-world experience working with IPT and IPC in training and implementation and continue to participate in their developments.

Expect to find inconsistencies between the chapters. We deliberately asked the authors to tell us about their experience in their words. While we edited chapters for brevity and clarity, we did not shape ideas. Although sections are organized by region, country, and different populations, we in no way assume homogeneity among national or diverse populations. Rather, we operate from an intersectional lens, which asserts that a multitude of identities (e.g., race, socioeconomic status, sexual orientation, migrant status) influences experiences with systems and shapes worldviews. Thus, cultural adaptations are not assumed to be implemented as a checklist, catchall solution or be prescriptive for any population. They instead highlight different practical approaches to tailoring and provide guideposts for adaptations that counselors can consider to better fit patients' values and worldviews. As contributors mention and we support, approaching delivery of any psychotherapy, including IPT, with a stance of cultural humility is paramount.

To be honest, psychotherapy, a psychosocial method, has always had "low status" on the scale of scientific treatment methods, seen by some as a last resort when nothing more is available. This belief seems to be changing. On May 12, 2022, *Nature*, a highly prestigious scientific journal, published an evaluation of randomized trials and reported the following: "Overall, the arms with psychosocial interventions were most cost effective, highlighting the value of including well designed psychosocial components and government-led multifaceted interventions for the extreme poor."[2] We would add that even the less poor or not at all poor can have psychosocial problems that limit their life and interactions with others.

The core of IPT is rooted in the observation that human attachments are critical to well-being. Their severance through death, disputes, life changes, or their absence are associated with psychological distress. This simple truth with different expressions holds across diverse cultures and reflects our common humanity. IPT is one of the psychosocial methods in an increasingly evidence-based toolbox to repair these human fractures when they occur.

REFERENCES

1. Woolston CA. Rush of inspiration. *Nature*. 2022;612:83–84.
2. Bossuroy T, Goldstein M, Karimou B, et al. Tackling psychosocial and capital constraints to alleviate poverty. *Nature*. 2022;605(7909):291–297.

ACKNOWLEDGMENTS

We first want to acknowledge our contributors from all over the world, including the United States. They freely and enthusiastically trusted us with their stories in a language that for some would not have been their first choice and sometimes apologetically having to delay because of COVID-19 or a humanitarian, global, regional, or local crisis. We thank the contributors for their dedication in addressing health disparities rooted in systemic and structural inequities that ultimately shape attachment and interpersonal experiences. We are grateful for your work to improve people's life experiences through creative implementation and adaptation of IPT to better fit diverse health system contexts, worldviews, and value systems. With little constraint of format and style, you have shared your story so others can learn from your experience.

We thank the clients and patients for being willing to take a chance with IPT and share their oftentimes most difficult life experiences with their therapists. For those who agreed to be a part of a research study and dedicated time and effort to discuss symptoms and experiences, your willingness has helped the many contributors of this book and others to better understand the benefits and limitations of IPT for different populations and settings. We thank you for that.

We thank Oxford Press and Sarah Harrington, who let us grow this book to more than double the size and who saw the value to the reader of the unknown and unexpected. We also thank them for moving our original contract for a traditional book, with a fixed price for those who can pay, to add an open access version that could be accessible to all.

We thank the originators and sustainers of the International Society of IPT (ISIPT), originated by several people and especially the Australian groups (Michael Robertson, Rebecca Reay, and C. M. Robinson), sustained by Scott Stuart as the first president, and carried forth by Holly Swartz, Paula Ravitz, Oguz Omay, John Markowitz, and Heather Flynn. These leaders worked tirelessly and imaginatively across the globe and as volunteers. The global reach would not have been possible without their efforts.

We thank Lena Verdeli for her continuing an excellent global program in IPT training. We thank Milton Wainberg for his imaginative implementation of IPT into healthcare all over the world.

We thank our university, Columbia, and the Department of Psychiatry in the Vagelos Columbia College of Physicians and Surgeons, as well as the affiliate New York State Psychiatric Institute, for supporting us throughout the book gestation as part of our regular research and teaching. This book was written nearly entirely through isolation of COVID when we worked remotely and talked by Zoom. In some ways, COVID has leveled the field as we communicated with global authors, whether our next-door colleagues or part of the global reach.

We thank the National Institute of Mental Health and others along the way for supporting through several mechanisms, the studies behind the evidence and the fellows who were trained in clinical trials and implementation science.

We thank our families who patiently tolerated our travels, off-hour Zoom calls, and dining room table takeover of papers, cell phones, and computers as part of this adventure across the globe. We are so fortunate to have family and colleagues who appreciate our common humanity and need for human attachments, even when outside world conditions challenge both.

A special thanks to Tenzin Yangchen. While still a graduate student, her brilliance promises an extraordinary future of innovation and achievement. She patiently took the fragments of paper as we passed them along and magically shaped them into a visual book.

Myrna M. Weissman, PhD, is Diane Goldman Kemper Family Professor of Epidemiology and Psychiatry, College of Physicians and Surgeons and the Mailman School of Public Health at Columbia University and co-director of the Division of Translational Epidemiology and Mental Health Equity at New York State Psychiatric Institute (NYSPI). She received her PhD in epidemiology from Yale University School of Medicine, where she also became a professor. Early in her career she began working with Gerald Klerman at Yale University on the development of what became interpersonal psychotherapy (IPT). Together they carried out this work, testing IPT in several clinical trials of maintenance and acute treatment of depression and a modification for primary care called interpersonal counseling (IPC). They published the first IPT manual in 1984 after there were 2 clinical trials supporting its efficacy. Dr. Weissman's research is on understanding mood and anxiety disorders in families using methods of epidemiology, genetics, neuroimaging, and the application of these findings to develop and test empirically based treatments and preventive intervention. She has received numerous awards for her research. She has been elected to the National Academy of Medicine, an arm of the National Academy of Science. In 2009, she was selected by the American College of Epidemiology as 1 of 10 epidemiologists in the United States who has had a major impact on public health. In 2016, she was listed among the 100 most cited researchers by Google Scholar Citations. In 2020, she received the Brain and Behavior Pardes Humanitarian Award. In 2021, she received the annual Research Award from the American Psychiatric Association. In 2022, she was ranked by Research Community as 34th female scientist globally and from all disciplines and 25th in the United States, based on the H-index meter of citations of work. In 2023, she received the Mood Disorder Research Award from the American College of Psychiatrists.

Jennifer J. Mootz, PhD, is a licensed psychologist, Assistant Professor of clinical Medical Psychology (in Psychiatry) at Columbia University and research scientist at the Research Foundation for Mental Hygiene/New York State Psychiatric Institute. She earned her PhD in counseling psychology from Texas Woman's University in 2015. She specializes in digitization of evidence-based treatments for task-shifted delivery by nonspecialized providers among marginalized populations. She has partnered with community and governmental agencies in low-resource and disaster-affected settings in low- and middle-income countries and the United States to conduct research on implementation of comprehensive mental health care scale-up and development of technology to improve delivery of mental health services. Comprehensive scale-up has included implementation of interpersonal counseling for common mental disorders. Jennifer has received a K23 Mentored Patient-Oriented Research Career Development Award from the National Institute of Mental Health to treat common mental disorders in women in Mozambique by addressing intimate partner violence in couples with couple-based IPT. As part of her role to lead development of technology for the Mental Wellness Equity Center in New York City, she is leading projects to adapt a provider-guided application developed in Mozambique for local task-shifted providers and develop an IPC mobile health tool that will include self-guided modules for adolescents and young adults. She has an interest in developing novel digitized methods technology to support training and supervision of nonspecialized providers in low-resource settings. Jennifer was honored to receive 2 awards from the American Psychological Association for her global research and was identified as 1 of 35 "emerging psychologists" across 22 different countries by the International Congress of Psychology.

CONTRIBUTORS

Niloofar Rafiei Alhosaini, MA
Department of Psychology, Najafabad
  Branch, Islamic Azad University,
  Najafabad, Iran

Timothy Anderson, PhD
Department of Psychology, Ohio
  University

Nazan Aydın, MD
Professor of Psychiatry, private practice, Istanbul, Turkey

Malin Bäck, PhD
Linköping University, Department
  of Behavioural Sciences and
  Learning (IBL)

Silvio Bellino, PhD
Department of Neuroscience,
  University of Turin, Italy

Charlotte Bernard, PhD
University of Bordeaux, National
  Institute for Health and Medical
  Research (INSERM), Research
  Institute for Sustainable
  Development (IRD), Bordeaux
  Population Health Research
  Centre, UMR 1219, Team GHiGS,
  Bordeaux, France

Sarah E. Bledsoe, PhD, MPhil, MSW
Associate Professor, School of Social
  Work, Co-Director National
  Initiative for Trauma Education and
  Workforce Development, University
  of North Carolina at Chapel
  Hill, 325 Pittsboro Street, Chapel
  Hill, NC

Marc Blom - Dr, PsyQ
Psychiatrist, Department of Mood
  Disorders, PsyQ, The Hague, The
  Netherlands

Kelsey A. Bonfils, PhD
Assistant Professor, Clinical
  Psychology Ph.D. Program, The
  University of Southern Mississippi

Paola Bozzatello
Department of Neuroscience,
  University of Turin, Italy

Eva-Lotta Brakemeier
Professor of Clinical Psychology
  and Psychotherapy; University of
  Greifswald

Santiago W. Bueno-López, PhD
Community Association of
  Progressive Dominicans (ACDP)

Natasha L. Burke, PhD
Assistant Professor, Department of
  Psychology, Fordham University,
  Bronx, NY, USA

Josephine Chase, PhD
School of Social Work, University of
  Georgia, Athens, GA

Sarah Chiao, MA
Research Assistant, Mental Wellness
  Equity Center, Columbia University

**Joseph Pui-yin Chung, MBBS,
MRCPsych, FHKCPsych,
FHKAM(Psychiatry)**
Associate Consultant, Department
  of Psychiatry, Pamela Youde
  Nethersole Eastern Hospital,

Hong Kong; Honorary Clinical
Assistant Professor, Department of
Psychiatry, Li Ka Shing Faculty of
Medicine, University of Hong Kong.
Department of Psychiatry, Pamela
Youde Nethersole Eastern Hospital,
Chai Wan, Hong Kong

Kathleen F. Clougherty, LCSW
Training Director, Global Mental
   Health Lab, Teachers College,
   Columbia University, USA

Kevin Croswell, PsyD
Department of Veterans Affairs Office
   of Mental Health and Suicide
   Prevention, United States

Pim Cuijpers, PhD
Department of Clinical, Neuro
   and Developmental Psychology,
   Amsterdam Public Health re-
   search institute, Vrije Universiteit
   Amsterdam, The Netherlands
WHO Collaborating Centre for
   Research and Dissemination of
   Psychological Interventions, Vrije
   Universiteit Amsterdam, The
   Netherlands
Babeş-Bolyai University, International
   Institute for Psychotherapy, Cluj-
   Napoca, Romania

Mary Curran, MSW
University of Washington School
   of Social Work & Department of
   Rehabilitation Medicine, Seattle,
   WA, USA

Marcelo Feijo de Mello, MD
Federal University of Sao Paulo,
   Faculdade Israelita de Ciências da
   Saúde Albert Einstein

Cindy-Lee Dennis, PhD
Professor and Women's Health
   Research Chair, [2] Department of

Psychiatry, Faculty of Medicine,
   Lawrence S Bloomberg Faculty of
   Nursing, University of Toronto, Li
   Ka Shing Knowledge Institute, St.
   Michael's Hospital, Toronto, Canada

Laura Dietz, PhD
Associate Professor, Department
   of Rehabilitation Science and
   Technology, University of Pittsburg,
   Department of Counseling and
   Behavioral Health, Pittsburg,
   PA, USA

Tara Donker, PhD
GGZ inGeest, Mental Health Care,
   Amsterdam, The Netherlands
Vrije Universiteit Amsterdam, Clinical,
   Neuro-, and Developmental
   Psychology. Amsterdam, The
   Netherlands

Els Dozeman, PhD
Amsterdam Public
   Health, Mental Health program,
   Amsterdam, The Netherlands
GGZ inGeest, Mental Health Care,
   Amsterdam, The Netherlands

Fiona Duffy, D.Clin.Psychol
University of Edinburgh, UK

David D. Ebert, PhD
Department of Clinical, Neuro
   and Developmental Psychology,
   Amsterdam Public Health re-
   search institute, Vrije Universiteit
   Amsterdam, The Netherlands
WHO Collaborating Centre for
   Research and Dissemination of
   Psychological Interventions, Vrije
   Universiteit Amsterdam, The
   Netherlands

Beyza Nur Ekşi, MsC
Psychologist, Neuroscience, private
   practice, Istanbul, Turkey

Jennifer Elkins, PHD, MSSW
Associate Professor, University of
Georgia School of Social Work

Zelde Espinel, MD, MPH
University of Miami, Miller School of
  Medicine

Paulino Feliciano, BA
Mozambique Ministry of Health

Linda Irvine Fitzpatrick, PhD
Strategic Programme Manager,
Thrive Edinburgh SRO, Edinburgh
Wellbeing Pact and Community
Mobilisation

Luis E. Flores, Jr, PhD
Assistant Professor, Queen's
  University, Humphrey Hall, 62 Arch
  Street, Kingston, ON, Canada

Heather A. Flynn, PhD
Professor and Chair, FSU College
  of Medicine, Department of
  Behavioral Sciences and Social
  Medicine, Director, FSU Center for
  Behavioral Health Integration

Glenda Garcia, MA
Project Coordinator, Division of
  Child and Adolescent Psychiatry,
  Columbia University Vagelos
  College of Physicians and Surgeons,
  New York State Psychiatric Institute,
  New York, New York

Michelle Garcia, LCSW
Community Association of
  Progressive Dominicans (ACDP)

Elisabeth Glatigny-Dallay, MsC
Clinical Psychologist, Centre
  Hospitalier Charles Perrens,
  Bordeaux, France

**Viktoriia Gorbunova, DSc Social
Psychology**
Zhytomyr State University, Zhytomyr,
  Ukraine

Patricia Graham, PhD
Department of Clinical Psychology,
NHS Lothian, Musselburgh, Scotland.

Sophie Grigoriadis, MD
Associate Professor of Psychiatry and
  Scientist; Head, Woman's mood
  and anxiety clinic: reproductive
  transitions; Department Psychiatry
  and Sunnybrook Research Institute,
  Sunnybrook Health Sciences
  Centre, Department of Psychiatry,
  Faculty of Medicine, University of
  Toronto, Canada

Nancy K. Grote, PhD (deceased)
University of Washington School of
  Social Work

Henok Hailu, MSCP, MA
Lecturer, Addis Ababa University

Mathias Harrer, MsC
Department of Clinical, Neuro
  and Developmental Psychology,
  Amsterdam Public Health re-
  search institute, Vrije Universiteit
  Amsterdam, The Netherlands
WHO Collaborating Centre for
  Research and Dissemination of
  Psychological Interventions, Vrije
  Universiteit Amsterdam, The
  Netherlands

**Maria Yellow Horse Brave
Heart, PhD**
Department of Psychiatry and
  Behavioral Sciences, University of
  New Mexico, Albuquerque, NM.
  Horse Nation Healing, Rapid City, SD

Bernadette D. Heckman, PhD
Department of Counseling and
  Human Development Services,
  University of Georgia

Timothy G. Heckman, PhD
College of Public Health, University of
  Georgia

Romi Hera
Candidate for Bachelor of Science
    Degree in Psychology with Minor
    in Business Administration at
    Northeastern University

Theodore Hovaguimian, MD
Retired psychiatrist and psycho-
    therapist (Geneva, Switzerland);
    Founder and former president of
    the Swiss Society of Interpersonal
    Therapy (SSPI)

Manli Huang, MD
Professor, Deputy Director of
    Psychiatry Department, Deputy
    Director of Key Laboratory of
    Mental Disorder Management of
    Zhejiang Province, First Affiliated
    Hospital of Zhejiang University
    School of Medicine, Zhejiang
    University, Hangzhou, China

Tonda L. Hughes, PhD, RN
Henrik H. Bendixen Professor
    of International Nursing (in
    Psychiatry), Associate Dean for
    Global Health, Columbia University
    School of Nursing, New York,
    NY, USA

Jennifer E. Johnson, PhD
C. S. Mott Endowed Professor of
    Public Health, Division of Public
    Health College of Human Medicine,
    Michigan State University, Flint,
    MI, USA

Kosse Jonker
Clinical Psychologist and
    Psychotherapist, Practice for mental
    health care LEV, Voorburg, The
    Netherlands

**Teresa Judge-Ellis, DNP, FNP-BC,
PMHNP-BC, APRN, FAANP**
University of Iowa College of Nursing,
    Associate Clinical Professor

Roma Kaczmarkiewicz, MA, EdM
Research Assistant, New York State
    Psychiatric Institute, New York,
    NY, USA

Eirini Karyotaki, PhD
Department of Clinical, Neuro
    and Developmental Psychology,
    Amsterdam Public Health re-
    search institute, Vrije Universiteit
    Amsterdam, The Netherlands
WHO Collaborating Centre for
    Research and Dissemination of
    Psychological Interventions, Vrije
    Universiteit Amsterdam, The
    Netherlands

Saida Khan, MA
Mozambique Ministry of Health

Jeremy D. Kidd, MD, MPH
Assistant Professor of Clinical
    Psychiatry, Columbia University
    and New York State Psychiatric
    Institute, New York, NY, USA

Anat Brunstein Klomek, PhD
Dean, Baruch Ivcher School
    of Psychology, Reichman
    University, Israel

**Vitalii Klymchuk, DSc Social
Psychology**
National Psychological Association,
    Kyiv, Ukraine

Claire Koljack, MD
Psychiatry Resident, Columbia
    University and New York State
    Psychiatric Institute, New York,
    NY, USA

Manasi Kumar, PhD
Brain and Mind Institute, Aga Khan
    University, Kenya

Susan Laitala
University of Helsinki, Helsinki,
    Finland, Department of Psychiatry,

Brain Center, Helsinki University Hospital

S. J. Langer, LCSW-R
Private Practice Psychotherapist, Faculty, Department of Art Therapy and Humanities and Sciences, School of Visual Arts, New York, NY, USA

Yael Latzer, DSc
Faculty of Social Welfare and Health Science, School of Social Work, University of Haifa,
Eating Disorders Institution, Psychiatric Division, Rambam, Health Care Campus, University of Haifa, Haifa, Israel

Benjamin Lavigne, MD
Psychiatrist, Lausanne University Hospitals, Lausanne, Switzerland

Roslyn Law, D.Clin.Psych
The Anna Freud National Centre for Children and Families, UK

Roberto Lewis-Fernández, MD
Professor of Clinical Psychiatry, Columbia University Vagelos College of Physicians and Surgeons, Director of the New York State (NYS) Center of Excellence for Cultural Competence and the Hispanic Treatment Program, Research Area Leader, Anxiety, Mood, Eating and Related Disorders, New York State Psychiatric Institute, Lecturer on Global Health and Social Medicine, Harvard University, New York, NY, USA

Weihui Li, MD, PhD
Professor, Director of Behavioral Medicine Department, The Mental Health Institute of Second Xiangya Hospital, Central South University, Changsha, Hunan Province, China

Xuejun Liu, MD
Professor and Vice President, The Brain Hospital of Hunan Province, Changsha, Hunan, China

Yanli Luo, MD
Professor, Director of Department of Psychological Medicine, Renji Hospital, Shanghai Jiao Tong University School of Medicine, Shanghai, China

Sue Luty, PhD
Psychiatrist, Mothers and Babies Service, Christchurch

Valasía Makridis, BA
Research Assistant, Division of Child and Adolescent Psychiatry, New York State Psychiatric Institute, New York, New York

Sandra Pardi Maradian, MPH
National Mental Health Programme, Ministry of Public Health, Lebanon

John C. Markowitz, MD
Professor of Clinical Psychiatry, Columbia Vagelos College of Physicians & Surgeons, Research Psychiatrist, New York State Psychiatric Institute, NY, USA

Jennifer Martin, PhD
Crisis Care Center, Rapid City, SD

Camila Matsuzaka, MD, PhD
Federal University of Sao Paulo, Faculdade Israelita de Ciências da Saúde Albert Einstein
Departamento de Psiquiatria, Universidade Federal de São Paulo, São Paulo, SP, Brazil

Sean Mayberry, MBA
Chief Executive Officer, StrongMinds, Kampala Uganda

Susan Meffert, MD, MPH
Professor, UCSF Department of
  Psychiatry, Affiliated Faculty, UCSF
  Global Health Sciences, USA

Marcelo Feijó Mello, MD, PhD
Full Professor School of Medicine,
  Faculdade Israelita de Ciências da
  Saúde Albert Einstein (FICSAE),
  Associate Professor Department of
  Psychiatry Federal University of Sao
  Paulo, Brazil

Milena Mello, MA
New York State Psychiatric Institute
Columbia University Department of
  Psychiatry

Clara Miguel, PhD
Department of Clinical, Neuro
  and Developmental Psychology,
  Amsterdam Public Health re-
  search institute, Vrije Universiteit
  Amsterdam, The Netherlands
WHO Collaborating Centre for
  Research and Dissemination of
  Psychological Interventions, Vrije
  Universiteit Amsterdam, The
  Netherlands

Kasperi Mikkonen, MA, PhD
University of Helsinki, Helsinki,
  Finland, Department of Psychiatry,
  Brain Center, Helsinki University
  Hospital

Hiroko Mizushima, MD, PhD
Director, Mental Health Clinic,
  Motoazabu, Minato-ku,
  Tokyo, Japan

Viivi Mondolin, MA, PhD
The FinnBrain Birth Cohort Study,
  Turku Brain and Mind Center,
  Department of Clinical Medicine,
  University of Turku, Department of
  Psychology and Speech-Language
  Pathology, University of Turku

Jennifer J. Mootz, PhD
New York State Psychiatric Institute
Columbia University Department of
  Psychiatry

Laura Mufson, PhD
Viola W. Bernard Professor of
  Medical Child Psychology,
  Associate Director, Division of
  Child and Adolescent Psychiatry,
  Columbia University Vagelos
  College of Physicians and Surgeons.
  Director of Clinical Psychology,
  New York State Psychiatric Institute,
  New York, New York 10032

Ibrahima Ndiaye, MD
Service de psychiatrie, CHNU de
  Fann, Dakar, Senegal

Delson Ngozo, BA
Mozambique Ministry of Health

Dawn Nolan, MSc
Clinical Nurse Specialist,
  Interpersonal Psychotherapist,
  Rangiora, New Zealand

Márta Novák
Department of Psychiatry, University
  of Toronto, Toronto, Canada

Danielle M. Novick, PhD
Evidence-based Psychotherapy
  Coordinator, Behavioral Health,
  Pittsburgh Veterans Affairs Medical
  Center, Pittsburgh, PA, USA

Oguz Omay, MD
Perinatal Psychiatrist, Les Toises
  Center for Psychiatry and
  Psychotherapy, Lausanne,
  Switzerland; Past President of ISIPT

Maria A. Oquendo, MD
Perelman School of Medicine,
  University of Pennsylvania

Nalan Öztürk, MD
Perinatal Psychiatrist, private practice, Istanbul, Turkey

Clare Pain, MD, FRCPI, DSc
Professor of Psychiatry, University of Toronto and Addis Ababa University

Sapana R. Patel, PhD
Associate Professor of Clinical Medical Psychology, Columbia University Vagelos College of Physicians and Surgeons, Director of Strategic Planning and Curriculum Development, Center for Practice Innovations, Director of Services and Implementation Research, Center for OCD and Related Disorders, New York State Psychiatric Institute, New York, NY, USA

Frenk Peeters, PhD
Professor of Clinical Psychology, Department of Clinical Psychological Science, Faculty of Psychology and Neuroscience, Maastricht University, Maastricht, The Netherlands

Xavier V. Pereira, MBBS, MPsyMed
Adjunct Professor, Taylor's University School of Medicine & Director of Health Equity Initiatives

Jorge Petit, MD
Services for the UnderServed (S:US)

Indira Pradhan, MA, M.Eda
Transcultural Psychosocial Organization Nepal, Kathmandu, Nepal

Klaus Ranta, M.D., Ph.D
Hospital District of Helsinki and Uusimaa

Paula Ravitz, MD
Department of Psychiatry, Faculty of Medicine, University of Toronto, Toronto, Canada
Sinai Health System, Department of Psychiatry, Toronto, Canada
Lunenfeld-Tanenbaum Research Institute, Sinai Health System, Toronto, Canada

Rebecca E. Reay, PhD
Senior Research Coordinator, Academic Unit of Psychiatry & Addiction Medicine, ANU Medical School Academic Unit of Psychiatry & Addiction Medicine, Canberra Hospital | Building 4, Level 4 | Medical School, Australia

Charles F. Reynolds III, MD
Distinguished Professor of Psychiatry and UPMC Endowed Professor in Geriatric Psychiatry, emeritus, University of Pittsburgh School of Medicine

Hasan Rezaei-Jamalouei, PhD
Department of Psychology, Najafabad Branch, Islamic Azad University, Najafabad, Iran

Sasha-Marie Robinson, Ed.D, LCSW, MA
Services for the UnderServed (S:US)

Kelly Rose-Clarke, MB, PhD
Department of Global Health & Social Medicine, King's College London, UK

Samuli I. Saarni, MD, M. Soc. Sc, PhD
University of Helsinki, Helsinki, Finland, Department of Psychiatry, Brain Center, Helsinki University Hospital

Suoma E. Saarni, MD, PhD
Tampere University, Faculty of
    Medicine and Health Technology

Nathalie Salomé, MD
Psychiatrist, Head of the
    Interpersonal Psychotherapy
    Unit, Centre Hospitalier Esquirol,
    Limoges, France

Palmira Santos, PhD
Mozambique Ministry of Health

Srishti Sardana, PhD, MSc
Global Mental Health Research
    Fellow - National Research Service
    Awardee (NIH)
Johns Hopkins Bloomberg School of
    Public Health

Tracy Sbrocco, PhD
Professor, Department of Medical and
    Clinical Psychology, Uniformed
    Services University of the
    Health Sciences, Bethesda, MD
    20814, USA

Amrah Y. Schotanus, PhD
Standard PhD Candidate,
    APH - Mental Health
Standard PhD Candidate,
    APH - Methodology
Standard PhD Candidate, Health
    Economics and Health
    Technology Assessment 2023

Jean-Marie Sengelen, MD
Psychiatrist, Head of the mental health
    department, Bernese Jura Hospital,
    Bienne, Switzerland

Moussa Seydi, MD
Service des maladies infectieuses et
    tropicales, CHNU de Fann, Dakar,
    Senegal

Lauren B. Shomaker, PhD
Associate Professor, Department of
    Human Development and Family

Studies, Colorado State University,
    Fort Collins, CO, USA

Pragya Shrestha, MA
Transcultural Psychosocial
    Organization Nepal,
    Kathmandu, Nepal

James M. Shultz, MSc, PhD
University of Miami, Miller School of
    Medicine

Daisy Radha Singla, PhD
Department of Psychiatry, Faculty of
    Medicine, University of Toronto,
    Toronto, Canada
Lunenfeld-Tanenbaum Research
    Institute, Sinai Health System,
    Toronto, Canada
Centre for Addiction and Mental
    Health, Toronto, Canada

Shahana Sittampalam
Research Coordinator

Cemile Ceren Sönmez, PhD
Koç University, College of Social
    Sciences and Humanities,
    Istanbul, Turkey

Adrienne Stauder, MD
Institute of Behavioral Sciences,
    Semmelweis University, Budapest,
    Hungary

Jennifer L. Steele, LCSW
VA IPT Trainer, National EBP
    Training Program, VISN 19 Clinical
    Resource Hub, Department of
    Veterans Affairs, IPT and IPC
    Trainer, International Society
    of Interpersonal Psychotherapy
    (ISIPT), USA

**Cindy Goodman Stulberg, DCS,
C.Psych**
Psychologist and Director, Institute
    for Interpersonal Psychotherapy,
    Ontario, M6C 3N! Canada

Antonio Suleman, MD
Mozambique Ministry of Health

Xia Sun, MS
Psychotherapist, Department
  of Psychological Medicine,
  Renji Hospital, Shanghai Jiao
  Tong University School of
  Medicine, China

Holly A. Swartz, MD
Professor of Psychiatry, University
  of Pittsburgh School of Medicine,
  Pittsburgh, PA USA; Past President
  of ISIPT

Annika C. Sweetland, DrPH, MSW
Department of Psychiatry, Columbia
  College of Physicians and Surgeons,
  New York State Psychiatric Institute,
  New York, New York, USA

Marian Tanofsky-Kraff, PhD
Professor, Departments of Medical
  and Clinical Psychology and
  Medicine, Uniformed Services
  University of the Health Sciences,
  Bethesda, MD, USA

William Tarrant, LCSW
Community Association of
  Progressive Dominicans (ACDP)

Miriam Tepper, MD
Columbia University/New York
  State Psychiatric Institute

Anneke van Schaik, MD, PhD
Amsterdam Public
  Health, Mental Health program,
  Amsterdam, The Netherlands
GGZ inGeest, Mental Health Care,
  Amsterdam, The Netherlands

Helen Verdeli, MSc, PhD
Teachers College, Columbia
  University, City of New York,
  USA

Sharuna Verghis, PhD
Senior Lecturer, Jeffrey Cheah School
  of Medicine and Health Sciences,
  Monash University Malaysia &
  Director of Health Equity Initiatives

Milton L. Wainberg, MD
New York State Psychiatric Institute
Columbia University Department of
  Psychiatry

Myrna M. Weissman, PhD
Diane Goldman Kemper Family
Professor of Epidemiology and
Psychiatry Columbia University
Vagelos College of Physicians
and Surgeons Chief, Division of
Translational Epidemiology & Mental
Health Equity, New York State
Psychiatric Institute

**Daniel Wesemann, DNP, MSW,
PMHNP-BC, APRN**
University of Iowa College of Nursing,
  Associate Clinical Professor,
  PMHNP-DNP Program Director

Dawit Wondimagegn, MD, MSc, MA
Consultant Psychiatrist, Associate
  Professor Addis Ababa University

Tenzin Yangchen, MA
Research Coordinator, New York
State Psychiatric Institute & Doctoral
Student, Brown University School of
Public Health

Obadia Yator, PhD
Department of Psychiatry University
  of Nairobi Kenya

Wanhong Zheng, MD
Professor, Program Director of
  Addiction Medicine Fellowship,
  Director of Chestnut Ridge Center
  Inpatient Services, Department of
  Behavioral Medicine and Psychiatry,
  Rockefeller Neuroscience
  Institute, West Virginia University,
  Morgantown, WV

Xiaoyi Zhou, MPhil
Psychotherapist, Psychiatry
    Department, First Affiliated
    Hospital of Zhejiang University
    School of Medicine, Hangzhou,
    Zhejiang Province, China

Salaheddine Ziadeh, PsyD
Global Mental Health Lab, Teachers
    College, Columbia University,
    New York, USA; Université
    Libanaise, Faculté de Santé
    Publique, Sidon, Lebanon

Introduction

History of Interpersonal Psychotherapy

Interpersonal psychotherapy (IPT) had a very humble origin in the 1970s, when it was first described as "high contact" because patients were seen for planned weekly sessions. The evidence for psychotherapy as a treatment rested largely on surmise. There were no psychotherapy manuals for training, no clinical trials, and therefore no demonstrated efficacy. Psychotropic medications were having great success with demonstrated efficacy in studies all over the world and with Food and Drug Administration approval in the United States. Nevertheless, the most common treatment for major nonpsychotic depression, if any treatment was given, was psychotherapy. It was a time of cognitive dissonance. Psychotherapists thought that medication might undo the effects of the transference. Pharmacologists thought that psychotherapy would upset the patient and interfere with the remission of symptoms. Many believed that psychotherapy could not be subjected to clinical trials as every patient and therapeutic relationship was unique.

It was against this background that Gerald Klerman, MD, a psychiatrist at Yale University, decided to test the efficacy of medication as a maintenance treatment for depression. There was good evidence for the efficacy of tricyclic antidepressants for acute treatment of depression, but how long to maintain patients on medication and prevent relapse was unknown. Psychotherapy had to be included in the study as a milieu effect, if only because most patients were receiving some form of psychotherapy in clinical practice. But which psychotherapy? It had to be what was commonly used in ambulatory psychiatric practice. Gerry admired Aaron Beck's beginning development of a manual for cognitive behavioral therapy (CBT), but behavioral therapy was not commonly used in clinics where medication was prescribed. Another alternative, psychoanalysis, also was not usually given with medication treatment and was not widely available.

Finally, "supportive" psychotherapy emerged as the most likely candidate. However, there were no manuals for supportive psychotherapy that could guide the therapy or the training of therapists. There was also no agreement on the content,

Introduction In: *Interpersonal Psychotherapy*. Edited by: Myrna M. Weissman and Jennifer J. Mootz, Oxford University Press.
© Oxford University Press 2024. DOI: 10.1093/oso/9780197652084.003.0001

procedures, or length of supportive psychotherapy. Gerry engaged me, an inexperienced social worker, to work with him to specify a psychotherapy that likely would
be practiced in a psychopharmacology clinic. We began developing a manual for
what we called high-contact psychotherapy. The underlying theoretical base came
from the writings of Harry Stack Sullivan, Adolph Meyer, and John Bowlby. The importance of human attachments, the effects of their disruption on well-being, and
the emergence of symptoms were key concepts. The life event methods, which were
being studied by the research team in relationship to depression, provided a way of
operationalizing the disruption in human attachment associated with depression.

  We were guided mostly by the works of Harry Stack Sullivan, with his focus
on the current interpersonal context of a psychiatric illness. Sullivan stated that
the interpersonal behaviors of others were the most significant events that trigger
emotions. Adolf Meyer put great emphasis on the patient's relationship to the interpersonal environment. John Bowlby emphasized that individuals make strong
affectional bonds, and that the separation of these bonds, or the threat of separation, gives rise to emotional distress and depression. We were also influenced
by the work on life events—both our own and others'—that showed, consistent
with these theoretical writings, that events that represented ruptures in social
attachments were associated with depression. The systematic study of life events
showed that a break in attachment through deaths, disputes, life changes, or the
absence of attachments and loneliness were often present before the onset of most
depressive episodes. In other cases, the patients' depression triggered these events.
The life events research later formed the basis of IPT. Our experience of beginning
medication trials with a diagnostic evaluation and a medical and psychosocial
history also determined the IPT manual content and the therapist training that
followed. For full details of the history of development of IPT, the theoretical base,
and the detailed manual, see Weissman, Markowitz, and Klerman.[1]

  In preparing the first draft of the high-contact psychotherapy manual, we decided
to begin by defining the dose and frequency of the treatment and the diagnostic process that became the first phase of IPT. This phase included a diagnostic evaluation;
a psychiatric history; patient education about depression, its symptoms, and treatment alternatives; an Interpersonal Inventory of important people currently in the
patient's life; the sick role allowing the patient to receive help; a discussion linking
symptom onset to interpersonal situations; and the identification of problem areas
associated with the onset of the depressive episode. Our experience in life events
research gave us the language to identify and define the key problem areas: grief and
complicated bereavement after a death; role disputes and conflicts with a significant
other in renegotiations, dissolution, or impasse; role transitions and changes in life
status (e.g., divorce, moving, retirement); and interpersonal deficits such as absence
of relationship, loneliness, or very few personal attachments.

  The maintenance trial, to our surprise, demonstrated the efficacy of high-
contact psychotherapy. Medication prevented symptom relapse, and psychotherapy enhanced social functioning, and patients on combined treatment
improved the most. With these positive findings, high-contact therapy was then
renamed Interpersonal Psychotherapy.

A GROWING IPT DATABASE EMERGES

Around the same time, Beck also published his clinical trials of CBT, and the field of evidence-based psychotherapy was launched. Gerry's untimely death in 1992 slowed the early flow of training and trials of IPT. The IPT field has caught up, especially with the adaptation of IPT in low-income countries, as we describe in this book.

In 2019, psychiatrist Paula Ravitz, MD, and colleagues published in the *Harvard Review of Psychiatry* a review covering from 1974 to 2017 of IPT trials.[2] They found 1119 English language articles and 133 randomized controlled clinical trials of IPT for depression, as well as for eating disorders, bipolar disorder, anxiety, post-traumatic stress disorder (PTSD), substance use, and comorbid medical illness in adults (see Chapter 2 on Efficacy). Since this review was completed, many clinical trials, including implementation studies, were launched, and another update should be forthcoming in a few years.

In 2018, we published an update of the IPT manual, adaptations, and clinical trials. IPT is now a part of recommended treatment guidelines for depression in the United States, United Kingdom, Canada, and Australia.[1] In February 2019, the US Preventive Services Task Force recommended IPT and CBT for the treatment and prevention of depression during pregnancy.[3] IPT has been adapted for groups, in brief formats, and web-based guided self-help and has been translated into several languages. There are numerous training programs and uses outside of universities or medical schools.

The most unexpected development has been the use and adaption of IPT in low-income countries. In 2001, our group at Columbia University was invited to participate in a study on the treatment of depression in Uganda. The civil war, social upheaval, HIV, and famine had left its citizens depleted. The village leaders and traditional healers asked for help in treating individuals with depression. Medication was not possible given the shortage of medical personnel and cost. The community leaders were interested in psychotherapy in groups since people in Uganda saw themselves as part of a family or group and did not trust individual treatment. Men and women had to be in separate groups to adhere to social norms. We simplified the language of the IPT manual and, as we engaged with local community leaders and learned more about the people and region, made changes in the manual.

The problem areas that IPT addressed—grief, death of a loved one, role disputes or disagreement, role transitions or life changes, and loneliness or social isolation—fit in well with community experience. Two members of our group, Lena Verdeli and Kathleen Clougherty, went to Uganda to train trainers, who would then train and supervise local community health workers. Lena and Kathleen have subsequently become world experts in global IPT training. A clinical trial led by Paul Bolton at Johns Hopkins University, using the manual we simplified, and our trainees was undertaken. The trial in 284 patients showed the efficacy of group IPT when compared with treatment as usual for depression and functioning improvement at both trial completion and 6-month follow-up. The results were published in the June 18, 2003, issue of *JAMA*. This was the first clinical trial of psychotherapy in Africa.[4]

Following the Uganda success, a humanitarian effort using the people we had trained in IPT was undertaken to treat women with depression in Uganda by Sean Mayberry through a nongovernmental organization (NGO) called StrongMinds. StrongMinds was rated by *Forbes* in 2019 as one of the most promising NGOs to support with donations. Since 2014, they have treated over 230,000 women and expanded to Zambia (see Chapter 21). In 2020, the therapists converted to teletherapy because of COVID-19. In 2022, Sean received the Brain and Behavior Humanitarian Honorary Tribute for his work in IPT. His IPT work in Africa has continued to receive international attention. See BBC, "People Fixing the World—The Power of Group Therapy"[5]; World Economic Forum, "Why We Should Invest in Mental Health in Africa";[6] *Vox*, "The Future of Mental Health Care Might Lie Beyond Psychiatry"[7]; and *Forbes*, "How Mental Health Charity StrongMinds Is Disrupting Depression in Africa."[8] Since the Uganda study, the International Society of IPT (ISIPT) which holds a meeting every other year, has supported global communication about IPT (see https://interpersonalpsychotherapy.org and chapters on the ISIPT). In 2021, the meeting of ISIPT, held remotely because of COVID, hosted scientists and clinicians from 28 countries. In 2024, the meeting of the society is in Newcastle upon Tyne in Northeast England.

There have been numerous expansions of IPT in clinical trials and for humanitarian purposes. For example, IPT training for clinical use or research has been carried out in China, Rwanda, Brazil, and Mozambique, among others. You will read about it in the chapters from the different regions of the world. Humanitarian efforts are ongoing in Lebanon with Syrian refugees. This work has been accelerated by the World Health Organization (WHO), when in 2016 they launched the Mental Health Gap Action Program (mhGAP) to determine how nonspecialist healthcare workers can treat people with mental disorders.[9] They developed a 100-page manual identifying priority neuropsychiatric disorders and evidence-based treatment and included IPT. In 2016, the WHO group IPT manual became a part of their World Mental Health Day. The WHO has translated the group manual into Arabic, Chinese, French, Russian, and Swahili.

In 2017, we were invited by a WHO group in Egypt to participate in their use of the IPT manual, which we simplified and called interpersonal counseling (IPC) for primary care patients in distress. This manual, which is available free, is being used in many parts of the world. Because of its simplicity, we have distributed this manual for adaptation in countries using community health workers, although many others are using it as well.[10]

COVID-19 AND LESSONS LEARNED

The COVID-19 pandemic and reported increase in rates of depression and other psychiatric disorders have hastened the development of more economical and briefer treatments to provide access to more people. There is a flurry of international activity in response to the COVID-19 pandemic, exemplified by an experience in Mozambique. Prior to COVID-19, Milton Wainberg and colleagues had trained 23 expert IPC national trainers, who, in turn, trained 15 mental health specialists and 70 primary care providers.[11]

In response to the pandemic, the Mozambique Ministry of Health implemented a free telephone service in which COVID-19-positive patients were referred to the mental health line as the first point of screening for psychiatric problems. About 100 mental health professionals across 10 provinces in Mozambique have been trained virtually to deliver IPC using a tablet-based application to guide facilitation is now in place, and a clinical trial as of this writing is being resumed (see Chapter 19 on Mozambique).

There are numerous other examples of the adaptation for the pandemic. Holly Swartz and colleagues at the University of Pittsburgh had been conducting a clinical trial using machine learning to better understand the patient-therapist mechanism of interaction during IPT when the pandemic caused them to move to telehealth. Now they will be able to assess the differences between in-person and telehealth-based therapy. Given the likely increase in telemedicine after the pandemic ends, this will be useful information for understanding the therapeutic alliance.

In response to COVID-19, StrongMinds has added educational material on anxiety disorders and pandemic-related stressors and have helped participants share their fears and identify specific life events related to lockdown. Moreover, as of this writing, Sean Mayberry is expanding his IPT methods to marginalized groups in the United States. His first program began in 2022 in Newark, New Jersey. To simplify and improve training, Ravitz and Singla and colleagues at the University of Toronto have created an online, case-based, self-directed IPT training course with interactive learning exercises and captioned demonstrations of the clinical principles. It is being piloted with psychiatry residents and will eventually be accessible globally to decrease barriers to IPT training (https://learnIPT.com).

John Markowitz, MD, has argued that IPT, which focuses on life events and social support, is an effective treatment for people adversely impacted by the pandemic, including the social and interpersonal upheaval of the lockdown, the stretching of social bonds with social distancing, the curtailing of usual pleasures, and the loss of a familiar daily structure and social supports. He has adapted the manual to deal with the aftermath of the pandemic.[12] He has shown clinically that persons under distress coming to medical clinics may receive relief from a brief guided psychosocial intervention, such as IPT or IPC[12] (see Chapter 52 on PTSD).

Access to care and not education or culture is the barrier to IPT dissemination. IPT is scalable. The task shifting to nonspecialist healthcare workers who are trained and supervised can be effective. Digital technology can be implemented in low-income as well as high-income countries because nearly everyone has a cell phone. These methods are being tested and used for teletherapy, training, guided, and self-administered approaches.

The evidence for the efficacy of IPT is strongest for major depression for adolescents, adults, and the elderly and for adjunctive treatment of bipolar disorder added to medication. There are fewer trials for PTSD, some eating disorders, and distress. IPT is negative for substance abuse thus far and is being tested with new adaptations. The use of IPT in groups and over the telephone is reasonably well supported by clinical trials and experience.

Dr. Klerman died on April 3, 1992, before most of these developments occurred. His seminal contributions continued to form the core of IPT, unchanged since its inception. Many other specialized manuals of IPT have appeared using the fundamental principles of IPT. Descriptions of the major adaptations can be found on the website of the ISIPT (https://interpersonalpsychotherapy.org). If interested in the history of IPT and recent growth, also see References 13 and 14.[13,14] The largest growth in IPT interest and use has been in low- and middle-income countries with use for refugee migration, civil war, natural disasters, and their aftermaths, which has prompted the writing of this book. It is likely that IPT is acceptable in diverse cultures because of the universality of the importance of human attachment. In this book, we update the latest developments and present the clinical experience of using IPT in diverse cultures and populations. Despite our enthusiasm, it also is important to note that this book only catches a moving snapshot. Moreover, allegiance to a single therapy has no place in the care of people, as no treatment works for everyone even with the same conditions. IPT should be seen as one of the several evidence-based psychotherapies in a clinician's toolbox.

REFERENCES

1. Weissman MM, Markowitz JC, Klerman GL. *The Guide to Interpersonal Psychotherapy: Updated and Expanded Edition*. Oxford University Press; 2018.
2. Ravitz P, Watson P, Lawson A, et al. Interpersonal psychotherapy: a scoping review and historical perspective (1974–2017). *Harv Rev Psychiatry*. 2019;27(3):165–180.
3. O'Connor E, Senger CA, Henninger ML, Coppola E, Gaynes BN. Interventions to prevent perinatal depression: evidence report and systematic review for the US Preventive Services Task Force. *JAMA*. 2019;321(6):588–601.
4. Bolton P, Bass J, Neugebauer R, et al. Group interpersonal psychotherapy for depression in rural Uganda: a randomized controlled trial. *JAMA*. 2003;289(23):3117–24.
5. BBC. People Fixing the World—The Power of Group Therapy. 2022. (Podcast). Accessed Sept 17, 2023. https://www.bbc.co.uk/programmes/w3ct3j2l.
6. World Economic Forum. Why We Should Invest in Mental Health in Africa. 2022. Accessed Sept 17, 2023. https://www.weforum.org/agenda/2022/09/why-we-sho uld-invest-in-mental-health-in-africa/.
7. Earthpages. The future of mental health care might lie beyond psychiatry—Vox. 2022. Accessed Sept 17, 2023. https://epages.wordpress.com/2022/11/30/the-fut ure-of-mental-health-care-might-lie-beyond-psychiatry-vox/.
8. Davide Banis. How Mental Health Charity StrongMinds Is Disrupting Depression in Africa. Forbes. 2019. Accessed Sept 17, 2023. https://www.forbes.com/sites/davi debanis/2019/02/18/how-mental-health-charity-strongminds-is-disrupting-dep ression-in-africa/?sh=7affc6d5167f. 2019.

9. World Health Organization and Columbia University. *Group Interpersonal Therapy (IPT) for Depression*. WHO; 2016. WHO generic field-trial version 1.0.

10. Weissman MM, Hankerson SH, Scorza P, Olfson M, Verdeli H, Shea S, Lantigua R, Wainberg M. Interpersonal Counseling (IPC) for Depression in Primary Care. *Am J Psychother*. 2014;68(4):359–83.

11. Wainberg ML, Gouveia ML, Stockton MA, et al. Technology and implementation science to forge the future of evidence-based psychotherapies: the PRIDE scale-up study. *BMJ Ment Health*. 2021;24(1):19–24.

12. Markowitz JC. *In the Aftermath of the Pandemic. Interpersonal Psychotherapy for Anxiety, Depression, and PTSD*. Oxford University Press; 2021.

13. Weissman MM. Interpersonal psychotherapy: history and future. *Am J Psychother*. 2020;73(1):3–7.

14. Weissman MM. IPT: from humble origins as "high contact therapy" to international adoption. *Psychiatric News*. 2021. https://psychnews.psychiatryonl ine.org/doi/full/10.1176/appi.pn.2021.5.4#:~:text=Now%20used%20worldw ide%2C%20interpersonal%20psychotherapy,as%20%E2%80%9Chigh%20cont act%E2%80%9D%20psychotherapy

Interpersonal Psychotherapy Methods in Brief

JENNIFER J. MOOTZ, TENZIN YANGCHEN,
AND MYRNA M. WEISSMAN ■

Interpersonal psychotherapy (IPT) is evidence-based, manualized psycho-therapy tested in numerous clinical trials. Originally developed to treat major depressive disorder among adults, the treatment has been extended to address several other disorders in multiple populations. The basic elements have remained distinctly similar throughout. A full description of IPT and the different adaptations are found detailed in the 2018 work by Weissman, Markowitz, and Klerman.[1] Numerous other adaptations have appeared over the years, including a publicly available group IPT version developed in collaboration with the World Health Organization[2] and the simplified version called interpersonal counseling (IPC).[3] Many other adaptations are described in the ensuing chapters.

The strategies, techniques, and goals of IPT and IPC[3] are similar. IPC was developed for therapists who did not have academic education in psychiatry, psychology, and other counseling professions. Thus, the examples and language were simplified. It was also developed to be used as a very brief treatment. Over the years, the descriptions of IPT and illustrations of IPC have blended, and there is a little difference between the two. We tend to call it IPC when the treatment is brief, 4 to 8 sessions or even fewer, and community health workers or others without professional mental health degrees are used. As this book goes to press, we are working on a simple session IPT. This is in recognition that some patients in distress do not want to be in regular psychotherapy, but clarification of the interpersonal context of their distress may provide a patient with new directions.

Jennifer J. Mootz, Tenzin Yangchen, and Myrna M. Weissman, *Interpersonal Psychotherapy Methods in Brief* In: *Interpersonal Psychotherapy*. Edited by: Myrna M. Weissman and Jennifer J. Mootz, Oxford University Press. © Oxford University Press 2024.
DOI: 10.1093/oso/9780197652084.003.0002

THE BASIC STRATEGIES OF IPT

The premise of IPT is that depression and other psychiatric disorders have an environmental, familial, and biological basis. However, whatever the ultimate "causes," the disorders occur in a social and interpersonal context. Understanding the development of symptoms in this context and finding better ways of handling them can help relieve symptoms. IPT is organized into three phases of treatment: initiation, middle, and termination. The number of sessions and the order in each phase may also vary depending on a patient's progress. The total number of treatment sessions will vary depending on the setting and resources.

THE INITIAL PHASE

In addition to establishing a strong working alliance with patients, in the initiation phase, therapists work with patients to complete several activities that will set the stage for future sessions.

1. Introduce the therapy, explain confidentiality, identify symptoms, and obtain a treatment history.
2. Explain the procedures of therapy.
3. Help patients understand that symptoms have a relationship to problems.
4. Assign a sick role.
5. Conduct an interpersonal inventory to identify important people in patients' lives.
6. Determine key problem areas.
7. Work with a patient to decide on the focus of treatment for the middle phase.

1. and 2. Introduce the therapy and explain procedures

The process begins with explaining the procedures of therapy and assessing patients' symptoms of distress. An initial assessment gives therapists an understanding of the severity of patients' level of distress and helps them track symptoms over the course of the treatment to describe when and how to conclude this time-limited intervention.

3. Conduct a timeline: Help patients understand that symptoms have a relationship to problems

Early evaluation of symptoms supports other initiation-phase activities, such as the *timeline*, wherein therapists connect patients' onset and fluctuations of symptoms of distress to interpersonal and life events. The completed timeline clarifies the course of distress and provides a psychoeducational tool that illustrates how changes in symptoms connect to interpersonal life events.

4. Assign a sick role

The idea behind the "sick role" is that the patient is someone with an illness that can be treated and is not a "defective" person but someone who needs care. The purpose of the concept is to reduce the patient's guilt about poor functioning, provide hope for solution, and ensure the patient receives care. Adopting the sick role strikes a balance between optimizing the environment and available social support networks for recovery and identifying activities that patients can do to feel better. Therapists assist patients in constructing a detailed plan for how to reach out to people they can spend time and talk with about their distress in addition to activities they might complete on their own or with others. Please note that we have eliminated the name "sick role" and now call it the "recovery role" due to objections by users. The concept and direction have not changed.

5. Conduct an interpersonal inventory

The interpersonal inventory gathers information about friends and family members connected to patients' well-being or distress. IPT therapists ask about and write down key relationships and how the relationships bring comfort to patients or are problematic. This interpersonal exploration pursues the roles that people have in patients' lives, whether the important people are living or deceased and how they are connected to the problem area(s). IPT therapists inquire about all aspects of the relationship and note ways that patients might want to change relationships.

6. Determine key problem areas

Doing a more structured *assessment of problem areas* in the initiation phase can aid therapists in understanding the different problems patients encounter and how patients prioritize those problems in relation to their distress. The following are the four core interpersonal problem areas as conceptualized in IPT and example questions to assess relevance of each area.

GRIEF—A loss following a death of someone important.

- Has someone who was close to you died?
- If yes, who was that person? When did [fill in name] die? Tell me a little about [name of person] and how he or she died.
- How are you dealing with the death?

DISPUTE—An argument with someone significant. Arguments can be open (e.g., fighting openly) or more hidden (becoming distant or cold).

- Are you and someone else having a strong disagreement or argument that is bringing you a great deal of pain? Identify the disagreement.
- Briefly tell me about the disagreement.
- Tell me more about how this disagreement has been affecting you.

TRANSITIONS (LIFE CHANGES)—Positive or negative transitions, already experienced or anticipated, in life.

- Have there been any changes in your life that have impacted you? Those changes could be good or bad. For example, important changes could be experiencing a divorce or separation, having a child, getting married, having an illness, or other changes that are important to you.
- Please describe how [name changes] have impacted you.

LONELINESS—An absence of close relationships, feelings of loneliness or emotional distance from others that could be lifelong or more recent.

- What are your relationships like? Do you have any close relationships?
- Tell me about any difficulties keeping close relationships.
- Has anything changed in your life so that now you feel lonely (but didn't before this change)?

7. Conduct an interpersonal formulation: Decide on focus of treatment

The interpersonal formulation is a summary of assessments and content discussed in the initiation phase. The components of the formulation are

- Summarize patients' symptoms of distress, including their onset and course.
- Describe the problem areas that patients have experienced.
- Connect the relationship of symptoms to those problem areas.
- Obtain feedback from patients about the formulation and decide on treatment focus.

Patients often have more than one interpersonal problem that may be linked to their distress. While it is preferable to focus on one problem area at a time, problem areas may be linked and/or change over time. In these cases, it is important to structure therapy such that patients experience the therapy as relevant to their current problem.

THE MIDDLE PHASE

Resolving the identified problem area(s) is the primary goal of the middle phase. In the middle sessions, therapists encourage patients to make changes and view the problem and their relationships from different perspectives. Understanding the details of daily events, problems, and relationships that work well can guide solutions.

Therapeutic goals

1. Review symptoms and problems since last session
2. Work on strategies for solving problem area(s)

1. REVIEW SYMPTOMS AND PROBLEMS SINCE LAST SESSION

Middle sessions start with tracking progress of symptoms through use of a standardized mental health questionnaire. Therapists also initiate sessions with a brief check-in about how patients' mood has been over the past week or since the last session. Therapists then hear from patients about their perception of how any changes in symptoms and mood might relate to their problem area(s) and social context. Continual emphasis on the connection between distress and the problem area(s) aids patients in gaining awareness about this connection and guides ideas about how and where patients want to make concrete changes that relate to their problem area(s).

2. WORK ON STRATEGIES FOR SOLVING PROBLEM AREA(S)

Table 1.1 provides strategies for working on problems.

THE TERMINATION PHASE

The time of the ending and the termination phase is usually negotiated and discussed in the initial phase.

Therapeutic goals

1. Deal with feelings about ending
2. Review progress and strategies for identifying and dealing with recurrences
3. Discuss options for future treatment if needed

1. DEAL WITH FEELINGS ABOUT ENDING

Help patients identify and discuss their feelings and thoughts about concluding treatment. Reminding patients early on about the time-limited nature of the

Table 1.1 STRATEGIES FOR PROBLEMS

Strategies for problems			
Grief	Disputes	Transitions/ life change	Loneliness and isolation
Mourn and accept loss by reconstructing relationship with deceased prior to, during, and after death Explore new or reestablish old interests and relationships	1. Identify disputes and their stage Renegotiation (parties arguing to find solution) Impasse (parties stopped communicating) Dissolution (one or both want to end relationship) 2. Explore options Renegotiation (determine issues, differences in expectations, and find alternatives) Impasse (open up communication and renegotiate) Dissolution (resolve ending in least harmful way)	Give up past and deal with loss by reconstructing what was lost Accept new role in as positive light possible Develop new skills and relationships to support change	Reduce isolation by understanding the origins and current encounters Encourage and assist in developing opportunities for relationships

intervention allows them to set realistic timelines for their treatment goals, begin emotionally preparing for termination, and plan for the future.

2. REVIEW PROGRESS AND STRATEGIES FOR IDENTIFYING AND DEALING WITH RECURRENCES

Therapists can summarize progress with help from the assessment results across sessions. Therapists then ask patients to summarize behaviors, communication, and strategies they have used to improve the problem area(s) and related distress. Therapists help patients plan for the future by imagining situations that could trigger distress and preemptively designing strategies to cope if those problems arise. Predetermining how patients will decide when they need to reach out for help from others or professional counseling can help build awareness if symptoms progressively worsen. For patients who are still symptomatic or who wish to continue to explore problem areas, alternative treatments or another course of IPT may be recommended.

3. DISCUSS OPTIONS FOR FUTURE TREATMENT, IF NEEDED

If treatment goals have not been met, therapists will discuss options for future treatment.

IPT techniques

Interpersonal psychotherapy therapists use techniques that are best practices to improve rapport and communication with patients. The IPT techniques are not new or different from those commonly used in clinical practice. For example, they elicit conversation through use of *open-ended questions* and *reflections* of patients' statements to check therapist understanding. They are also careful to *validate and normalize* patients' experiences so patients know they are not alone or in the wrong for how they feel about something. *Providing affirmations* and noticing patients' strengths supports patients' sense of self-efficacy to harness for improving interpersonal problems. Given the overarching interpersonal focus, emphasizing verbal and nonverbal communication and clarifying any discrepancies in communication is commonplace.

COMMUNICATION ANALYSIS

During communication analysis, therapists elicit a detailed account of a recent interaction between patients and a significant other to help them identify their communication patterns and modify distorted or unhelpful ones. This analysis engages patients in reporting and reflecting on the intentions that underlie communication, their affective responses, and what they believe the other person heard, understood, and felt. When assessing the quality of communication, therapists ask questions about the setting; verbal communication (what was said); nonverbal behaviors (body language, gestures, and facial expressions); and paraverbal cues (tone, pitch, and pace of voice) of the interactants. Therapists may then point out effective and maladaptive aspects of the communication patterns, encourage patients to consider another's perspective (e.g., how do you think the person felt when you said that?), and suggest ways of rectifying faulty communication that could have affected the outcome of the interaction and the accompanying feelings to help the client communicate more effectively.

DECISION ANALYSIS

As patients and therapists gain a deeper understanding of the interpersonal problem, including any maladaptive communication patterns, it can be helpful to explore alternative, more effective ways of communicating that could have resulted in a different outcome. When patients present an interpersonal problem, therapists ask patients how they would like to resolve it and encourage them to generate a list of possible solutions. Therapists may initially need to provide suggestions for some patients. Together with therapists, patients evaluate the pros and cons of each option and select one or a combination of choices that may lead to a better interpersonal interaction. If the solution that patients propose is not feasible, therapists can help them process that challenge.

ROLE PLAY

Role playing or acting out a recent or planned conversation allows patients to practice their newly established communication styles and receive constructive feedback on interpersonal skills and strategies before implementing them in real life. In role playing, patients generally play themselves or the significant other, while therapists play the opposite role. In some cases, patients may assume both roles (their own and the other person's). Rehearsing both ideal outcomes and less successful interactions helps patients solidify their newly learned adaptive communication strategies and prepares them to cope with any interpersonal interactions outside of therapy.

Adaptations

Over the years, numerous adaptations of IPT have been developed. This book describes some of them for different countries and diverse populations, different modalities, group, family, or couples, and digital. In all these adaptations, the basic principle, format, problem areas, and techniques as described here in brief have remained the same with minor exceptions.

REFERENCES

1. Weissman MM, Markowitz JC, Klerman GL. *The Guide to Interpersonal Psychotherapy: Updated and Expanded Edition*. Oxford University Press; 2018.
2. World Health Organization. *Group Interpersonal Therapy (IPT) for Depression*. World Health Organization; 2016.
3. Weissman MM, Hankerson SH, Scorza P, et al. Interpersonal counseling (IPC) for depression in primary care. *Am J Psychother*. 2014;68(4):359–383.

The Efficacy of Interpersonal Psychotherapy

PART 1

The Efficacy of Interpersonal
Psychotherapy

The Efficacy of Interpersonal Psychotherapy

MYRNA M. WEISSMAN AND JENNIFER J. MOOTZ ■

An important theme of our work and this book is the need for an evidence base for psychotherapy. In Chapter 1, "History of Interpersonal Psychotherapy," we described the origins of interpersonal therapy (IPT) and evidence from the first clinical trial when we called IPT "high contact." We also traced its historical developments, testing through clinical trials, and adaptations. In this section, we summarize the evidence from published scoping reviews and meta-analyses. Because information on clinical trials in low- and middle-income countries (LMICs) has been sparse and is recent, we have included a Chapter 2 by Cuijpers, a leader in meta-analyses, and colleagues, who provide information from LMICs specifically.

The reader may find this information on efficacy testing scattered. However, this is not different from what might be found for longer term testing of a medication. In the United States, for newly developed medications, efficacy must be established in several well-designed clinical trials to be released to the market. Then, testing of usage in different populations, doses, severity, comorbidities, as well as in different combinations of medications happens. Think about it in mathematical terms as a multidimensional, space matrix where it is impossible to fill all the possible combinations or, in math terms, make the matrix dense. Then what do you do? The solution is to let "a hundred flowers bloom." This scattered information becomes useful to specific groups, some of whom, we may learn, do not benefit from the treatment.

No treatment, no matter how efficacious, will work for everyone under every condition. Like many psychopharmacological medications, IPT has a solid evidence foundation based on controlled random assignment clinical trials, which gives legitimacy to its use and further testing. Against this background, we summarize the published overall data from a scoping review and meta-analyses so

Jennifer J. Mootz, Tenzin Yangchen, and Myrna M. Weissman, *The Efficacy of Interpersonal Psychotherapy* In: *Interpersonal Psychotherapy*. Edited by: Myrna M. Weissman and Jennifer J. Mootz, Oxford University Press.
© Oxford University Press 2024. DOI: 10.1093/oso/9780197652084.003.0003

that readers can have the IPT references and focus on what we think are the most relevant dimensions. Here is where the judgment of experienced people like our readers plays an important role.

SCOPING REVIEW

We begin this summary of evidence with the classic article by Ravitz et al., published in 2019 in *Harvard Review of Psychiatry*.[1] This article is a scoping review, which maps the main sources and types of evidence available to evaluate an area of research and underlying concepts.[2] Scoping reviews narratively summarize broad trends of evidence. Meta-analyses, which we also review, quantitatively evaluate outcomes across studies that are selected based on explicit parameters for inclusion and exclusion in the analysis.

The Ravitz et al. scoping review[1] summarizes the development of IPT and interpersonal counseling (IPC) for major depression, eating disorders, anxiety disorders, and bipolar disorders between 1974 and 2017. The database comes from published articles about IPT and IPC and depicts the historical developments, landmark studies, and shifting evolution. Their review covered 1109 articles, including 133 randomized controlled clinical trials (RCTs) and 131 nonrandomized, case-controlled studies, mainly on the treatment of adults with major depression. The interested scholar is encouraged to read this landmark article for the historical perspectives and scope of evidence. Here, we summarize the article and reflect on key points.

The first decade (1974–1984) is described as the founding years and the introduction of manuals and their use in RCTs testing IPT against medication and low-contact treatment (meeting only for monthly assessment), mostly to improve major depressive disorder. These studies led to the first publication of the IPT manual.[3] The treatment studies included a large multisite clinical trial, which included comparisons of IPT with cognitive behavioral therapy (CBT). This study showed that patients with high baseline severity did best on medication followed by IPT. CBT did not show a significant advantage to placebo in this trial,[4] a finding that, to our knowledge, has not been replicated in other published studies.

The first trial of IPT, led by Gerry Klerman, was not included in the review because IPT was then called "high contact," which meant that patients were seen weekly. It was a maintenance study of patients who had a reduction of symptoms with medication. The purpose was to see how to maintain remission after symptom reduction. This first study showed that high-contact treatment had effects on social functioning and medication on preventing return of depressive symptoms. The combination was the most effective.[4] High contact was later renamed IPT, and this first study became the impetus to continue IPT testing.

The second decade (1985–1994) saw an expansion of IPT to studies in Australia, United Kingdom, and Canada; studies in real-world settings, such as primary care and schools; studies across the life span from adolescence to late life[5,6]; and adaptations for eating disorders, as well as a brief version of IPT, termed interpersonal counseling (IPC).

The highlight of this period was a 3-year maintenance study by the Pittsburg group, Kupfer and Frank et al., to treat patients with highly recurrent depression who had responded to treatment with medication and IPT.[7] Patients were randomized to receive medication, placebo, monthly plus placebo maintenance IPT, or monthly IPT plus medication to see what worked best at preventing relapse over 3 years. Medication most effectively prevented relapse. However, IPT lengthened time to recurrence, whether alone or with medication. This work later showed remission could be sustained by monthly maintenance IPT in women who had improved with receiving IPT alone.[8]

The third decade (1995–2004) moved IPT into work in LMICs, particularly the first RCT of psychotherapy in Africa, the IPT study in Uganda. This study showed the feasibility and efficacy of group IPT for major depression in women, delivered by trained lay workers in a setting where traditional healing was the standard treatment.[9] These studies were later extended to northern Uganda and adolescents suffering from depression, under conditions of hardship. The results were stronger in adolescent girls than boys. These results gained the attention of the World Health Organization, who, with our permission, published and freely disseminated the group IPT manual. In the third decade, this work was followed by studies in South Africa, Sudan, India, Haiti, and Rwanda.

Other highlights of this period are further testing and refinement of the adolescent adaptations; development for perinatal depression; the further testing of IPT and IPC in primary care, with HIV patients, or for bulimia; further studies of the process and techniques; a broadening of interest in diverse, underserved populations; and finally a tiptoe into biological studies using magnetic resonance imaging, with little success.

Ravitz et al. covered 2005–2017 as the most recent epoch. During this period, there was more support for evidence-based treatments, and different parts of the world developed guidelines for clinical care.[10] The strengths of IPT in LMICs continued. Clinicians and researchers refined IPT for subpopulations of adolescents, pregnant women, families, elderly, people with obesity and medical illnesses, and mothers with depression who were raising children with mental health problems. The highlights of novelty were the adaptations and the RCTs of IPT for bipolar disorders, termed interpersonal and social rhythm therapy (IPSRT). The feature for patients with bipolar disorder were additions to regulate circadian rhythms and trace daily routines.[11] A series of studies demonstrated the efficacy of these adaptations for maintaining remission in bipolar disorder.

Whereas the early addiction studies of IPT for patients who were misusing opioids were not positive for IPT, pilot work has shown some promise for relapse prevention of alcohol misuse in female patients with depression. The studies of post-traumatic stress disorder (PTSD) using IPT compared to exposure-based (recount in detail the traumatic event) interventions, the gold standard in the field, began in this period. The results, much to the surprise of many involved with the treatment of PTSD, showed that IPT, which does not involve exposure work, was an option for patients adverse to describing traumatic memories.[12,13] Finally, there have been efforts to study the process and mechanism of IPT using sophisticated modeling and new methods of measurement and search for common factor sources versus specific intervention techniques and strategies. This work is in its infancy.

In this book, we extend the developments in IPT described in Ravitz's article[1] to report on developments in international organizations, technologies, adaptations, and training and implementation across the globe. Ravitz and her colleagues anticipated these developments in their final discussion. By the time this book is ready for the reader, the field will have moved forward from the developments we report, a good sign of a rapidly developing field that has reached across the globe and continues to grow in scope and depth. The reader is encouraged to read the Ravitz et al. article for fuller details of our summary.

META-ANALYSES

Numerous small and large meta-analyses of psychotherapy clinical trials, including IPT, have been carried out over the years. The most comprehensive and rigorous have been carried out by Pim Cuijpers and his group, who have made meta-analysis a special discipline. A free meta-analysis book with an accompanying course on meta-analysis is available for those who want to learn how to carry them out.[14]

The most comprehensive meta-analyses[15,16] that studied the effects of IPT were carried out in 2011 and 2016. The 2016 analysis included a variety of diagnoses and provided an update and extension of the study in 2011, which focused only on depression. After 2016, the studies focused on not only IPT but also large network analyses comparing eight types of psychotherapy, including IPT, as well as meta-analyses across different age groups[17,18] and studies on onset prevention.[19] What follows is a summary of these reports, usually taken directly from them.

The 2011 study included 38 RCTs (4356 patients) of IPT for depression, comparing IPT to a variety of conditions (no treatment, usual care, other treatments, psychotherapies, or medication, continuation with medication, maintenance treatment). The numbers of studies in each condition were small. We take this summary from them.[15(pp589-590)]

Compared with control groups, they noted a moderate to large effect of IPT in the acute treatment of depression and found some indications that IPT had less efficacy than SSRI (selective serotonin reuptake inhibitor) pharmacotherapy. However, the overall difference was small, not all analyses were significant, and the number of studies in this subsample was small. They noted indications that combination treatment with IPT and pharmacotherapy was somewhat more efficacious than pharmacotherapy alone. However, the effect size was also small.

They did not find that IPT had greater efficacy than other psychotherapies, including CBT, although the number of studies was too small to draw definite conclusions. IPT and CBT were the only psychotherapies for depression compared with control groups, other psychotherapies, antidepressant medication, and combination treatments. Therefore, in the 2011 article, they concluded that IPT and CBT were the best options for psychological treatments for depression. Both seemed equally effective overall.[15]

The number of studies examining the effects of maintenance IPT was small, Cuijpers et al. noted,[16] but had relatively high methodological quality. They concluded that maintenance IPT combined with pharmacotherapy reduced the relapse rate considerably compared with pharmacotherapy alone, and placebo plus IPT was more effective than placebo alone in reducing relapse rates. The superior effect of combination treatment over pharmacotherapy alone suggested that IPT has an additional effect on depression beyond the effects of pharmacotherapy, although they stated the effect size was small. They found that only 9 of 38 studies met all quality criteria. Despite these limitations, they concluded clear indications for the efficacy of IPT for unipolar depression and justified its inclusion in treatment guidelines.

The 2016 study[16(pp685–686)] included the depression trials in 2011, updated with new depression studies, and added trials of IPT for eating and anxiety disorders. The number of studies more than doubled to 90 studies (11,434 patients). The control conditions, ages, and designs were similar to the 2011 article. It should be noted in the spirit of transparency that Weissman was a coauthor of this article.

Two-thirds of the psychotherapy studies in the 2016 analysis aimed at treatment of depression, showing a moderate-to-large effect of IPT on depression compared with control groups, with smaller effects in older adults, in clinical samples, and in samples meeting diagnostic criteria for a depressive disorder. IPT was not significantly more or less effective than other psychotherapies for depression. There were some indications that pharmacotherapy may be somewhat more effective than IPT for acute-phase depression. They noted this finding may have been influenced by the high risk of bias in many of these trials.[16] Combined treatment was significantly more effective than IPT alone but not more effective than pharmacotherapy alone. These results are comparable to the earlier 2011 meta-analysis.

The IPT trials for eating disorders, anxiety disorders, substance misuse, and distress from general medical disorders showed some promising effects in the 2016 analysis. However, the authors cautioned that there was a high risk of bias in most trials and an insufficient number of trials. They concluded that IPT's focus on interpersonal experiences and problem areas, often triggers of a new episode, may provide an important alternative to pharmacotherapy or CBT.[16(p686)]

The next major article that included IPT is a more recent 2021 meta-analysis that covered 8 commonly used psychotherapies (IPT; CBT; psychodynamics; problem-solving; behavioral activation; life review; "third-wave" therapies, which included both acceptance and commitment therapy and mindfulness-based CBT; and nondirective supportive counseling) in different parts of the world as compared with each other, usual care, waiting list, and pill placebos.[17] This landmark article published in *World Psychiatry* has international authorship from Netherlands, Italy, Spain, and Japan, so that a range of therapies not commonly used in all countries is noted. The outcome was only for depression, and the focus was primarily on symptom reduction and remission. Social functioning and quality of life were not included as an outcome. Using a novel network method of analysis in 331 RCTs with 34,285 patients, they found that all therapies were more efficacious than usual care and a waiting list, and all therapies except nondirective supportive counseling and psychodynamic psychotherapy were more efficacious than pill placebo.

Only 90 studies had a 1-year follow-up, and they found the IPT, CBT, behavioral activation, problem-solving, and psychodynamic psychotherapy had significant effects compared to usual care, except for behavioral activation compared to waiting list. IPT was also significantly more effective than nondirective supportive counseling at 1-year follow-up. Considering bias, number of trials for each therapy, sensitivity analysis, follow-up, and differing patient population, including medically ill and elderly patients in some studies, the authors concluded that all these therapies except nondirective supportive counseling can be used in routine care. However, they suggested that "one important finding of this study is that several psychotherapies still have significant effects at one-year follow up, including CBT, behavioral activation therapy, problem solving therapy, interpersonal psychotherapy, and psychodynamic therapy."[17(p292)]

A separate meta-analysis was reported in 2016 on the effects of psychotherapy for depression on quality of life; it included 44 RCTs of psychotherapy for adults, including IPT.[18] Kolovos et al., including Cuijpers,[18] found that psychotherapy had a positive impact on the quality of life of patients with depression. Improvements in quality of life were not fully explained by improvement in depression symptoms. These findings echoed an earlier report, one also by the Cuijpers group, on social functioning outcome for depression.[19]

There are also meta-analyses of more detailed aspects of treatment available. A systematic search of RCT studies that tested the ability of interventions to prevent the onset of depression found 50 trials ($N = 12,606$ participants).[20] The 50 trials included 22 CBT, 8 IPT, 5 stepped care, 5 problem-solving, and 10 other, such as behavioral activation and acceptance and commitment therapy. The results of the therapies were pooled, but subgroup analyses found no major differences between IPT and the other interventions. The participants either had a history of depression or were patients with medical conditions, perinatal patients, or college students. The results showed that psychotherapy as compared to control reduced the risk of developing depression by 19%. The results were more significant in studies conducted in Europe or the United States, which may be due to a smaller number of non-Western studies (Australia, China, and India in 6 studies). We show in subsequent chapters the considerable increase in IPT use in non-Western countries. The authors concluded that psychotherapy may prevent the onset of depression in people who do not have the disorder at baseline. Many unanswered questions remain.[20]

Reviews of IPT clinical trials across age groups have also been completed.[21,22] Specific psychotherapies were not described. However, the results showed that the effects of psychotherapy were smaller in children and in adolescents than in adults. These results were repeated with depressed adolescents in 40 clinical trials ($N = 3779$ participants) and a variety of psychotherapies, including 6 IPT studies.

Again, they reported a moderate effect. Thirty-nine percent responded to psychotherapy at 1 to 2 months, and 24% responded to the control condition.

Two meta-analyses independently appeared in 2018 and 2019 and focused on IPT for adolescents (IPT-A).[23,24] The analyses included the same 10 RCTs ($N = 910$) and participants from the same parts of the world (United States, Uganda, Puerto Rico, Taiwan, and Australia).

Both studies concluded that IPT-A was an effective treatment for adolescent depression that demonstrated significant improvements in depression symptoms postintervention, with some evidence that improvements were maintained for up to 1 year. No interaction was found between group and individual delivery of IPT-A, indicating that both modalities could be delivered with good effects. However, there were fewer trials investigating group IPT-A; therefore, further exploration of this treatment format is needed.[24(p314)] There was a small significant effect in favor of IPT-A improving depressive symptoms in comparison to other active treatments, with this effect moderated by the type of intervention used as a control condition. When compared with CBT, there was no significant difference between the groups in postintervention depression symptoms. However, a medium significant effect was present when IPT-A was compared to less-structured interventions such as treatment as usual, clinical monitoring, and play therapy. These findings were mirrored by remission rates with IPT-A demonstrating significantly higher remission rates from depression postintervention when compared to non-CBT control conditions.[24] The authors expressed surprise that the effects were not stronger for relieving interpersonal difficulties for IPT or any of the other modalities and noted new studies of IPT with adolescents were ongoing. (See Chapter 44 by Mufson et al. for description.)

The last meta-analysis of psychotherapies from 2018 investigated whether psychotherapies (usually developed in Western, high-income countries, like IPT) were effective in LMICs and compared effects to those in high-income settings.[25] The meta-analysis included 253 studies ($N = 4607$ patients): 32 from LMICs and 221 from high-income countries. The LMIC countries included Uganda, China, Taiwan, Korea, Brazil, Iran, Japan, Mexico, Malaysia, Pakistan, Singapore, South Africa, Thailand, India, Israel, and Chile. They used the World Bank classification for income status. The studies from high-income countries were concentrated in North America, Europe, and Australia. Only 2 IPT studies from LMICs were included. Other included treatments were CBT, psychodynamic psychotherapy, and nondirective supportive counseling, among others.

The study[25] documented that psychotherapies for depression that have been developed in Western countries may also be effective in other countries. They even found indications that these therapies may be more effective in non-Western than in Western countries.

While these results are reassuring regarding the efficacy of psychotherapies (developed in high-income settings) in LMIC settings, the overall small number of studies per country and the inclusion of only 2 IPT studies from LMICs limit conclusions.[25] The results are important to have on IPT, given the large number of reports of IPT being used in other countries (see chapters on Africa, Asia and the Middle East, South America, and training experience in different countries. Chapter 3 by Cuijpers et al. provides a new meta-analysis of IPT for depression in LMICs compared to high-income countries.

For completeness, a network meta-analysis of the effects of psychotherapies, medication, and the combinations in the treatment of adult depression was carried out.[26] While the psychotherapies were not evaluated separately, IPT was included among 101 studies with 11,910 patients[26] with moderate to severe depression. Combined treatment was more effective than either treatment alone in achieving response at the end of treatment. There were no significant differences between medication and psychotherapy alone. Combined treatment and psychotherapy alone were more acceptable to patients than medication alone.

The scoping review and meta-analyses are presented to give the reader the background clinical trials that form the evidence to guide the use of IPT. As with medication, the overall efficacy has been established. Subsequent chapters show the application of IPT across numerous countries and settings. Emerging studies will determine the use of IPT under different conditions and may discover where IPT is not as useful or clinically indicated. This is how our knowledge of care is determined.

REFERENCES

1. Ravitz P, Watson P, Lawson A, et al. Interpersonal psychotherapy: A scoping review and historical perspective (1974–2017). *Harvard Rev Psychiatry*. 2019;27(3):165–180.
2. Pham MT, Rajic A, Greig JD, Sargeant JM, Papadopoulos A, McEwen SA. A scoping review of scoping reviews: Advancing the approach and enhancing the consistency. *Res Synth Methods*. 2014;5(4):371–385.
3. Klerman G, Weissman M, Rounsaville B, Chevron E. *Interpersonal Psychotherapy of Depression*. Basic; 1984.
4. Sotsky SM, Glass DR, Shea MT, et al. Patient predictors of response to psychotherapy and pharmacotherapy: Findings in the NIMH Treatment of Depression Collaborative Research Program. *Am J Psychiatry*. 1991;148(8):997–1008.
5. Mufson L, Weissman MM, Moreau D, Garfinkel R. Efficacy of interpersonal psychotherapy for depressed adolescents. *Arch Gen Psychiatry*. 1999;56(6):573–579.
6. Schulberg HC, Block MR, Madonia MJ, et al. Treating major depression in primary care practice. Eight-month clinical outcomes. *Arch Gen Psychiatry*. 1996;53(10):913–919.
7. Frank E, Kupfer DJ, Perel JM, et al. Three-year outcomes for maintenance therapies in recurrent depression. *Arch Gen Psychiatry*. 1990;47(12):1093–1099.
8. Frank E, Kupfer DJ, Buysse DJ, et al. Randomized trial of weekly, twice-monthly, and monthly interpersonal psychotherapy as maintenance treatment for women with recurrent depression. *Am J Psychiatry*. 2007;164(5):761–767.
9. Bolton P, Bass J, Neugebauer R, et al. Group interpersonal psychotherapy for depression in rural Uganda: A randomized controlled trial. *JAMA*. 2003;289(23):3117–3124.

10. Clark DM, Layard R, Smithies R, Richards DA, Suckling R, Wright B. Improving access to psychological therapy: Initial evaluation of two UK demonstration sites. *Behav Res Ther.* 2009;47(11):910–920.

11. Frank E, Swartz HA, Kupfer DJ. Interpersonal and social rhythm therapy: Managing the chaos of bipolar disorder. *Biol Psychiatry.* 2000;48(6):593–604.

12. Markowitz JC, Petkova E, Neria Y, et al. Is exposure necessary? A randomized clinical trial of interpersonal psychotherapy for PTSD. *Am J Psychiatry.* 2015;172(5):430–440.

13. Markowitz JC. *Interpersonal Psychotherapy for Posttraumatic Stress Disorder.* Oxford University Press; 2017.

14. Cuijpers P. *Meta-Analyses in Mental Health Research. A Practical Guide.* Vrije Universiteit Amsterdam; 2016.

15. Cuijpers P, Geraedts AS, van Oppen P, Andersson G, Markowitz JC, van Straten A. Interpersonal psychotherapy for depression: A meta-analysis. *Am J Psychiatry.* 2011;168(6):581–592.

16. Cuijpers P, Donker T, Weissman MM, Ravitz P, Cristea IA. Interpersonal psychotherapy for mental health problems: A comprehensive meta-analysis. *Am J Psychiatry.* 2016;173(7):680–687.

17. Cuijpers P, Quero S, Noma H, et al. Psychotherapies for depression: A network meta-analysis covering efficacy, acceptability and long-term outcomes of all main treatment types. *World Psychiatry.* 2021;20(2):283–293.

18. Kolovos S, Kleiboer A, Cuijpers P. Effect of psychotherapy for depression on quality of life: meta-analysis. *Br J Psychiatry.* 2016;209(6):460–468.

19. Renner F, Cuijpers P, Huibers MJ. The effect of psychotherapy for depression on improvements in social functioning: A meta-analysis. *Psychol Med.* 2014;44(14):2913–2926.

20. Cuijpers P, Pineda BS, Quero S, et al. Psychological interventions to prevent the onset of depressive disorders: A meta-analysis of randomized controlled trials. *Clin Psychol Rev.* 2021;83:101955.

21. Cuijpers P, Karyotaki E, Eckshtain D, et al. Psychotherapy for depression across different age groups: A systematic review and meta-analysis. *JAMA Psychiatry.* 2020;77(7):694–702.

22. Cuijpers P, Karyotaki E, Ciharova M, et al. The effects of psychological treatments of depression in children and adolescents on response, reliable change, and deterioration: A systematic review and meta-analysis. *Eur Child Adolesc Psychiatry.* 2023;32(1):177–192.

23. Mychailyszyn MP, Elson DM. Working through the blues: A meta-analysis on interpersonal psychotherapy for depressed adolescents (IPT-A). *Child Youth Serv Rev.* 2018;87:123–129.

24. Duffy F, Sharpe H, Schwannauer M. Review: The effectiveness of interpersonal psychotherapy for adolescents with depression—A systematic review and meta-analysis. *Child Adolesc Ment Health.* 2019;24(4):307–317.

25. Cuijpers P, Karyotaki E, Reijnders M, Purgato M, Barbui C. Psychotherapies for depression in low- and middle-income countries: A meta-analysis. *World Psychiatry.* 2018;17(1):90–101.

26. Cuijpers P, Noma H, Karyotaki E, Vinkers CH, Cipriani A, Furukawa TA. A network meta-analysis of the effects of psychotherapies, pharmacotherapies and their combination in treatment of adult depression. *World Psychiatry.* 2020;19(1):92–107.

3

Interpersonal Psychotherapy for Depression in Low- and Middle-Income Countries

A Meta-Analysis

PIM CUIJPERS, CLARA MIGUEL, MATHIAS HARRER, DAVID D. EBERT, AND EIRINI KARYOTAKI ■

INTRODUCTION

Almost a billion people suffered from a mental disorder in 2019; of these individuals, 82% lived in low- and middle-income countries (LMICs).[1] Depression is one of the most common disorders, with about 280 million people worldwide suffering from it. Depressive disorders not only are highly prevalent, but also result in considerable loss of quality of life in patients and their families.[2] Mental disorders are the leading cause of years lived with disability, accounting for about 15% of disability globally, and depression is responsible for about 40% of this disease burden.[1] Furthermore, depression is associated with increased morbidity and premature mortality[3] and with enormous economic costs.[4]

Several evidence-based interventions are available for the treatment of depression, including pharmacotherapy[5] and psychotherapies.[6] Pharmacotherapy is currently the first-line treatment for depression in most countries, although the evidence is increasing that psychotherapies are more effective in the longer term, and not prescribing antidepressants without combining then with psychotherapy should be considered.[7,8] Furthermore, the majority of patients with depression prefer psychotherapy over medications,[9] although research on patients'

Pim Cuijpers, Clara Miguel, Mathias Harrer, David D. Ebert, and Eirini Karyotaki, *Interpersonal Psychotherapy for Depression in Low- and Middle-Income Countries* In: *Interpersonal Psychotherapy.* Edited by: Myrna M. Weissman and Jennifer J. Mootz, Oxford University Press. © Oxford University Press 2024. DOI: 10.1093/oso/9780197652084.003.0004 preferences has largely been conducted in Western countries, and it is not clear whether this is also the case in LMICs.[10]

There are several psychotherapies that have been found to be effective in the treatment of depression. In a large network meta-analysis of psychotherapies for adult depression, we identified 8 main types of psychotherapy (cognitive behavioral, interpersonal, psychodynamic, problem-solving, behavioral activation, life-review and "third-wave" therapies, and nondirective supportive counseling).[11] This network meta-analysis indicated that all therapies are effective, and that there were no significant differences in effects between these therapies. Only nondirective counseling was found to be less effective, although that may be an artifact because this therapy is often used as a control condition for other therapies.

Most research on psychotherapies for depression have been conducted in Western high-income countries.[11] Since 2000, however, a growing number of trials were conducted in LMICs. This research showed that psychotherapies are at least as effective in LMICs as compared to high-income countries and maybe even more effective.[11] One major barrier to expand treatments of depression in LMICs is the lack of skilled mental health practitioners.[12] Task sharing to the front line (i.e., delegating care tasks to community or primary care–based nonspecialist workers) has been advocated to address this barrier.[13,14] A large, "individual patient data" meta-analysis showed that such task-sharing interventions have a small but significant effect on depression. To facilitate the implementation of task-sharing and other low-threshold interventions, the World Health Organization (WHO) developed several brief interventions that can be implemented easily, including Problem Management Plus (PM+),[15,16] Self-Help Plus (SH+),[17,18] and Step-by-Step, the digital version of PM+.[19,20]

Although task-sharing and other low-threshold interventions can improve access to psychological treatments in low-resourced settings, the effects are still modest, and many participants will not respond to these treatments. This means that more specialized treatments are still very much needed, also in low-resourced settings. Interpersonal psychotherapy (IPT) is one of these treatments that can be applied as not only a first-line treatment, but also in patients for whom other low-threshold interventions were not effective. IPT is recommended by WHO as a treatment of depression, and a manual of an 8-session group version of IPT has been published by WHO.[21] This manual is part of the Mental Health Gap Action Program (mhGAP) program of WHO, and it describes a simplified version of IPT that can be used by supervised facilitators who may not have received previous training in mental health. The manual is available in English, but it has also been translated into several other languages (Arabic, Chinese, Farsi, French, Russian, Spanish, and Swahili).

In this chapter, we give an updated overview of the research that has been conducted on IPT and conduct a meta-analysis of the effects of IPT for adult depression. We also focus on trials conducted in LMICs and compare these with the research on IPT in high-income countries. We use the data from a large meta-analytic project on psychotherapies for depression, which are openly available on the website of the project (https://www.metapsy.org).

METHODS

Identification and selection of studies

For this study we used the data of a larger meta-analytic project on psychological treatments of depression that was registered at the Open Science Framework,[22] and supplemental materials were available at the website of the project (https://www.metapsy.org). This database was used in a series of earlier published meta-analyses.[23]

The studies included in the current study were identified through the larger, already existing database of randomized trials on the psychological treatment of depression. For this database, we searched four major bibliographical databases (PubMed, PsycInfo, Embase, and the Cochrane Library) by combining index and free terms indicative of depression and psychotherapies, with filters for randomized controlled trials. The full search strings can be found at the project website (https://www.metapsy.org). Furthermore, we checked the references of earlier meta-analyses on psychological treatments of depression. The database is continuously updated and was developed through a comprehensive literature search (from 1966 to January 1, 2022). All records were screened by two independent researchers, and all papers that could possibly meet inclusion criteria according to one of the researchers were retrieved as full text. The decision to include or exclude a study in the database was also done by the two independent researchers, and disagreements were resolved through discussion.

For the current study, we selected randomized controlled trials in which IPT for adults with depression was compared with a control condition (wait list, care as usual, other). For a therapy to be defined as IPT, the authors have specifically referred to the most recent manuals.[21,24] Depression could be defined as meeting criteria for a depressive disorder according to a diagnostic interview or as a score above the cutoff on a self-report depression measure. We excluded studies in which two therapies were compared with each other and no control group was available as well as studies comparing IPT with pharmacotherapy. These results were published in a previous study.[25]

Quality assessment and data extraction

We assessed the validity of included studies using four criteria for the risk of bias (RoB) assessment tool, Version 1, developed by the Cochrane Collaboration.[26] We used Version 1 of this tool because this meta-analysis was included in the broader meta-analytic project of psychological treatments of depression.[27]

The RoB tool assesses possible sources of bias in randomized trials, including the adequate generation of allocation sequence; the concealment of allocation to conditions; the prevention of knowledge of the allocated intervention (masking of assessors); and dealing with incomplete outcome data (this was assessed as positive when intention-to-treat analyses were conducted, meaning that all randomized patients were included in the analyses). Assessment of the validity of the included studies was conducted by two independent researchers, and disagreements were solved through discussion.

We also coded participant characteristics (diagnostic method; recruitment method; target group; mean age; proportion of women); characteristics of IPT (treatment format; number of sessions); as well as general characteristics of the studies (type of control group; publication year; country where the study was conducted). The details and specific definitions of these characteristics can be found at the project website (https://www.metapsy.org).[28]

Outcome measures

For each comparison between a psychological treatment and a control condition, the effect size indicating the difference between the two groups at post-test was calculated (Hedges' g).[29] Effect sizes were calculated by subtracting (at posttest) the average score of the psychotherapy group from the average score of the control group and dividing the result by the pooled standard deviation. Because some studies were expected to have relatively small sample sizes, we corrected the effect size for small-sample bias. When means and standard deviations were not reported, we calculated the effect size using dichotomous outcomes or change scores; and if these also were not available, we used other statistics (e.g., t value or p value) to calculate the effect size.

Meta-analyses

Analyses were conducted using the metapsyTools28 package in R (Version 4.1.1) and RStudio (Version 1.1.463 for Mac). The metapsyTools package was specifically developed for the meta-analytic project, of which this study is part. The package imports functionality of the meta,[30] metafor,[31] and dmetar[32] packages.

We calculated the pooled effect sizes in several different ways, as implemented in the metapsy tools package, so that we could explore if different pooling methods resulted in different outcomes. In our main analysis model, all effect size data available for a comparison in a specific study were aggregated within that comparison first. These aggregated effects were then pooled across studies and comparisons. To aggregate effects within comparisons, an intrastudy correlation coefficient of $\rho = 0.5$ was assumed.

We conducted several other analyses to examine whether these main outcomes were robust. First, we estimated the pooled effect using a 3-level correlated and hierarchical effects (CHE) model, which was recently proposed by Pustejovsky and Tipton (2021)[33]; and parameter tests and confidence intervals (CIs), which were also calculated using robust variance estimation (RVE) to guard against model misspecification. We assumed an intrastudy correlation of $\rho = 0.5$ for this model. Second, we pooled effects while excluding outliers, using the "nonoverlapping confidence intervals" approach, in which a study is defined as an outlier when the 95% CI of the effect size does not overlap with the 95% CI of the pooled effect size.[28] Third, we pooled effects while excluding influential cases as defined by the diagnostics.[34] Fourth, we calculated the effect when only the smallest or largest effect in each study was considered. Fifth, we estimated the pooled effect using only studies with low RoB bias.

We also used three different methods to assess and adjust for potential publication bias[32,35]: Duval and Tweedie's trim and fill procedure,[36] Rücker's limit meta-analysis method,[37] and the selection model.[38,39]

A random-effects model was assumed for all analyses. Between-study heterogeneity variance (components) was estimated using restricted maximum likelihood. For models not fitted using RVE, we applied the Knapp-Hartung method to obtain robust CIs and significance tests of the overall effect.[39] As a test of homogeneity of effect sizes, we calculated the I^2 statistic and its 95% CI, which is an indicator of heterogeneity in percentages. A value of 0% indicates no observed heterogeneity, and larger values indicate increasing heterogeneity, with 25% as low, 50% as moderate, and 75% as high heterogeneity.[26] For the three-level model, we calculated a multilevel extension of I^2, which describes the amount of total variability attributable to heterogeneity within studies (level 2) and heterogeneity between studies (level 3).[32] Because I^2 cannot be interpreted as an absolute measure of the between-study heterogeneity, we also added the prediction interval (PI), which indicates the range in which the true effect size of 95% of all populations will fall.[40,41]

In addition to Hedge's g, we calculated the numbers needed to treat (NNT) for depression using the formulas provided in Reference 42, in which the control group's event rate was set at a conservative 17% (based on the pooled response rate of 50% reduction of symptoms across trials in psychotherapy for depression).[43]

We conducted a series of subgroup analyses. The main one was aimed at examining whether effect sizes found in studies in LMICs differed from those in high-income countries. In addition, we compared studies using different recruitment strategies; whether or not depression was established with a diagnostic interview; the target group (adults in general; women with perinatal depression; other specific target group); treatment format (individual; group; other/mixed); control group (care as usual; waitlist; other), and studies with low RoB (meeting all 4 criteria) versus other studies.

RESULTS

Selection and inclusion of studies

After examining a total of 30,889 records (21,563 after removal of duplicates), we retrieved 3,584 full-text papers for further consideration. A total of 878 studies were included in the database of trials on psychotherapies for adult depression. The data can be downloaded and analyzed at https://www.metapsy.org. A total of

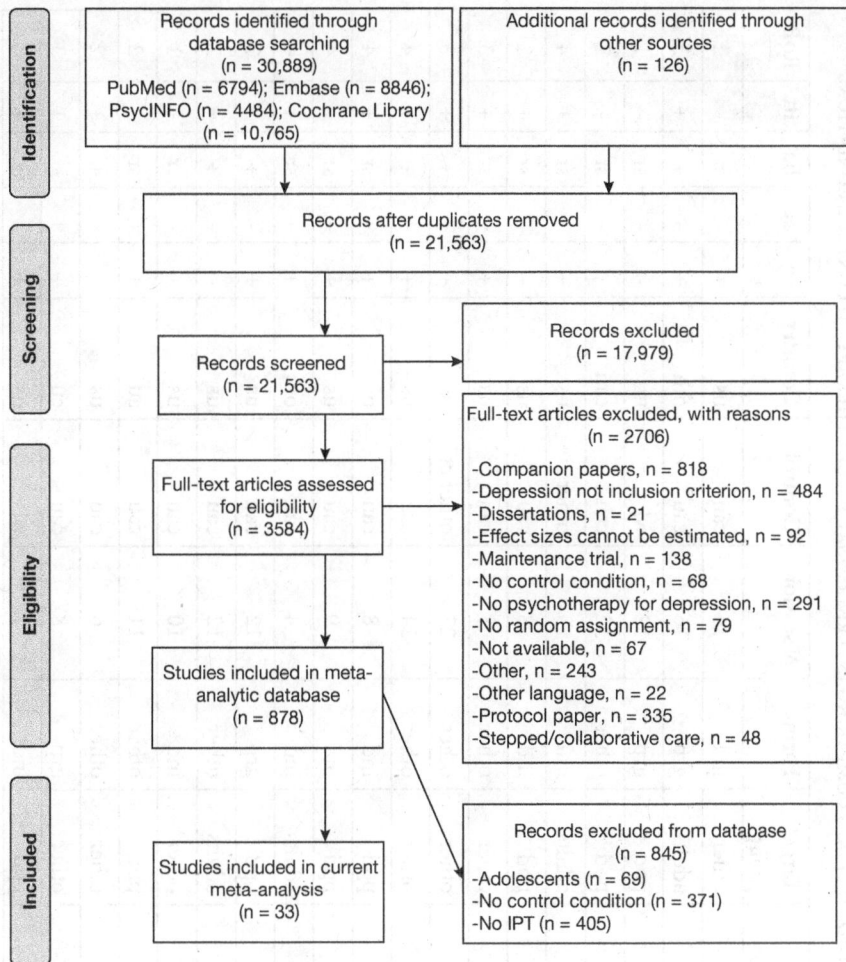

Figure 3.1 Flow chart of the inclusion of studies.

33 trials met the inclusion criteria for this meta-analysis. The PRISMA flow chart describing the inclusion process, including the reasons for exclusion, is presented in Figure 3.1.

Characteristics of included studies

A summary of key characteristics of the 33 included studies is presented in Table 3.1. In the trials, 2476 patients participated, 1245 in IPT and 1231 in the control conditions. Three trials were conducted in LMICs, one in a low-income country at the time of publication (Uganda: Bolton et al., 2003) and two in upper-middle-income countries (Brazil: Matsuzaka et al., 2017; and South Africa: Petersen et al., 2014). The other studies were conducted in high-income countries in North America (24), 5 in Europe, and 1 in Australia.

Table 3.1 SELECTED CHARACTERISTICS OF RANDOMIZED TRIALS COMPARING INTERPERSONAL PSYCHOTHERAPY TO CONTROL CONDITIONS

Study	Mood dis	Recr	Mean age	Prop women	Target group	Format	N sessions	Control	Country	sg	ac	ba	itt	RoB
Beeber, 2010	-	oth	26	1.00	other	ind	16	cau	us	+	-	sr	-	2
Bolton, 2003	+	oth	45	0.51	adults	grp	16	cau	oth	+	-	+	+	3
Clark, 2003	+	com	31	1.00	ppd	grp	12	wl	us	-	-	sr	-	1
Dennis, 2020	+	com	nr	1.00	ppd	other	12	cau	can	+	-	sr	-	2
Elkin, 1989	+	clin	35	0.70	adults	ind	13	other ctr	us	+	+	sr	+	4
Grote, 2009	-	oth	25	1.00	ppd	ind	8	cau	us	-	-	sr	+	2
Heckman, 2017	+	com	52	0.37	other	other	8	cau	us	+	-	sr	+	3
Johnson, 2012	+	oth	35	1.00	other	other	27	other ctr	us	-	+	+	+	3
Johnson, 2019	+	oth	39	0.35	other	other	24	cau	us	+	+	+	+	4
Lenze, 2017	+	com	27	1.00	ppd	ind	8	cau	us	+	+	sr	+	4
Lenze, 2020	+	com	26	1.00	ppd	ind	9	cau	us	+	+	sr	+	4
Matsuzaka, 2017	+	clin	44	0.94	adults	ind	4	cau	oth	+	+	sr	+	4
Mennen, 2021	-	oth	33	1.00	ppd	grp	12	cau	us	+	-	+	+	3
Miller, 2002	-	oth	32	1.00	adults	other	12	cau	us	-	-	+	+	2
Mossey, 1996	-	oth	71	0.78	other	ind	10	cau	us	-	-	sr	-	1
Mulcahy, 2010	+	clin	32	1.00	ppd	other	11	cau	au	+	-	sr	-	2
Neugebauer, 2006	-	oth	30	1.00	other	other	6	cau	us	-	-	+	+	2
Niedermoser, 2020	+	com	41	0.50	other	grp	8	cau	eu	+	+	-	+	3
O'Hara, 2000	+	oth	30	1.00	ppd	ind	12	wl	us	+	-	sr	+	3

Petersen, 2014	+	oth	37	0.74	other	grp	8	cau	oth	+	-	sr	-	2
Poleshuck, 2014	+	oth	37	1.00	other	ind	4	cau	us	+	-	-	+	2
Power, 2012	+	clin	36	0.62	adults	ind	16	wl	uk	-	-	sr	+	2
Ransom, 2008	+	com	44	0.16	other	other	6	cau	us	-	-	sr	+	2
Saloheimo, 2016	+	clin	42	0.72	adults	ind	13	cau	eu	+	+	+	-	3
Schramm, 2020	+	clin	47	0.79	other	grp	8	cau	eu	+	-	sr	+	3
Schulberg, 1996	+	clin	38	0.83	adults	ind	16	cau	us	-	-	+	+	2
Spinelli, 2003	+	com	29	1.00	ppd	ind	16	other ctr	us	-	-	-	+	1
Spinelli, 2013	+	oth	30	1.00	ppd	ind	12	other ctr	us	+	-	-	-	1
Swartz, 2008	+	com	43	1.00	other	ind	9	cau	us	-	-	-	-	0
Talbot, 2011	+	clin	36	1.00	other	ind	13	cau	us	-	-	-	+	1
van Schaik, 2006	+	clin	68	0.69	other	ind	8	cau	eu	+	-	+	+	3
Vigod, 2021	-	com	33	1.00	ppd	grp	10	wl	can	-	-	+	+	2
Weissman, 1979	+	clin	nr	nr	adults	ind	16	other ctr	us	-	-	+	-	1

In most studies' (26/33) participants met criteria for a depressive disorder according to a clinical interview, while in the other 7 studies participants scored above a cutoff on a self-rating scale. In 10 studies, participants were recruited through the community; in 10 studies through clinical referrals; and 13 studies used other recruitment methods. Eight studies were aimed at adults in general, 11 at women with perinatal depression; the other 14 were aimed at other specific target groups. The interventions in 18 studies had an individual format; 7 had a group format; 19 had a guided self-help format; and the remaining 8 studies had a mixed format. The number of sessions ranged from 4 to 27, with the majority (27 studies) between 8 and 16 sessions. In 24 studies, usual care was used as control group; 4 studies used a wait-list control group; and the 5 remaining studies used another control group.

Nineteen of the 33 studies reported an adequate sequence generation (57.6%); 8 reported allocation to conditions by an independent party (24.2%); 9 reported using blinded outcome assessors (27.3%); 23 used only self-report outcomes (69.7%); and in one study blinding of outcome assessors was unclear. In 23 studies, intent-to-treat analyses were conducted (69.7%). Four studies (12.1%) met all criteria for low RoB, 21 studies (63.6%) met 2 or 3 criteria, and 7 met 1 or none of the criteria (21.2%).

Overall effects of IPT on depression

The overall effects of IPT as well as the sensitivity analyses are reported in Table 3.2, and the forest plot is presented in Figure 3.2. The overall effect size for the 33 studies was $g = 0.50$ (95% CI: 0.34; 0.65), with high heterogeneity ($I^2 = 76$; 95% CI: 66; 83), and a broad PI (-0.26; 1.26). The NNT was 6.49. Most sensitivity analyses resulted in comparable outcomes (Table 3.2). When 5 outliers were removed the effect size was somewhat smaller ($g = 0.35$; 95% CI: 0.24; 0.47), but heterogeneity was low ($I^2 = 30$; 95% CI: 0; 56) and the PI was narrower and did not include zero (0.05; 0.66). The number of studies with low RoB was small and pooling these studies while excluding other studies resulted in a small and nonsignificant effect size. Egger's test did not indicate significant publication bias ($P = .79$), and the three models adjusting for this bias indicated results that were comparable to the main analyses and with comparable levels of heterogeneity.

Effects of IPT in LMICs compared with high-income countries

A subgroup analysis comparing the effects found in trials in LMICs compared with high-income countries found no significant difference (Table 3.3). The effects in the three LMICs were somewhat larger ($g = 0.75$; 95% CI: -0.95; 2.45) than in high-income countries, but they were not significant, and heterogeneity

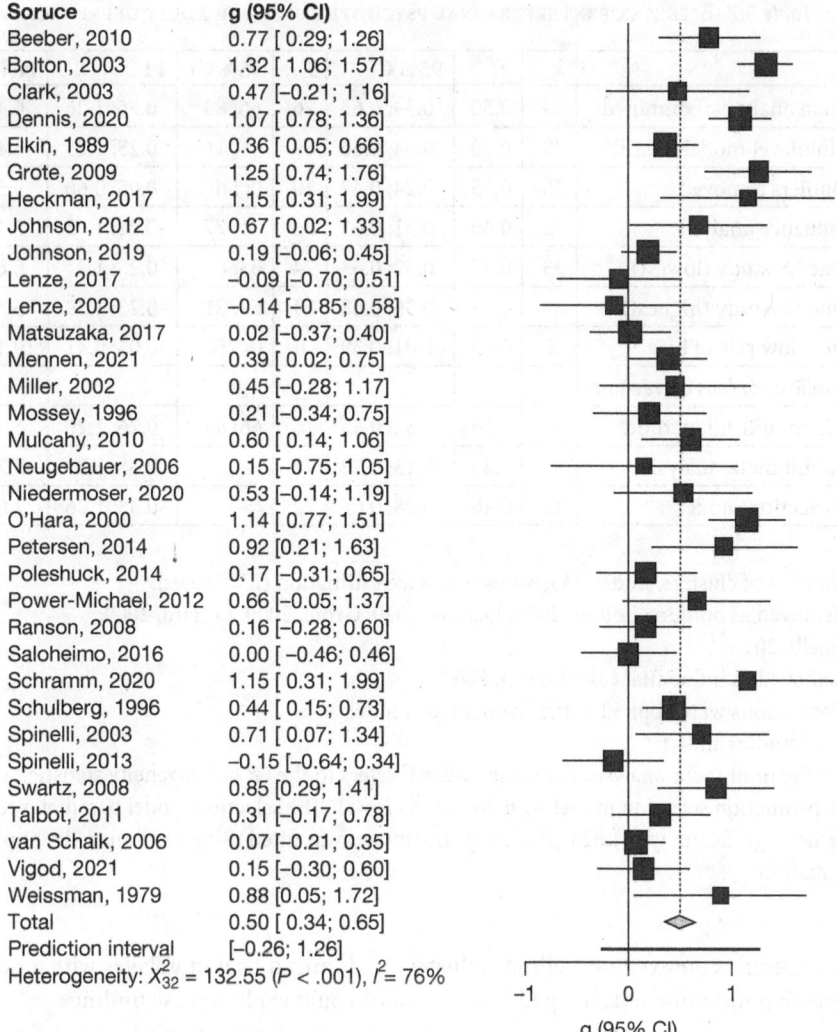

Figure 3.2 Forest plot.

was very high (I^2 = 94; 95% CI: 84; 97). It should be noted that statistical power is notoriously low in subgroup analyses,[43] meaning that it is not clear whether the effects of IPT in LMICs are smaller, comparable, or larger than in high-income countries.

The high level of heterogeneity among the three studies in LMICs can be explained by the very large effect size found in Bolton et al. (g = 1.32; 95% CI: 1.06; 1.57), the very small effect size found by Matsuzaka et al. (g = 0.02; 95% CI: -0.37; 0.40) and the effect size found in Petersen et al. in between (g = 0.92; 95% CI: 0.21; 1.63). Furthermore, the study by Bolton et al. was an outlier in the main analyses, and it was also identified as the only influential study according to the criteria of Viechtbauer and Cheung.[34] It is not clear why this study was an outlier, but perhaps

Table 3.2 EFFECTS OF INTERPERSONAL PSYCHOTHERAPY FOR ADULT DEPRESSION

	k	g	95% CI	I^2	95% CI	PI	NNT
Main analyses: combined	33	0.50	0.34; 0.65	76	66; 83	-0.26; 1.26	6.49
Multilevel model (CHE)[a]	49	0.50	0.34; 0.66	69	-	-0.25; 1.25	6.47
Outliers removed[b]	28	0.35	0.24; 0.47	30	0; 56	0.05; 0.66	9.59
Influence analysis[c]	32	0.46	0.31; 0.61	66	51; 77	-0.21; 1.13	7.12
One ES/study (lowest)	33	0.47	0.32; 0.63	74	63; 81	-0.28; 1.23	6.88
One ES/study (highest)	33	0.52	0.36; 0.68	74	63; 81	-0.25; 1.29	6.16
Only low risk of bias	6	0.19	-0.01; 0.39	0	0; 75	-0.03; 0.41	19.16
Publication bias correction[d]							
- Trim-and-fill method[e]	33	0.50	0.34; 0.65	76	66; 83	-0.26; 1.26	6.49
- Limit meta-analysis[f]	33	0.43	0.13; 0.72	77	-	-0.38; 1.23	7.76
- Selection model[g]	33	0.46	0.28; 0.65	72	-	-0.33; 1.26	7.06

[a] Number of clusters/studies: 33; robust variance estimation (RVE) used.
[b] Removed as outliers: Bolton, 2003; Dennis, 2020; Grote, 2009; O'Hara, 2000; Spinelli, 2013.
[c] Removed as influential case: Bolton, 2003.
[d] Corrections were applied to the "combined" model.
[e] Zero studies added.
[f] For the limit meta-analysis, the value under I^2 refers to the G^2 heterogeneity statistic.
[g] Step-function selection model with cut points $P = .1$. The selection model parameter test was not significant: $\chi^2 = 1.624$ ($P = .203$). The model was fitted using maximum likelihood estimation.

the specific context and methods (cluster-randomized trial in villages with a depression instrument developed for this study) could explain these findings.

Other subgroup analyses

The results of the other subgroup analyses are reported in Table 3.3. We found no indication that the type of recruitment, a diagnosis versus a cutoff, the target group, the format, or the type of control group was associated with significantly larger or smaller effect sizes. We did find that studies with low RoB had significantly smaller effect sizes than the other studies.

DISCUSSION

We conducted a meta-analysis of randomized trials comparing IPT with control groups in high-income and LMICs and found that IPT had a significant effect on

Table 3.3 Subgroup analyses

Variable	Level	n_{comp}	g	CI	I^2	CI	NNT	P
Main subgroup analysis								
Country	Western	30	0.47	0.31; 0.62	66	50; 77	6.94	.48
	Non-Western	3	0.75	-0.95; 2.45	94	84; 97	4.01	
Other subgroup analyses								
Recruitment	Community	10	0.49	0.16; 0.82	69	41; 84	6.61	.26
	Clinical	10	0.33	0.11; 0.55	43	0; 73	10.39	
	Other	13	0.59	0.3; 0.89	83	73; 90	5.32	
Diagnosis	Mood disorder	26	0.50	0.32; 0.68	79	70; 85	6.46	
	Cutoff score	7	0.50	0.12; 0.88	57	0; 81	6.46	.99
Target group	Adults	8	0.51	0.12; 0.89	86	74; 92	6.31	.85
	Perinatal	11	0.52	0.17; 0.87	79	63; 88	6.17	
	Other	14	0.43	0.22; 0.64	45	0; 71	7.69	
Format	Individual	18	0.40	0.19; 0.62	70	51; 81	8.35	.31
	Group	7	0.70	0.28; 1.12	81	60; 90	4.35	
	Other/mixed	8	0.55	0.22; 0.88	73	44; 87	5.78	
Control	Care as usual	24	0.49	0.3; 0.68	79	69; 86	6.61	.77
	Wait list	4	0.62	-0.09; 1.33	74	29; 91	5.02	
	Other control	5	0.42	-0.07; 0.91	48	0; 81	7.90	
Low risk of bias	Yes	6	0.19	-0.01; 0.39	0	0; 75	19.09	<.001
	No	27	0.58	0.41; 0.75	76	65; 83	5.43	

depression. This was supported in a series of sensitivity analyses, although the significant effects were not confirmed in the small set of studies with low RoB.

We also compared the studies conducted in LMICs with those conducted in high-income countries. We did not find a significant difference between these two groups of studies, but unfortunately the number of studies in LMICs was very small, and subgroup analyses are notoriously underpowered when the number of studies is small. We also found that one of the three studies was an outlier with much larger effect sizes than the other studies on IPT. This means that we cannot be certain whether IPT is also effective in LMICs.

In a large meta-analysis on psychological treatments of adult depression in which we also included other types of psychotherapy, we found that psychotherapies in LMICs were at least as effective as those in high-income countries.[10] We even found that the effects were somewhat larger in LMICs, but that could be an artifact related to the low quality of many studies or, for example, differences in what usual care is between high-income countries and LMICs. This suggests that our findings on IPT are in line with other research findings suggesting that psychotherapies are at least as effective in LMICs.

It is worrying that only a limited number of trials met all criteria for low RoB. In the broader field of psychotherapies for depression, it is also found that less than 25% of trials have low RoB.[43] Just like in the current meta-analyses, it is usually also found that the effects found for studies with low RoB are smaller than other studies. This means that the effects of IPT and other psychotherapies, such as cognitive behavior therapy, behavioral activation, problem-solving, and psychodynamic therapies, are probably overestimated.

The results of this study should be considered with caution because of several important limitations. First, the number of studies, especially in LMICs, was small. Second, as already indicated, the number of studies with low RoB was small, making all outcomes uncertain. Third, we did not look at longer term outcomes or comparisons with other therapies or pharmacotherapy.

Despite these limitations, we can conclude that IPT is probably an effective treatment of adult depression, and that there is no reason to assume that the effects are smaller in LMICs, although more research, especially high-quality research, is needed to verify that.

REFERENCES

1. World Health Organization. *World Mental Health Report: Transforming Mental Health for All.* World Health Organization; 2022.
2. Herrman H, Patel V, Kieling C, et al. Time for united action on depression: a Lancet–World Psychiatric Association Commission. *Lancet.* 2022;399(10328):957–1022.
3. Cuijpers P, Vogelzangs N, Twisk J, Kleiboer A, Li J, Penninx B. Comprehensive meta-analysis of excess mortality in depression in the general community versus patients with specific illnesses. *Am J Psychiatry.* 2014;171(4):453–462.
4. Chisholm D, Sweeny K, Sheehan P, et al. Scaling-up treatment of depression and anxiety: a global return on investment analysis. *Lancet Psychiatry.* 2016;3(5):415–424.
5. Cipriani A, Furukawa TA, Salanti G, et al. Comparative efficacy and acceptability of 21 antidepressant drugs for the acute treatment of adults with major depressive disorder: a systematic review and network meta-analysis. *Lancet.* 2018;391:1357–1366.
6. Cuijpers P, Karyotaki E, Ciharova M, Miguel C, Noma H, Furukawa TA. The effects of psychotherapies for depression on response, remission, reliable change, and deterioration: a meta-analysis. *Acta Psychiatr Scand.* 2021;144(3):288–299.
7. Cuijpers P, Noma H, Karyotaki E, Vinkers CH, Cipriani A, Furukawa TA. A network meta-analysis of the effects of psychotherapies, pharmacotherapies and their combination in the treatment of adult depression. *World Psychiatry.* 2020;19(1):92–107.
8. Furukawa TA, Shinohara K, Sahker E, et al. Initial treatment choices to achieve sustained response in major depression: a systematic review and network meta-analysis. *World Psychiatry.* 2021;20:387–396.
9. McHugh RK, Whitton SW, Peckham AD, Welge JA, Otto MW. Patient preference for psychological vs. pharmacologic treatment of psychiatric disorders: a meta-analytic review. *J Clin Psychiatry.* 2013;74:595–602.

10. Cuijpers P, Karyotaki E, Reijnders M, Purgato M, Barbui C. Psychotherapies for depression in low- and middle-income countries: a meta-analysis. *World Psychiatry*. 2018;17:90–101.
11. Cuijpers P, Griffin JW, Furukawa TA. The lack of statistical power of subgroup analyses in meta-analyses: a cautionary note. *Epidemiol Psychiatr Sci*. 2021;30:e78.
12. Patel V. Mental health: in the spotlight but a long way to go. *Int Health*. 2019;11(5):324–326.
13. Karyotaki E, Araya R, Kessler RC, et al. Association of task-shared psychological interventions with depression outcomes in low- and middle-income countries: a systematic review and individual patient data meta-analysis. *JAMA Psychiatry*. 2022;79(5):430–443. Erratum in: *JAMA Psychiatry*. 2022;79(12):1241.
14. Papola D, Purgato M, Gastaldon C, et al. Psychological and social interventions for the prevention of mental disorders in people living in low-and middle-income countries affected by humanitarian crises. *Cochrane Database Syst Rev*. 2020;9(9):CD012417.
15. Rahman A, Hamdani SU, Awan NR, et al. Effect of a multicomponent behavioral intervention in adults impaired by psychological distress in a conflict-affected area of Pakistan: a randomized clinical trial. *JAMA*. 2016;316(24):2609–2617.
16. Bryant RA, Schafer A, Dawson KS, et al. Effectiveness of a brief behavioural intervention on psychological distress among women with a history of gender-based violence in urban Kenya: a randomised clinical trial. *PLoS Med*. 2017;14(8):e1002371.
17. Purgato M, Carswell K, Tedeschi F, et al. Effectiveness of self-help plus in preventing mental disorders in refugees and asylum seekers in Western Europe: a multinational randomized controlled trial. *Psychother Psychosom*. 2021;90(6):403–414.
18. Acarturk C, Uygun E, Ilkkursun Z, et al. Effectiveness of a WHO self-help psychological intervention for preventing mental disorders among Syrian refugees in Turkey: a randomized controlled trial. *World Psychiatry*. 2022;21(1):88–95.
19. Cuijpers P, Heim E, Abi Ramia J, et al. Effects of a WHO-guided digital health intervention for depression in Syrian refugees in Lebanon: a randomized controlled trial. *PLoS Med*. 2022;19(6):e1004025.
20. Cuijpers P, Heim E, Abi Ramia J, et al. Guided digital health intervention for depression in Lebanon: randomised trial. *BMJ Ment Health*. 2022;25(e1):e34–e40.
21. World Health Organization and Columbia University. *Group Interpersonal Therapy (IPT) for Depression (WHO Generic Field-Trial Version 1.0)*. World Health Organization; 2016.
22. Cuijpers P, Karyotaki E, de Wit L, Ebert DD. The effects of fifteen evidence-supported therapies for adult depression: a meta-analytic review. *Psychother Res*. 2020;30(3):279–293.
23. Cuijpers P. Four decades of outcome research on psychotherapies for adult depression: an overview of a series of meta-analyses. *Can Psychol*. 2017;58(1):7.
24. Weissman MM, Markowitz JC, Klerman GL. *The Guide to Interpersonal Psychotherapy*. Oxford Press; 2018.
25. Cuijpers P, Cristea IA, Karyotaki E, Reijnders M, Huibers MJ. How effective are cognitive behavior therapies for major depression and anxiety disorders? A meta-analytic update of the evidence. *World Psychiatry*. 2016;15(3):245–258.
26. Higgins JP, Altman DG, Gøtzsche PC, et al. The Cochrane Collaboration's tool for assessing risk of bias in randomised trials. *BMJ*. 2011;343.

27. Sterne JA, Savović J, Page MJ, et al. RoB 2: a revised tool for assessing risk of bias in randomised trials. *BMJ*. 2019;366:l4898.
28. Harrer M, Kuper P, Cuijpers P. metapsyTools: several R helper functions for the "metapsy" database. R package version 0.3.2.2022. https://tools.metapsy.org. 2022. Accessed August 18, 2022.
29. Hedges LV, Olkin I. *Statistical Methods for Meta-analysis*. Academic Press; 2014.
30. Balduzzi S, Rücker G, Schwarzer G. How to perform a meta-analysis with R: a practical tutorial. *BMJ Ment Health*. 2019;22(4):153–160.
31. Viechtbauer W. Conducting meta-analyses in R with the metafor package. *J StatiSoftw*. 2010;36(3):1–48.
32. Harrer M, Cuijpers P, Furukawa TA, Ebert DD. *Doing meta-analysis with R: a hands-on guide*. Chapman & Hall/CRC Press; 2021.
33. Pustejovsky JE, Tipton E. Meta-analysis with robust variance estimation: expanding the range of working models. *Prev Sci*. 2022;23(3):425–438.
34. Viechtbauer W, Cheung MW. Outlier and influence diagnostics for meta-analysis. *Res Synth Methods*. 2010;1(2):112–125.
35. Maier M, VanderWeele TJ, Mathur MB. Using selection models to assess sensitivity to publication bias: a tutorial and call for more routine use. *Campbell Syst Rev*. 2022;18(3):e1256.
36. Duval S, Tweedie R. Trim and fill: a simple funnel-plot–based method of testing and adjusting for publication bias in meta-analysis. *Biometrics*. 2000;56(2):455–463.
37. Rücker G, Schwarzer G, Carpenter JR, Binder H, Schumacher M. Treatment-effect estimates adjusted for small-study effects via a limit meta-analysis. *Biostatistics*. 2011;12(1):122–142.
38. McShane BB, Böckenholt U, Hansen KT. Adjusting for publication bias in meta-analysis: an evaluation of selection methods and some cautionary notes. *Perspect Psychol Sci*. 2016;11(5):730–749.
39. Carter EC, Schönbrodt FD, Gervais WM, Hilgard J. Correcting for bias in psychology: a comparison of meta-analytic methods. *Adv Methods Pract Psychol Sci*. 2019;2(2):115–144.
40. IntHout J, Ioannidis JP, Borm GF. The Hartung-Knapp-Sidik-Jonkman method for random effects meta-analysis is straightforward and considerably outperforms the standard DerSimonian-Laird method. *BMC Med Res Methodol*. 2014;14:1–2.
41. Borenstein M, Higgins JP, Hedges LV, Rothstein HR. Basics of meta-analysis: I2 is not an absolute measure of heterogeneity. *Res Synth Methods*. 2017;8(1):5–18.
42. Furukawa TA. From effect size into number needed to treat. *Lancet*. 1999;353(9165):1680.
43. Cuijpers P, Quero S, Noma H, et al. Psychotherapies for depression: a network meta-analysis covering efficacy, acceptability and long-term outcomes of all main treatment types. *World Psychiatry*. 2021;20:283–293.

International Society of Interpersonal Psychotherapy

4

International Society of Interpersonal Psychotherapy (ISIPT)

JOHN C. MARKOWITZ ■

Designed and first tested in the 1970s by M. M. Weissman, the late G. L. Klerman, and their colleagues at Yale and Harvard Universities, interpersonal psychotherapy (IPT[1]) became a research success as a novel, time-limited treatment for patients with major depression.[1,2] Dissemination of IPT proceeded more slowly. As IPT spread, however, the need arose for an organization to bring clinicians and researchers together. This is the brief history of a still small society, the International Society of Interpersonal Psychotherapy (ISIPT; https://interperson alpsychotherapy.org/).

Drs. Klerman and Weissman developed IPT as a research treatment in the context of a clinical trial.[2,3] When IPT showed both efficacy[3] for depression and a gain in social functioning that antidepressant medication lacked,[4] several investigators tested its efficacy in randomized controlled clinical trials for major depression and other disorders. Klerman and Weissman took a relatively cautious approach to dissemination, first ensuring that the treatment actually worked. For years, IPT researchers joked that there were more published papers on IPT than there were IPT therapists. Moreover, most of those scarce therapists were engaged in clinical research trials rather than community practice. Then in 1992, soon after IPT had gained recognition for its outcomes in landmark studies like the National Institute of Mental Health Treatment of Depression Collaborative Research Program,[5,6] Dr. Klerman prematurely died, derailing the spread of the treatment. Research on IPT continued,[1] but it took years for it to reach clinicians through clinical training programs and continuing education courses. Even today, only a minority of healthcare professional programs provide instruction and clinical supervision in IPT despite impressive supporting evidence for its efficacy.[7,8]

John C. Markowitz, *International Society of Interpersonal Psychotherapy (ISIPT)* In: *Interpersonal Psychotherapy.* Edited by: Myrna M. Weissman and Jennifer J. Mootz, Oxford University Press. © Oxford University Press 2024. DOI: 10.1093/oso/9780197652084.003.0005

FORMATION OF THE ISIPT

In the late 20th century, IPT researchers and clinicians began to meet informally at national and international conferences, particularly at the American Psychiatric Association (APA) annual meetings. In May 2000, at an APA meeting in Chicago, a small group of us in a hotel conference room agreed to form an informal IPT organization. Participants attended from Australia, Canada, Germany, Great Britain, Iceland, Luxembourg, New Zealand, the United States, and other countries. That same year in Australia, Michael Robertson, led the formation of the International Society *for* Interpersonal Psychotherapy, headquartered in Australia, with three chapters in North America, the United Kingdom/Europe, and Australasia. He and Rebecca Reay, in Australia emailed a helpful news bulletin. The original ISIPT goals, which mirror those today, included the following:

- Disseminating IPT as a therapeutic modality
- Promoting training in IPT
- Promoting international cooperation in IPT research, training, and delivery
- Promoting dialogue among clinicians in order to further evolve IPT in various research and clinical settings
- Establishing training and accreditation pathways for IPT

Interpersonal psychotherapy therapists and clinicians began to stay in touch. In June 2004, Ellen Frank, and David Kupfer, organized the first ISIPT meeting in Pittsburgh, Pennsylvania, a 3-day event bringing together researchers and clinicians from several continents. International meetings have since continued roughly every 2 years, in Toronto, New York, Amsterdam, Iowa City, London, Toronto (again), Budapest, and most recently a November 2021 COVID-year virtual conference beamed from Florida. The 10th annual conference will be held in Newcastle Upon Tyne, United Kingdom, in 2024.

At one early gathering, Scott Stuart, from Iowa City, Iowa, was unanimously chosen as the first ISIPT president by a small group of IPTers, a role he retained for more than a decade. During this time, IPT training spread while the ISIPT remained a loosely knit, informal organization. In 2011, the ISIPT board transferred the ISIPT organizational base from Australia to Iowa City, Iowa, where it was again incorporated as a nonprofit institution. In 2015, the ISIPT membership held its first formal elections, electing Holly Swartz, from Pittsburgh, Pennsylvania, to a 2-year term as president (2015–2017), with Paula Ravitz, of Toronto, Canada, as vice president. Also elected were a treasurer, secretary, and an elected executive council, which held monthly meetings. Bylaws were approved, and the organization was reincorporated in 2016 as the International Society *of* Interpersonal Psychotherapy in Brentwood, Tennessee. Regular elections for officers and executive council members continue. Subsequent presidents have been Dr. Ravitz (2017–2019); Oguz Omay (2019–2021); and now myself (2021–2023). Heather Flynn, is the vice president and president-elect.

THE CURRENT ORGANIZATION

Since its 2015 reorganization, the ISIPT has become an active, far-flung, vibrant, solvent, if still small organization. It remains "a multidisciplinary, non-commercial, international organization committed to the advancement of interpersonal psychotherapy (IPT) through scientific research, training and dissemination. The ISIPT sees the broad application of IPT by therapists worldwide as one of the valuable means for alleviating human suffering due to mental disorders" (https:// interpersonalpsychotherapy.org/about-isipt/mission-vision). ISIPT membership spans 6 continents. In addition to its individual members, ISIPT embraces national and regional chapters (Brazil, China, and Turkey, with other countries and regional groups in the wings) and maintains cordial informal affiliation with independent, nonchapter national IPT organizations (e.g., IPT-UK; Dutch, German, and Swedish IPT groups). Dr. Omay deserves credit for the innovation of the national and regional chapters.

Members communicate through an active listserv and via the frequently updated website, which was curated first by Dr. Gokben Hizli Sayar of Turkey and now by Malin Bäck of Sweden. Based on membership dues, dedicated teaching workshops, and proceeds of the biennial international meetings, the ISIPT has built a modest treasury to support its training, certification, and advocacy efforts.

The executive council meets monthly by Zoom. It comprises the president, vice president, secretary, treasurer, 6 council members (currently from four continents), and 2 nonvoting council members: Dr. Weissman as the inventor of IPT and Dr. Swartz as parliamentarian. The ISIPT component committees generally reflect the organization's initiatives. Their liaisons report to the executive council (see Figure 4.1).

Interpersonal psychotherapy remains underutilized as a treatment considering its therapist and patient friendliness and its proven efficacy for psychiatric conditions, ranging from unipolar to bipolar mood disorders, eating disorders, and post-traumatic stress disorder.[1,8] In recent years, under the dynamic leadership

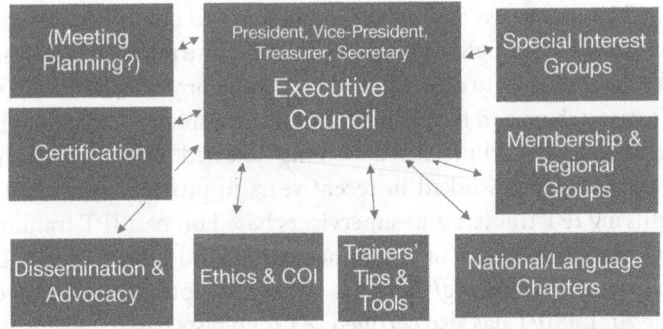

Figure 4.1 Structure of the International Society of Interpersonal Psychotherapy current goals.

of Drs. Swartz, Ravitz, and Omay, ISIPT has mobilized to conduct several important initiatives.

1. *Promoting IPT and ISIPT membership.* Most psychotherapists begin training by learning a cognitive behavioral, supportive, or psychodynamic approach. Too few psychiatric residencies and psychology and social work programs provide IPT training.[7] (The ISIPT is currently resurveying the extent of IPT training across North American programs.) IPT is thus supplemental training for most therapists. ISIPT sponsors training workshops, to which IPT experts donate their time and energy to orient participants to IPT principles and practice. Workshop profits support the organization, and it is hoped many of these new IPT users will eventually join ISIPT.

The ISIPT supports its members through its active global listserv and website. The website offers the outside world information about IPT and the ISIPT. Its Members Only section presents videotape and PowerPoint training materials, IPT assessments, past meeting presentations, a "Tips and Trainers" educational section, member directory, and other resources. The listserv provides the opportunity to learn about and discuss with experts new developments in IPT clinical practice and research. Since 2001 a special interest group initiative has attracted great member interest. To date there have been meetings for those interested in IPT for adolescent, peripartum, and bipolar patients. ISIPT membership affords discounts to ISIPT meetings and for ISIPT certification.

Initially developed in the United States, IPT has now spread widely in Europe, Australasia, and South America and increasingly into Africa and Asia. We have been pleased to see IPT, and by extension ISIPT, disseminated well beyond America. There have been studies and large training projects in Uganda, Kenya, Ethiopia, Mozambique, and South Africa, as well as in Japan, Korea, Hong Kong, and now mainland China. Researchers from 28 countries on 6 continents attended the last ISIPT biennial meeting. ISIPT membership is rising but remains too sparse considering its global spread. Readers interested in the organization are encouraged to join ISIPT (https://interpersonalpsychotherapy.org/membership/join-now/), which offers reduced rates to clinicians from LMICs and to students.

2. *Promoting IPT research.* IPT began as a research treatment. Its range has been defined by its success and failure in randomized controlled clinical trials.[1,8] Although research has taught us much about IPT, more remains to be learned. The ISIPT lacks the resources to directly fund psychotherapy research, but it brings together IPT researchers and fosters the funding atmosphere where possible.

3. *Certification.* IPT clinicians have long yearned for proof of their skills training, and ISIPT has worked in recent years to provide that. In 2020, ISIPT began certifying IPT trainers and supervisors based on past IPT training and supervisory experience, letters of recommendation, and other criteria (https://interpersonalpsychotherapy.org/therapists-trainers/isipt-certification-requirements/). Since 2021, ISIPT has also certified IPT therapists based on educational and clinical data. Goals of certification include maintaining the integrity of training

and practice and identifying IPT experts around the world. Certification requires ISIPT membership.

4. *Advocacy for patients and for psychotherapy.* A relatively new organizational facet has been to promote IPT and psychotherapy more generally to ensure patient access to effective treatment and thus reduce suffering. ISIPT has written to correct bias in treatment practice guidelines, to promote psychotherapy to US congressional panels, to critique inaccurate newspaper articles with letters to editors, and to advocate for clinical research funding. A particular problem IPT has faced is that the US National Institute of Mental Health, historically the richest source of clinical research funding in the world, in the past decade has essentially reduced clinical research grants in favor of neuroscience studies.[9,10] Because there is strength in numbers, ISIPT has begun to collaborate on advocacy with cognitive behavioral and psychoanalytic organizations, and with national societies such as the American Psychiatric Association, to promote access to care and patient safety where needed.

This short chapter cannot fully describe the workings and benefits of our growing organization, but it is hoped it conveys some of the vibrancy of the ISIPT. If you have not already done so, please go to the website (https://interpersonalps ychotherapy.org/) and see for yourself.

ACKNOWLEDGMENT

I thank Rebecca Reay and Michael Robertson for their help in reconstructing the early history of ISIPT.

REFERENCES

1. Weissman MM, Markowitz JC, Klerman GL. *The Guide to Interpersonal Psychotherapy.* Oxford University Press; 2018.
2. Markowitz JC, Weissman MM. IPT: past, present, and future. *Clin Psychol Psychother.* 2012;19:99–105.
3. Klerman GL, Dimascio A, Weissman M, Prusoff B, Paykel ES. Treatment of depression by drugs and psychotherapy. *Am J Psychiatry.* 1974;131:186–191.
4. Weissman MM, Klerman GL, Paykel ES, Prusoff B, Hanson B. Treatment effects on the social adjustment of depressed patients. *Arch Gen Psychiatry.* 1974;30:771–778.
5. Elkin I, Parloff MB, Hadley SW, Autry JH. NIMH Treatment of Depression Collaborative Research Program. Background and research plan. *Arch Gen Psychiatry.* 1985;42:305–316.
6. Elkin I, Shea MT, Watkins JT, et al. National Institute of Mental Health Treatment of Depression Collaborative Research Program. General effectiveness of treatments. *Arch Gen Psychiatry.* 1989;46:971–982.
7. Weissman MM, Verdeli H, Gameroff MJ, et al. National survey of psychotherapy training in psychiatry, psychology, and social work. *Arch Gen Psychiatry.* 2006;63:925–934.

8. Cuijpers P, Donker T, Weissman MM, Ravitz P, Cristea IA. Interpersonal psychotherapy for mental health problems: A comprehensive meta-analysis. *Am J Psychiatry*. 2016;173:680–687.

9. Markowitz JC, Friedman RA. NIMH's straight and neural path: The road to killing clinical psychiatric research. *Psychiatr Serv*. 2020;71:1096–1097.

10. Torrey EF, Simmons WW, Hancq ES, Snook J. The continuing decline of clinical research on serious mental illnesses at NIMH. *Psychiatr Serv*. 2021;72:1342–1344.

International Society of Interpersonal Psychotherapy Certification Program

CINDY GOODMAN STULBERG AND HEATHER A. FLYNN ■

Discussion regarding whether and how to create a certification process for IPT trainers, supervisors, and psychotherapists within the International Society of Interpersonal Psychotherapy (ISIPT) began around the inception of the organization in 2000. The issue of certification within the organization was an ongoing topic at the biannual meetings, on the ISIPT listserv, and among the ISIPT committees.

Some of the concerns raised by members included issues around ISIPT organization having to accept professional responsibility for certified members as well as the size of the organization. ISIPT had been a relatively small organization that did not historically have the infrastructure to implement the certification program. Support for certification from members centered on the need for ISIPT to create processes and supports for high-quality dissemination of interpersonal psychotherapy (IPT) globally. The organization also saw other psychotherapy models offering certification, and this contributed to the dissemination of those models. Requests for certification were particularly strong from members living in countries where their governing bodies and governments that sometimes paid for counseling services were asking for certified clinicians.

In 2015, an ISIPT Certification Committee was charged with systematically exploring whether and how to create a certification process for ISIPT. The committee comprised 10 ISIPT members from different parts of the world, representing diverse disciplines (e.g., psychologists, psychiatrists, social workers, etc.) and roles, including clinicians, researchers, and academics. The committee was first established to explore and develop processes for trainer

Cindy Goodman Stulberg and Heather A. Flynn, *International Society of Interpersonal Psychotherapy Certification Program*
In: *Interpersonal Psychotherapy*. Edited by: Myrna M. Weissman and Jennifer J. Mootz, Oxford University Press.
© Oxford University Press 2024. DOI: 10.1093/oso/9780197652084.003.0006

and supervisor certification, with a plan to develop psychotherapist certification later.

By design, the committee was inclusive of different points of view and encouraged participants to share their professional experiences to get a thorough picture of the needs of clinicians from around the world. The mission of the committee was to "develop standards and processes supporting continued educational development and voluntary certification of IPT trainers and supervisors." The implementation of the mission included standards and processes that support excellence in training professionals in IPT. The accomplishment of the mission included identifying a range of options for obtaining the most effective experience for IPT certification process and criteria, eliciting expertise and informing the ISIPT members, and working closely with the ISIPT Executive Committee and ISIPT membership on these options and associated recommendations. Implementation of the mission also outlined that guidelines and standards for trainer development and training competencies would be agreed on by consensus and would be iterative. That is, the process would evolve based on emerging empirical evidence and training wisdom.

In addition to determining a mission for the certification committee, a set of guiding principles was developed, based on consensus, to support training effectiveness, dissemination, as well as ongoing IPT trainer development. These principles included the following:

- Trainer certification criteria will reflect the mission of the ISIPT and will support trainer development.
- Any standards, criteria, and/or processes should be linked, where feasible, to training quality and outcomes.
- Certification will be voluntary in that ISIPT members may choose whether or not to pursue certification.
- There are multiple pathways to trainer development and to being able to meet certification criteria, accommodating multiple styles, roles, resources, cultures, and contexts.
- Trainer certification should be feasible for any ISIPT member to pursue, regardless of culture, geographic location, or resources
- Any established standards and processes will be evaluated continually and informed by new knowledge (e.g., IPT mechanisms of action).
- Any process must be feasible and sustainable for ISIPT to implement and sustain.

Once the mission and guiding principles were established, a number of developmental, foundational activities were completed by the certification committee in order to carefully determine consensus as well as a preliminary certification process. These activities included the following:

- Regular committee conference calls
- A qualitative study of IPT experts' perspectives on certification

- An ISIPT member survey about member perspectives on trainer and supervisor certification
- Compilation of key issues related to other comparable models of trainer/ supervisor certification and development
- Compilation of other existing IPT certification and training programs globally
- Compiled/reviewed existing models of IPT trainer development and materials
- Ongoing consultations with the ISIPT Executive Committee
- Expert consensus on IPT trainer competencies linked to quality in conjunction with review of existing trainer quality rating tools
- Devised process of refinement of key elements of the trainer development and certification competencies based on targeted ISIPT member input

Based on these developmental activities, an initial ISIPT certification process for IPT trainers and supervisors was developed. The initial offering of certification was implemented as a "grandfathering" stage. This process was developed to accommodate and certify very experienced trainers and supervisors, including the originators, early leaders, and those who historically launched IPT training and supervision globally. Applicants certified in this grandfathering or "legacy" stage included members from many different countries, including Brazil, Japan, China, France, Italy, Netherlands, Israel, Lebanon, Canada, and the United States. A broad group of members was initially certified as trainers and/or supervisors, including psychiatrists, general practitioners, psychologists, social workers, and psychiatric nurses providing training and supervision in many different languages in low-, middle-, and high-income countries, to children, adolescents, adults, and older adults.

Since the initial implementation of trainer and supervisor certification (Figure 5.1), over 95% of applicants have been certified by ISIPT. Fees for the application review process will be implemented with financial support offered to low-income countries.

The challenges that presented during the initial implementation of trainer and supervisor certification included creating a pool of volunteer application reviewers from the ISIPT organization and providing clear instructions around how to apply the review criteria. As well, we needed to create a fair and timely process to follow up with applicants who needed to provide additional information if their submissions were insufficient. Creating the infrastructure required collecting and distributing the application information and notifying applicants once a review had been completed had to be established without allocated funds. Once applicants are certified, they are listed on the ISIPT website.

The ISIPT has also now followed an analogous pathway and created a process for psychotherapist certification. As we move forward, we are creating supports and

Figure 5.1 Ad for ISIPT certification. Credit: International Society of Interpersonal Psychotherapy.

guidance for ongoing trainer, supervisor, and therapist development. Examples of current ISIPT member ongoing development questions include

- Is there adequate and equitable access to ongoing IPT training for therapists, trainers, and supervisors?
- Can we create mentorship programs to build expert certified trainers?
- Can we offer ongoing professional development so certified clinicians can continue to offer high-quality service?
- What requirements should be set for recertification and over how long a period of time?

Interpersonal psychotherapy is a highly effective researched psychotherapy model that has been utilized all over the world and delivered to many different individuals, groups, families, and couples for many years. IPT clinicians, trainers and supervisors, researchers, and academics are passionate about helping others and providing excellent therapy to as many people as they can. Certification should always support this effort in every way it can.

IPT TRAINING

Interpersonal psychotherapy training is a broad, international effort to disseminate IPT around the world so as many people as possible can have access to this highly recommended, effective model of psychotherapy.

There is no central organization that coordinates or oversees IPT training, although the ISIPT organization has begun to provide certification for IPT therapists, trainers, and supervisors. IPT training has evolved over many years, originating with what might be called a mentorship and research-based process.

Drs. Klerman and Weissman, who initiated the first clinical research trials of IPT in the 1970s, trained clinicians to provide IPT as part of the research. This was continued as research studies were done. As information about IPT spread through articles on the research results, clinicians and researchers sought training.

As the work progressed and publications cited IPT as a researched model of psychotherapy for depression, other clinicians/researchers began to adapt the model to work with clients with other disorders, and different ages and modalities (e.g., eating disorders, dysthymia, adolescents, group therapy). Clinicians/researchers saw the efficacy of the model and began to seek training from those who had been previously trained and expand and enhance the use of IPT.

Clinicians who had been trained by the original developers and those subsequently trained began to use the model and develop training programs in their own countries. Some of these training programs tied to university programs, the Veterans Administration program in the United States; government-funded programs (e.g., in the United Kingdom); and private practice clinicians in different countries (e.g., the Institute for Interpersonal Psychotherapy based in Canada).

Training was offered, over the years, at the American Psychiatric Association conference and at the venue once the ISIPT began having biannual conferences. Training was unregulated and traditionally began with a 5-day training schedule, composed of didactic information stressing the core components and effective delivery of the model. It included opportunities to practice skills and to receive feedback from trainers as well as case videos and descriptions of case examples. This was typically a beginner's introduction to IPT but provided enough information for a clinician to begin to deliver the therapy. Supervision following training was encouraged, but not always done based primarily on cost, time, and trainer availability.

Over the years, the length of training time was changed in some settings, anywhere from 2 to 5 days in total. Virtual training began to be offered during COVID, which had the advantage of allowing access to clinicians at greater distance and reducing travel costs for participants. Some online programs are available as well.

Training is now being provided at an introductory and more advanced level and for many IPT adaptations, including perinatal, older adults, couples, and post-traumatic stress disorder (PTSD). IPT training is being provided to graduate psychology and psychiatry students as well as in psychology and psychiatry programs. There are many training opportunities around the world, and English-speaking trainers have used translators to teach in other countries. Training is being done in Brazil, China, Lebanon, Africa, and elsewhere. IPT books and training materials have been translated in many different languages.

The following is an example of an IPT training and supervision program in Brazil.

TRAINING AND SUPERVISION IN INTERPERSONAL PSYCHOTHERAPY

IPT-Brazil-Federal University of São Paulo Group
Euthymia Prado

Training was initiated in 2007 by Prof. Marcelo Feijó de Mello, associate professor at the Department of Psychiatry at the Federal University of São Paulo. He initially formed a group of psychiatrists and psychotherapists (Fernando S. Lacaz, Aline F. Schoedl, Mariana Pupo, and Rosaly F. Braga), who went on to provide training and supervision under his leadership, creating the Interpersonal Therapy Clinic (C-TIP).

Between 2007 and 2011, courses with theoretical classes and seminars were held annually, totaling 30 hours. An additional 30 hours of supervision occurred in each course, supervising groups of 3 to 4 students who presented at least 2 cases each. Around 100 students participated and were certified, including psychiatrists and psychotherapists. At the end, each student presented a detailed written report of supervised cases. The criteria for approval were attendance of at least 75%, participation in seminars, and a final paper to be presented orally.

In 2012, Euthymia Prado and Rosaly Braga started coordinating a weekly 2-hour meeting that included theoretical training and case supervision of members of the department's staff. Graduate students and interested residents also participated. In 2015, an online course was developed, using the distance learning platform of the Assistance and Research Program in Violence of the Department of Psychiatry of the University of São Paulo, in collaboration with the Center for Studies and Research of the same department. The platform allows organized, dynamic, and collaborative visual interaction, with material available every week, totaling 6 weeks, and the student can complete it in up to 12 weeks. In addition to video-recorded classes, there are vignettes of clinical cases that address the foci of interpersonal therapy, theoretical texts, and questionnaires at the end of each module to evaluate the learning of the content. After completing the theoretical course, students can request supervision of cases handled in the service or in other workplaces. As of 2021, Mariana Pupo, Thays Mello, Mario Diniz, and Marcelo Mello guided discussions and weekly supervision for psychiatry residents who participated in these online courses throughout the school year, while maintaining the online course for the public outside the university.

Several IPT research and clinical applications have been carried out over the years in eating disorders, depression, schizophrenia, PTSD among rape victims, IPT group for PTSD among adolescents, and interpersonal counseling in depression in a community setting have also been included.

FURTHER READING

Klerman GL Weissman MM, Rousaville BJ, Chevron ES. *Interpersonal Psychotherapy of Depression*. Basic Books; 1984.

Rousaville BJ, Chevron ES, Weissman MM. Specification of technicians in interpersonal psychotherapy. In Williams JBW, Spitzer RL, eds. *Psychotherapy Research: Where Are We and Where Should We Go?* Guilford Press; 1984:160–172.

Stuart S, Robertson M. *Interpersonal Psychotherapy: A Clinician's Guide*. Arnold Hodder; 2013.

Weissman MM, Markowitz JC, Klerman GL. *A Clinician's Quick Guide to Interpersonal Psychotherapy*. Oxford University Press; 2006.

Weissman MM, Markowitz JC, Klerman GL. *Comprehensive Guide to Interpersonal Psychotherapy*. Basic Books; 2000.

Weissman MM, Markowitz JC, Klerman GL. *The Guide to Interpersonal Psychotherapy: Updated and Expanded Edition*. Oxford University Press; 2018.

Weissman MM, Rousaville BJ, Chevron ES. Training psychotherapists to participate in psychotherapy outcomes studies. *Am J Psychiatry*. 1982;139:1442–1446.

International Society of Interpersonal Psychotherapy Chapters

OGUZ OMAY AND HOLLY A. SWARTZ ■

The International Society of Interpersonal Psychotherapy (ISIPT) is a not-for-profit, global organization with members located in over 25 countries. ISIPT membership provides access to interpersonal psychotherapy (IPT) knowledge experts, ISIPT certification procedures, and IPT training support. Despite the expansive mission and membership of ISIPT, there remain unmet needs within the IPT practitioner community. Specifically, groups of IPT clinicians who affiliate around shared language, cultural, or geographic identities may lack either the infrastructure or capacity to ally with the ISIPT, thereby missing out on opportunities for professional support, networking, and knowledge transfer. As this book illustrates, there have been many groups in different countries and regions engaged in IPT research and training. In 2021, ISIPT took a step further and decided to create formal ISIPT chapters to better include and represent our global community.

Formal ISIPT chapters are formed by IPT practitioners who represent specific regional, national, or language-based IPT interests. Some organizations define their chapters based solely on nationality or country; however, ISIPT permits chapters to self-define based on other relevant identity features. For instance, French-speaking IPT therapists reside in many countries, including France, Canada, Belgium, Tunisia, and Morocco. A francophone ISIPT chapter is planned based on shared linguistic rather than geographic ties, whereas the Brazilian chapter, even though their members share a common language with Portuguese colleagues, opted to define itself on national terms because of its specific challenges and priorities in terms of training and national dissemination.

Oguz Omay and Holly A. Swartz, *International Society of Interpersonal Psychotherapy Chapters* In: *Interpersonal Psychotherapy*. Edited by: Myrna M. Weissman and Jennifer J. Mootz, Oxford University Press. © Oxford University Press 2024. DOI: 10.1093/oso/9780197652084.003.0007

The ISIPT chapters share the same mission as the parent ISIPT organization, but they work toward these goals within a smaller or more homogeneous group. Thus, all ISIPT chapters abide by the ISIPT Mission Statement: a commitment to the advancement of IPT by scientific research, training, and dissemination. Each ISIPT chapter shares with ISIPT these fundamental values, although individual chapters may have additional goals or objectives beyond their primary ISIPT directive. Affiliated chapters of ISIPT function according to the purposes and principals of ISIPT while operating as financially, legally, and administratively independent arms of the society.

Clinicians and researchers interested in and involved with IPT have the option of belonging to local ISIPT chapters as well as to the international umbrella organization, the ISIPT. Either or both may provide attractive options for interested individuals. Thus, the availability of ISIPT chapters facilitates another part of the ISIPT mission: broad application of IPT by therapists worldwide as one of the valuable means by which human suffering due to mental disorders can be alleviated.

Chapter formation is also part of a strategic plan to grow ISIPT. ISIPT is an English language organization with roots in North American and European academic medical centers. These features of ISIPT may not meet the needs of all IPT practitioners, especially those who are non-English speaking or those whose priorities are hyperlocal (i.e., specific refugee communities, non-Western cultural foci, etc.). Chapters pull together individuals with shared objectives and concerns, providing infrastructure that links smaller IPT practitioner groups to the broader ISIPT family. If they have an ISIPT-certified trainer in their group or association, chapters are empowered to certify local IPT therapists, thereby expanding the pool of trained IPT clinicians in areas that may not have access to broader ISIPT initiatives (including formal ISIPT therapist training/certification) for reasons of language, geography, or finances. New IPT therapists are encouraged to join their local ISIPT chapter, thereby providing a pathway for ISIPT engagement and growth, especially among non-English-speaking and culturally distinct IPT learning communities.

ISIPT CHAPTER REQUIREMENTS AND BENEFITS

The ISIPT chapters are formed by groups pursuing a comprehensive IPT-related mission (education, training, advocacy, mentorship) and linked by geographic or linguistic commonalities. Entities whose sole mission is profit-based IPT training, such as IPT training academies or schools, are not eligible to form ISIPT chapters.

Requirements for groups who wish to form ISIPT chapters include

- A minimum of 10 members in the group, at least 5 of whom who are full, dues-paying members of ISIPT
- Completion of an application (available on the ISIPT website) and payment of an application fee

- Payment of annual fees to maintain ISIPT affiliation (reduced fee schedules available to chapters organized in low- and middle-income countries) and provision of yearly updates to ISIPT leadership

The ISIPT chapter members enjoy all the benefits of their individual groups as well as some general ones, ISIPT benefits. Benefits of chapter affiliation include

- Listing of the chapter's name, website, officers, and brief description of the chapter on the ISIPT website
- Opportunity to list/advertise chapter events and trainings on the ISIPT website
- Right to use the ISIPT logo on chapter materials and website
- Registration of chapter members at reduced rates for all ISIPT trainings and conferences
- Option for affiliate chapter members to apply for full ISIPT membership (with full ISIPT benefits)
- If chapters include ISIPT certified trainers/supervisors, those individuals may certify therapists through the chapter according to ISIPT certification guidelines (note that these locally certified individuals do not immediately qualify for ISIPT therapist certification, but they can easily use chapter-based training as part of their ISIPT therapist certification application should they become full ISIPT members)

Unless individual ISIPT chapter members are also ISIPT members, they are not entitled to some ISIPT benefits, such as online training tools/resources (members-only section of the website), the ISIPT listserv, the right to vote in ISIPT elections, and individual listings on the ISIPT website as a certified IPT therapist, supervisor, or trainer.

RECOGNIZED ISIPT CHAPTERS

As of September 2022, there were 5 recognized ISIPT chapters. In order of date of initial affiliation, they are IPT-Turkey, IPT-China, IPT-Swiss, IPT-Brazil, and IPT Sub-Saharan Africa.

It is interesting to note considerable differences between the chapters, indicating variability in pathways to chapter status. The Turkish, Swiss, and Brazilian chapters represent the culmination of several decades of effort by local professionals engaged in IPT research or training. The Chinese and sub-Saharan African chapters have been created de novo in response to relatively recent training initiatives in their regions. While IPT-China tries to federate a huge country with hundreds of interested or trained professionals, the sub-Saharan African chapter brings together professionals from several countries seeking to make a difference in patient outcomes by sharing and expanding regional expertise.

Some countries in which IPT is well established—like the United Kingdom or the Netherlands—may choose to focus on their own well-developed IPT training infrastructure rather than formally partnering with ISIPT as chapters. Other regions or countries, however, are considering creation of formal affiliated chapters. For instance, a planned French-speaking federation of IPT may apply for affiliated ISIPT chapter status, seeking to unite different countries through their shared language.

SUMMARY

The ISIPT chapters foster global cooperation among IPT researchers, trainers, and practitioners. They advance ISIPT's goal of extending the reach of IPT worldwide as one of the valuable means for alleviating human suffering due to mental disorders. ISIPT welcomes chapter applications from all interested and qualified groups.

PART III

Training in Interpersonal Psychotherapy

7

Interpersonal Psychotherapy Training—Digital, Online Educational Formats

PAULA RAVITZ, SHAHANA SITTAMPALAM,
MALIN BÄCK, KEVIN CROSWELL, HOLLY A. SWARTZ,
AND DAISY RADHA SINGLA ∎

Access to interpersonal psychotherapy (IPT) is limited despite its strong evidentiary base.[1,2] This is due to not only systemic barriers to mental health (MH) care,[3] but also insufficient numbers of health providers with IPT expertise. There is an imperative to scale access to evidence-supported psychotherapies that may in part be addressed with low-barrier access to training.[1,4] This chapter reviews digital IPT courses for readers interested in IPT training. Digital, online, computer-, or smartphone app-assisted, Internet-based educational formats have potential to improve training access and overcome geographic and practical barriers, at lower cost, with the convenience for learners of open enrollment and participation at their own pace.[5-8]

Curricular design innovations of competency-based health education have advanced digital, Internet-based pedagogy, including psychotherapy training for mental healthcare providers (Figure 7.1).[7,9-13] Specific to psychotherapy training, digital courses feature didactic and interactive case-based teaching with videotaped demonstrations of therapeutic strategies. The creation and implementation of these courses requires modality-specific psychotherapy experts, instructional designers with expertise in best e-learning practices, learning management system (LMS) programmers, secure web hosting, and course administration processes for learner enrollment and communications. In addition, accredited course planning involves conducting learning needs assessments, creating actionable learning objectives with an inclusive planning committee that represents

Paula Ravitz, Shahana Sittampalam, Malin Bäck, Kevin Croswell, Holly A. Swartz, and Daisy Radha Singla, *Interpersonal Psychotherapy Training—Digital, Online Educational Formats* In: *Interpersonal Psychotherapy.* Edited by: Myrna M. Weissman and Jennifer J. Mootz, Oxford University Press. © Oxford University Press 2024. DOI: 10.1093/oso/9780197652084.003.0008

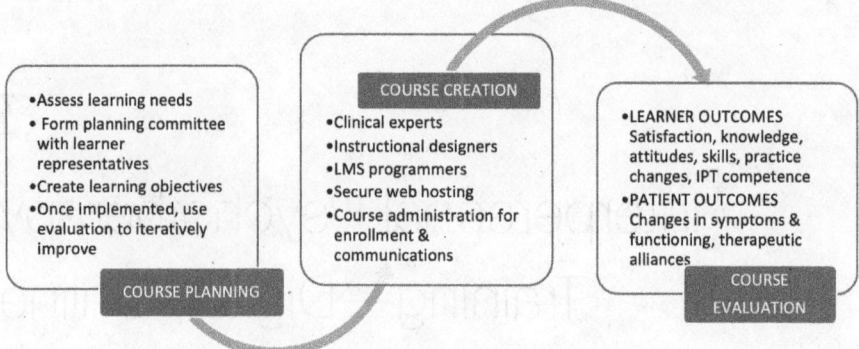

Figure 7.1 Tasks, experts, and supports needed to plan, create, implement, and evaluate digital courses.

Table 7.1 INTERACTIVE DIGITAL IPT TRAINING COURSES

Digital IPT training courses	Access
1. http://www.ipttraining.net[22]	Commercially available
2. https://www.IPSRT.org[23]	Open access
3. https://pter.mcmaster.ca[24]	Commercially available; free by request to LMIC settings
4. https://www.relatera.net [25]	Open to psychology students at Linköping University and members of the IPT Swedish society
5. US Department of Veterans Affairs[26]	Available to therapists working in the US Department of Veterans Affairs facilities
6. https://www.LearnIPT.com[27,28]	Open access through University of Toronto, Temerty Faculty of Medicine "Learn Interpersonal Psychotherapy" Coursera Course, and for university-affiliated faculty through the e-Campus Ontario virtual library

diverse learners, and creating agendas that balance didactic teaching with interactive learning.[14,15] Measurement of learning outcomes and the acquisition of psychotherapy competence can include associated changes in knowledge, skills, or patient outcomes resulting from clinical practice.[16–18]

Digital IPT educational materials range from didactic instructional videos and webinars to highly interactive, case-based digital courses for self-directed online learning or in combination with skills training workshops. We searched for and identified six IPT digital courses that were described in the literature and/ or presented at conferences and that provided foundational didactic training to prepare learners for IPT clinical practice (Table 7.1). Additional educational materials are also available online through the International Society of IPT (ISIPT) website (https://www.interpersonalpsychotherapy.org) to members with slide presentations, webinars, and teaching videos demonstrating therapeutic techniques[19,20] from varied IPT communities of practitioners (e.g., in the United Kingdom, Israel, Ethiopia, and China). In addition, Kumar et al. in Kenya engaged multiple stakeholders to culturally adapt and inform future instructional design for digital training of nonspecialist providers of IPT in global low-income settings.[21] This chapter reviews six case-based, interactive digital IPT training courses:

1. http://www.ipttraining.net is an online, digital IPT training program piloted with community-based clinicians and MH trainees by Kobak et al. (United States) that is now commercialized. It has three components: a 3- to 4-hour, web-based tutorial on concepts and techniques of IPT; a videoconferenced live training session (45–60 minutes) with case formulation and skills practicing using a role play with an IPT expert trainer portraying a simulated patient; and post-training facilitation with practice reminders to support IPT adherence and measurement-based quality care.[22] There are modules that cover principles of IPT and its purported mechanisms of change and modules on each of the 4 IPT problem areas of grief, social role transitions, role disputes, and interpersonal deficits. The program features interactive exercises, animations, graphical illustrations, and clinical vignettes. The program was evaluated with 26 community-based clinician learners with around 10 years of clinical experience and found high levels of learner satisfaction with significant improvement in IPT knowledge.[22]

2. Interpersonal and social rhythm therapy (IPSRT) is an adaptation of IPT for individuals with bipolar disorder. Ellen Frank and Holly Swartz created an open-access, online, 8-hour training course in IPSRT (https://www.IPSRT.org/). It incorporates videotaped interviews with IPSRT experts, downloadable IPSRT tracking tools, patient handouts, instruments for assessing symptoms of bipolar disorder, a message board for knowledge exchange, and links to IPSRT-related websites. An educational pilot study was conducted using this web-based IPSRT training with 36 clinicians and their 136 patients from 5 MH centers.[23] The clinicians were randomly allocated to in-person training with local supervision or online training with an online learning collaborative supported by expert clinicians. Significant post-training differences were found between the live and online training groups, favoring the latter, in the extent to which patients reported on the clinicians' use of 19 IPSRT techniques.[23]

3. Psychotherapy Training e-Resources (PTeR; https://pter.mcmaster.ca/) is a collection of accredited psychotherapy training e-resources on a commercialized website; the collection is free to low-income country settings to assist with psychotherapy education. It features differing kinds of psychotherapy, including a module on IPT for interprofessional graduate, postgraduate, and continuing education (CE) training. PTeR

was created and has been updated by Weerasekera and colleagues at McMaster University (Canada) over the past 22 years.[24] The training modules contain videotaped demonstrations with simulated patients portrayed by faculty, psychiatry residents or staff; quizzes; and interactive components with a "virtual therapist" for clinical skills teaching. In addition, and related to the curriculum on IPT, an introductory course on psychotherapies demonstrates the application of four different psychotherapies for treating grief with the same simulated patient: IPT, cognitive behavioral therapy (CBT), psychodynamic psychotherapy, and emotion-focused therapy. A 2017 survey of PTeR users revealed high levels of satisfaction and educational value (personal communication with Weerasekera).

4. IPT is included in the national depression treatment guidelines in Sweden, and national IPT therapist certification guidelines require a 4-day workshop followed by clinically supervised casework. There are limited IPT training opportunities at universities or CE programs in Sweden. Thus, a Swedish-language digital IPT training platform was developed by Bäck for university and CE teaching. It began with migrating extant curriculum to a digital format with uploaded recorded lectures and slides for asynchronous access and assignments using a "flipped-classroom" educational process.[29] The lectures include IPT history, research, clinical skills, and theories, with case-based teaching and simulated demonstrations with a patient portrayed by a colleague.[25] The course is offered in a hybrid format, combining asynchronous online self-study with virtual online classroom discussions and as a stand-alone distance educational course with access to online discussions and instructor feedback (https://www.relatera.net). Postgraduate trainees have endorsed finding the hybrid format of online self-study combined with live online discussion with instructor feedback as helpful to facilitate learning.

5. The US Department of Veterans Affairs (VA) has scaled up access to evidence-based psychotherapies for veterans care, including IPT. IPT training of hundreds of licensed VA MH practitioners migrated from in-person workshops led by IPT experts Kathleen Clougherty and Greg Hinrichson to a hybrid format of live online group workshops combined with a digital interactive self-study simulation program. The trainings are followed by 6 months of once-weekly, live, distance, case-based consultations. The 5-day hybrid IPT training agenda features live online morning lectures (delivered through Adobe Connect), early afternoons of protected time on a digital interactive self-directed software learning program, and group-based live online skills practicing consolidating learning in the late afternoons. The digital curriculum includes many videotaped clinical demonstrations, with branching scenarios for learners to virtually practice with computer-programmed feedback on poor, better, and best IPT responses. This online curriculum

takes around 6 hours to complete. Learners reported that the self-directed online branching scenarios increased their understanding of and confidence to deliver IPT. Of note, the cases and standardized patients, portrayed by actors or computer simulations, are diverse and inclusive of differing races, ages, and gender identities. The VA's program evaluation framework for competency-based training utilizes various sources of information to examine viability and effectiveness. Success of this training model was demonstrated by IPT knowledge checks (including self-study performance feedback), qualitative ratings from participant-learners, consultant ratings of participant progress based on session recording ratings of IPT fidelity, and patient outcomes of depression symptom changes, quality of life, and therapeutic alliances.[30] A recent internal VA report on the shift to digital and Internet learning revealed comparable positive learning outcomes and changes in trainee competence and patient outcomes when compared to the in-person training format.[26]

6. The Learn IPT website https://www.LearnIPT.com) is a case-based, asynchronous, self-directed digital training course created by Paula Ravitz with IPT experts, instructional designers and LMS programmers.[28] The target learner audience is interprofessional MH trainees and providers. A mixed-methods, single-blind, randomized controlled design compared feasibility, acceptability, and preliminary effectiveness of the asynchronous self-directed digital training to live large-group online workshop training as usual for postgraduate psychiatry residents. Both the online and live workshops were case based and highly interactive. The trainings were followed by clinically supervised casework, with tracking of patient and learner outcomes. Qualitative semistructured interviews revealed high levels of overall satisfaction and an appreciation of the diverse identities represented in the clinical cases included in the online course. In alignment with the learning objectives, learners reported becoming more attuned to relational aspects of patient experiences. The interactive 5-module curriculum takes around 6 hours to complete and covers the IPT phase- and focus-specific therapeutic tasks for the beginning, middle, and termination sessions, with additional emphasis on individual patient differences, such as cultural aspects of identity, therapeutic alliances, and attachment patterns of relating. The course's videotaped simulated demonstrations with trained actors portraying standardized patients are captioned to identify the therapist's deliberate application of IPT strategies. A forthcoming evaluation will examine both learner and patient outcomes with an IPT knowledge quiz, formative feedback on IPT clinical skills in an observed simulated clinical encounter (OSCE)[18,31] with a standardized patient, and externally rated competence of actual IPT sessions with consenting patients whose symptom changes will be tracked.[23]

These case-based digital training curricula focus on teaching manual-adherent IPT using demonstrations of IPT with patients portrayed by actors, trained simulated patients, faculty, or trainees. Some of the simulations have voice-over comments or captions to illustrate principles in practice at therapeutic choice points. Most of the evaluation frameworks examine learner satisfaction and knowledge. Several have also evaluated competency-based digital training with patient outcomes or applied IPT clinical skills in real practice, such as the IPSRT course, the US VA course, and https://www.LearnIPT.com. Measuring patient outcomes and applied practices of clinical educational programs is challenging. However, it represents the most rigorous and highest level of educational program evaluation.[17] It is also important to use the feedback and evaluation data to improve future iterations of training curriculum. These digital IPT courses all employ case-based, interactive learning with varying levels of instructor feedback. To consolidate expertise, clinically supervised casework is needed following the foundational digital training.

Increased access to IPT training is needed for scaling up of IPT globally. Greater attention to cultural adaptations of IPT and inclusion of faculty and patients with diverse intersectional identities will enhance the salience for a broad group of learners. Digital web-based courses are expanding access to training, with potential to advance the implementation of IPT and ultimately improve patients' access to and outcomes of evidence-supported mental healthcare.

ACKNOWLEDGMENTS

The website https://www.LearnIPT.com was funded by a University Health Network and Sinai Health System Academic Health Science Centre Innovation Award to Paula Ravitz and Daisy Singla; the "Learn Interpersonal Psychotherapy" Coursera MOOC was funded by the University of Toronto Open Course Initiative Fund, the Temerty Faculty of Medicine, and Sinai Health System, Department of Psychiatry.

DECLARATION OF INTERESTS

Authors S. S., M. B., and D. R. S. report no disclosures or financial relationships with any organizations that might have an interest in the submitted work in the previous 3 years and no other relationships or activities that could appear to have influenced the submitted work. P. R. receives royalties for WW Norton. K. C. is employed by the US Department of Veterans Affairs. D. R. S. is partly supported with an Academic Scholars Award from the Department of Psychiatry at the University of Toronto. H. A. S. reports receiving an editorial stipend and royalties from American Psychiatric Association Press, royalties from Wolters Kluwer, and consultant fees from Intracellular Therapeutics, WebMD, and Novus Medical Education.

REFERENCES

1. World Health Organization. *mhGAP Intervention Guide for Mental, Neurological and Substance Use Disorders in Non-Specialized Health Settings: Mental Health Gap Action Programme (mhGAP)*. World Health Organization; 2010.

2. Cuijpers P, Donker T, Weissman MM, Ravitz P, Cristea IA. Interpersonal psychotherapy for mental health problems: A comprehensive meta-analysis. *Am J Psychiatry*. 2016;173(7):680–687.

3. Fonagy P, Luyten P. Socioeconomic and sociocultural factors affecting access to psychotherapies: The way forward. *World Psychiatry*. 2021;20(3):315–316.

4. Singla DR, Raviola G, Patel V. Scaling up psychological treatments for common mental disorders: A call to action. *World Psychiatry*. 2018;17(2):226–227.

5. Fairburn CG, Allen E, Bailey-Straebler S, O'Connor ME, Cooper Z. Scaling up psychological treatments: A countrywide test of the online training of therapists. *J Med Internet Res*. 2017;19(6):6.

6. Cooper Z, Bailey-Straebler S, Morgan KE, et al. Using the Internet to train therapists: Randomized comparison of two scalable methods. *J Med Internet Res*. 2017;19(10):9.

7. O'Connor M, Morgan KE, Bailey-Straebler S, Fairburn CG, Cooper Z. Increasing the availability of psychological treatments: A multinational study of a scalable method for training therapists. *J Med Internet Res*. 2018;20(6):e10386. doi:10.2196/10386. PMID: 29884606; PMCID: PMC6015265.

8. Naslund JA, Tugnawat D, Anand A, et al. Digital training for non-specialist health workers to deliver a brief psychological treatment for depression in India: Protocol for a three-arm randomized controlled trial. *Contemporary Clinical Trials*. 2021;102:106267. doi:10.1016/j.cct.2021.106267. Epub 2021 Jan 6. PMID: 33421650.

9. Weingardt KR. The role of instructional design and technology in the dissemination of empirically supported, manual-based therapies. *Clin Psychol Sci Pract*. 2004;11(3):313–331.

10. Frank HE, Becker-Haimes EM, Kendall PC. Therapist training in evidence-based interventions for mental health: A systematic review of training approaches and outcomes. *Clin Psychol Sci Pract*. 2020;27(3):30.

11. Ravitz P, Wondimagegn D, Pain C, et al. Psychotherapy knowledge translation and interpersonal psychotherapy: Using best-education practices to transform mental health care in Canada and Ethiopia. *Am J Psychother*. 2014;68(4):463–488.

12. Ravitz P, Cooke RG, Mitchell S, et al. Continuing education to go: Capacity building in psychotherapies for front-line mental health workers in underserviced communities. *Can J Psychiatry*. 2013;58(6):335–343.

13. Murphy D, Slovak P, Thieme A, Jackson D, Olivier P, Fitzpatrick G. Developing technology to enhance learning interpersonal skills in counsellor education. *Br J Guid Couns*. 2019;47(3):328–341.

14. Ruggeri K, Farrington C, Brayne C. A global model for effective use and evaluation of e-learning in health. *Telemedicine J E Health*. 2013;19(4):312–321.

15. Centers for Disease Control and Prevention. ADDIE Model 2018. 2018. Accessed September 18, 2023. https://www.cdc.gov/training/development/addie-model.html

16. Kirkpatrick DL. *Evaluating Training Programs: The Four Levels.* Berrett-Koehler; 1994.

17. Kirkpatrick DL, Kirkpatrick JD. *Implementing the Four Levels: A Practical Guide for Effective Evaluation of Training Programs.* Berrett-Koehler Publishers; 2007.

18. Ottman KE, Kohrt BA, Pedersen GA, Schafer A. Use of role plays to assess therapist competency and its association with client outcomes in psychological interventions: A scoping review and competency research agenda. *Behav Res Ther.* 2020;130:103531. doi:10.1016/j.brat.2019.103531. Epub 2019 Dec 14. PMID: 31902517; PMCID: PMC7293551.

19. Mufson L, Verdeli H, Clougherty KF, Weissman M. *Interpersonal Psychotherapy for Depression.* Columbia University; 2006.

20. Ravitz P, Watson P, Grigoriadis S. *Psychotherapy Essentials to Go: Interpersonal Psychotherapy for Depression.* Ravitz P, Maunder R, eds. WW Norton; 2013.

21. Kumar M, Macharia P, Nyongesa V, et al. Human-centered design exploration with Kenyan health workers on proposed digital mental health screening and intervention training development: Thematic analysis of user preferences and needs. *Digit Health.* 2022;8:1–13.

22. Kobak KA, Lipsitz JD, Markowitz JC, Bleiberg KL. Web-based therapist training in interpersonal psychotherapy for depression: Pilot Study. *J Med Internet Res.* 2017;19(7):e257.

23. Stein BD, Celedonia KL, Swartz HA, et al. Implementing a web-based intervention to train community clinicians in an evidence-based psychotherapy: A pilot study. *Psychiatr Serv.* 2015;66(9):988–991.

24. Weerasekera P. Psychotherapy Training e-Resources (PTeR): On-line psychotherapy education. *Academic Psychiatry.* 2013;37(1):51–54.

25. Bäck M. Learning IPT from distance—ten years of experience in teaching and supervise IPT-therapists online. Presented at International Society of Interpersonal Psychotherapy 9th Biennial conference; 2021.

26. Prevention Department of Veterans Affairs Office of Mental Health and Suicide Prevention. *National Evidence-Based Psychotherapy Training Program: Interpersonal Psychotherapy for Depression Program Evaluation Report.* Department of Veterans Affairs Office of Mental Health and Suicide Prevention; 2018.

27. NIH US National Library of Medicine. Increasing access to evidence-based treatments for depression. 2020. Accessed September 18, 2023. https://clinicaltrials.gov/ct2/show/NCT04619615

28. Ravitz P, Singla DR, Lawson A, et al. Increasing access to evidence-based treatments for depression—The development and evaluation of a digital training platform for interpersonal psychotherapy. International Society of Interpersonal Psychotherapy 9th Biennial Conference; November 2021.

29. O'Flaherty J, Phillips C. The use of flipped classrooms in higher education: A scoping review. *Internet and Higher Education.* 2015;25:85–95.

30. Stewart MO, Raffa SD, Steele JL, et al. National dissemination of interpersonal psychotherapy for depression in veterans: Therapist and patient-level outcomes. *J Consult Clin Psychol.* 2014;82(6):1201–1206.

31. McNaughton N, Ravitz P, Wadell A, Hodges BD. Psychiatric education and simulation: A review of the literature. *Can J Psychiatry.* 2008;53(2):85–93.

8

Interpersonal Psychotherapy and Interpersonal Counseling

Digital Training Tools in Finland

KASPERI MIKKONEN, VIIVI MONDOLIN, SUSAN LAITALA,
SAMULI I. SAARNI, AND SUOMA E. SAARNI ■

It is a challenge to realize the outcomes of clinical trials in naturalistic environments. The demand for evidence-based practices like interpersonal psychotherapy (IPT) and interpersonal counseling (IPC) often exceeds health systems' possibilities for training, implementing, supervising, and sustaining services. These challenges are not limited to evidence-based practices for mental health and have been approached successfully with digital tools in many fields of service. We briefly describe the Finnish approach for using digital tools in trying to close the service gap for IPT and IPC.

FIRST-LINE THERAPIES INITIATIVE IN FINLAND

The *first-line therapies* initiative is a comprehensive program for providing early, evidence-based practices for mental health to all according to need in Finland. National implementation of IPT and IPC is included, as they are recommended treatments for adult and adolescent depression and have been found feasible in small regional pilots.[1,2]

The initiative takes a holistic view of digitally supported implementation of evidence-based practices for mental health. It includes, for example, a 24/7 service platform for psychoeducation, with over 30 self-help programs, a digitally supported system for assessing therapy needs (the *Finnish Therapy Navigator*[3]) and implementing stepped care, a large variety of online therapy services, a

Kasperi Mikkonen, Viivi Mondolin, Susan Laitala, Samuli I. Saarni, and Suoma E. Saarni, *Interpersonal Psychotherapy and Interpersonal Counseling* In: *Interpersonal Psychotherapy*. Edited by: Myrna M. Weissman and Jennifer J. Mootz, Oxford University Press. © Oxford University Press 2024. DOI: 10.1093/oso/9780197652084.003.0009 support portal for professionals, a tool for individual- and system-level outcome measurement (the *Finnish Psychotherapy Quality Registry*[4]), and a digitally aided training model for large-scale training and supervising of evidence-based therapeutic modalities, as described here.

Our approach is based on the proposition that a successful implementation of IPT and IPC requires permanently fixing the processes *around* treatment provision. Training many therapists alone is unlikely to translate into permanent clinical gains or treatment provision. The work processes need to be changed to enable early identification of the right patients, timely provision of IPC and IPC, and ongoing support for fidelity. Digital solutions excel in standardizing and scaling processes and in shortening routine tasks. This makes large-scale implementation of new therapies faster and can make new ways of working "stick" much better than nondigital approaches.

DIGITAL FRONTIER OF THERAPIST TRAINING

A necessary step in ensuring continuity of IPT and IPC services is the continuous training of therapists in volumes that match population needs and personnel turnover (currently about 10% in Finland). Scalable training that considers individual learning styles can be achieved using digital solutions and modern e-learning principles. E-learning can be defined as a theoretical framework that combines educational theories and technology.[5] It is used synonymously with digital learning but is differentiated from distance learning, such as Zoom lectures.[6]

Digital learning has been evaluated in the context of therapist training with encouraging results. In a wait-list-controlled randomized controlled trial, a digital training alone significantly improved the participants' subjective and objective knowledge of an evidence-based trauma therapy, self-rated competencies, and willingness to conduct the therapy.[7] In another trial, in-person training and digital training were compared in the training of skills in dialectical behavior therapy. In-person training outperformed digital training in trainee satisfaction, self-efficacy, and motivation, but digital training was superior in increasing knowledge. There were no differences between training methods in observer-rated clinical proficiency or self-reported clinical use.[8] Digital training has also been used previously in the context of IPT with a reported support for its feasibility and efficacy.[9] Over a decade ago, Bennett-Levy and Perry from Australia reviewed the overall potential of digital training, stating that most of the didactic, modeling, and self-experiential elements of therapist training can be undertaken via digital training, allowing the in-person training to focus on skills practice and role play. They estimated that digital training can reduce trainer time required by at least 50%.[10] Since then, digital trainings have been a staple in national-level therapist training in Australia.[11] A systematic review including 20 studies reported that digital trainings were associated with improvements in both knowledge and skill levels, which are generally comparable with in-person training, and concluded that digital training is a way to increase the reach and cost-effectiveness of therapist training programs.[12]

THE MODEL OF DIGITALLY AIDED IPT AND IPC TRAINING IN FINLAND

In the first-line therapies initiative, focus on digitally supported training has been the spearhead in the strategy of national dissemination of evidence-based practices, including IPT and IPC. Based on the literature presented above, digital training is seen as a solution for increasing flexibility and training volumes without compromising the learning outcomes. Because of this, we chose to build a centrally operated digital learning platform and a digitally aided model of therapist training and make this open for all publicly funded healthcare providers.

Our system aims to secure high-quality, standardized IPT and IPC training permanently available in Finland in needed volumes. A centrally operated digital platform, a shared knowledge base, and a combination of digital and in-person training modalities form our training model of IPT and IPC. The digital platform is an open-source, Drupal-based learning management system operated by Helsinki University Hospital. The system allows the creation of versatile digital trainings, user progress monitoring, and automatic evaluation through exams. The content hosted in the system has a modular structure, which means that it can easily be used in multiple trainings. For example, a module consisting of interpersonal development during adolescence included in IPT for Adolescents (IPT-A) training can be used in other training programs with similar needs. The knowledge base defines the learning objectives, learning methods, and evaluative processes used in the training (e.g., what is included in the training, who can act as a supervisor, what the supervision involves).

The IPT and IPC trainings consist of learning activities in the described learning platform and supervised interventions. All theoretical content included in the trainings is delivered via the platform and consists of various modalities (e.g., text, videos, tables, graphs) and interactive assignments (e.g., multiple-choice questions, essays with automated feedback) and are based on standard manuals of IPT and IPC, which have been translated and adapted for Finland.[13-16] This adaptation included, for example, filming of 15 video demonstrations of techniques with professional actors and formulating case vignettes that reflect the Finnish healthcare system. Training is approved by the Finnish society for dynamic and interpersonal psychotherapy. Passing the IPC training requires completing the digital training with a multiple-choice exam (approximately 15 hours), attending supervision (15 hours), and conducting 3 IPC interventions from 2 problem areas and monitoring the interventions with selected patient-reported outcome and experience measures. The IPT training is similar but includes a more profound digital training (approximately 25 hours) and more supervision (21 hours). As with IPC, the IPT trainee must conduct 3 interventions from 2 different problem areas with outcome monitoring. The adolescent versions of the digital trainings have the same structure as the adult counterparts but include content about adolescent depression and development as well as videos and vignettes with adolescents. The structure and content of the supervision is standardized so that every session includes skills training, role play, and facilitation of feedback-informed treatment using the measures gathered during the interventions.

RESULTS AND EXPERIENCES SO FAR

The first version of the digital platform was built in 2021. Digital trainings for IPC-A and IPT-A were created first with adult versions a year later. During the first year, 300 IPC-trainees and 70 IPT-trainees completed the digital training with an estimated 1000-2000 new trainees nationally for 2023-2024. After a year of experience, it is evident that digitally aided IPT and IPC trainings are feasible and well-accepted solutions for trainees, supervisors, and organizations.

For trainees, digital training offers flexibility in learning. Trainees can progress in the course at their own pace, and learning can occur in small units. This is suggested to reduce the cognitive load of the training.[17] The content can be used as an interactive manual after the training, and the system itself includes all the necessary materials for conducting the interventions (e.g., symptom measures, various documents used during the interventions).

For supervisors, the platform helps to ensure that a specific level of theoretical understanding has been achieved before moving forward in the training. Thus, all the time used for in-person training can be used to practice skills and conduct role play. The role of the supervisor is to confirm that every trainee takes an active part during the supervisions and that everyone reaches a desired skill level. Digital trainings are also created to train and support beginner-level supervisors.

For organizations, digitally aided training is a tool to strengthen the level of employee competence in IPT and IPC and to maintain a specific service level. Digital solutions reduce costs associated with training employees and allow the training to be optimized to the organization's needs and timetables. For example, new employees can begin the training as a part of their onboarding period, and those who have completed the training can be assigned periodic booster training and skills tests automatically. Standardizing the training and the supervision also helps the organization train and move employees toward supervisor roles more promptly. With standardized models, organizations can more aptly predict the resources needed to train the employees in a given time.

SUMMARY

The first-line therapies digital learning environment will allow us to train a substantial number of IPT and IPC clinicians. Our model of continuous training aims to permanently increase the availability of the interventions and help maintain competence and fidelity in the long term. Other digital tools provided will help place IPT and IPC in their ideal positions within a stepped care framework. The only plausible way to answer the high demand for evidence-based practices in mental health is to apply digital tools in all parts of the process: training therapists, implementing treatment methods, following outcomes, and sustaining best practices.

REFERENCES

1. Ranta K, Parhiala P, Law R, Marttunen M. Treating adolescent depression in multi-professional school services with IPC-A. Implementation results from the national pilot trial. *Psychiatria Fennica.* 2022;53:36–55.
2. Kontunen J, Timonen M, Muotka J, Liukkonen T. Is interpersonal counselling (IPC) sufficient treatment for depression in primary care patients? A pilot study comparing IPC and interpersonal psychotherapy (IPT). *J Affect Disord.* 2016;189:89–93.
3. Saarni S, Nurminen S, Mikkonen K, et al. The Finnish therapy navigator—digital support system for introducing stepped care in Finland. *Psychiatria Fennica.* 2022;53:120–137.
4. Saarni SE, Rosenström T, Stenberg JH, et al. Finnish Psychotherapy Quality Register: rationale, development, and baseline results. *Nord J Psychiatry.* 2023 Jul;77(5):455–466. doi:10.1080/08039488.2022.2150788. Epub 2022 Dec 21. PMID: 36541920.
5. Choudhury S, Pattnaik S. Emerging themes in e-learning: a review from the stakeholders' perspective. *Comput Educ.* 2020;144:103657.
6. Guri-Rosenblit S. "Distance education" and "e-learning": not the same thing. *High Educ.* 2005;49:467–493. https://doi.org/10.1007/s10734-004-0040-0
7. Sansen LM, Saupe LB, Steidl A, Fegert JM, Hoffmann U, Neuner F. Development and randomized-controlled evaluation of a web-based training in evidence-based trauma therapy. *Prof Psychol: Res Pract.* 2020;51(2):115.
8. Dimeff LA, Harned MS, Woodcock EA, Skutch JM, Koerner K, Linehan MM. Investigating bang for your training buck: a randomized controlled trial comparing three methods of training clinicians in two core strategies of dialectical behavior therapy. *Behav Ther.* 2015;46(3):283–295.
9. Kobak KA, Lipsitz JD, Markowitz JC, Bleiberg KL. Web-based therapist training in interpersonal psychotherapy for depression: pilot study. *J Med Internet Res.* 2017;19(7):e257.
10. Bennett-Levy J, Perry H. The promise of online cognitive behavioural therapy training for rural and remote mental health professionals. *Australas Psychiatry.* 2009;17(Suppl):S121–S124.
11. Bennett-Levy J, Hawkins R, Perry H, Cromarty P, Mills J. Online cognitive behavioural therapy training for therapists: outcomes, acceptability, and impact of support. *Aust Psychol.* 2012;47(3):174–182.
12. Frank HE, Becker-Haimes EM, Kendall PC. Therapist training in evidence-based interventions for mental health: a systematic review of training approaches and outcomes. *Clin Psychol Sci Pract.* 2020;27(3):20.
13. Weissman MM, Markowitz JC, Klerman GL. *The Guide to Interpersonal Psychotherapy*: Updated *and* Expanded Edition. Oxford University Press; 2017.
14. Weissman MM, Verdeli H. *Interpersonal Counseling for Primary Care.* Columbia University College of Physicians and Surgeons; 2018.

15. Wilkinson P, Cestaro V, Weismann MM. *IPC for Adolescents Manual*; 2019.

16. Mufson L, Dorta KP, Moreau D, Weissman MM. *Interpersonal Psychotherapy for Depressed Adolescents*. 2nd ed. Guilford Press; 2011.

17. Young JQ, Van Merrienboer J, Durning S, Ten Cate O. Cognitive load theory: implications for medical education: AMEE Guide No. 86. Med Teach. 2014;36(5):371–384.

Interpersonal Psychotherapy Training in Mainland China

WANHONG ZHENG, XUEJUN LIU, YANLI LUO, MANLI HUANG, AND WEIHUI LI ■

Although interpersonal psychotherapy (IPT) has been widely practiced in Western countries for more than half a century, this therapy modality remained virtually unknown in China until recently. One of the earliest efforts to disseminate IPT knowledge to practitioners in China was initiated by Wanhong Zheng, a psychiatrist practicing at West Virginia University. In August 2017, Zheng and Xuejun Liu, a general psychiatrist and vice president of the Hunan Brain Hospital, invited Holly Swartz, 2015–2016 president of the International Society of Interpersonal Psychotherapy (ISIPT), to give the keynote address at the first China-America Xiaoxiang Summit on Psychiatry and Clinical Psychology. Over 600 mental health clinicians from several provinces in central China attended, among them psychiatrists, primary care physicians, nurses, and psychological counselors. Swartz gave a 60-minute introductory lecture on IPT, describing the framework, supporting clinical evidence, and target populations. Much of the audience expressed great interest in learning more about IPT.

A year later, Mark Miller, a frequently published author and expert on IPT in the geriatric population, gave a 300-minute course on IPT to over 800 mental health clinicians at the second summit meeting in Changsha. In this 3-session course, after providing a comparative review of short-term psychotherapeutic modalities, Miller discussed the context in which IPT was developed, taught the principles of IPT, and explained the rationale for using IPT as a practical toolbox of techniques for handling common life problems. He clearly delineated the sequence of steps for implementation and discussed the 4 IPT problem areas in depth, using clinical vignettes to illustrate each problem area and demonstrating specific techniques to help audiences understand IPT practice. The course also included an overview

Wanhong Zheng, Xuejun Liu, Yanli Luo, Manli Huang, and Weihui Li, *Interpersonal Psychotherapy Training in Mainland China* In: *Interpersonal Psychotherapy*. Edited by: Myrna M. Weissman and Jennifer J. Mootz, Oxford University Press.
© Oxford University Press 2024. DOI: 10.1093/oso/9780197652084.003.0010

of IPT expansion for use in different settings and with various psychopathologies and a discussion of adaptations for using IPT in different cultures. He later taught the same course at a hospital in Zhejiang Province.

In October 2018, Paula Ravitz (president of ISIPT 2017–2018) and Holly Swartz successfully ran 2 IPT workshops in China, each lasting 2½ days. Over 150 people attended these workshops, which were delivered in English with onstage Chinese translation. Ravitz and Swartz presented case vignettes and illustrated IPT techniques using faculty and video demonstrations.

Feedback reports from a sample of 278 audience members showed that 72% of attendees were female, 73% were between 26 and 45 years old, 39% were associated with teaching hospitals, and 32% were associated with community hospitals.[1] In terms of profession, 41% were psychiatrists, 2% were primary care physicians, 36% were counselors, and 9% were nurses. None had a background in social work.

While some of the respondents reported that the live translation from English affected the learning process, most indicated a high level of satisfaction with the training. On a 10-point Likert scale, with 1 being "the least" and 10 being "the most," the mean score for effectiveness of the lecture/workshop in articulating the principles and techniques of IPT was 8.14. Other mean ratings included 7.39 for the relevance of the case vignettes to Chinese culture, 8.70 for the likelihood that the respondent would consider using IPT with their own patients, and 8.52 for interest in receiving more training in IPT.

At almost the same time, Diana Koszycki, a professor at the University of Ottawa, and Scott Stuart, a former president of ISIPT, also began offering IPT courses, workshops, and case supervisions at Renji Hospital in Shanghai. Yanli Luo, the director of psychological services of Renji Hospital, initiated and hosted these trainings. From 2018 to 2022, over 600 people received IPT training in Shanghai; 20 went on to complete online case supervision.

One of the critical steps for making IPT training more available in China was the translation of IPT training manuals into the native language. As part of this effort, in 2018 Zheng and colleagues translated the World Health Organization (WHO) manual *Group Interpersonal Therapy (IPT) for Depression*[2] into Chinese, followed later by Weissman, Markowitz, and Klerman's (2018) book[3] *The Guide to Interpersonal Psychotherapy*. As many therapists and patients prefer short-term psychotherapy, in 2020 Manli Huang and colleagues translated Swartz and colleagues' (2004) *Brief Interpersonal Psychotherapy (IPT-B) Training Manual*[4] into Chinese. The combination of these translated resources and the newly available courses and workshops prepared trainees for hands-on training sessions and ongoing case supervisions.

In 2019, experienced therapists (n = 24) who had attended the IPT training courses and workshops were selected to receive case supervision in IPT over Zoom from 6 IPT experts from the United States, Canada, and Israel. The trainees were divided into 6 groups and participated in weekly 75-minute virtual case supervision sessions for 16 weeks. As part of this program, Zheng and his colleagues compiled a 49-page manual in English, with Chinese translation, that included instruction for IPT therapists; information about the 6 IPT case supervisors; a brief IPT session summary (BISS); the Patient Health Questionnaire-9 (PHQ-9); and an IPT clinical reference companion written by Paula Ravitz. Each group had one interpreter and one designated group leader who coordinated the schedule and communication between sessions. Supervisees took turns presenting their cases and listening to the case presentations of other students. The case supervisor reviewed the cases at the end and provided immediate feedback and instruction. Supervisors and supervisees addressed questions about cases that arose between sessions via email. Immediately following each IPT session, supervisees were asked to complete the IPT Therapy Self-Report Checklist (SRC) and the BISS. Throughout the supervision period, the supervisors encouraged supervisees to consider the specific cultural contexts of the patients receiving IPT. Examples of questions discussed during the case supervision sessions include the following:

- What local Chinese traditions or practices surround each of the four core IPT interpersonal problem areas: grief, social role transitions, role disputes, and interpersonal deficits?
- How do the proposed IPT approaches to improving resolution of each of the four interpersonal problem areas differ from traditional Chinese practices of managing stressful life events?
- What triggers or factors do Chinese people traditionally consider to be the causes of depression symptoms?
- How might stigma dissuade participation in IPT?

As the supervisors were not licensed as practitioners in China, the goal of the IPT supervision sessions was to teach supervisees to translate specific IPT skills into practice rather than to oversee the actual clinical care of patients. The outcome was very satisfactory. All trainees enjoyed the learning experience and felt that IPT was very helpful to their patients. Most of the supervisors also gave very positive feedback, describing supervisees, for example, as "knowledgeable and warm, empathic and eager to learn," and, in another instance, saying that a supervisee had "leadership characteristics and would be very influential as an IPT supervisor and presenter or trainer."

In a recent article, Zheng et al. (2021) described a phased strategic plan for promoting IPT in China.[1] As with the process described above, the strategy starts with inviting IPT experts to present introductory lectures. These introductory lectures are then expanded in lecture series and workshops that include case demonstrations. Trainees with previous therapy experience are then selected for case supervision. Those supervisees can then implement IPT in practice and train other practitioners in IPT in their own native Chinese language. The strategy of initially training experienced Chinese therapists in IPT to become trainers for other practitioners facilitates fast and effective dissemination of IPT in a country whose native language is not English and whose practitioners have no prior familiarity with IPT.

As part of the strategic plan for the dissemination of knowledge about IPT in China, the ISIPT Chinese chapter (IPT China) was established in 2021. Since then, IPT China has sponsored a group supervision program and a 2-day online IPT workshop.

The challenges of providing IPT training in China are multifold. The most obvious has been language. As most trainees have limited fluency in English, problems can arise with comprehension in teaching and supervision. Therefore, translators are always needed in the early stage lectures and supervision. With the rapid development of language-translation software, it is possible that an electronic device may, in the future, be available to instantaneously translate the content to Chinese IPT trainees.

The facilitation of communication between trainers and trainees has been another challenge. Until now, case supervision has been provided through the videoconferencing tool Zoom, with a bilingual intermediary playing a major role in the supervision meetings. Between supervision meetings, email has served as the main communication channel between trainer and trainees. Though quick and easy, email also has a few drawbacks, including time delay, limited clarity, and concerns regarding data privacy. We initially encountered some challenges in scheduling supervision meetings because of differences in time zones, which we resolved through the compromise of meeting after working hours in China.

In addition, limited resources have made it difficult to meet the need for case supervision, as only a few attendees of IPT lectures and workshops have received case supervision, although many had a clear desire to receive further training.

To maintain high standards and consistency in the practice of IPT, ISIPT recently initiated a certification process and completed the first round of certifying IPT trainers. Numerous trainees in our courses and workshops in China have asked where and how one can be certified. Creation of a formal certification process in IPT training in China is, indeed, a priority: first, because it is a way to validate trainees' mastery of IPT skills and knowledge and their ability to apply them in daily practice; second, because passing a test for recognition of an achievement is ingrained in Chinese culture, having originated from Confucius's teachings promoting meritocracy more than a thousand years ago.[5] Along with the present government certification process for counseling, a formal IPT certification would not only help therapists be recognized for their expertise in IPT but also increase their chances of employment. A major challenge, of course, is the current lack of ISIPT-certified trainers or supervisors who can provide training to Chinese-speaking therapists without need of translation. Some of the therapists who completed our first round of training and supervision classes have applied for ISIPT supervisor certification. One practitioner in Hong Kong, Joseph Chung, has already obtained this certification. It is our hope that more bilingual clinicians can be certified by ISIPT soon to facilitate the dissemination of IPT in China through training and supervision. Ultimately, our goal is to collaborate with ISIPT to establish a Chinese certification system designed for Chinese-speaking clinicians who want to integrate IPT into their practice.

Another potential challenge to further dissemination of IPT in China is cost to the trainees. We have noted that most of the trainees thus far have had to pay out of pocket for IPT training, including the costs of travel, meals, and lodging. The process of getting approval and reimbursement for continuing medical education hours in China differs from that in Western countries, and only a few trainees have had grant funding or support from their employers. With our experience, especially the success from remote case supervision, one way to address this challenge could be using more online trainings in the future.

Finally, it is imperative that trainees practice IPT in real life after completing training. Since 2013, Chinese mental health law has restricted psychologists' practice of "psychotherapy" in mainland China to hospital settings only, while allowing "counseling" services to be offered elsewhere.[6] Psychotherapy in China is therefore distinguished from "psychological counseling" in that the former is only available for people with at least one clinical psychiatric diagnosis made by a licensed psychiatrist. The law, however, does not define what constitutes a "psychological counselor," what specific types of treatment are considered psychotherapy, or even what type of training is required for a practitioner to provide psychotherapy, making it difficult to implement therapy services.[7] As a result, some local governments were authorized to take specific measures to make up for the deficits in the national mental health law and have drafted more detailed operational guidelines to encourage evidence-based psychotherapy practices and support training for practitioners.[8] Many patients have seen the benefit of psychotherapy and thus are willing to pay for these services out of pocket. Certainly, keeping up to date on current mental health policies, legal considerations, and insurance coverage will pose challenges for therapists who complete IPT training and want to begin to practice in China; however, given the economic boom and increasing demand for better mental health services, the potential for the successful dissemination and practice of IPT in China is great.

REFERENCES

1. Zheng W, Liu X, Chandran DN, et al. Interpersonal psychotherapy knowledge dissemination in China. *Heart and Mind*. 2021;5(4):144.
2. World Health Organization and Columbia University Group Interpersonal Therapy (IPT) for Depression (WHO generic field-trial version 1.0). Geneva, WHO, 2016.
3. Weissman MM, Markowitz JC, Klerman GL. *The Guide to Interpersonal Psychotherapy: Updated and Expanded Edition*. Oxford University Press; 2018.
4. Swartz H, Grote NK, Frank E, Bledsoe SE, Fleming MA, Shear K. Brief interpersonal psychotherapy (IPT-B): a treatment manual [Unpublished manual]. Department of Psychiatry, University of Pittsburgh School of Medicine, Western Psychiatric Institute and Clinic; 2004.
5. Stephens M. China's gruelling exam culture under question. *Western Independent*. October 4, 2022. Accessed September 18, 2023.https://westernindependent.com.au/2018/10/04/chinas-gruelling-exam-culture-under-question/
6. Clay RA. Psychotherapy in China. *Monitor on Psychology*. 2019;50(9):26. Accessed September 18, 2023. https://www.apa.org/monitor/2019/10/psychotherapy-china

7. Chen HH, Phillips MR, Cheng H, et al. Mental Health Law of the People's Republic of China (English translation with annotations): translated and annotated version of China's new Mental Health Law. *Shanghai Archives of Psychiatry.* 2012;24(6):305.
8. Shao Y, Wang J, Xie B. The first mental health law of China. *Asian Journal of Psychiatry.* 2015;13:72–74.

10

Interpersonal Psychotherapy Training in France

OGUZ OMAY, ELISABETH GLATIGNY-DALLAY,
BENJAMIN LAVIGNE, NATHALIE SALOMÉ, AND
JEAN-MARIE SENGELEN ■

INTRODUCTION OF IPT IN FRANCE

Interpersonal psychotherapy (IPT) was introduced in France at the end of the 2000s in 2 different ways and by 2 groups of professionals who first worked separately before combining forces.

CREATIP

A small group of French psychiatrists wishing to discover new approaches in the treatment of depression noted that IPT, regularly cited in international recommendations, was neither sufficiently known nor taught in France. The group organized to receive training in New York from Lena Verdeli, Kathleen Clougherty, and Myrna Weissman in 2004 and 2006. In 2005, the 9 members founded CREATIP,[1] a nonprofit association for teaching and promoting IPT in France. At first, the group proposed complementary medical education activities, presenting the basics and the functioning of IPT to practicing psychiatrists in various French regions during stand-alone conferences.

Gradually, the interest in more comprehensive training became apparent. In 2009, the CREATIP IPT training course was launched. It was organized in Paris. The cycle consisted of 10 days of training spread over a year. In addition to adult psychiatry, aspects specific to the elderly and adolescents were

Oguz Omay, Elisabeth Glatigny-Dallay, Benjamin Lavigne, Nathalie Salomé, and Jean-Marie Sengelen, *Interpersonal Psychotherapy Training in France* In: *Interpersonal Psychotherapy*. Edited by: Myrna M. Weissman and Jennifer J. Mootz, Oxford University Press. © Oxford University Press 2024. DOI: 10.1093/oso/9780197652084.003.0011 covered. Interpersonal and social rhythm therapy (IPSRT) was also covered by Thierry Bottai, who was introduced to it by Ellen Frank and Holly Swartz.[1-3] Each year, the CREATIP training bring together about 20 students from various backgrounds: not only psychiatrists, psychologists, psychiatry residents, but also general practitioners and nurses. In 2014, CREATIP created a partnership with the *Association Française et Fédérative des Etudiants en Psychiatrie* (AFFEP), an association of psychiatry residents in France. This partnership facilitates the access of young psychiatrists to IPT.

PERINATAL CIRCLES — THE FRANCOPHONE MARCÉ SOCIETY AND ARIP

At the same time as CREATIP came to be, another way of introducing IPT in France was initiated by Oguz Omay, a perinatal psychiatrist working at the time at La Teppe Medical Center, in Tain l'Hermitage, a small town in Southern France. Oguz Omay discovered IPT, which is well adapted to perinatal work, through reading Weissman and Markowitz's manual[4] in 2002. This reading alone transformed his practice, and in 2008 he had the chance to receive specific training in Australia, during the International Marcé Society Congress with Mike O'Hara, Scott Stuart, and Rebecca Reay. From that moment, his mission was to introduce and develop this approach in France. He organized the first training at La Teppe in June 2009 with Scott Stuart, president of ISIPT at the time.

Oguz Omay was supported from the start by Elisabeth Glatigny-Dallay, a perinatal psychologist in Bordeaux, and by Michel Dugnat, a perinatal psychiatrist in Avignon. These three professionals were strongly involved in the emerging perinatal psychiatry in France and were active members of the executive board of the Société Marcé Francophone (SMF), a linguistic and regional chapter of the International Marcé Society for Perinatal Mental Health. Michel Dugnat is the president of Association pour la Recherche et l'(In)formation en Périnatalité (ARIP), a French association working for the promotion of perinatal mental health.

Supervised by French-speaking Canadian IPT teams, Oguz Omay and Elisabeth Glatigny, joined by Ingrid Lacaze, a perinatal psychologist in Bordeaux, trained to become accredited IPT supervisors and trainers, enabling them to offer their own training courses from 2012 on. This training has been supported from the beginning and still today by the SMF and ARIP, allowing IPT to develop among perinatal care professionals in France and in neighboring French-speaking countries such as Switzerland and Belgium. From 2014, Oguz Omay joined CREATIP as a trainer in their training cycle in Paris. Many synergies have been created between these two groups of professionals to promote IPT in France and foster links with the international IPT community.

IPT HUBS IN FRANCE

La Teppe—The Woodstock moment

From 2009 to 2017, at La Teppe Medical Center, Oguz Omay ran IPT courses, and international experts led seminars. In a countryside atmosphere, over 3, 5, or 7 days, various workshops were organized, with extensive informal time spent together in groups fostering interpersonal relationships. These international seminars attracted not only French professionals but also participants from around the world.

The trainers, in chronological order of appearance, were Scott Stuart, Simon Patry, Holly Swartz, Ellen Frank, Paula Ravitz, Anat Burnstein-Klomek, Heather Flynn, John Markowitz, and Barbara Milrod, with many international experts among the audience. In 2016 and 2017, the seminar series was named IPT-Week France and received strong international exposure.

It is difficult to distinguish precisely between perinatal and IPT training within the many seminars offered during this period at La Teppe as the interpersonal approach affected the clinical approach in perinatal care that was taught there. As a general indicator, training organized by Oguz Omay between 2009 and 2017 attracted 1337 people, including 1183 French participants and 154 foreign participants from all healthcare professions, mostly from the perinatal sector. Foreign participants came from 24 different countries from Europe and the United States, Canada, Brazil, Australia, New Zealand, Turkey, Israel, and Japan.

Today, this period evokes in its enthusiasm, energy, and naiveté, as well as the nostalgic memories cherished by many participants, a real "Woodstock" moment of IPT in France. These actions have given visibility to France in the world of IPT, probably facilitating the election of Oguz Omay as vice president/president elect of ISIPT between 2017 and 2019 and president between 2019 and 2021.

Limoges—Where IPT took root in France

Limoges, another small provincial town in central France, is another illustration of IPT expansion in France. In 2012, Jean-Albert Meynard, a psychiatrist and one of the founding members of CREATIP, gave a lecture to psychiatrists at the Esquirol Hospital. This was the beginning of a fundamental movement within this institution. Starting in 2012, several psychiatrists from Limoges trained in IPT with CREATIP in Paris. They progressively built up a pool of trained professionals gathered in the same institution. These professionals took advantage of their number to create peer supervision. Then they created training spaces to train their collaborators, especially nurses, in the basics of IPT. A specific seminar was also created for psychiatry residents at Esquirol Hospital over 4 half-days, led by psychiatrists trained at CREATIP.

In 2015, there were 20 professionals (psychiatrists, psychologists, social workers, and nurses) who received either basic or full training in IPT at the Esquirol Hospital in Limoges.

In 2016, Benjamin Lavigne, Nathalie Salomé, and Elodie Audebert, all psychiatrists and second-generation IPT therapists from CREATIP, created a dedicated IPT care unit at the Esquirol Hospital.

Two nurses were trained in the full CREATIP IPT curriculum so that they could form the core of the unit, under the supervision of IPT-trained psychiatrists. Charlène Gorse and Nicolas Besse became the 2 nurses of the IPT-IPSRT unit, directed by Benjamin Lavigne at first, then by Nathalie Salomé when Benjamin left Limoges for Switzerland.

This unit has been a great success and continues to this day, now under additional supervision from Oguz Omay, reinforcing the skills of the professionals who work there. Charlene Gorse and Nicolas Besse also contribute to the online training spaces created by Oguz Omay, Nathalie Salomé, and Elisabeth Glatigny by offering their clinical experience as an example to professionals who are training in IPT.

IPT TRAINING IN FRANCE

Since 2009, CREATIP has been offering comprehensive IPT training in Paris for 10 days a year. This model has provided solid training for practitioners to work with diverse populations: adults, adolescents, elderly subjects, and IPSRT. CREATIP training was suspended by the COVID pandemic in 2020, with the hope of resuming the original format in 2023. However, this has not yet been possible.

From the original CREATIP group or their students, other associations or training institutes have been created based on the CREATIP model, with similar names: AFTIP[2] and IFTIP. Though they are not connected to the international IPT community, these groups contribute to the visibility of IPT through their publications and the training courses they offer in Paris.

For their part, Oguz Omay and his collaborators offer introductory training over 2 consecutive days, internationally listed as level A or level 1. In addition to training sessions in La Teppe, numerous training sessions have been held in different French cities, as precongress trainings before SMF or ARIP perinatal congresses: in Bordeaux (2013), Limoges (2014), Marseille (2015), Lyon (2018), Limoges (2021)—and since 2015 almost every year in Avignon (ARIP).

Since 2020, several online sessions per year of this training is offered by ARIP, reaching French, Belgian, and Swiss practitioners. To extend the training, Oguz Omay has created an additional 8-day level 2 training, following level 1. These in-depth cycles have taken place twice in La Teppe (2016 and 2017) and once in Lausanne, Switzerland (2019). An online version of this in-depth training is currently under consideration. In addition, Oguz Omay, Elisabeth Glatigny, and Nathalie Salomé have been co-facilitating monthly online peer supervision sessions since April 2021, hosting participants from France, Switzerland, and Belgium.

Another IPT training hub is located in Bordeaux. Psychologists Elisabeth Glatigny-Dallay and Ingrid Lacaze teach IPT courses at the University of Bordeaux: within the University Diploma of Initial Training in Psychotherapeutic Practices, within the framework of the Master 2 courses in psychology, courses for advanced practice nurses, and courses for psychiatry residents. It should be noted that from 2023 onward, psychiatry residents will benefit from a 2-day introductory training in IPT, to our knowledge the only training of this type offered formally by the university to psychiatric residents in France to date, integrated into their undergraduate training.

Also in Bordeaux, IRCCADE,[3] provides an introduction to IPT to all its cognitive behavioral therapy (CBT) students. This 2-day training has been provided in Bordeaux since 2018 by Elisabeth Glatigny Dallay and Ingrid Lacaze, following previous interventions in the same setting by Theodore Hovaguimian,[5-7] another pioneer of IPT in French-speaking Switzerland.

If we turn to university teaching, the university diplomas (DUs) of perinatal mental health have been an ideal entry point for initiations to IPT. Antoine and Nicole Guedeney, a couple of renowned Parisian child psychiatrists involved in the field of attachment and early childhood, took an early interest in the work carried out at La Teppe, where Nicole Guedeney came to train. These pioneers in the teaching of attachment theory in France integrated a yearly 2-day training course on IPT, led by Oguz Omay, into the programs of the DU of perinatal psychopathology and the DU of attachment that they supervise at the Paris Cité University, Faculty of Medicine. Their support has helped introduce many classes of students to IPT since 2015.

In Bordeaux, Anne-Laure Sutter integrates IPT into the DU in perinatal psychiatry for which she is responsible. Elisabeth Glatigny-Dallay and Ingrid Lacaze have given 2 days of initiation every year since 2016 to interested students in this setting. Nevertheless, despite these valuable forays into university teaching, it must be noted that IPT does not receive the attention it deserves in the pregraduate training of either psychiatrists or psychologists in France.

Beyond France, we note that CREATIP has organized training outside France in Morocco and Tunisia. Oguz Omay facilitated training involving several hundred professionals in Montreal and Sherbrook, Québec, Canada, in 2017 and 2018, in collaboration with child psychiatrist Anna Bourgeois and psychiatrist Stephane Richard-Devantoy.

Three people among the authors of this chapter, Benjamin Lavigne, Jean Marie Sengelen, and Oguz Omay emigrated to Switzerland in 2017–2018, the professional links existing between them facilitating this grouped migration. They are now active in the Swiss Society of Interpersonal Psychotherapy (see chapter 11 in this volume). Nevertheless, they continue to give occasional or regular training in France. Oguz Omay is also strongly influenced by his experience as a trainer with his Turkish colleagues, his country of origin, where he was able to contribute to the diffusion of IPT.

Regarding the future, the idea is gaining ground to unite all IPT trainers in French-speaking countries (France; Switzerland; Québec Province in Canada, among others) in a federation that would become an affiliated chapter of ISIPT and could enable the coordination of training and development efforts deployed by all in their respective countries.

PUBLICATIONS: BOOKS AND ARTICLES

The self-published book by Simon Patry (Canada), no longer available for sale, and the introductory book by Théodore Hovagimian (Switzerland)[6] were the first publications useful to French-speaking readers, as well as the special issue of the Canadian French-language journal *Santé Mentale* in Québec.[7] There is now a translation of an IPT manual into French.[8]

Thanks to CREATIP, several medical theses have been written on IPT by residents completing their studies in psychiatry.[9-11] Original books have been published by AFTIP[12] and IFTIP[13,14] trainers, facilitating their training efforts. Other articles[15-20]or chapters in specialized books[8,9] have traced the efforts of development or adaptations of IPT to specific disorders in French.[21,22]

Finally, several communications have been made by all the professionals mentioned in this article in the framework of national and international congresses, including the ISIPT congresses in Amsterdam (2011); Iowa City, United States (2013); London (2015); and Budapest (2019).

IPT PRACTICE IN FRANCE AND LOCAL ADAPTATIONS

Limoges and La Teppe were two places where teams practiced IPT in public psychiatry care institutions in the outpatient setting. Limoges is still very active, but the team of La Teppe unfortunately dispersed after Oguz Omay's departure from this institution.

Today, it is not easy to have a clear indication of how IPT is practiced in France. There are of course individual professionals very much engaged in IPT, some in private practice and some in public services. As has been detailed in this chapter, IPT has been rarely integrated into undergraduate training in psychiatry, psychology, or social work. Training has been mostly in the setting of continuing education, enabled by nonprofit organizations. It must be noted that although CREATIP trained mainly psychiatrists, psychologists, and psychiatry nurses, training courses organized by Oguz Omay have included not only these core professions but also general practitioners, midwives, social workers, child care nurses, pediatricians, gynecologists, and many other professions.[23] Even mothers with lived experience working with *Maman Blues*—a peer support group for perinatal care in France—have been trained in the model.

The challenge has been how to ingrain core competences into the practice of professionals with little training time available, to make a precious difference in practice resulting in tangible outcomes. To reach this aim, Oguz Omay has developed his concept of interpersonal virtuosity, *la virtuosité relationnelle* in French.[24] Interpersonal virtuosity is defined as the capacity to pay attention to interpersonal interactions and use them to alleviate the patient's suffering. An example may best illustrate this challenge: In 2013, an experienced pediatrician took one of our 2-day IPT training courses. We as trainers weren't sure what she would make of it, as she was not planning to exercise psychotherapy. At the end of the course, when she was asked what she would do differently from now on, she said:

> I see mothers who lose their babies at the end of the pregnancy. In our hospital, the day after giving birth, they go to meet and spend time with the lifeless baby in a special room. I will now ask them: *Is there a person who you would like to have beside you when you meet your baby?*

This subtle attention to interpersonal resources, and of course the tone of the voice, the caring nonverbal interaction when this question is asked, might make a difference for the grieving mother or the parents. IPT training in France has tried to nourish the interpersonal virtuosity of trainees, and this emphasis has been a trademark of the perinatal group. Oguz Omay gave a keynote talk during the ISIPT congress in Budapest on this topic, sharing his approach with the international IPT community.[24]

NOTES

1. The name CREATIP is the abbreviation of *Cercle de Recherches et d'Etudes Appliquées à la Thérapie InterPersonnelle*. For description, see Rahioui H, Blecha L, Bottai T, et al. [Interpersonal psychotherapy from research to practice]. *Encephale*. 2015;41(2):184–189. The founding members were Michel Biloa Tang, Thierry Bottai, Sophie Christophe, Carole Dupuy, Laurent Jacquesy, Frederic Kochman, Jean-Albert Meynard, Didier Papeta, and Hassan Rahioui.
2. AFTIP: Association Française de Thérapie Interpersonnelle, founded in 2013 by Hassan Rahioui. IFTIP: Institut de Formation en Thérapies InterPersonnelles, founded by Nicolas Neveux.
3. IRCCADE: Institut de Recherche Comportementale et Cognitive sur l'Anxiété et la Dépression: association offering training in the field of cognitive behavioral therapies (CBTs) since 1993 in the Bordeaux area.

REFERENCES

1. Rahioui H, Blecha L, Bottai T, et al. Interpersonal psychotherapy from research to practice. *L'encephale*. 2014;41(2):184–189.
2. Bottai T, Biloa-Tang M, Christophe S, et al. Interpersonal and social rhythm therapy (IPSRT). *L'encephale*. 2010;36:S206–S217.

3. Pringuey D, Fakra E, Cherikh F, et al. Affective disorders: news in chronobiological models. *L'encephale*. 2010;36:S157–S166.

4. Weissman MM, Markowitz JC, Klerman G. *Comprehensive Guide to Interpersonal Psychotherapy*. Basic Books; 2008.

5. Hovaguimian T, Markowitz J. La formation en psychothérapie interpersonnelle. De sa conception aux USA à son adaptation à Genève. *Psychothérapies*. 2006;26(4):221–232.

6. Hovaguimian T. La psychothérapie interpersonnelle de la dépression. *Médecine et Hygiène*. 2003:103.

7. Leblanc J, Streit U. Origines et description de la Psychothérapie interpersonnelle (PTI). *Santé mentale au Québec*. 2009;33(2):31–47.

8. Stuart S., Robertson M. *Psychothérapie interpersonnelle. Guide du clinicien*. Traduction par Oguz O, Carmona G. Erès édition; 2021.

9. Lavigne B. *Adaptation de la thérapie InterPersonnelle avec Aménagement des Rythmes Sociaux à un groupe ambulatoire de patients bipolaires*. Université de Limoges; 2015.

10. Klein L. *Intérêt de la thérapie interpersonnelle dans la prise en charge de la dépression du sujet âgé*. Université de Besançon; 2020.

11. Paulovics D. *Thérapie interpersonnelle et d'aménagement des rythmes sociaux en groupe*. Sciences du Vivant [q-bio]. 2020.

12. Rahioui H. *La thérapie interpersonnelle*. PUF editor; 2016.

13. Neveux N. *Pratiquer la TIP - Thérapie Interpersonnelle, Les ateliers du praticien*. 2nd ed. Dunod; 2017.

14. Neveux N. *Prendre en charge la dépression avec la thérapie interpersonnelle*. Les ateliers du praticien. Dunod; 2022.

15. Bottai T, Biloa-Tang M, Christophe S, et al. Thérapie interpersonnelle et aménagement des rythmes sociaux (TIPARS): du concept anglo-saxon à l'expérience française. Interpersonal and social rhythm therapy (IPSRT). *L'Encéphale*. 2010;36:S206–S217.

16. Glatigny-Dallay E, Barandon S, Lacaze I, Omay O, Sutter AL. Psychothérapie interpersonnelle et périnatalité, de l'anté- au post-natal. *Vocation Sage-femme*. 2017;(128):35–38.

17. Glatigny-Dallay E, Omay O. Psychothérapie interpersonnelle en périnatalité. In Sous la direction de Benoit Bayle ed., *Psychiatrie et Psychopathologie Périnatales*. Aide-mémoire. Dunod. 2017:397–403.

18. Glatigny-Dallay E. La psychothérapie Interpersonnelle pour les pères? dans : Nine M.-C. Glangeaud-Freudenthal éd., *Accueillir les pères en périnatalité*. La vie de l'enfant. Eres; 2017:217–220.

19. Bottai T, Aubin V, Loftus J, Swartz HA. *Interpersonal and social rhythm therapy (IPSRT) ou thérapie interpersonnelle et d'aménagement des rythmes sociaux (TIPARS). Les troubles bipolaires*. Lavoisier; 2014:512–526.

20. Bottai T, Jacquesy L, Kochman F. *Psychothérapie interpersonnelle. Actualités sur les maladies dépressives*. Lavoisier; 2018:478–487.

21. Sengelen J-M, Lavigne B, Omay O, Bottai T. La Thérapie Interpersonnelle dans la dépression. *Santé Mentale*. 2017;215:42–47.

22. Lavigne B, Audebert-Mérilhou E, Buisson G, Kochman F, Clément JP, Olliac B. Interpersonal Therapy (IPT) in child and adolescent psychiatry. *Encephale*. 2016;42(6):535–539.

23. Omay O, Hizli Sayar G. Superimposed psychological suffering, *Journal of Neurobehavioral Sciences*. 2018;5(1):1–2.

24. Omay O. Interpersonal virtuosity: nourish or perish. Keynote at: 8th International Conference of International Society of Interpersonal Psychotherapy (ISIPT); November 2019; Budapest, Hungary.

11

Interpersonal Psychotherapy Training in Switzerland

THEODORE HOVAGUIMIAN AND OGUZ OMAY ■

THE HISTORY OF INTERPERSONAL THERAPY IN GENEVA

Geographical context

Switzerland is a multilingual federation of 26 German-, French-, and Italian-speaking cantons, among which, located in the far southwest, lies Geneva, a French-speaking city-canton. With a modest area of less than 1% of Switzerland, Geneva canton still ranks second, along with Zürich and Basel, among the three most important cantons in the country. Because of its high demographic density, the canton serves a large population of about 510,000 permanent inhabitants added during weekdays with the flows of cross-border workers from neighboring France and commuters from neighboring Swiss cantons (which amount to more than 100,000 nonresident persons coming to the city daily). In addition, Geneva canton is home to many international organizations, including the United Nations, the World Health Organization (WHO), the World Trade Organization, and the International Labor Office, among others, which contribute to its international influence.

Although the quality of life has declined in recent years, Geneva remains in the top 10 of the most pleasant cities in the world.[1] Yet the rate of depression is higher there than in most Swiss cantons and very much so in comparison with almost all European countries.[2] This paradox is probably explained by the high rate of uprooted persons, who account for up to 40% of the canton's resident population. Indeed, according to a recent survey in Switzerland, people who cannot rely on strong social support have twice the risk of developing mental

Theodore Hovaguimian and Oguz Omay, *Interpersonal Psychotherapy Training in Switzerland* In: *Interpersonal Psychotherapy.* Edited by: Myrna M. Weissman and Jennifer J. Mootz, Oxford University Press. © Oxford University Press 2024. DOI: 10.1093/oso/9780197652084.003.0012 health problems (16% to 26%) than those benefitting from this protective factor (8% to 13%).[2]

The academic recognition of interpersonal psychotherapy in Geneva

Theodore Hovaguimian, a psychiatrist from Geneva, was trained in interpersonal psychotherapy (IPT) in 1996 by John Markowitz. Impressed by the pragmatic aspect of this approach, he enthusiastically imported it to Geneva, where he was a lecturer at the university and a consulting supervisor of Geneva's University Hospitals Department of Psychiatry. Thus, this university became one of the first European centers to teach IPT. This introduction was facilitated by the recognition of the evidence-based cost-effectiveness of IPT at a time when pressure to diminish healthcare expenditure was beginning to be exerted on physicians. The Department of Psychiatry could not ignore managed care and evidence-based medicine despite the controversy that surrounded these movements.[3]

Another factor that promoted the introduction of IPT was that, in the early 2000s, WHO, based in Geneva, put mental health on the agenda of the health policy and started to support its member states in taking initiatives aimed at preserving and promoting mental health and supporting the social and professional integration of the concerned persons.[4] Theodore Hovaguimian had worked with the WHO Division of Mental Health as a temporary advisor, and this new priority created opportunities for him to promote IPT further in the university.

TRAINING IN IPT IN SWITZERLAND

In July 2000, based on the experiences reported in Geneva and on publications in the international literature, the federal regulating authority of medical education and specializations validated postgraduate training in IPT as a possible option for obtaining the title of specialist in psychiatry and psychotherapy. This recognition enabled psychiatrists working in university institutions to select this approach among other choices offered to them during their academic training. Some of them even chose IPT as the theme of their doctoral dissertations.

Publication of a manual in French

Encouraged by this success, Hovaguimian, in collaboration with Markowitz, published an introductory booklet to IPT in French in 2002.[5] This booklet was the only IPT reference in the French language until 2006, when a Canadian translation of the IPT manual was published by Simon Patry. The Hovaguimian-Markowitz booklet helped introduce IPT and support IPT training in the French-speaking Swiss cantons and in France.

The Swiss Society of Interpersonal Psychotherapy and its training target groups

In 2006, together with several colleagues involved in IPT, Theodore Hovaguimian founded the Swiss Society of Interpersonal Psychotherapy (SSPI) with the mission to serve all practitioners trained or receiving training in this method. Over the years, IPT has spread from academic circles to clinicians in private practice. More particularly, in Geneva the method also attracted a good number of primary care doctors because it was part of a medical model, relatively easy to apply, and could be associated with the pharmacotherapy of depression.

In 2014, reaching retirement age after a very active period within Geneva University Hospitals, Hovaguimian stopped the teaching of medical students and supervision of residents, but continued with the society to organize yearly workshops focused on IPT, contributing to the continuing education of private practice psychiatrists and primary care doctors. Hence, the experience in Geneva was based on the training of three distinct populations of medical doctors. The first group included psychiatrists working in university hospitals who chose IPT among other tools during their postgraduate training. The second group was composed of primary care doctors in private practice who had experience in treating depressed patients mainly with antidepressants, and the third group were psychiatrists already settled in private practice who wanted to acquire IPT as part of their continuing education.

Adaptation of teaching according to status in career

In the first group of academic trainees, the teaching of IPT focused on the common grounds and essential differences between this approach and the three other schools of psychotherapies offered to them: the psychodynamic, cognitive behavioral, and systemic therapies.

Adaptation of supervision according to specialization

As for the second and third groups, the variety of backgrounds allowed us to make the following interesting observations, stemming from *supervision*, mostly in line with what was published by Markowitz et al.[6]

Primary care doctors were naturally more comfortable than psychiatrists with a technique that put more therapeutic emphasis on changing pathogenic situations in the here and now than on understanding their root cause. As a result, they were easily able to focus on current interpersonal problems and relate them to the patient's depression rather than seeking to explore their childhood. Also, primary care doctors were generally keen on taking an active stance, siding with patients and advocating their cause against a "blamable medical illness," while some of the psychiatrists were more used to remaining neutral (especially in Switzerland) in order to promote patients' insight and autonomy. Then, the supervisor had to moderate the excessive interventionism of some primary care doctors, while with some withdrawn psychiatrists, the supervisor had to prompt a more active posture. Psychiatrists were more adept at identifying previous sensitizations and patterns of behaviors dating to the past. However, depressed patients benefit from focusing on the current problematic aspects of their life. Therefore, some psychiatrists had to be reminded not to dwell too much on early childhood patterns given the time-limited nature of IPT. They sometimes needed more help to focus their interventions on connecting the depressive episode to the targeted problem area.

Finally, knowing that improvement tends to be attributed to medication rather than to psychotherapy when used in combination, we made the usual recommendation to beginning therapists to refrain, whenever possible, from prescribing antidepressants to their patients to gain confidence that IPT alone could reduce depression. Psychiatrists, here, were more comfortable with this rule than primary care doctors, for whom talk therapy alone was unusual in their practice. They required more encouragement to tolerate and even use the expression of negative affect during the sessions instead of prescribing "a pill for every ill."

DISCUSSION

Geneva was among the first centers in Europe to recognize the validity of IPT and to disseminate its teaching into the university curricula at the pre- and postgraduate levels, as well as in continuing education of private practitioners. This latest mission was pursued by the SSPI.[6]

Among the private practitioners, a special emphasis has been placed on the training of primary care doctors who, like elsewhere, are the first line of intervention in most cases of depression. In Switzerland, although the tendency to consult a psychiatrist directly is increasing for young adults, primary care doctors remain the privileged caretakers of mood disorders, especially for the older age group. But as they lack psychotherapeutic tools, they can only rely heavily on medication.[7] According to the latest figures from the Federal Office of Statistics, half of the total number of antidepressant prescriptions is attributed to them.[7]

Our experience in Geneva in training primary care doctors has been quite positive. The high motivation and familiarity with depression management that characterized the preselection of this group probably reflected the ease of training them and the good results obtained with most of them. This outcome is like that of the early developers of IPT, who published an 85% rate of certified competent therapists at the end of their training.[8]

Recently, because of the special effort that was made to open IPT trainings to primary care doctors, Doctor Johanna Sommer, Professor of Primary Care Medicine, trained by Hovaguimian as a qualified IPT trainer and on her way to becoming supervisor, has formally included this approach in a continuing education program designed for primary care physicians working with psychosomatic patients.

FUTURE DEVELOPMENTS

In 2018, as Hovaguimian was preparing for retirement, Oguz Omay, a psychiatrist working in neighboring France, immigrated to Switzerland and began working in Les Toises Psychiatry and Psychotherapy Center in Lausanne. Oguz Omay was at that point the president of the International Society of Interpersonal Psychotherapy (ISIPT). He had contact with Hovaguimian before his installation in Switzerland and was kindly invited to join the executive committee of SSPI as early as 2017. Nominated president-elect of SSPI in 2019, he then took over the presidency of this association in 2020, helped by Gregoire Rubovszky, the vice president. He brought with him his international experience as the former ISIPT president and helped the SSPI become the third affiliated chapter of ISIPT, after Turkey and China, in 2021.

The importance given to psychotherapy in Switzerland attracted two other well-trained IPT therapists and trainers from France to Switzerland during the same period: Jean-Marie Sengelen (Bienne, Canton Bern) and Benjamin Lavigne (Lausanne, Canton Vaud). They joined the SSIP in 2021 with the aim of opening the mainly Geneva-based society to other French-speaking cantons. A further aim is to extend the reach of the association to German- and Italian-speaking cantons.

AND NOW?

After a period of slow down related to the COVID-19 pandemic, the SSPI resumed its training activity in 2022. The continuing use of online training after the pandemic has also opened new possibilities. It is now possible to imagine training courses where professionals from all French-speaking Swiss cantons, France, Belgium, and French-speaking Canada may participate. Guided by this observation, Oguz Omay, Simon Patry (Canada), and their colleagues are now working on creating a French-speaking chapter of ISIPT. At the same time, IPT Swiss, as the association is now called, nourishes its historic ties with primary care doctors and envisages more training in their direction with the help of Johanna Sommer and Scheherazade Fischberg, both primary care doctors and active members of IPT Swiss.

REFERENCES

1. Economist Intelligence Unit. The Global Liveability Index. 2021. Accessed September 5, 2022 https://www.eiu.com/n/campaigns/global-liveability-index-2021
2. Schuler D, Tuch A, Peter C. La santé psychique en Suisse, Monitorage 2020, Éditeur Observatoire suisse de la santé (Obsan). *Neuchâtel.* 2020;2(2):33–39.
3. Hovaguimian T. Cherish or perish—the values of private psychiatry. In Guimon J, Sartorius N, eds. *Manage or Perish? The Challenges of Managed Mental Health in Europe.* Kluwer Academic/Plenum Publishers; 1999:227–230.

4. World Health Organization. *The World Health Report 2001: Mental Health: New Understanding, New Hope*. 2001. Bulletin of the World Health Organization 20079:1085–1085.

5. Hovaguimian T, Markowitz J. *La Psychothérapie Interpersonnelle de la Dépression* (2nd edn). Médecine et Hygiène; 2002.

6. Markowitz JC, Svartberg M, Swartz HA. Is IPT time-limited psychodynamic psycho-therapy? *J Psychother Pract Res.* 1998;7(3):185–195.

7. Hovaguimian T, Markowitz J. La formation en psychothérapie interpersonnelle: de sa conception aux USA à son adaptation à Genève. *Psychothérapies.* 2006;26(4):221–232.

8. Office fédéral de la santé publique. *Avenir de la psychiatrie en* Suisse. Rapport en réponse au postulat de Philipp Stähelin (10.3255). Confédération Suisse. 2016:29.

12

Interpersonal Psychotherapy Training in Turkey

NAZAN AYDIN, OGUZ OMAY, NALAN ÖZTÜRK,
AND BEYZA NUR EKŞI ■

INTRODUCTION

The Harbor Bridge to Turkey

The story of interpersonal psychotherapy (IPT) in Turkey began unexpectedly in 2008 in Sydney, Australia, where Oguz Omay and Nazan Aydın met for the first time during an International Marcé Society congress. Both were psychiatrists with a keen interest in perinatal psychiatry. Oguz is of Turkish origin, but he had been trained in France, where at the time he had been working for 20 years. He had lost nearly all contact with Turkey and could hardly speak Turkish in a professional setting. Nazan was working at the Atatürk University, Erzurum, in the eastern part of Turkey. Both realized the limits of their clinical tools and were looking for better ways to treat perinatal women. Oguz had just taken his first formal IPT course and spoke enthusiastically to Nazan about his desire to learn more and to disseminate IPT in his perinatal circles in France. IPT, as evidence has shown, is precisely adapted to perinatal women. Nazan joined him in his desire and encouraged him to come and teach also in Turkey.

So, the Harbor Bridge in Sydney became a bridge connecting these two people, whose friendship and collaboration were to lay the foundations of IPT in Turkey. They kept in touch, both investing their time and energy in IPT, and finally Nazan organized an IPT training course given by Oguz in July 2012 in Erzurum, at her university. This course was followed by another one in Istanbul, Turkey, with the support of the Turkish Association for Psychopharmacology.

Nazan Aydın, Oguz Omay, Nalan Öztürk, and Beyza Nur Ekşi, *Interpersonal Psychotherapy Training in Turkey* In: *Interpersonal Psychotherapy*. Edited by: Myrna M. Weissman and Jennifer J. Mootz, Oxford University Press. © Oxford University Press 2024.
DOI: 10.1093/oso/9780197652084.003.0013

The initial courses were received well. Oguz, who had become a fledgling IPT trainer at the time, was struck by the enthusiasm of Turkish colleagues. The Turkish Association for Psychopharmacology was reaching out to many psychiatrists; attendance was from all over Turkey. To these trainees who were mostly psychiatrists, Nazan and Oguz added midwives and clinical nurses from the beginning. In April 2013, Scott Stuart, the president of the International Society of Interpersonal Psychotherapy (ISIPT) at the time, and Oguz Omay gave another series of training courses. These initial steps paved the way to regular courses and supervision in the country with ever-deepening collaboration between Nazan Aydın, Haluk Savaş, and Oguz Omay.

FROM TURKISH ASSOCIATION FOR INTERPERSONAL PSYCHOTHERAPY TO IPT-TURKEY

As Turkish clinicians and academics were introduced to IPT, their demand to learn more and practice IPT increased significantly. With this encouragement and her desire for dissemination, Nazan Aydın established the Turkish Association for Interpersonal Psychotherapy (KIPT-DER) in 2013. The mission of KIPT-DER is to create a team of highly educated and certified IPT clinicians, supervisors, and trainers and to ensure that IPT is disseminated and provided in compliance with the model. As of 2022, KIPT-DER (hereafter *IPT Turkey*) has been active for nearly 10 years and became the first formally affiliated national chapter of ISIPT in 2021. Nazan Aydın is still the president of this association and is now working with a new generation of IPTers, two of whom are also coauthors of this chapter.

In line with ISIPT guidelines, IPT Turkey can certify therapists; it has had two ISIPT-certified trainers: Nazan Aydın and the late Haluk Savaş. They were among the first 70 grandfathered certified trainers of ISIPT internationally in 2019, having built a strong curriculum of activities as trainers. The early loss of Haluk Savaş has been deeply regretted. His style had an important influence on cultural adaptations of IPT to Turkey during the initial training sessions. Oguz Omay, an ISIPT certified trainer, also trains with IPT-Turkey, even though he is now based in Switzerland.

IPT TRAINING IN TURKEY

As of July 2022, a total of 954 mental health workers have attended the IPT courses organized in Turkey by IPT Turkey. Examining the professions of the trainees, 53% were psychiatrists, 28% psychologists, 6% nurses, 5% child and adolescent psychiatrists, 2% psychological counseling practitioners, 1% midwives, 1% social workers, and 4% other diverse professions.

Level A training programs

The level A training programs are courses that last 2 days/16 hours and represent a general introduction to IPT. Theoretical aspects of IPT, the evidence base, as well as clinical practice tools are presented. Small-group discussions, role playing, and analyses of audio/videorecordings are used with a strong experiential component.

Modular training

Modular training provides advanced-level training courses that last 8 days/64 hours. They are composed of 4r separate modules of 2 days each. The aim of these courses is to provide advanced theoretical knowledge and clinical skills with more time to practice compared to the classical level A training. In recent years, approximately 4 modular courses per year have been organized by IPT Turkey. Although there have been some face-to-face modular courses in many Turkish cities, such as Erzurum, Balikesir, and Denizli, most have been carried out in bigger cities, such as Ankara and Istanbul, to reach a larger audience. Since the COVID-19 pandemic, training has moved to online platforms. The silver lining has been that the courses remained as experiential as before, and it was ensured that IPT reached more people in every part of the country.

Teaching at a university setting

Gokben Hizli Sayar, now a professor of psychiatry, introduced to IPT by Oguz Omay, Haluk Savaş, and Nazan Aydın has been one of the most active second-generation IPT enthusiasts in Turkey. Her efforts have moved IPT training forward in Turkey after a pause in 2016. She has organized a modular IPT training at the University of Üsküdar in Istanbul. She has also given hundreds of hours of IPT courses to her students at the Psychology Department, establishing the first IPT courses integrated into undergraduate training from 2017 on. She has conceptualized the IPT-Touch with Oguz Omay and included it in the undergraduate training of social workers, midwives, nurses, child development specialists, and even dialysis and anesthesia technicians trained at her university.

Gokben Hizli Sayar, still a professor of psychiatry, has also become a standup comedian and is unique in her career developments in the world of IPT. Although she is not so active in the field today, her energy and creativity have raised awareness of IPT among many young students of psychology and other professions.

INTERPERSONAL AND SOCIAL RHYTHM THERAPY TRAINING

Interpersonal and Social Rhythm Therapy (IPSRT), which has evidence-based efficacy for treating bipolar disorder, has also attracted the attention of clinicians in

Turkey. To gain more knowledge and experience in this approach, three psychiatry professors (Mesut Cetin, Haluk Savaş, and Nazan Aydın) participated in a 3-day training course organized by the University of Pittsburgh School of Medicine in 2013. Haluk Savaş and Nazan Aydın started giving IPSRT courses from 2015 on, and as of 2022, six IPSRT courses have been organized in Turkey, and they are followed with interest by professionals.

SUPERVISION AND THERAPIST CERTIFICATION PROCESS

Professionals who have completed modular IPT training can already use IPT techniques in their clinical practice. But to qualify formally as an IPT therapist, they are required to complete a clinical supervision training course. IPT Turkey recommends that supervisions be based on audio recordings of sessions.

Individual supervision

The supervisee and supervisor work on the recordings of 2 complete case studies, with at least 8 sessions recorded for each case for a total of 16 sessions. The golden rule is that the supervisee and the supervisor listen to the whole audio recording of each consultation (1 hour). Then the consultation is discussed for approximately 1 hour. For each case, a portfolio consisting of a summary of each session and forms measuring compliance with what needs to be done are prepared and presented to the supervisor at the end of the therapy.

Even if individual supervision by listening to the recordings of whole sessions is considered the gold standard, the increasing demand and the scarcity of supervisor availability have led IPT Turkey to design a specific online group supervision format, in place since the end of 2021. This new model enables more practitioners to access supervision and is also a hub of skill sharing in the IPT community.

ONLINE GROUP SUPERVISION

The aim of online group supervision is to work individually with each supervisee but make the exchange an opportunity for other trainees to contribute and learn. A group of 12 participants meet with 2 supervisors (Nazan Aydın and Oguz Omay) every month online for 3 hours. Recordings of 2 therapy sessions are presented by 2 different supervisees and are discussed by one supervisor. The group listens and contributes by written chat or by live discussion. Every supervisee gets the chance to have a personal supervision while the group benefits from being exposed to different patients and different therapist styles and to the work of 2 different supervisors.

In preparation, the participants send their audio recordings with the *Preliminary Consideration Form* for preliminary assessment. These forms are examined, and 2 audio recordings are selected for the supervision. The supervisor and the supervisee listen to the whole recording before the supervision. The presenting participant indicates the work done in accordance with IPT techniques, noting *what has been done well* and *what may have been better* in the *Detailed Work Form*. Several days before the supervision, the information in the Preliminary Consideration Form and the Detailed Work Form is shared with all participants so that they are ready to discuss the case.

During the 3-hour online supervision meeting, one supervisor conducts an individual supervision in front of the group, with the supervisee presenting the audio recording. Meanwhile, other participants listen actively with cameras and microphones turned off and take notes. Certain parts of the recording are played and analyzed together with the participants. The chat is used to generate questions and remarks. After a break, the same procedures are performed with another therapist and the second supervisor on the second case. The session is completed with a general discussion between all participants.

To get full certification as an IPT therapist, each supervisee is required to complete 72 hours of group supervision lasting a total of 24 months, preferably by attending 4 consecutive 6-month group supervision training periods. During this 24-month period, each participant presents 2 patients and 4 recordings (i.e., 2 recordings from different moments of the therapy of each patient). At the same time, during this period, the participant gets the chance to listen to 44 different recordings from 22 different patients by 11 different therapists.

PUBLICATIONS

Given the increasing interest and need for resources, *The Clinician's Guide to IPT* by Stuart and Robertson was translated into Turkish in 2012. This out-of-print book remains an essential resource for those clinicians who wish to learn and practice IPT in Turkey.[1]

The 2019 special issue of the scientific journal *Türkiye Klinikleri Psychiatry— Special Topics* is the first resource on IPT written in Turkish.[2] Published as a book, edited by Nazan Aydın and Oguz Omay, this special issue consists of sections written by invited authors who are specialists in different aspects of IPT. Several IPT resource booklets, books, and manuals have been translated into Turkish.[3-7] There are also book chapters,[8,9] articles,[10-14] and academic theses[15-17] on IPT in Turkish.

REFERENCES

1. Stuart S, Robertson M. *Kişilerarası İlişkiler Psikoterapisi: Klinisyen Klavuzu*. Omay O, Aydın N, eds. Aydın N, Oral M, Aras N, trans. Yerküre Press; 2014.
2. Aydın N, Omay O, eds. *Kişilerarası İlişkiler Psikoterapisi*. Türkiye Klinikleri Yayınları; 2019.

3. Stuart S, Schultz J. *Gruplar İçin Kişilerarası İlişkiler Psikoterapisi*. Omay O, Hızlı Sayar G, Aydın N, trans. 2019.

4. Stuart S, Schultz J, McCann E. *Kişilerarası İlişkiler Psikoterapisi Klinisyen El Kitabı*. Omay O, Hızlı Sayar G, Aydın N, trans. 2019.

5. Weissman M, Verdeli H. *Birinci Basamak Sağlık Hizmetlerinde Kişilerarası Danışmanlık*. Hizli Sayar G, Omay O, Aydın N, Dönmez M, trans. Kapak gorseli: Irfan Sayar; 2019.

6. Frank E, Levenson JC. *Kişilerarası Psikoterapi*. Gonca Akkaya, trans. Okuyan Us Yayınları; 2015.

7. Frank E. *Bipolar Bozukluğu Tedavi Etmek: Kişilerarası ve Sosyal Ritim Terapisi Rehberi*. Savaş H, trans. Yerküre Press; 2014.

8. Aydın N, Omay O, Savaş H. Kişilerarası İlişkiler Psikoterapisi. In Köroğlu E, eds. *Psikoterapi Yöntemleri: Kuramlar ve Uygulama Yönergeleri*. 3th ed. Boylam Psikiyatri Press; 2017:347–364.

9. Aydın P, Aydın N. Gebelikte ve Doğum Sonrası Dönemde Kişilerarası İlişkiler Psikoterapisi. In Aydın N, Akdeniz F, Aydın P, eds. *Gebelikte ve Doğum Sonrası Dönemde Ruhsal Bozuklukların Sağaltım Kılavuzu*. Turkish Psychiatry Association Press; 2021:281–291.

10. Yuksel G, Aydın N, Omay O. IPT in postpartum depression. *Clin Mother Child Health*. 2015;12(4):11–12.

11. Okanlı A, Durmaz H, Oral M. Interpersonal psychotherapy as an integrative approach for caregivers of individuals with mental illness: a case report. *Turkish J Integrative Med*. 2015;3(2):83–85.

12. Ozer U, Yuksel G. Interpersonal psychotherapy in the treatment of perinatal complicated grief: a case who experienced intrauterine loss of twins. *J Mood Disord*. 2016;6:20–24.

13. Oral M, Tuncay T. Majör Depresyon Tanısı Almış Kadınlarda Kişilerarası İlişkiler Terapisi Yaklaşımına Dayalı Grupla Sosyal Hizmet Uygulamasının Depresyon ve Sosyal Problem Çözme Düzeyleri Üzerine Etkisi: Bir Karma Yöntem Araştırması. *Toplum ve Sosyal Hizmet*. 2018;29(2):114–143.

14. Sükrü F, Öztürk M, Kilic O, Guneytepe S, Ucok A. The impact of a six-month interpersonal group psychotherapy on functionality of patients with schizophrenia in a community mental health center. *Anadolu Psikiyatri Dergisi*. 2018;19(6):559–566.

15. Durmaz H. *Effects of Interpersonal Psychotherapy (IPT) Techniques and Psychoeducation on Self-Efficacy and Care Burden in Families of Patients with Schizophrenia*. PhD thesis. Atatürk University; 2015.

16. Kurultay C. *Effects of Interpersonal Psychotherapy Training on Mental Wellness, Social and Emotional Intelligence*. Master's thesis. Üsküdar University; 2018.

17. Varol C. *The Effects of Interpersonal Psychotherapy Training on Subjective Happiness, Empathy, Expressing Emotions and Experiences in Close Relationships*. Master's thesis. Üsküdar University; 2018.

13

Interpersonal Psychotherapy Training and Accreditation in the United Kingdom

ROSLYN LAW AND FIONA DUFFY ■

CONTEXT OF WORK

Interpersonal Psychotherapy (IPT) training in the United Kingdom covers four nations (England, Scotland, Northern Ireland, and Wales) and their respective healthcare systems. The protocols for training, supervision, and accreditation are standardized by Interpersonal Psychotherapy United Kingdom (IPTUK), the IPT therapist membership and training regulating body in the UK, allowing a broadly consistent approach despite different funding streams. In England, IPT and IPT-A (IPT for adolescents) dissemination is mostly, but not exclusively, supported by UK government funding and delivered through the Improving Access to Psychological Therapy (IAPT) and Children and Young People's IAPT (CYP IAPT) programmes. Funding supports approximately 115 practitioner and 30 supervisor training places each year, based on a national needs assessment conducted by Health Education England (HEE). IPT has been part of IAPT training since 2008, and IPT-A was added to CYP IAPT training in 2012. These programs increase public access to evidence-based treatments for common mental health disorders. IAPT training targets the existing psychological therapies workforce, and CYP IAPT recruits into new posts with IPT-A training provided. IAPT services provide treatments recommended in the National Institute for Health and Care Excellence (NICE) guidelines for depression in adults[1] and young people.[2]

In Northern Ireland, practitioner training is funded biannually by the Department of Health for up to 10 trainees, drawn from the existing workforce. In Northern Ireland, psychotherapy has historically been poorly resourced, and

Roslyn Law and Fiona Duffy, *Interpersonal Psychotherapy Training and Accreditation in the United Kingdom* In: *Interpersonal Psychotherapy*. Edited by: Myrna M. Weissman and Jennifer J. Mootz, Oxford University Press. © Oxford University Press 2024. DOI: 10.1093/oso/9780197652084.003.0014 consequently therapists complete training in their own time. To date there has only been one funded IPT post in the region.

In Scotland, the University of Edinburgh (UoE) delivers IPT training for 3 target audiences—NHS clinicians completing training based on a centralized strategic needs assessment, clinicians accruing credit as part of an MSc in psychological therapies (UoE), and final year trainee clinical psychologists at the Universities of Edinburgh and Glasgow. Training is either self-funded or funded through National Health Service (NHS) Education Scotland (NES). Approximately 15–20 participants work toward accredited practitioner status following training each year.

In Wales, IPT training is available in the South Wales NHS. Approximately 6 participants from across South Wales can access practitioner training annually and are supported directly or indirectly with NHS funding. Each participating service is supported to develop a sustainable IPT pathway with in-house IPT supervision.

MODEL OF TRAINING

Practitioner

The IPT practitioner training is delivered by 3 training centers in England and 1 training center each in Wales, Northern Ireland, and Scotland. In Scotland, the practitioner course provides combined training for IPT and IPT-A trainees. Practitioner training is delivered over a minimum of 5 days plus 12 months of weekly supervision provided by an IPTUK accredited supervisor. Most supervision in the United Kingdom is delivered remotely, by either telephone or videoconferencing. This allows courses to be supported by a national network of supervisors, frequently working across the country to support trainees' learning. All government- or NHS-funded training includes didactic teaching and supervised casework, which can also be accessed with nongovernment funding. Each trainee is required to complete 4 cases of IPT or IPT-A, reflecting work in at least 2 focal areas. A minimum of 12 hours of recorded therapy sessions are self-assessed and formally rated using a competency-based assessment based on[3] participants in training are mostly qualified therapists from a range of training backgrounds, such as counseling, clinical psychology, and Cognitive Behavioral Therapy (CBT). Participants receive varying degrees of service-level support, ranging from completing training in their own time to having at least 1 day of protected work time for the duration of training.

The IPT-A training in the CYP IAPT program is delivered as a postgraduate diploma combining training in core therapeutic skills and one modality or clinical specialism of choice, including IPT-A. The post-graduate diploma is available through University College London and the Anna Freud Center and aims to upskill the pre- and post-qualification workforce serving young people with common mental health difficulties across England. IPT-A training may also be accessed as a 5-day training following by 12 months of supervised practice through the AFC and as part of CYP IAPT post-graduate certificate programme delivered in conjunction with core skills training at the University of Manchester.

Supervisor

Government-funded supervisor training is available in England and Scotland for IPTUK-accredited practitioners. In England, 6 days of supervisor training are delivered over 12–18 months, combining didactic teaching, advanced practice casework, and experience working as a peer and primary supervisor. Following successful completion of expert-facilitated and peer-supervised advance practice, the trainee supervisor works with a novice IPT or IPT-A practitioner under the continued supervision of an accredited IPTUK supervisor.

In Scotland, the UoE 2-day IPT supervisor course follows completion of the comprehensive and cross modality 3-day NES psychological therapy supervisor course, available to individuals 2 years postqualification. This is followed by 2 advanced practice IPT cases and supervision of supervised practice. Approximately 10 places are funded biannually.

ADAPTATIONS TO IPT TRAINING AND SUPERVISION

Interpersonal Psychotherapy training in the United Kingdom primarily focuses on a 16 weekly session model of IPT for depression[3] and a 12 weekly session model of IPT-A for adolescents, with additional sessions with parents and caregivers.[4] Didactic training is also available in family-based IPT[5] and IPT-A Skills Training[6] particularly targeting a new strand of the mental health workforce, the school-based educational mental health practitioners (EMHPs).

Pilot research has supported the development of small Interpersonal Counseling (IPC) and IPT-Group (IPT-G) training and supervision programs. IPC has been evaluated with young people supported in nonspecialist services,[7] with depressed women during pregnancy,[8] and in IAPT primary care services. In collaboration with the Columbia University Global Mental Health Lab, IPT-G is being piloted in perinatal, health psychology, and military settings. Guidelines are being developed by IPTUK for CPD training in empirically supported adaptations of IPT not currently included in the NICE guidelines.

CONTENT AND PROCESS ADAPTATIONS

Three distinct areas of emphasis in UK trainings are (1) focus on clinicians providing detailed formulations, clearly aligned with focal areas; and (2) promotion of the routine use of the interpersonal sensitivities focus area (originally known as interpersonal deficits); and (3) emphasis on mentalizing and reestablishing social learning.

Use of the interpersonal sensitivities focus has been the subject of debate in the IPT literature. Historically, it has been discouraged[3] with people experiencing long-standing interpersonal difficulties and with few current supports, argued to be less responsive to short-term interventions. This view has not resonated in the United Kingdom, where all 4 focal areas are routinely used. Comparative outcomes across focal areas were reviewed in a recent survey of 130 IPT training cases conducted over 2 years in IAPT services (Figure 13.1).[9] Interpersonal sensitivities was the second most chosen focus, accounting for 24% of the casework. Of the sensitivities group, 62% achieved recovery by the end of therapy, and 72% reported reliable improvement on the Patient Health Questionnaire-9 (PHQ-9). The routine collection of session-by-session outcome data during IPT training in the United Kingdom allows empirical questions to be explored, and results are fed back into the training discussion.

Mentalizing, the ability to accurately reflect on one's own intentions and feelings and those of the people around us, reinforces the positive attachment cycle from which it emerged. Being understood promotes self-understanding and encourages us to see others as useful and trustworthy sources of information and support, fostering epistemic trust. This ability is inhibited under conditions of social threat and by many mental health conditions, including depression.[10] Lapses in mentalizing increase social alienation—losing sight of oneself and others, at least temporarily. This psychological isolation is fertile ground for the interpersonal difficulties to flourish that are the focal areas of IPT, conflict, unresolved change, and loss. The mentalizing framework has been incorporated as a potential mediator of change in IPT training, facilitating a nuanced formulation of the nature of the interpersonal missteps that surround depression. Unlike mentalization-based therapies, in which the therapeutic relation is an explicit focus, IPT conducted with consideration of mentalizing processes remains primarily focused on the person's social network, navigating the consequences of a breakdown in social learning and consequent interpersonal hypervigilance. Mentalizing also provides a framework for the explicitly reflective practice necessary when social learning

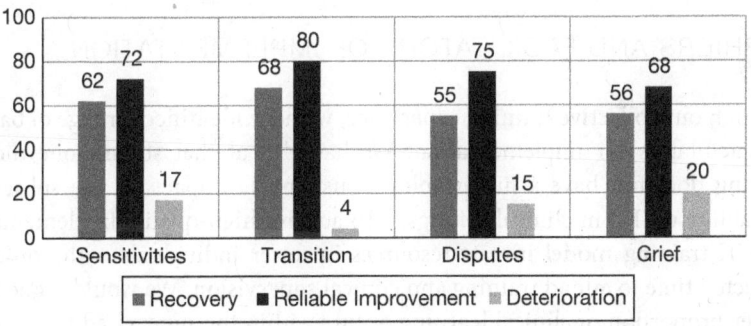

Figure 13.1 Outcomes by focal areas (IAPT sample).

falters within the therapeutic alliance, as illustrated in the case example in this chapter. Mentalizing has been widely incorporated into practitioner, supervisor, and CPD training in the United Kingdom alongside underpinning attachment and contemporary interpersonal theory.[11,12,13]

CULTURAL ADAPTATIONS

Further adaptations to core training currently in process in the United Kingdom reflect the multidisciplinary training cohorts providing and multicultural populations served by IPT. Some elements of the standard IPT protocol (e.g., medical model, sick role, diagnosis) do not easily translate across disciplines and cultural groups. The United Kingdom training courses are currently undertaking a detailed review of our curricula to ensure they embrace a Multicultural Orientation Framework.[14] This commits us to adopting a stance of cultural humility, exploring cultural opportunities, and attending to cultural discomfort in implementation and adherence to the IPT model across professional and cultural groups.

   Also, IPTUK has given explicit attention to equity of training opportunities across therapists from different ethnic backgrounds. A recent survey of the IPTUK membership revealed that while training numbers at practitioner level reflect national population figures, this is not true as trainees move to practitioner, supervisor, and trainer accreditation. Practitioners from non-White backgrounds are underrepresented at higher levels of training. IPTUK is consulting with the membership to identify barriers to progression for clinicians of colour, including lack of representation at higher levels of the IPTUK executive, unnecessary systemic barriers (e.g., previous requirement to be an IPT supervisor to be eligible to chair IPTUK), conscious and unconscious bias in supervision, and a lack of management support for advanced training in the workplace. IPTUK has explicitly committed to improving, including enhancing understanding of cultural and racial bias in selection and training programs for practitioner and supervisors, with the aim of increasing opportunities for advanced training and accreditation across all members.

BARRIERS AND FACILITATORS OF IMPLEMENTATION

Through our collective training experience, we have identified a range of barriers and facilitators for implementation. We have learnt that stand-alone didactic training does not have a discernible or sustainable impact on the subsequent availability of IPT in clinical settings.[15] To achieve high-quality implementation, the UK training model invests resources in fewer individuals with confirmed protected time to attend training and clinical supervision. We would argue that a higher proportion of clinical learning occurs within the supervised practice that follows didactic training than in the training course itself, albeit this is valuable for implementation. We recommend that training and clinical supervision be conducted within a clear accreditation framework to maintain quality standards and in collaboration with a national funding or training body providing strategic oversight of national training needs. High-quality clinical practice in IPT is dependent on clinical supervision inclusive of continual self-assessment and competency-based feedback. While acknowledging the contribution of continuing education in evidence-based approaches, supervision, and feedback monitoring, Rousmanier et al.[16] argued for the necessity of moving from routine performance and passive learning to deliberate practice involving "repetitively practicing specific skills with continuous corrective feedback" to generate a cycle of excellence. This approach to implementation of IPT reflects enhanced focus on equitable formal accreditation of psychological therapists from multiple training and ethnic backgrounds and core consideration of adherence to an established competency framework in the United Kingdom.

FUTURE PLANS

The IPTUK is currently undertaking a review of the accreditation process to widen access to training for the expanding low-intensity workforce, such as Child Well-being Practitioners (CWPs) and EMHPs with experience in low-intensity, manualized interventions. Low-intensity training is being developed across both the adult and child and adolescent workforce. This is inclusive of IPC and more formal training, and accreditation standards are currently being developed to support implementation in a standardized way.

CASE EXAMPLE

Sylvia is a 63-year-old White woman living in a small rural village in the southeast of England. Sylvia referred herself to a local IAPT service because she felt lonely and isolated following the death of her partner of 12 years, Emma, 4 years earlier. Sylvia describes having no friends and not having felt the need for anyone else when she and Emma were together. Since her bereavement, Sylvia has tried to make friends but thinks she is "too intense" and other people back off, leaving her feeling even more alone and helpless. She describes this as a lifelong pattern, with Emma being the only person she felt understood and accepted her. Sylvia explains she is frequently sad and tearful, especially in the evening when she finds it difficult to distract herself. She often feels agitated and has difficulty concentrating and taking care of herself. Her appetite is minimal, often resulting in missed meals, and she routinely feels tired and lethargic following poor sleep. She is not suicidal but experiences no pleasure in her life. Sylvia's symptoms are rated on the PHQ-9 each week and tracked in supervision.

Sylvia has been in contact with mental health services throughout most of her adult life, including two short periods of inpatient care, once in her early 20s following workplace bullying and again in her mid-30s following the end of a close relationship. She had attended multiple counseling sessions and group interventions, including 1 year of grief-focused counseling following Emma's death. She self-referred to her local IAPT service soon after completing her last episode of care. She believes therapy helped temporarily, but she finds endings very difficult, and depression quickly returns. Sylvia had been prescribed several antidepressants since adolescence but had not found them helpful and has stopped taking them on each occasion.

Sylvia begins her IPT by asking what else will be offered when it ends, highlighting the urgency of her wish for support. It is clear she finds her loneliness intolerable, made worse by the loss of her relationship with Emma. When drawing a timeline of depression in the first session, it becomes apparent that the relationship with Emma offered a partial but not complete reprieve from the loneliness and sadness Sylvia has experienced since childhood and that had been felt very deeply following her loss. It appears that on several occasions, before, during, and since her relationship with Emma, Sylvia has used therapy to fulfill her need for someone to listen to her and felt devastated each time it ended. The IPT therapist uses weekly IPT supervision to discuss how to work with the long-term nature of Sylvia's difficulties in a time-limited treatment and the emotional impact of the urgency of the demand Sylvia expresses. Supervision helped to guide the therapist back to focusing on the here-and-now focus of IPT and the rationale of focusing on current interpersonal relationships to relieve immediate depressive symptoms. The experience of forming a therapeutic relationship with Sylvia was also used to inform thinking about potential focal areas.

Sylvia's Interpersonal Inventory is sparsely populated, with no contact with her family of origin, who disapproved of her sexuality, and minimal contact with Emma's children from her marriage prior to being with Sylvia. Sylvia has had occasional contact with an LGBTQ+ (lesbian, gay, bisexual, transgender, queer/questioning+) support group in recent years but is disappointed by what she perceives as their focus on younger people and has not maintained contact. Sylvia explains that Emma had poor physical health throughout their relationship, and Sylvia acted as carer and partner for most of their time together. She welcomed this role and was good at it, having worked as a nursing assistant for 30 years. However, in her most insecure moments she fears Emma was with her because she couldn't manage on her own rather than because it was what she really wanted. Sylvia never expressed this fear to Emma. Sylvia describes two short, intense friendships that both began and ended badly in the context of support groups in the last 2 years, which she experiences as rejections.

Throughout the assessment phase the importance of losing Emma is acknowledged, and the recurring difficulty of establishing and maintaining relationships, which pre-dated and followed that relationship, is also a central focus of discussion. Ways of understanding Sylvia's current interpersonal difficulties and how to frame the IPT work are discussed weekly in supervision. A written formulation is discussed in supervision prior to sharing the proposed focus with Sylvia. In session 4, a formulation, collaboratively developed with Sylvia over the first 3 sessions, is tentatively shared and discussed. Sylvia acknowledges that she started therapy assuming the focus would be on losing Emma but recognizes that this is an opportunity to understand the broader context of her continuing struggle to connect with other people, which is at the heart of her depression. It is agreed that a sensitivities focus will be used to capture the recurring nature of Sylvia's interpersonal difficulties, and this will include attention to the way in which her relationship with Emma replicated and avoided the patterns that are powerful in maintaining her current depression. Recorded clips of the therapy are reviewed weekly, and a full-session recording of the formulation session with a competency-based self-assessment is shared with the IPT supervisor, who provides detailed written and verbal feedback.

Following Klerman et al.'s guidance,[17] the early middle phase sessions are used to review a selection of relationships, each of which involved a pattern of intense engagement and then painful ending that Sylvia described occurring several times in her life. This review includes the friendships that broke down during the last 4 years and further examples that pre-dated Sylvia's relationship with Emma, which had been the longest relationship of her life. Sylvia's relationship with Emma is used as comparison to try to understand what worked successfully and to clarify which aspects of maintaining a wider network of relationships have proven so difficult for Sylvia. Each relationship is discussed in terms of how it began, how the acquaintance developed, who initiated contact, what worked well, and where the challenges lay. Given the significance of ending for Sylvia, this is discussed in detail for each example. This review exercise, conducted over 2 sessions, is used to develop a simple representation of a recurring interpersonal pattern that had been significant in maintaining Sylvia's depression over decades of her life (Figure 13.2). It is helpful to capture this pattern visually, in the way that a single example might be captured in a depression circle, to focus attention and create an essential tool for subsequent sessions. Creating a diagram of the recurring pattern helps to interrupt the well-practiced narrative of idealized and rejecting relationships that Sylvia initially expresses and prompts her to become curious about how each step in the cycle leads to the next and in so doing maintains her depression. This also provided a way to navigate current choices when Sylvia explores opportunities for interpersonal contact through a volunteering role she has taken up and the way in which the pattern plays out in therapy.

Mapping the pattern on a page supports Sylvia to revisit what had been discussed in a more concrete way than she has been able to do when previous discussions were forgotten or overshadowed by a change in mood. Having a stable visual representation allows her to work with support to consider different perspectives and identify specific options at each stage of the cycle, integrating core IPT strategies into the discussion as relevant. These include developing a more nuanced recognition and expression of her feelings, using decision analysis and communication analysis to plan when and how to approach those occasions when she would have previously been too intense due to the urgency of her wish for connection. New interactions are carefully planned, creating and role-playing simple scripts. Sessions are used to help Sylvia tolerate and process the

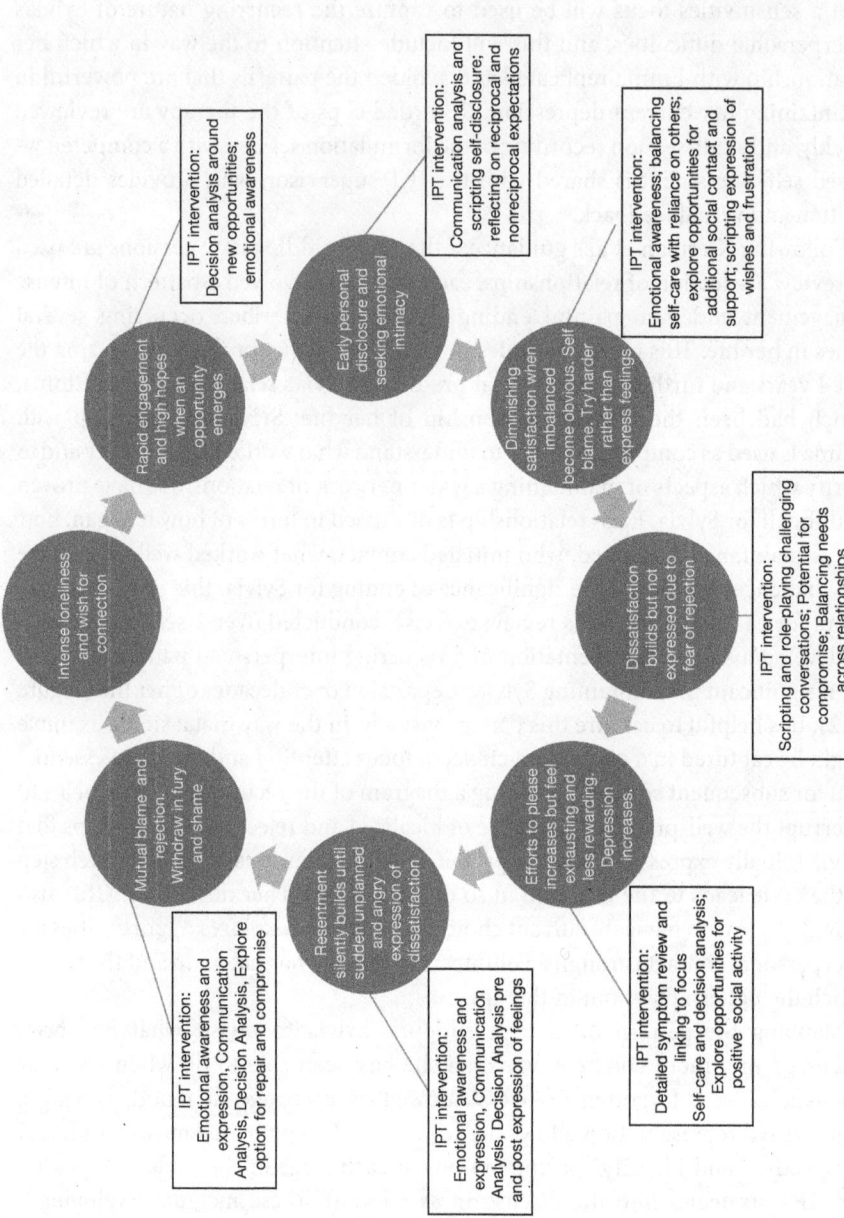

Figure 13.2 Diagram of recurring pattern.

IPT intervention:
Decision analysis around
new opportunities;
emotional awareness

IPT intervention:
Communication analysis and
scripting self-disclosure;
reflecting on reciprocal and
nonreciprocal expectations

IPT intervention:
Emotional awareness; balancing
self-care with reliance on others;
explore opportunities for
additional social contact and
support; scripting expression of
wishes and frustration

IPT intervention:
Scripting and role-playing challenging
conversations; Potential for
compromise; Balancing needs
across relationships

IPT intervention:
Detailed symptom review and
linking to focus
Self-care and decision analysis;
Explore opportunities for
positive social activity

IPT intervention:
Emotional awareness and
expression, Communication
Analysis, Decision Analysis pre
and post expression of feelings

IPT intervention:
Emotional awareness and
expression, Communication
Analysis, Decision Analysis, Explore
option for repair and compromise

Rapid engagement
and high hopes
when an
opportunity
emerges

Early personal
disclosure and
seeking emotional
intimacy

Diminishing
satisfaction when
imbalanced
become obvious. Self
blame. Try harder
rather than
express feelings

Dissatisfaction
builds but not
expressed due to
fear of rejection

Efforts to please
increases but feel
exhausting and
less rewarding.
Depression
increases.

Resentment
silently builds until
sudden unplanned
and angry
expression of
dissatisfaction

Mutual blame and
rejection.
Withdraw in fury
and shame

Intense loneliness
and wish for
connection

frustration and disappointment she feels when the opportunities available to her offer some but far from all of what she wishes for in terms of connection and support, including therapy itself. The visual diagrams are used in supervision to support reflective practice, focusing on the core interpersonal patterns, how they perpetuated the depression, choice of specific IPT techniques that may be helpful and how these interpersonal patterns are evident and can be managed in the therapeutic relationship.

The progress in these sessions is slow, something that is characteristic of sensitivities work. At times, the frustration arising from trying to redirect efforts away from the all-or-nothing pattern that has characterized Sylvia's interpersonal style flares up in therapy, temporarily transforming it from being helpful and offering new insights to being too little and too slow with the end of therapy rapidly approaching like another inevitable rejection. Having the pattern mapped out on a page is useful to support Sylvia to consider how the recurring sequence is playing out in therapy. Each example is examined carefully to repair the rupture and inform how to navigate comparable experiences or setback outside of therapy. As this move in and out, a deliberate reflective position became more practiced, Sylvia's confidence in her ability to influence the course of interactions increased, something she had not previously experienced. Previously, she said she felt like she was repeatedly racing toward another inevitable collision, and now she had more ideas about how to steer and pace her own journey. This process of lapse and recovery is mirrored in weekly supervision to build the novice IPT therapist's confidence as an explicitly reflective practitioner within the model.

Part of the IAPT model involves routine outcome monitoring, allowing Sylvia to track the impact of the work she is doing against her weekly PHQ-9 scores and how she rates progress toward her individual goals, set at the time of agreeing to the focus. Both show good progress, with PHQ9 scores gradually reducing week on week from session 7 onward and goals-based outcome charting setbacks and successes in an overall positive trajectory. By the end of therapy, Sylvia's depression scores are within the healthy range, and she has moved more than halfway toward her individual goals.

Given the significance of endings in Sylvia's relationship history, the prospect of ending is consistently held in mind and given explicit attention over the final 4 sessions. Sylvia's feelings about ending are discussed during each session and care is taken in capturing the work that had been done and how this could be sustained in the weeks and months ahead. Sylvia's volunteer role in a local community kitchen has gone well, and she felt supported by people who understand vulnerable mental health and are positive about her ability to help others. This provides an opportunity for Sylvia to share her nurturing side, which had been so important in the success of her career and relationship with Emma. Sylvia can talk about therapy ending with the volunteer coordinator and makes posttherapy plans that relate to her own resources rather than relying on further therapy to sustain her progress. Sylvia accepts the end of therapy and expresses a pragmatic view that something useful had been started and will need more practice to consolidate. For the first time, she does not want to be referred for more therapy as she feels able to continue with the help of her map and current support.

REFERENCES

1. National Institute for Health and Care Excellence. Depression in adults: recognition and management. 2009. https://www.nice.org.uk/guidance/cg90. Accessed June 8, 2022.
2. National Institute for Health and Care Excellence. Depression in children and young people: identification and management. 2019. https://www.nice.org.uk/guidance/ng134. Accessed June 8, 2022.
3. Lemma A, Roth A, Pilling S. The competences required to deliver effective interpersonal psychotherapy (IPT). 2009. https://www.ucl.ac.uk/clinical-psychology//CORE/IPT%20competences%20Oct%202010/IPT%20clinician%20guide.pdf. Accessed June 8, 2022.
4. Weissman MM, Markowitz JC, Klerman GL. *The Guide to Interpersonal Psychotherapy: Updated and Expanded Edition*. Oxford University Press; 2017.
5. Mufson L, Pollack DK, Moreau D, Weissman MM. *Interpersonal Psychotherapy for Depressed Adolescent*. 2nd ed. Guilford Press; 2004.
6. Dietz LJ, Mufson L, Weinberg RJ. *Family-Based Interpersonal Psychotherapy for Depressed Preadolescents*. Oxford University Press; 2018.
7. Young JF, Mufson L, Schueler CM. *Preventing Adolescent Depression: Interpersonal Psychotherapy–Adolescent Skills Training*. Oxford University Press; 2016.
8. Wilkinson PO, Cestaro V, Pinchen I. Pilot mixed-methods evaluation of interpersonal counselling for young people with depressive symptoms in non-specialist services. *BMJ Ment Health*. 2018;21(4):134–138.
9. Ingram J, Johnson D, Johnson S, et al. Protocol for a feasibility randomised trial of low-intensity interventions for antenatal depression: ADAGIO trial comparing interpersonal counselling with cognitive behavioural therapy. *BMJ Open*. 2019;9(8):e032649.
10. Law R. Internal review of IAPT IPT training cases 2019–2022. 2022. IPTUK network meeting.
11. Fischer-Kern M, Fonagy P, Kapusta ND, et al. Mentalizing in female inpatients with major depressive disorder. *J Nerv Ment Dis*. 2013;201(3):202–207.
12. Ravitz P, Maunder R, McBride C. Attachment, contemporary interpersonal theory and IPT: an integration of theoretical, clinical, and empirical perspectives. *J Contemp Psychother*. 2008;38:11–21.
13. Law R, Ravitz P, Pain C, Fonagy P. Interpersonal psychotherapy and mentalizing—synergies in clinical practice. *Am J Psychother*. 2022;75(1):44–50.
14. Davis DE, DeBlaere C, Owen J, et al. The multicultural orientation framework: a narrative review. *Psychotherapy*. 2018;55(1):89.
15. Miller SD, Hubble MA, Chow DL, Seidel JA. The outcome of psychotherapy: yesterday, today, and tomorrow. *Psychotherapy*. 2013;50(1):88–97.
16. Rousmaniere T, Goodyear RK, Miller SD, Wampold BE, eds. *The Cycle of Excellence: Using Deliberate Practice to Improve Supervision and Training*. John Wiley & Sons; 2017.

17. Klerman GL, Weissman MM, Rounsaville BJ, Chevron E. *Interpersonal Psychotherapy of Depression: A Brief, Focused, Specific Strategy*. Basic Books; 1984.

IMPLEMENTATION RESOURCES

IPTUK website and associated accreditation standards. https://www.iptuk.net

IAPT data set reports. https://digital.nhs.uk/data-and-information/data-collections-and-data-sets/data-sets/improving-access-to-psychological-therapies-data-set/improving-access-to-psychological-therapies-data-set-reports. Accessed June 8, 2022.

IAPT manual. https://www.rcpsych.ac.uk/docs/default-source/improving-care/nccmh/iapt/nccmh-iapt-manual-appendices-helpful-resources-v2.pdf?sfvrsn=a607ef5_4. Accessed June 8, 2022.

14

Interpersonal Psychotherapy Training in Graduate and Residency Programs in the United States

LUIS E. FLORES, JR., KELSEY A. BONFILS,
SARAH E. BLEDSOE, AND DANIELLE M. NOVICK ■

Evidence supports the efficacy of interpersonal psychotherapy (IPT) for treating a variety of disorders across populations and age groups.[1-8] Thus, IPT is designated as an evidence-based treatment (EBT)[9,10] and is included in prominent clinical practice guidelines, especially for the treatment of depression.[11-14]

Despite their inclusion in influential guidelines, EBTs such as IPT have not been universally adopted for inclusion in curricula by training programs for mental health professionals.[10,15,16] Evidence suggests IPT has not been disseminated as effectively as other EBTs, such as cognitive behavioral therapy (CBT). Indeed, in the United States, CBT is the predominant psychotherapeutic paradigm taught in clinical training programs, including clinical psychology, psychiatry, and social work.[16] In recent years, graduate curricula generally have come to focus disproportionately on CBT and psychodynamic approaches, leaving few opportunities for IPT training.[17] These disparities signal the need to investigate current training efforts in IPT and how they differ across disciplines that provide training in psychotherapy, including psychiatry, psychology, social work, counseling, and psychiatric mental health nurse practitioner (PMHNP) programs.

Luis E. Flores, Jr., Kelsey A. Bonfils, Sarah E. Bledsoe, and Danielle M. Novick, *Interpersonal Psychotherapy Training in Graduate and Residency Programs in the United States* In: *Interpersonal Psychotherapy*. Edited by: Myrna M. Weissman and Jennifer J. Mootz, Oxford University Press. © Oxford University Press 2024. DOI: 10.1093/oso/9780197652084.003.0015

PSYCHOTHERAPY TRAINING

In recent decades, many disciplines that deliver psychotherapy have had their accrediting bodies add stipulations that training programs must provide foundational training in core areas of psychotherapy. Accreditation sets quality standards for entry into a field by promoting accountability and consistency in goals and expectations for training and education. Guidelines for psychotherapy training vary vastly across professional degree programs, meaning that their graduates will likely vary in their preparedness to deliver psychotherapy, as outlined below[18–22]:

- Psychiatric residents—competence in applying brief and long-term supportive, psychodynamic, and cognitive behavioral psychotherapies.[18]
- Clinical and counseling psychology doctoral trainees—competence in assessment and intervention; the training program must demonstrate that practice is evidence based and that evidence is practice informed.[19]
- Social work master's degree trainees—competence in selecting appropriate intervention strategies based on research knowledge; knowledge of evidence-informed interventions.[20]
- Master's degrees in psychology and counseling trainees—competence in evidence-based theories and practice of counseling and psychotherapy; ability to plan and implement interventions utilizing at least one consistent theoretical orientation.[21]
- PMHNP doctoral students—competence in psychotherapy; the training program must teach psychotherapy skills.[22]

The "gold standard" for learning and developing psychotherapy competency is a combination of didactics and supervised clinical work.[16,23] Yet, no discipline's accreditation guidelines explicitly include this as requisite for EBT training. That is, many programs do not require their students to complete didactics and supervised clinical work in an EBT to graduate.

NATIONAL PSYCHOTHERAPY TRAINING SURVEY-I

In 2006, Weissman and colleagues published the results of their National Psychotherapy Training Survey (NPTS-I) based on a probability sample of all accredited psychiatry, clinical psychology (PhD and PsyD), and social work master's programs in the United States.[16] The NPTS-I was a unique multidisciplinary effort that included leaders from psychiatry, psychology, and social work, focused on what was taught in training programs and practicums across disciplines. Its objective was to determine how commonly each EBT was offered in accredited training programs in psychiatry, clinical psychology, and social work. The original survey also gathered data on whether training was elective or required and provided through didactic training and/or clinical supervision.[16]

Original survey methods

The cross-sectional survey asked directors of clinical training (or persons with equivalent job duties) to indicate (1) whether particular psychotherapeutic approaches were taught, (2) if they were required or elective, and (3) if they were discussed in lectures/coursework (didactic) and/or supervised clinical work. The survey ran from May 2004 to December 2004, achieving over a 70% response rate.

Accreditation rosters were used to identify 552 training programs (182 psychiatric residencies, 150 clinical psychology PhD programs, 55 PsyD psychology programs, and 165 social work programs). Programs were divided by discipline and region (West, South, Midwest, Northeast), and a random sample of 300 programs (54.4%) was selected. Selection criteria were based on stratified random sampling with proportional allocation among the 16 disciplines by region strata to ensure meaningful comparisons of programs across stratification variables.

Programs that met the gold standard for training in psychotherapy were those that required all students to receive didactic training and clinical supervision in the psychotherapy in question. Rates among programs were presented as weighted percentages, with 95% confidence intervals to account for the sampling design.

Summary of results

Although many programs across all disciplines offered IPT training, CBT was the predominant psychotherapy training modality. Among disciplines, psychiatry residency programs reported the highest percentage *offering* didactic training in IPT (70%), although other disciplines also offered didactic training in IPT at moderate rates (60% of PsyD programs; 56% of clinical psychology PhD programs; 55% of social work programs). Compared to offering IPT didactic training, slightly fewer psychiatry residency programs *required* IPT didactic training (60%). However, percentages were much lower at about a quarter to a third for other types of training programs (37% of PsyD programs; 29% of clinical psychology PhD programs; and 28% of social work programs). In contrast, most training programs required didactic training in CBT (99% of psychiatry residency programs; 96% of PsyD programs; 89% of clinical psychology PhD programs; and 80% of social work programs). Strikingly, all disciplines—apart from clinical psychology PhD programs—had higher percentages of programs requiring didactic training in at least one non-EBT than those requiring didactic training in IPT.

A similar pattern appeared for supervised clinical work in IPT. Most psychiatry (65%), clinical psychology PhD (66%), and PsyD (60%) programs *offered* clinical supervision in IPT, while the rate was lower for social work programs (43%). In contrast, CBT supervision was offered in most training programs across all disciplines (psychiatry, 94%; clinical psychology PhD, 97%; PsyD, 76%; social work, 66%). Relatively few training programs *required* clinical supervision in IPT across disciplines (psychiatry, 29%; PsyD, 24%; clinical psychology, 11%; social work, 7%). In contrast, most training programs in psychiatry (93%) and clinical psychology (53%) required clinical supervision in CBT. About 20% of PsyD and social work programs required clinical supervision in CBT. Similar to results for didactics, programs from all disciplines offered or required clinical supervision of at least one non-EBT at a higher rate than for IPT. Together, these results highlight the available opportunities to increase IPT didactic and clinical supervision training opportunities across disciplines.

NATIONAL PSYCHOTHERAPY TRAINING SURVEY-II

Since NPTS-I was conducted in 2004, IPT researchers, clinicians, and educators have continued IPT dissemination efforts. These have included the establishment and growth of the International Society of Interpersonal Psychotherapy (ISIPT), continued publication of IPT research and training materials,[24-28] adaptation of IPT for other disorders,[29] and increased availability of IPT trainings.[30] Although these efforts should have increased the availability of IPT didactics and clinical supervision in training programs, they coincided with the emergence and dissemination of other now-popular EBTs, such as acceptance and commitment therapy (ACT), mindfulness-based therapies, and motivational interviewing.[31-33] Given training programs' limited resources and increased demand for varied training in multiple EBTs, it is as of yet unclear whether training opportunities in IPT have increased, despite great efforts in the field. Thus, reassessment of the availability of IPT didactic training and clinical supervision across disciplines is needed.

The original NPTS-I survey was expanded to NPTS-II to include counseling (i.e., counseling and counseling psychology) and PMHNP programs, which is critical given that they train a large proportion of practicing therapists.[34-36] Similar to NPTS-I, all accredited training programs in the United States were identified for the disciplines of interest: clinical psychology (PhD and PsyD, American Psychological Association accredited); counseling (master's, Masters in Psychology and Counseling Accreditation Council accredited; PhD or PsyD, American Psychological Association accredited); PMHNP (master's; postgraduate certificate, doctor of nursing practice; Accreditation Commission for Education in Nursing accredited); psychiatry residency (American Psychiatric Association-accredited); and social work (master of social work; Council on Social Work Education accredited). Stratified random sampling was conducted to select 50% of programs in each discipline in four US regions (Midwest, Northeast, South, West), yielding a total of 574 training programs. Training directors (or equivalent) and their contact information were identified via program websites. Data collection began in October 2021 and is ongoing. Preliminary descriptive statistics presented here reflect data as of April 2022. Email notifications were sent in 1-week intervals for the first 3 weeks of data collection. Subsequent phone and email reminders have been made in 2- to 4-week intervals.

As of April 2022, training directors (or their equivalent) of 167 training programs have completed the survey, providing a 29.1% overall response rate so far. Response rates by discipline were 41.0% clinical psychology PhD; 33.3%

clinical psychology PsyD; 42.4% counseling; 27.3% PMHNP; 29.2% psychiatry; and 17.6% social work. The total number of training programs with completed responses (and percentage of total completed responses) by discipline were 34 clinical psychology PhD (20.4% of 167 completed survey responses); 13 clinical psychology PsyD (7.8%); 25 counseling (15.0%); 30 PMHNP (18.0%); 38 psychiatry (22.8%); and 27 social work (16.2%).

Preliminary findings of NPTS-II indicate the availability of IPT in training programs (all percentages reported below are of training programs with completed responses). Of 167 training programs with completed responses, 73.7% of programs *offered* and 53.3% of programs *required* didactic training (e.g., graduate course or workshop; lectures/readings/coursework) in IPT. Didactic training ranged from 3 hours or less (e.g., an introductory lecture) to 30 hours or more (e.g., a semester-long graduate course). ISIPT requires at least 16 hours of didactic training for therapist certification, and in the past 3 years 19.8% of training programs with completed responses have offered didactic training that meets this requirement. Thus, although about half of programs required didactic training in IPT, and only one-fifth offered sufficient didactic training for ISIPT therapist certification. In contrast to IPT didactic training rates, 73.1% of training programs *offered* and 16.2% *required* IPT clinical supervision.

Most training programs *offered both* didactic training and clinical supervision (63.5%), while only a minority of training programs *required both* (13.2%). These preliminary findings are similar to results of the original survey based on weighted means across the four disciplines reported: 60.8% of programs *offered* and 39.9% *required* IPT didactic training; 58.2% *offered* and 17.1% *required* IPT clinical supervision. Thus, the prevalence of IPT offerings and requirements in training programs may have remained stable or slightly increased in the past 17 years.

CONCLUSION

In NPTS-I, it was found that didactic training and clinical supervision in IPT was widely offered across training programs in the United States, despite being offered at fewer programs than some other EBTs, like CBT. Preliminary findings of NPTS-II suggested that didactic training and clinical supervision in IPT continue to be offered at most training programs in the United States. The availability of IPT training may have slightly increased from 2004 to 2022, but full results await the completion of the 2022 survey. This possible increase may be attributable to ongoing IPT research and dissemination efforts, as well as many disciplines' accrediting bodies requiring their training programs to provide foundational training in psychotherapy. Because the current preliminary and future finalized results have limited generalizability outside the United States, an international replication would enhance understanding of the availability of IPT training internationally and aid researchers', clinicians', and educators' IPT dissemination efforts.

REFERENCES

1. Althobaiti S, Kazantzis N, Ofori-Asenso R, et al. Efficacy of interpersonal psychotherapy for post-traumatic stress disorder: a systematic review and meta-analysis. *J Affect Disord.* 2020;264:286–294.

2. Cuijpers P, Geraedts AS, van Oppen P, Andersson G, Markowitz JC, van Straten A. Interpersonal psychotherapy for depression: a meta-analysis. *Am J Psychiatry.* 2011;168(6):581–592.

3. Cuijpers P, Donker T, Weissman MM, Ravitz P, Cristea IA. Interpersonal psychotherapy for mental health problems: a comprehensive meta-analysis. *Am J Psychiatry.* 2016;173(7):680–687.

4. Duffy F, Sharpe H, Schwannauer M. The effectiveness of interpersonal psychotherapy for adolescents with depression—a systematic review and meta-analysis. *J Child Adolesc Ment Health.* 2019;24(4):307–317.

5. Mychailyszyn MP, Elson DM. Working through the blues: a meta-analysis on interpersonal psychotherapy for depressed adolescents (IPT-A). *Child Youth Serv Rev.* 2018;87:123–129.

6. Pu J, Zhou X, Liu L, et al. Efficacy and acceptability of interpersonal psychotherapy for depression in adolescents: a meta-analysis of randomized controlled trials. *Psychiatry Res.* 2017;253:226–232.

7. Sockol LE. A systematic review and meta-analysis of interpersonal psychotherapy for perinatal women. *J Affect Disord.* 2018;232:316–328.

8. Whiston A, Bockting CL, Semkovska M. Towards personalising treatment: a systematic review and meta-analysis of face-to-face efficacy moderators of cognitive-behavioral therapy and interpersonal psychotherapy for major depressive disorder. *Psychol Med.* 2019;49(16):2657–2668.

9. Chambless DL, Hollon SD. Defining empirically supported therapies. *J Consult Clin Psychol.* 1998;66(1):7–18.

10. Tolin DF, McKay D, Forman EM, Klonsky ED, Thombs BD. Empirically supported treatment: recommendations for a new model. *Clin Psychol Sci Pract.* 2015;22(4):317–338.

11. American Psychological Association. *APA Clinical Practice Guideline for the Treatment of Depression Across Three Age Cohorts.* American Psychological Association; 2019.

12. American Psychiatric Association. *Practice Guideline for the Treatment of Patients with Major Depressive Disorder (No. 3).* American Psychiatric Association; 2010.

13. The Management of Major Depressive Disorder Working Group. *VA/DoD Clinical Practice Guideline for the Management of Major Depressive Disorder (No. 3).* Department of Veterans Affairs and the Department of Defense; 2016.

14. NICE Clinical Guidelines. *Depression in Adults: Recognition and Management.* National Institute for Health and Care Excellence (NICE); 2009. https://www.fundacion-salto.org/wp-content/uploads/2018/09/Depression-in-adults.pdf. Accessed May 31, 2022.

15. Stewart RE, Stirman SW, Chambless DL. A qualitative investigation of practicing psychologists' attitudes toward research-informed practice: implications for dissemination strategies. *Prof Psychol Res Pr.* 2012;43(2):100–109.

16. Weissman MM, Verdeli H, Gameroff MJ, et al. National survey of psychotherapy training in psychiatry, psychology, and social work. *Arch Gen Psychiatry*. 2006;63(8):925–934.

17. Heatherington L, Messer SB, Angus L, Strauman TJ, Friedlander ML, Kolden GG. The narrowing of theoretical orientations in clinical psychology doctoral training. *Clin Psychol Sci Pract*. 2012;19(4):364–374.

18. Accreditation Council for Graduate Medical Education. ACGME program requirements for graduate medical education in psychiatry. Approved June 13, 2021. Accessed April 11, 2022. https://www.acgme.org/globalassets/pfassets/programrequirements/400_psychiatry_2021.pdf

19. American Psychological Association. Standards of accreditation for health service psychology. Approved February 2015. Accessed April 11, 2022. https://www.apa.org/ed/accreditation/about/policies/standards-of-accreditation.pdf

20. Council on Social Work Education (CSWE) Commission on Accreditation. Educational policy and accreditation standards. Accessed April 11, 2022. https://www.cswe.org/getattachment/Accreditation/Standards-and-Policies/2015-EPAS/2015EPASandGlossary.pdf

21. Masters in Psychology and Counseling Accreditation Council (MPCAC). Accreditation manual. April 217. Revised September 2021. Accessed April 11, 2022. http://mpcacaccreditation.org/wp-content/uploads/2021/10/MPCAC2017AccreditationManual-revised-September-2021.pdf

22. National Panel for Psychiatric-Mental Health NP Competencies. Psychiatric-mental health nurse practitioner competencies. 2003. Accessed April 11, 2022. https://cdn.ymaws.com/www.nonpf.org/resource/resmgr/imported/PMHNPcomps03.pdf

23. Division 12 Task Force on Teaching Evidence Based Practice in Clinical Psychology. Models for the graduate curricula in clinical psychology. Accessed April 11, 2022. https://div12.org/principles-for-training-in-evidence-based-psychology/

24. Weissman M, Markowitz J, Klerman G. *The Guide to Interpersonal Psychotherapy: Updated and Expanded Edition*. Oxford University Press; 2017.

25. Markowitz JC, Weissman MM (eds.). *Casebook of Interpersonal Psychotherapy*. Oxford University Press; 2012.

26. Frank E, Levenson JC. *Interpersonal Psychotherapy*. American Psychological Association; 2011.

27. Ravitz P, Watson P, Grigoriadis S. *Psychotherapy Essentials to Go: Interpersonal Psychotherapy for Depression*. WW Norton & Company; 2013.

28. Stuart S, Robertson M. *Interpersonal Psychotherapy: A Clinician's Guide*. 2nd ed. CRC Press; 2012.

29. Ravitz P, Watson P, Lawson A, et al. Interpersonal psychotherapy: a scoping review and historical perspective (1974–2017). *Harv Rev Psychiatry*. 2019;27(3):165–180.

30. Weissman MM. Interpersonal psychotherapy: history and future. *Am J Psychother*. 2020;73(1):3–7.

31. Luoma JB, Hayes SC, Walser RD. *Learning ACT: An Acceptance and Commitment Therapy Skills-Training Manual for Therapists*. New Harbinger Publications; 2007.

32. Khoury B, Lecomte T, Fortin G, et al. Mindfulness-based therapy: a comprehensive meta-analysis. *Clin Psychol Rev*. 2013;33(6):763–771.

33. Rubak S, Sandbæk A, Lauritzen T, Christensen B. Motivational interviewing: a systematic review and meta-analysis. *Br J Gen Pract*. 2005;55(513):305–312.

34. Rush AJ. Making therapy widely available: clinical research triumph or existential catastrophe? *Am J Psychiatry*. 2022;179(2):79–82.

35. Tadman D, Olfson M. Trends in outpatient psychotherapy provision by US psychiatrists: 1996–2016. *Am J Psychiatry*. 2022;179(2):110–121.

36. American Psychiatric Nurses Association. *Expanding Mental Health Care Services in America: The Pivotal Role of Psychiatric-Mental Health Nurses*. American Psychiatric Nurses Association; 2019.

15

Interpersonal Psychotherapy Training in the Veterans Health Administration in the United States

KATHLEEN F. CLOUGHERTY, JENNIFER L. STEELE, AND KEVIN CROSWELL ■

The Veterans Health Administration's (VHA's) evidence-based provider psycho-therapy training program in interpersonal psychotherapy (IPT) is among the largest competency-based IPT training programs in the United States. This chapter describes how the provider training initiative came about, how IPT training was developed and disseminated, the changes made over time, and lessons learned. This may serve as a guide to the development of future large-scale IPT training projects.

The VHA is America's largest integrated healthcare system, providing care at 1298 healthcare facilities, including 171 medical centers and 1113 outpatient sites of care, to more than 9 million veterans enrolled in the VA healthcare pro-gram. Mental healthcare at these facilities is provided by a multidisciplinary cadre of mental health professionals, including, but not limited to, psychiatrists, psychologists, social workers, and psychiatric nurses. Among the most common psychiatric diagnoses for veterans include anxiety, post-traumatic stress dis-order (PTSD), depression, and substance use disorders, with high levels of comorbidity.[1]

In 2002, the president's New Freedom Commission on Mental Health conducted a study of the nation's mental health care.[2] The commission's final report emphasized the importance of mental health in overall wellness and concluded that healthcare providers should improve patient access, offer collabo-rative care, and implement research-based best practices. Based on this guidance,

Kathleen F. Clougherty, Jennifer L. Steele, and Kevin Croswell, *Interpersonal Psychotherapy Training in the Veterans Health Administration in the United States* In: *Interpersonal Psychotherapy*. Edited by: Myrna M. Weissman and Jennifer J. Mootz, Oxford University Press. © Oxford University Press 2024. DOI: 10.1093/oso/9780197652084.003.0016 the Department of Defense and Department of Veterans Affairs created a strategic plan to transform VA mental health care. As part of the strategic plan, VHA developed a national evidence-based psychotherapy (EBP) provider training program. The goal of the program is to improve veteran outcomes by mitigating gaps in the clinical workforce's ability to competently provide veterans with EBPs to ensure they have access to high-quality mental health care regardless of location or circumstance.

Initial training programs, starting in 2006, focused on meeting the needs of veterans with PTSD by training providers in cognitive processing therapy and/ or prolonged exposure therapy, both of which were supported by robust effectiveness data as well as successful community implementation trials. The training model was competency based and required trainees to attend an experientially based workshop (3–5 days), participate in weekly consultation calls with a national expert (1.5 hours/week for 6 months), submit audio recordings of sessions, meet criteria on rating scales, and complete a set number of cases and sessions. There was variability between training programs.[3]

The VHA's handbook[4] required that veterans have access to EBPs shown to be effective for specific mental health or behavioral health conditions. Originally, this included PTSD, depression, and other serious mental illness. The handbook specified that veterans with depression must have access to EBPs for depression. Training initiatives included competency-based clinical training in cognitive behavioral therapy, acceptance and commitment Therapy, and IPT. The VA currently also provides competency-based training in EBPs for chronic pain, relationship distress, insomnia, substance use disorders, and suicide prevention. All VA provider training initiatives are consistent with the training recommendations of evidence reviews and the latest updated evidence synthesis by Frank and colleagues demonstrating that didactic and experiential training components followed by consultation improve provider competence and intervention use.[5]

DEVELOPMENT OF THE IPT TRAINING PROGRAM

In 2011, two external IPT subject matter experts, Kathleen Clougherty and Gregory Hinrichsen, were asked to develop a veteran specific IPT training program, which would be competency based and would become self-sustaining. The task included designing a 3-day didactic/experiential IPT training workshop template; writing a veteran-specific treatment manual[6] that was based on the original IPT manual developed by Weissman, Markowitz, and Klerman[7]; and developing a therapist adherence measure[8] and a veteran-specific training film.[9] The subject matter experts were advised by Jennifer Steele and Michael Stewart, the internal veteran therapist experts. Because of the high rates of suicidality among veterans, the internal experts also added a suicide safety protocol to the IPT training workshop, and since veterans can initially be difficult to engage in psychotherapy, the internal experts also added a half-day motivational interviewing component.

THERAPIST TRAININGS

In-person workshops began in 2011. The aim was to hold 4 to 5 trainings per year, although in some years there were fewer. Trainees included 30 to 40 licensed psychiatrists, psychologists, social workers, and psychiatric health nurses per workshop. Four to 7 external IPT experts were invited to lead breakout groups during the training. They later became supervisors (called "IPT consultants" at the VA).

After the workshop, each trainee was assigned to a consultation group with an expert consultant and 3 other trainees. The group met weekly for 1.5 hours for 6 months. Prior to the session, trainees sent their audiotaped IPT sessions to the consultant for full review. Trainees had to attend 75% of the consultation sessions and achieve an adherence score over 2.5 out of 4 over 2 cases. Due to funding issues, trainees were supervised on 2 cases, rather than the standard 3. The experts agreed to reevaluate the need for an additional training case, based on adherence and competency indicators, after the first training cohort completed their 2 cases. When the experts reviewed the therapist and veteran outcome ratings on these first 124 trainees, they determined that supervision on 2 cases was sufficient to reach competence.

Trainees were expected to complete at least 12 sessions, including all phases of treatment for their primary case and at least 8 sessions for their secondary case. They were to demonstrate an understanding of strategies and techniques for the problem areas that were the focus of their veteran cases. Supervision requirements have changed over time. Originally, 12 complete tapes over 2 cases were reviewed using the Interpersonal Psychotherapy Rating Scale (IPTRS). Currently, consultants review 10 recorded sessions over 2 cases.

An analysis of the first 124 trainees found that IPT was effective in reducing depression in veterans, improved their quality of life over multiple domains, and was well received. Trainees found the training and supervision to be helpful in their practice. Over 85% of all trainees successfully completed their training and were adherent based on the IPTRS.[10]

EXTERNAL CONSULTANTS' TRAINING

A major hurdle in bringing IPT to the VA was that there was only 1 internal IPT consultant to supervise the trainees. The first 10 consultants were IPT experts from outside the VA. Most of them had been trained to treat patients in IPT research trials and had been supervising IPT clinicians for many years. To ensure fidelity of supervision, there was a 2-day consultation workshop during which consultants listened to and rated veteran IPT sessions for each problem area, across all phases of treatment, using the IPTRS. The internal experts provided guidance to the consultants on the needs and issues of veterans. Twice-monthly calls were held with the consultants to discuss questions about using IPT with veterans and issues that arose during their consultation calls.

As VA therapists completed IPT training, they began to take the place of the external consultants. To become internal VA consultants, the VA therapists completed 3 additional supervised IPT cases, supervised trainees on 3 cases under the supervision of an existing consultant, and attended the consultants' training workshop. By 2014, there were 12 potential internal VA consultants in varying stages of training. In 2022, all training and consultation was provided by VA staff. In total, there were 8 trainers and 28 consultants.

Changes to the IPT training program

In 2016, the VA's IPT program became a fully functioning training program that no longer relied on external experts. The initial program evaluation data demonstrated the training model was successful and feasible based on measures of participant learning and veteran self-reported benefits.[10] Since then, the program has continued to evolve. The VA replaced its in-person IPT workshops with 5-day online workshops. Serendipitously, this meant that when the COVID pandemic struck, training could continue. The program has also adapted in response to participant feedback. For example, the workshop week now includes a daily 30-minute "Ask the Trainers" Q&A (question-and-answer) session.

The VA contracted with a software design company to create an online learning tool to complement the workshops and consultation. The company worked for 2 years with the VA's lead IPT trainers, Kevin Croswell and Leila Zwelling, and program coordinator, Hani Shabana, to develop a variety of IPT simulation options. The VA IPT Interactive Training Program was published online and put into practice at the beginning of 2019 as part of the workshop.[11] The guided self-study offers a variety of IPT-specific clinical simulations for trainees to apply their knowledge of IPT to different scenarios and get computer-based feedback and instruction based on their answers. The self-study program includes interactive conversations, as well as videos for participants to evaluate, and it covers all 3 phases of IPT.

The VA incorporated the self-study training into the virtual workshop so trainees could learn from didactic sessions in the morning, practice skills in the self-study, and then participate in breakout groups in the afternoon. Trainees consistently reported that the self-study allowed them to practice on their own and get important feedback before practicing in the consultation group. Consultants found that the self-study made trainees more prepared, less nervous, and more engaged in the breakout sessions. All training sessions are conducted over video calls, which help to keep participants engaged and allow consultants to incorporate visual components into their training.

The VA also turned a VA IPT training video into an online continuing education unit course available to all VA staff and providers.[12] This course is an excellent introduction for trainees or professionals new to IPT because they can watch the video demonstrations and begin to learn basics of IPT. In addition, it can be a helpful resource for IPT-trained clinicians, who can review specific IPT topics with clinical descriptions and video demonstrations.

In 2018, the VA, in an unpublished program evaluation, reported on the national IPT training program evaluation data from 2011 to 2018. The report compared the first 12 in-person workshops with audio consultation (2011–2015) to the first 6 virtual workshops with consultation (2016–2018). In both cohorts, the report found significant increases in therapist competence in delivering IPT, large overall reductions in depression among patients, and improvements in veterans' quality of life and therapeutic alliance. Virtual training did not result in significantly different participant ratings, completion rates were similar, and there were no differences in patient outcomes on any measure. The report strongly supported the continued viability and effectiveness of IPT dissemination and training within the VHA.[13]

To date, the VA has trained over 800 mental health professionals and treated thousands of veterans across its healthcare system. While aspects of the training have changed over the past 10 years, the model remains essentially intact. Even in the original in-person training model, the supervision and ongoing feedback were delivered remotely. The current virtual training model retains the structure of synchronous training followed by remote small group/one-on-one supervision.

LESSONS LEARNED

This project would not have been possible without VHA support. Despite many obstacles, the external experts were allowed to develop a rich IPT training model that met the training needs of the VA therapists. A good working relationship with the funding organization is essential. It takes time to train to internal independence—time to develop expertise among employees in sufficient numbers to ensure system-wide, high-quality IPT clinicians; time to develop supervisors from those who were interested and skilled enough in IPT to move on to become supervisors; and time to mentor some of those supervisors as they become trainers. It usually takes from 3 to 5 years. This is expensive, and many organizations cannot fund this. But developing a fully functional, internal IPT training program more quickly is not realistic. Organizations will initially need to hire external consultants and train them to understand the population to be treated. The first training round should be used to gather information to see which adaptations need to be made to the basic IPT model.

After the first round of consultation, the experts reviewed consultation notes to see if any changes needed to be made to the basic IPT protocol. With that information, the external experts wrote the IPT for veterans manual.[14] There were only 2 aspects of IPT that needed adaptation. The first was the sick role. Many veterans did not relate the idea of an impairing medical condition in which they should "take activities off their plate" while recovering. Instead, therapists help veterans recognize that when they are depressed, they are not able to function as well as they normally would. The therapists help them temporarily adjust expectations for themselves while they focus on recovery.

The second change was in how interpersonal deficits were conceptualized. Deficits fell into 2 categories: first, veterans who entered service with interpersonal deficits and second veterans who did not exhibit deficits prior to deployment, but who experienced newfound chronic loneliness and isolation on returning to civilian life. In the latter group, it became clear that experiences of deployment stymied the veterans' use of interpersonal skills they possessed prior to deployment. For the first group of veterans, the task was to help build interpersonal skills; for the second group, the task was to help veterans retrieve skills that were there, but for various reasons became dormant after return from deployment. Based on this experience, the experts adapted how interpersonal deficits were taught to the trainees.

REFERENCES

1. *National Academies of Sciences, Engineering, and Medicine, Health and Medicine Division, Board on Health Care Services, Committee to Evaluate the Department of Veterans Affairs Mental Health Services.* Evaluation of the Department of Veterans Affairs Mental Health Services. National Academies Press; 2018.
2. New Freedom Commission on Mental Health. *Achieving the Promise: Transforming Mental Health Care in America. Final report.* US Department of Health and Human Services; 2003. Publication no. SMA-03-3832.
3. Karlin BE, Cross G. From the laboratory to the therapy room: National dissemination and implementation of evidence-based psychotherapies in the US Department of Veterans Affairs Health Care System. *Am Psychol.* 2014;69(1):19.
4. US Department of Veterans Affairs. *Uniform Mental Health Services in VA Medical Centers and Clinics.* US Department of Veterans Affairs; 2008. VHA Handbook 1160.01.
5. Frank HE, Becker-Haimes EM, Kendall PC. Therapist training in evidence-based interventions for mental health: a systematic review of training approaches and outcomes. *Clin Psychol: Sci Pract.* 2020;27(3):20.
6. Clougherty KF, Hinrichsen GA, Steele JL, et al. *Therapist Guide to Interpersonal Psychotherapy for Depression in Veterans.* US Department of Veterans Affairs; 2014.
7. Clougherty KF, Hinrichsen GA, Stewart MO, Raffa SD, Steele J, Karlin BE. *Interpersonal Psychotherapy Rating Scale.* Department of Veterans Affairs; 2012.
8. US Department of Veterans Affairs. *Interpersonal Psychotherapy for Depression in Veterans.* DVD. Employee Education System; 2013.
9. Weissman MM, Markowitz JC, Klerman G. *Comprehensive Guide to Interpersonal Psychotherapy.* Basic Books; 2008.
10. Stewart MO, Raffa SD, Steele JL, et al. National dissemination of interpersonal psychotherapy for depression in veterans: therapist and patient-level outcomes. *J Consult Clin Psychol.* 2014;82(6):1201.
11. Croswell K, Zwelling L, Clougherty K, Hinrichsen G. *VA Interpersonal Psychotherapy for Depression (IPT-D) Interactive Training.* US Department of Veterans Affairs; 2019.
12. Croswell K, Zwelling L, Clougherty K, Hinrichsen G. *Interpersonal Psychotherapy (IPT) for Depression in Veterans.* US Department of Veterans Affairs; 2019. VA TMS Item #38034.

13. Department of Veterans Affairs Office of Mental Health and Suicide Prevention, National Evidence-Based Psychotherapy Training Program. Interpersonal Psychotherapy for Depression Program evaluation report. US Department of Veteran Affairs; 2018.
14. Clougherty KF, Hinrichsen GA, Steele JL, et al. *Therapist Guide to Interpersonal Psychotherapy for Depression in Veterans*. US Department of Veterans Affairs; 2014.

Interpersonal Psychotherapy
in Africa

Interpersonal Psychotherapy
in Africa

16

Interpersonal Psychotherapy in Ethiopia (IPT-E)

DAWIT WONDIMAGEGN, HENOK HAILU,
PAULA RAVITZ, AND CLARE PAIN ∎

Interpersonal psychotherapy (IPT) was adapted by Ethiopian psychiatrists to the local culture and context (IPT-E) and subsequently taught more broadly to provide access to services for Ethiopian patients with common mental disorders (CMDs). This chapter describes the country background and healthcare context, along with the history, the process, and facilitators of and barriers to the cultural adaptation and implementation of IPT-E.

COUNTRY CONTEXT

The Federal Democratic Republic of Ethiopia, located in the horn of Africa, has a population of 120 million.[1] It is a landlocked country, and most Ethiopians live rurally as subsistence farmers, accounting for 78.3% of the adult population in 2020. Ethiopia is a multiethnic country with over 80 nationalities and languages and hundreds of dialects. The religion of most Ethiopians is Orthodox Christian (43.8%), followed by Muslim (31.3%) and Protestant (22.8%). Basic infrastructure, communication, and services are limited, and access to healthcare can be challenging. Ethiopia remains a low-income country, with a Human Development Index value in 2019 of 0.485, placing the country in the bottom 10% at 173 out of 189 countries and territories.[2]

Primary healthcare in Ethiopia has grown significantly in the last 10 years, and healthy life expectancy has gradually improved over the last 3 decades, largely because of successful efforts to reduce infant, child, and maternal morbidity. However, the Ethiopian health system continues to struggle under the triple

Dawit Wondimagegn, Henok Hailu, Paula Ravitz, and Clare Pain, *Interpersonal Psychotherapy in Ethiopia (IPT-E)*
In: *Interpersonal Psychotherapy*. Edited by: Myrna M. Weissman and Jennifer J. Mootz, Oxford University Press.
© Oxford University Press 2024. DOI: 10.1093/oso/9780197652084.003.0017

burden of communicable diseases, noncommunicable diseases, and the results of physical injuries from accidents.

MENTAL HEALTH SERVICES

With few Western-trained mental health practitioners together with a well-established and highly respected network of religious and traditional healers who provide care and healing for health disorders throughout the country, it is only recently that mental health has reached a level of priority in health policy. According to the government of Ethiopia, 26% of health facilities provided mental health services in 2021. While this is a significant improvement from even a decade ago, the coverage for priority mental health conditions remains very low. For example, treatment for those with psychotic conditions is 10%, while treatment coverage for child and adolescent mental health conditions is 1%. In general, the treatment of mental health problems is limited to pharmacotherapy with inconsistent medication supplies.[3] The prevalence of mental health disorders in Ethiopia ranges from 14.9% to 27.6% in a variety of populations, with higher rates among women.[4-7]

THE TORONTO ADDIS ABABA PSYCHIATRY PROGRAM

In 2003 the University of Toronto (UofT) in Canada and Addis Ababa University (AAU) in Ethiopia launched an educational partnership named the Toronto Addis Ababa Psychiatry Project (TAAPP). The aims of TAAPP were to assist with opening the first psychiatry residency training program in the country and to promote the development of capacity and sustainability of mental health education and clinical services. The major contribution by UofT continues to be month-long on-site teaching and supervision for up to 3 times annually (https://taaac.ca/psy chiatry).[8,9] Prior to the establishment of the AAU psychiatry residency training program in Ethiopia, there were about 500 psychiatric inpatient beds in one facility providing custodial care for long-stay forensic psychiatric patients and one outpatient mental health clinic to serve the entire population. There were only 11 psychiatrists in the country, all of whom had trained abroad, as well as about 100 psychiatric nurses with one university-affiliated Department of Psychiatry located at AAU. With the assistance of TAAPP, the scenario has changed significantly, and now Ethiopia has over 100 psychiatrists. TAAPP has also been involved training in the only clinical psychology program in the country; there are now about 50 graduates. Ethiopia has scores of psychiatric nurses; several master's trained mental health officers are similar to clinical psychologists but with limited training in psychological treatments who provide services for the mentally ill across the health system.

One of the milestone achievements of TAAPP was the introduction of psychotherapy to the Ethiopian health system. In 2006, TAAPP taught the first 1-month IPT training in the psychiatry residency training program at AAU. It introduced the entirely new idea that "talk therapy" is a modality of treatment for CMDs in Ethiopia. There was neither the knowledge nor the culture of "talk as therapy" in Ethiopia. Thus, the history of the introduction of IPT in Ethiopia is also the history of the introduction of psychotherapy. As such, it had to meet and continues to meet all the challenges of any novel treatment modality in a new context, while at the same time paving the way for other forms of psychotherapy to make inroads into Ethiopian mental health education and service development.

The ontology of suffering in Ethiopia is recognized as relational in a culture where daily life is organized around the centrality of community.[10] Whereas mental illness as understood by Ethiopians refers to florid psychotic disorders, most obviously for example, a homeless man behaving bizarrely, such as directing traffic while naked in public. The symptoms and difficulties of CMDs, such as anxiety, depression, and somatoform problems, are recognized as relatively frequent, private, and part of the burden of life. The idea in IPT that both the struggles that lead to psychological distress and how a person recovers are a function of their social relationships and are congruent with local understandings. As a result, when IPT was introduced as a modality of treatment, it had an instant appeal to providers, trainees, and patients as intuitively familiar.

Although talking to a trusted other such as a family member or a village elder is helpful and valued, it is not considered a form of therapy or a medical service. Healthcare workers (HCWs) are expected to tend to the sick with medications or procedures, not with psychotherapy, and no HCW from primary care to tertiary specialists were trained or expected to provide therapy as a modality of treatment. As the psychiatry residency program matured, senior residents and newly qualified psychiatrists became increasingly interested in psychotherapy because the use of medications, especially for those with CMDs, provided disappointing results, and medication supply chains are unreliable.

IPT-ETHIOPIA ADAPTATIONS

One of the barriers to IPT at the time of its introduction to Ethiopia was that the only evidence for the cultural adaptation of IPT was for group therapy by trained lay providers in Uganda.[11,12] This lack was an obstacle to academic teaching and a stimulus to adapt individual IPT for teaching and practice in Ethiopia.

Multiple TAAPP month-long IPT trainings have occurred over several years since 2006. Following the first training, there were initial attempts to practice IPT with distance supervision from UofT faculty, which failed for a variety of logistic and systemic reasons. In 2011, we conducted a large focus group consultation with over 40 psychiatrists for cultural adaptation purposes sponsored by the Ethiopian Psychiatric Association. There was widespread recognition that local languages did not have words that mapped directly or easily onto the Western concept of depression. Differences in the cultural experiences of anguish and distress meant that the literal translation of English words into local languages would be misleading. In response, the decision was made to change the language of therapeutic communications within the phase- or focus-specific IPT clinical guidelines to incorporate local sayings and phrases to make IPT concepts make sense and be more acceptable to patients.

Through this process we were able to incorporate some of existing and familiar cultural practices as part of our recommendation for IPT adaptation.[13] Examples included the use of "Shemegelena," a local process of interpersonal conflict resolution through soliciting counsel from a respected member of the community and the recognition of Ethiopian postpartum rituals that were shown to protect against the development of CMDs.[14] Another example is the inclusion of two Amharic sayings that are relevant to Ethiopian patients with regard to talking about their emotional experiences: *Hulun beyawerut hode bado yekeral* ("If you speak all that you have, then you will be empty inside"). If the patient cites this concern, the counselor can reply, *Kalemenager Deje Azmachent yekeral* ("If you don't speak up, you might miss out on moving ahead"), conveying that there is benefit to the expression of emotions. In this way patients are gently encouraged to describe their experiences, speak about their problems, and give voice to their wishes and feelings, which is important to the therapeutic process.

The original IPT manual instructs therapists to provide psychoeducation, informing the patient they have a medical illness called depression in order to alleviate self-stigma, legitimize the patient's need for help, and reframe their difficulties as the "sick role," with the intent of instilling hope.[15] However, explaining the diagnosis with a medical explanatory model of depression as a disorder or illness in Ethiopia is associated with life-threatening conditions and experienced as frightening and peculiar rather than helpful; thus, this needed to be adapted as described in the case vignette in this chapter.

The "dose" of 12–16 sessions of the IPT model as it was originally designed is not possible because most patients cannot afford the time off work or the travel costs to come for therapy for multiple sessions. We reduced the number of IPT sessions to 4 (8 were rarely feasible). In keeping with other global mental health packages of care and subsequent adaptations of IPT in low- and middle-income country settings, this dose of IPT helped to address potential barriers, logistical challenges, and opportunity costs that patients faced.[16,17]

Following the above process, in 2012 and beyond, we secured funding from Grand Challenges Canada for the "Biaber Project" to adapt and test the possibility of introducing IPT-E into primary care within the Ethiopian health system. The project name was inspired by the Ethiopian proverb *Der Biaber Ambassa Yassir*, which means "Alone we are a spider's web; together the web becomes a rope to capture the lion." This evoked the spirit of collectively addressing a threat—in this case, underrecognized and undertreated CMDs—and gave us the opportunity to iteratively adapt and implement the model further.

Prior to the Biaber Project, there were no mental health services available in primary healthcare. Primary care health clinics are staffed by general nurses who do not receive training in mental health. To address this, we followed a train-the-trainers model and task shifted the delivery of IPT-E to the general nurses who run the health centers.[18] We first trained psychiatrists, who then trained midlevel mental health professionals (psychiatric nurses and clinical psychologists, etc.), who together trained primary care nurses to identify and treat CMDs with IPT-E. Supervision and mentorship were provided by the midlevel mental health professionals on a weekly basis to the newly trained general nurses in the health centers. The counselors had all passed the IPT-E course examination in their classroom training and were equipped with an Amharic checklist to ensure they remembered what to do in each phase of treatment when they worked clinically. With weekly direct and indirect supervision by their mentors on site, it became evident which of the counselors needed extra help and who had moved easily into using IPT-E. Those who needed more help to feel confident and competent were given it. It was never mandatory for the primary HCWs to screen and deliver IPT-E; up to 75% of all trained personnel continued to provide these mental health services, which suggests those who were able to deliver the services adequately continued to do so.

In all, we developed 8 Amharic and English language training modules to scale up screening and treatment of CMDs using IPT-E with 4 modules specific to IPT and additional modules on introducing mental health into primary care covering such topics as stigma, screening, safety, domestic and sexual violence, substance use, building resilience, and project protocols. Teaching videos with captioned demonstrations of IPT strategies were used with interactive case-based skills practicing in live workshops. In addition, an "antistigma" and a "recovery is possible" video were created and screened in primary care waiting rooms of all the health centers involved, and banners were placed in the health centers advertising the availability of mental health care.

We have now trained over 900 health professionals and front-line workers in IPT-E through 3 scale-up projects across 23 health centers and 5 regions of Ethiopia, including 2 refugee camps in Western Ethiopia and university student health centers in Wolaita Sodo University.[19] We have screened more than 30,000 patients for CMDs, and those individuals recognized as able to benefit from IPT-E and who were available for treatment were referred for up to 4 sessions of IPT-E ($N = >1700$ patients).

BARRIERS, FACILITATORS, AND NEXT STEPS FOR IMPLEMENTATION

The most significant barrier for the widespread implementation of IPT-E is the novelty of talk therapy to the clinical culture, and the ongoing idea that mental illness is a psychotic disorder that can best be managed by medications. This has been addressed in the psychiatry and family medicine residency training programs and in clinical psychology master's programs by the regular teaching and practice of IPT-E and other relevant models of psychotherapy.

However, within primary healthcare, the sheer burden of service provision because of a limited number of health workers who cater to large numbers of patients makes the idea of spending 45 minutes with 1 patient in therapy at best a misplaced luxury and at worst a complete waste of time. Understandably, resistance comes from hospital administrators, who are pressed for "efficiency," and HCWs who have a large quota of patients to see and whose availability is compromised by the length of time an IPT session takes. However, following the trainings, we were struck by the willingness of primary care nurses to use IPT-E to treat patients, despite time constraints and patient quotas. The nurses were very positive about how IPT-E helped their patients, and they felt empowered and grateful for the training and mentoring they received. Similar findings have been found in health providers for distressed students at Wolaita Sodo University, Ethiopia.[20] The Ethiopian government has recognized the need to provide mental health services in primary health clinics by placing one psychiatric nurse or equivalent into each health center. At present, this individual sees all people with mental health problems and provides medications but no therapy.

It is ironic that as we try to continue to introduce IPT-E into Ethiopia, the prevailing model of mental health services in the West coincides with a widespread move toward medications and away from psychotherapies.[21] However, to make IPT-E more accessible to Ethiopians, we believe the introduction of IPT-E training into all appropriate healthcare education programs is the path to long-term change. So far, IPT training has been successfully introduced into Ethiopian psychiatry and family medicine residency training programs and into the clinical psychology masters' program at AAU. To enable IPT-E to be available as an accessible treatment for CMDs in Ethiopia, the training needs to be introduced into all nursing programs, as well as all master's level mental health programming in the country. It has been heartening to see what an excellent model IPT is for Ethiopia. It is intuitively relevant and relatively easy to adapt and train nonmedical practitioners to perform. That it will take considerably more time to provide a scaling up of services has become an incentive for our Ethiopian colleagues to persevere.

CASE EXAMPLE

Almaz is a 28-year-old married mother of 2 young children. She lives with her husband and extended family and works part-time as a waitress. Her third child died after a brief illness 5 months ago. She came to the primary healthcare clinic because of a severe headache, with complaints of frequent tearfulness and sadness, trouble sleeping, and a lack appetite. She had lost 5 pounds in the prior 2 months. She had missed several days of work over the last few weeks and struggled to manage her chores, sometimes wishing she was not alive and could be with her dead child in heaven. She took no medication and had no known medical conditions or history of psychological problems. She screened positive for a CMD and was interested and able to come for IPT-E therapy.

Telling other patients with similar problems that they had an illness called depression had not helped the other patients with similar problems, assisted them to feel validated in a sick role, or relieved them of feelings of personal blame for their condition. In fact, the thought that Almaz might have a mental illness (understood as a severe psychotic illness and sign of God's disapproval) would keep most patients like Almaz from coming to the clinic and increase her sense of stigma. As well, in Ethiopia an illness is usually an acute infectious disease and a frequent cause of death. As well, there are no words in the commonly used Ethiopian language of Amharic for depression. "Sadness without a cause," which some people use, is not useful in IPT because linking cause and symptoms is of fundamental importance. Of interest, the structure of the verbs in Amharic are such that experiences are felt to be done to one (e.g., the sun hits me, the rain drums on me, the world/God strikes me by taking my daughter). So, agency is seen as coming from an external source and the question of weakness or self-blame is not common, whereas CMDs with depressive, anxious, and somatic symptoms are considered a common price to pay for the burden of life. A patient's attendance at the clinic tends to validate their distress as legitimate and not imaginary.

Rather than emphasizing the sick role, the link in IPT-E was made with the death of Almaz's daughter and the onset of her symptoms, which makes sense and engenders relief, strengthening the therapeutic bond with the health worker. This achieves the same effect that IPT aims for in the West with psychoeducation with regard to depression. The IPT-E provider proceeded to deliver the treatment with a focus on loss, helping Almaz to connect with supportive others and to benefit from traditional bereavement practices, and the patients' symptoms resolved.

REFERENCES

1. Ethiopia population. https://www.worldometers.info/world-population/ethiopia-population/
2. Human development report. United Nations Development Program; 2020.
3. Ethiopia Country Strategic Plan. *A summary of program-specific strategic plans/ roadmaps of the Health Sector Policy, Plan, Monitoring and Evaluation Directorate (PPMED)*. 2020.
4. Hunduma G, Girma M, Digaffe T, Weldegebreal F, Tola A. Prevalence and determinants of common mental illness among adult residents of Harari Regional State, Eastern Ethiopia. *Pan Afr Med J*. 2017;28(1).
5. Habtamu Y, Admasu K, Tullu M, Kebede A. Magnitude of common mental disorders and factors associated among people living in Addis Ababa, Ethiopia 2018: community based cross-sectional study. *BMC Psychiatry*. 2022;22(1):1–10.
6. Yimam K, Kebede Y, Azale T. Prevalence of common mental disorders and associated factors among adults in Kombolcha Town, Northeast Ethiopia. *J Depress Anxiety*. S:007. 2014;S1:007.
7. Habtamu K, Minaye A, Zeleke WA. Prevalence and associated factors of common mental disorders among Ethiopian migrant returnees from the Middle East and South Africa. *BMC Psychiatry*. 2017;17(1):144.
8. Wondimagegn D, Pain C, Baheretibeb Y, Toronto Addis Ababa Academic Collaboration. A relational, partnership model for building educational capacity between a high-and low-income university. *Acad Med*. 2018;93:1795–1801.

9. Shuchman M, Wondimagegn D, Pain C, Alem A. Partnering with local scientists should be mandatory. *Nat Med*. 2014;20(1):12.

10. Kleinman A, Benson P. Anthropology in the clinic: the problem of cultural competency and how to fix it. *PLoS Med*. 2006;3(10):e294.

11. Bolton P, Bass J, Neugebauer R, et al. Group interpersonal psychotherapy for depression in rural Uganda: a randomized controlled trial. *JAMA*. 2003;289(23):3117–3124.

12. Bolton P, Bass J, Betancourt T, et al. Interventions for depression symptoms among adolescent survivors of war and displacement in northern Uganda: a randomized controlled trial. *JAMA*. 2007;298(5):519–527.

13. Ravitz P, Wondimagegn D, Pain C, et al. Psychotherapy knowledge translation and interpersonal psychotherapy: using best-education practices to transform mental health care in Canada and Ethiopia. *Am J Psychother*. 2014;68(4):463–488.

14. Hanlon C, Medhin G, Alem A, et al. Sociocultural practices in Ethiopia: association with onset and persistence of postnatal common mental disorders. *Br J Psychiatry*. 2010;197(6):468–475.

15. Weissman M, Markowitz J, Klerman GL. *The Guide to Interpersonal Psychotherapy*. Oxford University Press; 2018.

16. Patel V, Weiss HA, Chowdhary N, et al. Effectiveness of an intervention led by lay health counsellors for depressive and anxiety disorders in primary care in Goa, India (MANAS): a cluster randomised controlled trial. *Lancet*. 2010;376(9758):2086–2095.

17. Chowdhary N, Jotheeswaran AT, Nadkarni A, et al. The methods and outcomes of cultural adaptations of psychological treatments for depressive disorders: a systematic review. *Psychol Med*. 2014;44(6):1131–1146.

18. Van Ginneken N, Tharyan P, Lewin S, et al. Non-specialist health worker interventions for the care of mental, neurological and substance-abuse disorders in low- and middle-income countries. *Cochrane Database Syst Rev*. 2013;(11):CD009149.

19. Negash A, Khan MA, Medhin G, Wondimagegn D, Pain C, Araya M. Feasibility and acceptability of brief individual interpersonal psychotherapy among university students with mental distress in Ethiopia. *BMC Psychol*. 2021;9(1):64.

20. Negash A, Khan MA, Medhin G, Wondimagegn D, Araya M. Mental distress, perceived need, and barriers to receive professional mental health care among university students in Ethiopia. *BMC Psychiatry*. 2020;20(1):1–5.

21. Tadmon D, Olfson M. Trends in outpatient psychotherapy provision by US psychiatrists: 1996–2016. *Am J Psychiatry*. 2022;179(2):110–121.

17

Interpersonal Psychotherapy
in Kenya

OBADIA YATOR AND MANASI KUMAR ■

African-centered psychology is a reawakening, a road towards emancipa-
tion, a project that encompasses emotional, cognitive, cultural, political
and economic attitudes and practices. . . . it is a knowledge that begins with
an inward-looking process, with speaking not about yourself but about the
world as you have come to know it.

—RATELE, 2019[1]

SITUATING KENYA

In non-Western societies, families and extended community networks become
vital to an individual sense of identity and well-being. Interpersonal relationships
extend to social and community ties, and these inform the subjective sense of
well-being.[2] The choice of applying interpersonal psychotherapy (IPT) in Kenya
was also determined by the need to strengthen communication and connection
between individuals and families that gets disrupted due to extreme adversities,
stress, and pressures of modern living. Kenya is an East African country that the
World Bank classifies as a low- and middle-income country (with a population
of over 54 million and per capita income of 4370 PPP dollars).[3,4] About 30% of
Kenyans live in urban centers, and urban living implies disconnection from traditional ways of living and disrupted social networks and protection mechanisms.
Over 32.4% of Kenyans live in absolute poverty (according to 2021 World Bank
estimates).[5] Therefore, the struggle for livelihoods, taking care of basic health, education, and other essential services remains the primary concern. Under such

Obadia Yator and Manasi Kumar, *Interpersonal Psychotherapy in Kenya* In: *Interpersonal Psychotherapy.*
Edited by: Myrna M. Weissman and Jennifer J. Mootz, Oxford University Press. © Oxford University Press 2024.
DOI: 10.1093/oso/9780197652084.003.0018

prolonged stress, families experience sadness, loss of control, distanced ties, and their interpersonal life begins to suffer.

In sub-Saharan Africa, maternal, adolescent, and child mental health remain poorly understood. The burden of disease is high; the supportive services, psychotherapy and specialist psychiatric services, are unevenly distributed, with urban centers receiving the most support and rural the most marginalized. The human development index score of .601 implies medium human development.[6] There are improvements in the key indicators of mean years of schooling, expected years of schooling, life expectancy at birth, and gross national income per capita over time.

INTERPERSONAL PSYCHOTHERAPY AS A FRAMEWORK TO UNDERSTAND THE SUBJECTIVE EXPERIENCE OF DISTRESS IN KENYA

The above context provides a sense of challenge and deprivation that a large populace experiences in Kenya. In addressing adverse social determinants of health and well-being, individuals and families are experiencing greater noncommunicable disease burden as the shift in health disparities moves from infectious diseases; cancer, cardiovascular, metabolic diseases, and mental and substance use disorders are on the rise.[7]

Interpersonal theory offers a unique opportunity to begin to understand how socioemotional communication, social communication, and family stress factors that impact help-seeking behaviors and how health, prevention, promotion, and treatment issues are discussed and managed in a relationship context.

Relationships from an African perspective are defined in interconnectedness, interdependence, sense of solidarity, and belongingness,[8] and to be human is to be in the community, participating in beliefs, ceremonies, rituals, and festivals that give a sense of belonging.[9] It has also been suggested that in unearthing the reasons for the importance of relationships points toward a dialectic pattern of African individualism–collectivism in which independent and interdependent orientations flow together.[9]

Life events predispose persons to mood changes, and if an unpleasant event is persistent, the interpersonal distress sets in and an individual may then experience depressive symptoms. Among our perinatal population, we realized that role transition and role conflict scores high. The age of the mother at the time of pregnancy, levels of partner involvement, reaction of the immediate family members toward pregnancy, and prior expectation of the concerned mother are some of the key determinants of the levels of depressive symptoms. We found out that unplanned and unwanted pregnancy, low levels of education, lack of male partner/family support, and low social economic ability are some of the common variables that influence the levels of interpersonal distress among perinatal women.[10] The drivers of a range of adverse social determinants of health, such as poverty, disengagement from school and education, poor healthcare access, and poor family support and well-being in the context of young girls and women can be situated within interpersonal and family context using the interpersonal framework that IPT extends.

TASK SHARING, TASK SHIFTING, AND MENTAL ILLNESS STIGMA REDUCTION

Our efforts at offering IPT have been devoted toward leveraging limited human resources in formal health services and using nonspecialist and lay health workers to offer therapy with continuous supportive supervision. This practice, also called "task shifting/sharing," from specialists to nonspecialists or lay health workers is one of the innovations of global mental health that has enabled narrowing the mental health treatment gap.

Mental health stigma is so rampant that, in addition to working with community health workers (CHWs) and primary care staff, a process of normalizing mental health treatment has to be initiated. This normalizing process is the only way of mitigating mental health stigma—the stigma of being seen as "mentally disabled," "mad," "bewitched," or "having an incurable disease." One of the ways of addressing stigma in the communities and in seeking services in primary and specialist care is to offer an open, transparent process. Therapy offered in groups has the potential not only to mitigate stigma and put things out in the open, but also reach out to many needy individuals at one time. Individual psychotherapy does not have any sort of traction as it still maintains the perception that the recipient of the intervention is "out of joint."

Group IPT has taken the form of a community of practice that engages in meaning making around the link between depression and life events: addressing adversities and relationship setbacks, offering opportunities for group members to learn and intervene with one another. We have added to this another innovation, which is to have two facilitators, preferably a male and female work together to allow a well-synergized exchange between group members that is moderated by the therapists (or facilitators). Having two lay health workers (CHWs) work in tandem gives them confidence to rehearse and act on IPT principles together. Variance in age among the two facilitators is another area worth exploring considering some participants prefer to share their setback experiences openly on specific areas of their lives when prompted by a facilitator of a certain age group, such as issues to do with marital conflict for the elder facilitators and matters on teenage pregnancies for the young facilitators. In an African context, discussing sex is a rare topic within family the setup, and adolescents mostly learn from their peers leaving them more vulnerable to sexually transmitted diseases and in some instances unplanned, unwanted teenage pregnancies. According to the 2014 Kenya Demographic and Health Survey, women's median age at first birth was reported to be 20.3 years, similar to the median age of 20.2 years at the time of marriage[11]; hence, the adolescent population requires an evidence-based mental health intervention at the primary services level.

HEALTHCARE WORKER CAPACITY BUILDING AND
TRAINING IN INTERPERSONAL SKILLS

We spend over 2–3 months training the lay and nonspecialist health workers, first beginning by introducing principles of the World Health Organization's WHO's Mental Health Gap Action Program (mhGAP),[12] which stipulates mental health as a global good and a fundamental human right. It also stipulates that the mental health treatment gap needs action from communities, health facilities, schools, as well as other civil society institutions. We train the health workers in mental disorders, basic management, and attitudes towards mental health care, including preventing spread of stigma, addressing needs of vulnerable populations, and more. This training is then followed by IPT training, which lasts 2 weeks. In these 2 weeks, basic principles of IPT are offered along with preparing the team for group IPT. These trainings are followed intensely with practice sessions, role plays, and simple assessment of key skills and knowledge of IPT. A 2-day training for those intending to be supervisors (usually social workers, higher level health managers, psychiatric nurses, and clinical psychologists) is organized to keep a supervisory pipeline running to oversee the groups and facilitators in action. WHO's group style has been used, but over time adapted along the following domains and along content-versus-process modification:[13,14] with what, by whom, context, and level of delivery.[15,16] These trainings have been finessed over time. However, for HIV-positive adolescent mothers, Yator et al. have laid out a detailed plan of action.[17] Figure 17.1 provides an overview of recommended adaptations that the team has made in contextualizing IPT (more has been written on it).[10,16]

For our team, the implementation of IPT has also meant adopting a top-up and bottom-down approach to sustainably build capacity and interest in talk therapy. The top-up approach enables higher level managers, policymakers, senior program officers, and clinicians to become aware of the benefits of IPT and dividends on maintaining a supervisory pipeline and investment in IPT. The bottom-down approach enages the community and individuals with lived experience and works closely with lay and nonspecialist health workers. Both approaches are important and allow forbetter penetration of ideas across the community and health system.

Offering IPT in routine services, including training postgraduate students in psychiatry and clinical psychology, offers a good opportunity for uptake of it in specialist service delivery and medical education programs. This approach has helped us identify barriers to and facilitators of IPT within clinical settings, which has enabled us to sensitize the stakeholders on feasible ways toward scaling up IPT. The perinatal women who have received IPT have also become agents of change within their neighborhood, and this is very encouraging. We reach out to the underserved population of perinatal women with a view to indirectly transfer the benefits of IPT to the unborn child. Attachment and bonding for young children is often dependent on the mother-child relationship as the primary point of reference; hence, a happy mother enhances emotional stability among the young children.

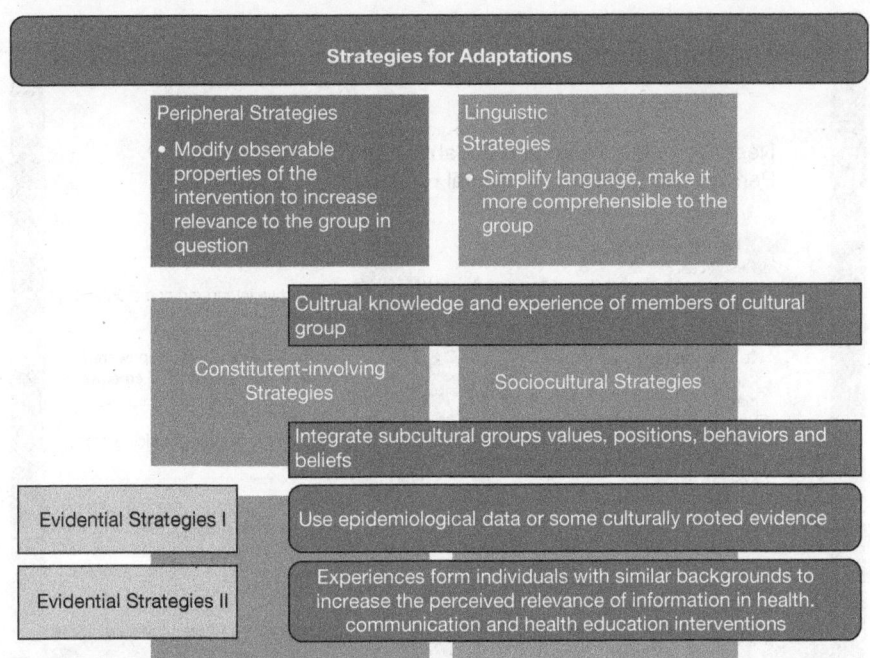

Figure 17.1 Top-down and bottom-up mobilization of key stakeholders for mental health integration in routine services.
SOURCE: Barrera M Jr, Castro FG, Strycker LA, Toobert DJ. (2013).

The community and health system must work together to improve outcomes for individuals in need. The national, regional, and local resources and policies are shaped by community participation and mobilization. At least in democratic systems, individuals and communities are empowered to play that role. Health systems in the African context are being encouraged to develop family and self-management support and enhance delivery system design and decision support in multiple ways: integrating digital, real-time monitoring to task-shifted mechanisms. With the pandemic, the impetus for strengthening clinical information systems became stronger than before. These two systems in themselves promote an integrated community and informed, active, empowered individuals and families, thus enhancing the ability of the practice teams to become more resilient, engaged, and "mental health friendly."

Potential to build capacity of IPT delivered by individuals with lived experience and for health promotion

Our group has expertise in offering IPT in groups to children and young people ages 10–19 years as well as to pregnant and parenting adolescents, including young mothers living with HIV and adult women with postpartum or maternal depression (Figure 17.2). Our efforts now are directed toward engaging

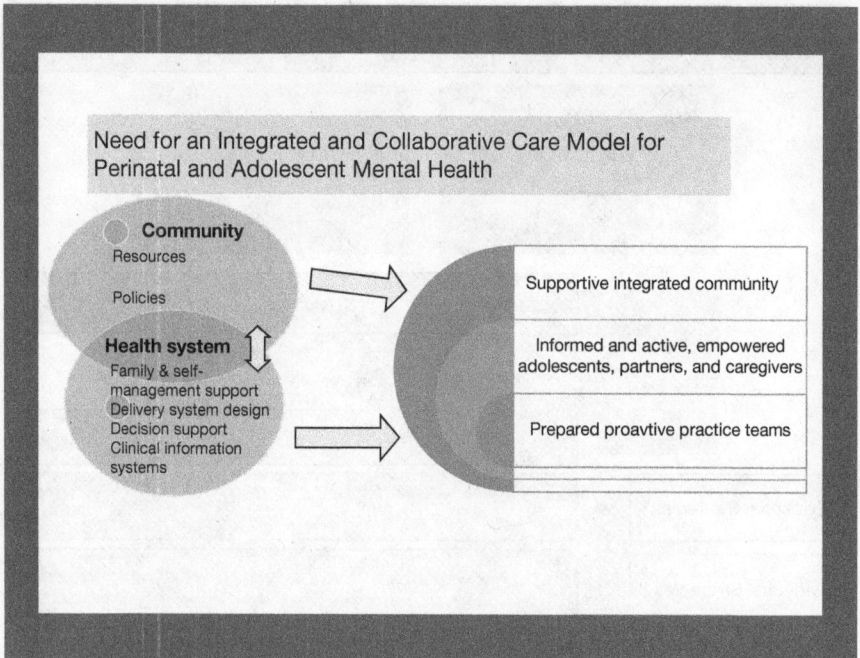

Figure 17.2 Integrated and collaborative care model where IPT is embedded as an EBI.
CREDIT: WHO 2016 integrated care model.

with young adolescents and women who receive treatment to not only become champions of IPT but also train in offering it in groups or individually. We have focused our attention on refining the supervisory pipeline and planning high-risk referrals that provide services associated with medical or social service to individuals nonresponsive to IPT or with complex needs.

Continuous supportive supervision is what we have adopted, and we can report that this has worked well for us in training CHWs in IPT and overseeing them as they deliver the intervention in a primary healthcare setting.[18] In our past IPT intervention studies, we have also empowered CHWs on termination IPT to link the participants to community-based organizations (CBOs) and other programs providing livelihood skills. Those with persistent depressive symptoms are referred to a mental health specialist for further assessment and treatment. In one of the previous studies, we were able to link most of the young adolescent mothers living with HIV to some existing CBOs, where they were enrolled in programs targeting family strengthening, parenting and caregiver programming, and social economic support services.

Our other efforts are devoted toward offering IPT in a prevention-focused program. We believe IPT can be used in our setting to address adverse childhood-associated trauma experiences and interpersonal and gender-based violence exposures given that each of these risks includes a dysfunctional relationship pattern that can change if role transitions, expectations, and communication strategies are better aligned. In these programs, IPT is being used in secondary and tertiary prevention. The CHWs we have trained have been able to pass their knowledge acquired within the community to address issues of loss and grief, life changes, interpersonal conflicts, and interpersonal deficits, which are the common problems affecting the general population within low-resource settings. On termination of IPT, some participants have opted to form a self-help group given the positive impact on their livelihood.

IPT's acceptability as a context-sensitive, evidence-based intervention

Our experience with IPT delivered by CHWs efficiently makes this intervention appropriate for Kenya to expand the coverage of mental health intervention among this vulnerable populace. Group IPT as an intervention with 8 sessions on a weekly basis for a duration of 90 minutes makes it adaptable within primary healthcare. The context of IPT delivery is flexible and can be conducted in a room, tent, or even under a tree, which makes it easy to roll out with few resources. The positive outcomes among depressed perinatal women after receiving IPT were improved social functioning, better communication, and improved social interaction. Thus, the intervention was highly recommended for scaling up.

REFERENCES

1. Ratele K. *The World Looks Like This From Here: Thoughts on African Psychology.* Wits University Press; 2019.
2. Fernando S. Mental health and mental illness in non-Western countries. In *Mental Health Worldwide: Culture, Globalization and Development*; 2014:45–62.
3. World Bank. Data: low & middle income. 2020. https://data.worldbank.org/country/XO
4. United Nations Population Fund. *International Conference on Population and Development Programme of Action.* 20th anniversary ed. United Nations Population Fund; 2014. https://www.unfpa.org/publications/international-conference-population-and-development-programme-action
5. World Bank. Property and equity brief. April 2020. https://databank.worldbank.org/data/download/poverty/33EF03BB-9722-4AE2-ABC7-AA2972D68AFE/Global_POVEQ_KEN.pdf
6. United Nations Development Program (UNDP) Human Development Reports. Human development NT insights. Briefing note: Kenya. 2020. https://hdr.undp.org/sites/default/files/Country-Profiles/KEN.pdf
7. Achoki T, Miller-Petrie MK, Glenn SD, et al. Health disparities across the counties of Kenya and implications for policy makers, 1990–2016: a systematic analysis for the Global Burden of Disease Study 2016. *Lancet Glob Health.* 2019;7(1):e81–e95.

8. Samuel K, Alkire S, Zavaleta D, Mills C, Hammock J. Social isolation and its relationship to multidimensional poverty. *Oxf Dev Stud*. 2018;46(1):83–97.

9. Wissing MP, Wilson Fadiji A, Schutte L, Chigeza S, Schutte WD, Temane QM. Motivations for relationships as sources of meaning: Ghanaian and South African experiences. *Front Psychol*. 2019:11.

10. Kumar M, Yator O, Nyongesa V, et al. Interpersonal psychotherapy's problem areas as an organizing framework to understand depression and sexual and reproductive health needs of Kenyan pregnant and parenting adolescents: a qualitative study. *BMC Pregnancy Childbirth*. 2022b;22(1):940.

11. Kenya Demographic and Health Survey. Kenya 2014 Democratic and Health Survey key findings. 2014:61-:24. https://www.dhsprogram.com/pubs/pdf/sr227/sr227.pdf

12. World Health Organization. mhGAP Intervention Guide for Mental, Neurological and Substance Use Disorders in Non-Specialized Health Settings: Mental Health Gap Action Programme (mhGAP). MhGAP Intervention Guide for Mental, Neurological and Substance Use Disorders in Non-Specialized Health Settings: Mental Health Gap Action Programme (MhGAP). 2010:1–121. https://www.who.int/publications/i/item/9789241549790

13. World Health Organization. *Group Interpersonal Therapy (IPT) for Depression.* World Health Organization; 2016. http://apps.who.int/iris/bitstream/handle/10665/250219/WHO-MSD-MER-16.4-pg. eng.pdf;jsessionid=713E2FF0ECC3B0 42136E1C3F33910A75?sequence=1

14. Aarons GA, Sklar M, Mustanski B, Benbow N, Brown CH. "Scaling-out" evidence-based interventions to new populations or new health care delivery systems. *Implement Sci*. 2017;12:1–3.

15. Wiltsey Stirman S, Baumann AA, Miller CJ. The FRAME: an expanded framework for reporting adaptations and modifications to evidence-based interventions. *Implement Sci*. 2019;14(58).

16. Kumar M, Verdeli H, Saxena S, et al. Modifying group interpersonal psychotherapy for peripartum adolescents in sub-Saharan African context: reviewing differential contextual and implementation considerations. *Clin Med Insights Psychiatry*. 2022;13:11795573221075573.

17. Yator O, Kagoya M, Khasakhala L, John-Stewart G, Kumar M. Task-sharing and piloting WHO group interpersonal psychotherapy (IPT-G) for adolescent mothers living with HIV in Nairobi primary health care centers: a process paper. *AIDS Care*. 2021;33(7):873–878.

18. Yator O, Khasakhala L, Stewart GJ, Kumar M. Acceptability and impact of group interpersonal therapy (IPT-G) on Kenyan adolescent mothers living with human immunodeficiency virus (HIV): a qualitative analysis. *BMC Womens Health*. 2022;22(1):240.

18

Interpersonal Psychotherapy
in East Africa

The Nyanza Region of Kenya

SUSAN MEFFERT ∎

KENYAN CONTEXT

Background

Our team tests strategies for delivering and scaling up evidence-based mental health treatment for the most common adult disorders in East Africa, which include depression (major depressive disorder [MDD]) and trauma-related disorders such as post-traumatic stress disorder (PTSD). Our first studies in the region were with Sudanese (Darfur) refugees living in Cairo, Egypt. We began with a qualitative assessment of mental health care needs and hypothesized that the findings would direct us to some type of trauma-informed cognitive behavioral therapy (e.g., exposure therapy, cognitive processing therapy), which were leading PTSD psychological treatments at the time. Instead, we found a high prevalence of interpersonal distress and intimate partner violence.[1] Those findings, in combination with data emerging at that time showing success with interpersonal psychotherapy (IPT) for treating PTSD,[2-4] led to our decision to use IPT delivered by nonspecialists in our subsequent treatment study.[1,5] Our work in the Nyanza region of western Kenya began in 2010 with HIV-positive women, among whom there was (and is) a very high prevalence of gender-based violence.[6-9] Again, our qualitative data showed that interpersonal relationships were, overwhelmingly, the dominant source of emotional distress, and that social support was the primary coping mechanism in the region—supporting the idea that IPT would be culturally syntonic.[10] Our subsequent nonspecialist IPT study was highly

Susan Meffert, *Interpersonal Psychotherapy in East Africa* In: *Interpersonal Psychotherapy*. Edited by: Myrna M. Weissman and Jennifer J. Mootz, Oxford University Press. © Oxford University Press 2024. DOI: 10.1093/oso/9780197652084.003.0019 effective for MDD and PTSD and reduction of disability and violent victimization of HIV-positive women.[11] Our current study is SMART-DAPPER, a collaboration between the University of California–San Francisco and the University of Nairobi, funded by the National Institute of Mental Health (R01MH115512, R01MH113722): a Sequential, Multiple Assignment Randomized Trial (SMART) for nonspecialist treatment of common mental disorders in Kenya and the Depression and Primary-Care Partnership for Effectiveness-Implementation Research Project (DAPPER).[12]

Study populations

We focus on underserved public-sector populations in East Africa and integrate mental health care with existing priority care platforms, such as HIV or primary care. As implementation scientists, we try to approximate "real-world" conditions as much as possible to optimize the relevance of our study findings to local practice. As such, we use nonaggressive recruitment strategies, such as providing a talk regarding the study in priority care waiting areas and providing study contact information for self-referrals. Using methods such as these, most of our study participants are women between the ages of 30 and 50 years old. Common biopsychosocial stressors for our target populations include HIV infection (reaching 20% of the general population at some study sites), domestic violence, traumatic deaths of family members from motor vehicle accidents or disease, violence related to elections, and financial distress.

ADAPTATIONS: TRAINING, SUPERVISION, AND DELIVERY OF IPT

IPT therapists

Testing strategies that can be sustained with local personnel and scaled to similar settings is crucial to effective impact on population mental health. As such, we train nonspecialists to deliver IPT. While we require successful completion of training and competency assessment, we have not required that IPT therapists have more than a diploma (equivalent to US high school education) or specific healthcare training. We have developed a process of posting IPT nonspecialist job opportunities, emphasizing that successful completion of IPT training and competitive selection are necessary for final hire. We then screen applications, focusing on those with strong interpersonal skills and emotional intelligence and accept at least twice as many to the training as we will need for study tasks. We have found that overinclusion of trainees/prospective IPT therapists is helpful in many ways: It provides community education on the existence of effective mental health care for common disorders, and it allows for self-selection/attrition. As trainees learn more about the process of providing

IPT, some conclude that the work is emotionally overwhelming or otherwise impossible and drop out.

IPT TRAINING

Content and process

As our studies and refresher trainings proceed, we have shifted increasingly toward interactive training, using didactic content of no more than 30 minutes interspersed with frequent, small-group breakout sessions to practice IPT phases and techniques (e.g., interpersonal inventory, communication analysis). As our group of local IPT experts has expanded, they have led an increasing amount of the training and are now solely responsible for peer supervision. We have also shortened the overall duration of the formal training period to 5 days and have extended the (highly monitored) IPT practice case period. We provide extensive education on vicarious trauma of the therapist, incorporate regular supplemental trainings on vicarious trauma; it is a standing agenda item for local, weekly IPT supervision groups.

COMPETENCY ASSESSMENT

The competence of prospective IPT therapists is evaluated in many ways. The first is at the conclusion of the didactic training, at which time they must successfully model an example of each IPT phase (initial, middle, end) to graduate from the didactics and be eligible for advancement to IPT practice clients with weekly in-person or telephone supervision from a psychiatrist who is expert in using IPT in the region. Each IPT practice case session is scored on 8–10 items specific to the protocol of each IPT phase, using a 0–10 Likert scale (poor IPT protocol adherence [0] to optimal adherence [10]). Only those participants who consistently score 9 or higher on every item for every session may continue to see IPT patients with on-site group supervision led by local IPT experts who have gone through the same training and advanced to supervisory roles with ongoing support from psychiatrists. Participation in weekly, local IPT group supervision is mandatory for all IPT therapists. On-site IPT supervisors continue IPT teaching and adherence monitoring (adherence forms required for every session), provide crucial emotional support for new IPT therapists, and individual supervision for any therapists who have trouble maintaining high adherence to IPT protocol or are struggling with vicarious trauma. In addition, all study therapists undergo at least annual IPT refresher training, often taking the form of joining a didactic training for new, prospective IPT therapists and supporting their learning while refreshing IPT skills. To date, we have maintained the traditional 12 weekly IPT session format. We are now conducting symptom assessments at week 6 to determine if the same gains might be achieved with fewer sessions, which would make IPT more scalable in this region given healthcare budget constraints. Maintenance of gains would have to be evaluated, of course.

BARRIERS AND FACILITATORS

One challenge with using IPT in this setting was to effectively communicate about the type of healthcare provider-patient relationship necessary to achieve a successful therapeutic alliance. Specifically, we noted that a hierarchical interaction in which the provider gives advice and the patient listens (little dialogue) would be suboptimal for achieving psychotherapy goals in general and IPT goals in particular. We used strategies such as reminding prospective IPT therapists that their role was not to give advice to participants but rather to help participants find their own answers and frequently reiterating the idea that participants should be talking far more than IPT therapists in every session.

First and foremost, IPT appears to be an excellent fit with the experience of depression and PTSD for our target populations. Not only are interpersonal issues typically a dominant source of distress, but local communities contain a wealth of long-established social support structures (e.g., money-borrowing groups, church groups, frequent gatherings of extended family, HIV support groups, and broad friendship networks) and a sophisticated understanding of how social connection facilitates human thriving. Our strategy of overrecruiting prospective IPT therapists with more attention to interpersonal skills and empathy than to exact educational background has been quite successful for finding talented IPT therapists, providing education to interested community members and allowing for self-selection of IPT therapists. We have also had success promoting those who are talented and experienced into supervisory roles. Rigorous training and adherence monitoring during the initial phases, with ongoing supervision and adherence monitoring after training completion has likely been essential for maintaining the quality of IPT and the integrity and morale of the therapist group. Likewise, education and ongoing attention to self-care for IPT therapists is crucial for avoiding vicarious trauma.

RECOMMENDATIONS FOR FUTURE IPT WORK

Our current study was launched in 2020, during the coronavirus disease 2019 (COVID-19) pandemic. As a result, we offered IPT via telehealth to protect the health of participants and staff. Telehealth consisted of telephone (audio-only) IPT using a "flip phone" without video capabilities. While cell phone penetrance is extremely high in Kenya (>80% have access to a cell phone), currently only those of relatively high social-economic status have access to a smartphone, while the majority have access to a flip phone. Given the focus of our research on public-sector patients, most of our study populations have flip phone access, and few have smartphones. Therefore, we drew on early literature demonstrating psychotherapy efficacy when delivered via phone, as well as newer literature demonstrating success with telephone IPT.[13-17] Telephone IPT was widely accepted by study participants, with approximately 30% selecting mHealth delivery of care at baseline and an increasing number switching to mHealth over the course of the 12 sessions. IPT therapists also liked providing treatment via phone. We saw no increase of adverse events or other safety issues related to use of IPT mHealth. Overall, we found that nonspecialist IPT delivered partially or exclusively via mHealth was feasible, acceptable, and safe. If our forthcoming analyses demonstrate that IPT mHealth is also effective, then we think an important future direction for nonspecialist IPT scale up should include mHealth options via either smartphone or flip phone. This could go a significant distance toward providing evidence-based mental health care for populations with little access to high-quality, in-person treatment, particularly in low- and middle-income countries where flip phones remain prevalent in underserved populations.

COMMON SCENARIOS FOR IPT CASES

Every case is unique of course. However, in our work with populations living in the Nyanza region of Kenya, we do often see IPT cases in which the study participant is a married, middle-aged woman with children who has a suboptimal marital relationship involving infidelity, physical/emotional/sexual violence, blame for HIV infection, and/or financial or emotional neglect.[18] Women in these situations can be isolated, in part because of a common cultural practice in which married couples live on a homestead located on the husband's parents' property. In the setting of marital conflict, some parents support their son's view and participate in violence toward their son's wife. Thus, many of the women in our studies who have conflict in their marriages have little to no support (or worse) at home. These cases may lead to a formulation involving IPT role conflict. We have seen repeated success using IPT role conflict to improve marital (and in-law) communication, reduce violence, and help women recruit healthy social support outside their homes. The last often leads to economic opportunities, which improves their ability to sustain themselves and their children independently of husbands, making financial neglect less dangerous.

ACKNOWLEDGMENTS

The studies described in this chapter are products of a dedicated team of talented individuals, without whom they are not possible. We call particular attention to the multiple principal investigator of the SMART DAPPER study, Dr. Muthoni Mathai at the University of Nairobi, Dr. Linnet Ongeri (Co-I) at the Kenya Medical Research Institute (KEMRI), and our talented local IPT team leads: Ms. Elizabeth Opiyo and Mr. Dennis Oluoch.

REFERENCES

1. Meffert SM, Marmar CR. Darfur refugees in Cairo: mental health and interpersonal conflict in the aftermath of genocide. *J Interpers Violence.* 2009;24(11):1835–1848.
2. Bleiberg KL, Markowitz JC. A pilot study of interpersonal psychotherapy for posttraumatic stress disorder. *Am J Psychiatry.* 2005;162(1):181–183.
3. Markowitz JC, Milrod B, Bleiberg K, Marshall RD. Interpersonal factors in understanding and treating posttraumatic stress disorder. *J Psychiatr Pract.* 2009;15(2):133–140.
4. Markowitz JC. IPT and PTSD. *Depress anxiety.* 2010;27(10):879–881.
5. Meffert SM, Abdo AO, Alla OAA, et al. Sudanese refugees in Cairo, Egypt: a randomized controlled trial of interpersonal psychotherapy for trauma, depression and interpersonal violence. *Psychol Trauma.* 2011;6(3):240–249.
6. Meffert SM, Musalo K, Abdo AO, et al. Feelings of betrayal by the united nations high commissioner for refugees and emotionally distressed Sudanese refugees in Cairo. *Med Confl Surviv.* 2010;26(2):160–172.
7. Campbell JC, Baty ML, Ghandour RM, Stockman JK, Francisco L, Wagman J. The intersection of intimate partner violence against women and HIV/AIDS: a review. *Int J Inj Contr Saf Promot.* 2008;15(4):221–231.
8. Decker MR, Seage GR 3rd, Hemenway D, et al. Intimate partner violence functions as both a risk marker and risk factor for women's HIV infection: findings from Indian husband-wife dyads. *J Acquir Immune Defic Syndr.* 2009;51(5):593–600.
9. Li Y, Marshall CM, Rees HC, Nunez A, Ezeanolue EE, Ehiri JE. Intimate partner violence and HIV infection among women: a systematic review and meta-analysis. *J Int AIDS Soc.* 2014;17:18845.
10. Zunner B, Dworkin SL, Neylan TC, et al. HIV, violence and women: unmet mental health care needs. *J Affect Disord.* 2015;174:619–626.
11. Onu C, Ongeri L, Bukusi E, et al. Interpersonal psychotherapy for depression and posttraumatic stress disorder among HIV-positive women in Kisumu, Kenya: study protocol for a randomized controlled trial. *Trials.* 2016;17:64.
12. Levy R, Mathai M, Chatterjee P, et al. Implementation research for public sector mental health care scale-up (SMART-DAPPER): a sequential multiple, assignment randomized trial (SMART) of non-specialist-delivered psychotherapy and/or medication for major depressive disorder and posttraumatic stress disorder (DAPPER) integrated with outpatient care clinics at a county hospital in Kenya. *BMC Psychiatry.* 2019;19(1):424.
13. Mohr DC, Ho J, Duffecy J, et al. Effect of telephone-administered vs face-to-face cognitive behavioral therapy on adherence to therapy and depression outcomes among primary care patients: a randomized trial. *JAMA.* 2012;307(21):2278–2285.
14. Dennis CL, Grigoriadis S, Zupancic J, Kiss A, Ravitz P. Telephone-based nurse-delivered interpersonal psychotherapy for postpartum depression: nationwide randomised controlled trial. *Br J Psychiatry.* 2020;216(4):189–196.
15. Guille C, Douglas E. Telephone delivery of interpersonal psychotherapy by certified nurse-midwives may help reduce symptoms of postpartum depression. *Evid Based Nurs.* 2017;20(1):12–13.
16. Miller L, Weissman M. Interpersonal psychotherapy delivered over the telephone to recurrent depressives. A pilot study. *Depress Anxiety.* 2002;16(3):114–117.

17. Miniati M, Marzetti F, Palagini L, et al. Telephone-delivered interpersonal psycho-therapy: a systematic review. *CNS Spectr*. 2023;28(1):16–28.
18. Opiyo E, Ongeri L, Rota G, Verdeli H, Neylan T, Meffert S. Collaborative inter-personal psychotherapy for HIV-positive women in Kenya: a case study from the Mental Health, HIV and Domestic Violence (MIND) study. *J Clin Psychol*. 2016;72(8):779–783.

Interpersonal Counseling Scale-Up in Mozambique

SAIDA KHAN, PAULINO FELICIANO, MILTON L. WAINBERG, ANTONIO SULEMAN, PALMIRA SANTOS, DELSON NGOZO, KATHLEEN F. CLOUGHERTY, CAMILA MATSUZAKA, MILENA MELLO, MARIA A. OQUENDO, MARCELO FEIJO DE MELLO, AND JENNIFER J. MOOTZ ■

Mental disorders consistently rank in the top 10 leading causes of burden globally.[1] This burden is disproportionately experienced in low- and middle-income countries (LMICs) where access to mental health treatment services is poorest.[2] Common mental disorders (depression, anxiety, and post-traumatic stress disorder; CMDs) are pervasive worldwide among both men and women and cause the highest disability-adjusted life-years.[1] The presence of depressive disorders is particularly high (4540 cases per 100,000 people) in sub-Saharan Africa, where few resources exist for mental health services.[1]

Mozambique, located in the southeast region of sub-Saharan Africa, is the seventh least developed country in the world[3] and suffers from high rates of CMDs.[4,5] Over 60% of the population lives in rural areas with no access to mental health care.[6] Mozambique has 11 provinces with a population of approximately 30 million people. Mozambique has just 18 psychiatrists and 439 psychologists to serve its 29 million people and has a significant mental health treatment gap.[7,8]

Responding to this scarcity, the Mozambican Ministry of Health has taken impressive initiative to reduce the mental health treatment gap by integrating mental health treatment into primary care through task shifting (teaching nonspecialized providers to deliver mental health care). Two decades ago, the Ministry of Health began training psychiatric technicians, who now number 336 and practice in all 135 districts, to provide psychiatric services at primary care clinics. Psychiatric technicians complete a 2.5-year technical degree following secondary school.

Saida Khan, Paulino Feliciano, Milton L. Wainberg, Antonio Suleman, Palmira Santos, Delson Ngozo, Kathleen F. Clougherty, Camila Matsuzaka, Milena Mello, Maria A. Oquendo, Marcelo Feijo de Mello, and Jennifer J. Mootz, *Interpersonal Counseling Scale-Up in Mozambique* In: *Interpersonal Psychotherapy*. Edited by: Myrna M. Weissman and Jennifer J. Mootz, Oxford University Press. © Oxford University Press 2024. DOI: 10.1093/oso/9780197652084.003.0020

They can prescribe psychopharmalogic medications under supervision of a psychiatrist. However, there are still just 2.6 mental health providers for every 100,000 people, and a treatment gap remains. In this chapter, we describe a national scale-up program of interpersonal counseling (IPC) for the treatment of common mental disorders to reduce the treatment gap in access to care.

TRAINING IN IPC

Training in IPC began in March 2016 as part of a US National Institute of Mental Health (NIMH)/Fogarty-funded D43 training program called PALOP (Paises Africanos de Lingua Oficial Portuguesa) Mental Health Implementation Research Training (principal investigators are Drs. Milton Wainberg and Maria Oquendo). Camila Matsuzaka and Rosaly Braga Ferreira from Brazil facilitated a 4-day IPC training for 20 Mozambican mental health professionals. The training process also concerned addressing the language nuances (Brazilian Portuguese of the trainers is slightly different from Mozambican Portuguese), cultural views, and comprehension of interpersonal problems commonly presented by Mozambican patients.

Some barriers experienced during the training were that trainees varied widely in terms of experience in psychotherapy, and there was a need to reorient counseling as an empathic process that facilitates client reflection and engagement rather than as a process where providers give advice. Facilitators of training were having Portuguese-speaking trainers, having preselected professionals known by the ministry to be competent and enthusiastic, using active learning strategies throughout the training, and using of local case examples as models. The trained professionals embraced IPC as a facilitator for their clinical practice and were enthusiastic about training others in IPC.

DEVELOPING A NATIONAL CADRE OF IPC TRAINERS

Two expert supervisors, Camila Matsuzaka from Brazil and Kathleen Cloughterty from the United States, facilitated a second 5-day training in IPC in November 2017 to develop a national cadre of 23 IPC expert trainers from 4 provinces (Nampula, Gaza, Sofala, and Maputo) to lead future training and supervision for a task-shifted (nonspecialized in mental health) workforce. To achieve certification in facilitation of IPC, trainers needed to complete an IPC course of treatment with 3 patients. To become supervisors, they completed an additional 2 cases. With 130, ninety-minute virtual supervision calls, groups held weekly consultations that ranged in number from 18 (smaller groups) to 52. Supervision sessions also focused on training supervisors how to supervise each other on their cases. The 23 counselors and supervisors provided IPC to 160 patients ($n = 130$ women; $n = 30$ men). They saw on average 6 IPC patients with a range from 1 to 11. Results based on the *Patient Health Questionnaire-9* (PHQ-9) showed that most patients improved in just 4 sessions.

There were some barriers to supervising this national cadre. One group had an English-speaking supervisor, and their calls needed translation, which required more time and at times could be challenging to translate and communicate complex therapeutic concepts. Most supervisors also had demanding workloads with the healthcare system, and fitting supervision consultations into workday schedules could be difficult. Many patients lived in rural areas, and it was not feasible for them to travel to health centers for weekly psychotherapy. It therefore often took longer to complete IPC than the expected 4 weeks. Finally, Internet connectivity was poor and regularly interfered with supervision calls, which were virtual.

To offset challenges, having Portuguese-speaking supervisors facilitated communication. The supervisees held a meeting prior to convening supervision to organize discussion of cases, which helped more efficiently make use of supervision time. In addition, having a "champion," someone who engaged and encouraged others, among the supervisees made supervision more effective and increased group participation. Observing improvement in the patients' symptoms increased trainees' enthusiasm to participate. Many patients reported feeling relief at the end of treatment with IPC.

NATIONAL SCALE-UP OF MENTAL HEALTH SERVICES IN PRIMARY CARE

Funded by the US NIMH, the Research Partnerships to Implement and Disseminate Expanded and Sustainable Evidence-Based Practices in Sub-Saharan Africa (called PRIDE) started in 2016. PRIDE was a collaborative implementation scale-up study with the Mozambique Ministry of Health, South Africa, Brazil, and Columbia University in the United States (principal investigators were Drs. Milton Wainberg and Maria Oquendo). The objective of PRIDE was to determine the most effective pathway for delivering task-shifted comprehensive mental health care. The 3 examined service delivery pathways were treatment as usual (psychiatric technicians at the district level), delivery of mental health care by primary care providers in clinics, and delivery of mental health care by community health workers in community settings. Using the apprenticeship model of training and supervision,[9] the Ministry of Health selected 6 IPC champions (i.e., IPC Workgroup) from the national cadre of trainers to train a nonspecialized workforce of 228 community health workers, 25 psychiatric technicians, and 71 primary care providers.[10]

IPC APPLICATION

Members of our team (IPC Workgroup and Columbia University faculty) developed a provider-guided mobile health (mHealth) app to aid nonspecialized providers in their facilitation of IPC (see Figure 19.1). The team first collaborated to adapt the manual Interpersonal Counseling for Primary Care[11] into Interpersonal

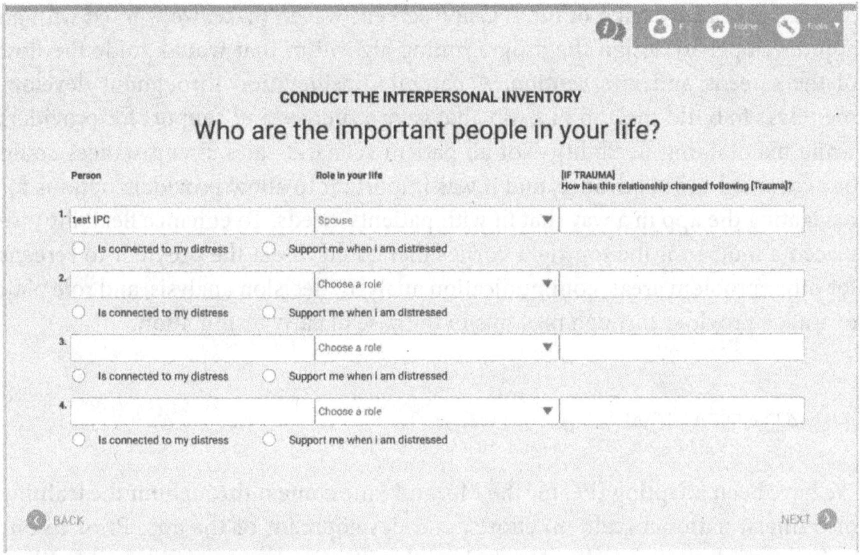

Figure 19.1 Example IPC app screen.
CREDIT: Members of the authors of this chapter (IPC Workgroup and Columbia University faculty) developed a provider-guided mHealth app to aid nonspecialized providers in their facilitation of IPC.

Counseling for Primary Care and Community Health Workers—Tablet Version.[12] Some examples of adaptations were continued simplification of sample script to guide nonspecialized providers like community health workers, whose education requirement is to have completed secondary education. We expanded IPC to address more comprehensively common mental disorders and included analogies and language (e.g., conceptualizing symptoms as distress rather than a specific disorder) that were more congruent with Mozambican cultural norms and values.

The revised manual became the basis for the content of the app. Our team first worked with a graphic designer to determine iconography (e.g., to represent interpersonal problem areas) that was culturally congruent for the Mozambique context and guided the designer in the concepts that should be represented with iconography. The graphic designer provided several initial examples, and the IPC Workgroup responded with feedback and selected final icons for inclusion through an iterative process. Design tasks also consisted of determining the text (needed to be minimal so providers would not spend a lot of time reading screens) to be placed on each screen. We constructed categories of possible responses to discussion prompts, where possible, so providers could select buttons that would record responses for exportable health record session summaries. For example, at-home activities were grouped into relational, physical, community, and other. Something that helped the adaptation process was to present pregenerated examples to the IPC Workgroup rather than start from scratch. Another facilitator was recording workgroup discussions or having the graphic designer attend meetings to hear feedback about the design and could follow up with questions.

Once the basic design of the IPC app screens was in place, we worked with an app developer to design the programming algorithm that would guide the flow of the screens and intervention. A central consideration throughout development was to build the app in a way that gave structure and support for providers while maintaining flexibility. Not all patient scenarios and circumstances could be accounted for in advance, and it was important to allow providers options for navigating the app in a way that fit with patients' needs. To enhance flexibility, we placed a toolbar at the top right corner that could direct the provider to screens for other problem areas, communication analysis, decision analysis, and role play, or walk a provider through prompts in the case of early termination.

IPC ADAPTATION

We have been adapting IPC for the Mozambique context throughout the training of trainers, national scale-up efforts, and development of the app. Prior to our trainings with nonspecialized providers, the IPC Workgroup, led by Saida Khan and Paulino Feliciano, presented the manual to psychiatric technicians and psychologists from Maputo, Gaza, Sofala, and Nampula. We then collected feedback from psychiatric technicians and primary care providers during their IPC training.

Many of these adaptations consisted of continued changes from Brazilian Portuguese to Mozambican Portuguese. We also made minor adaptations to address the interpersonal problem areas in culturally relevant ways. Most of the strategies for grief were retained without much modification. Given that the Mozambique population comprises multiple ethnic groups with various customs for dealing with grief and loss, our overarching principle was to ask about and respect traditional ways of mourning.

Another important consideration when working with grief was how to help women who lost a husband. In some provinces, women's in-laws may attempt to acquire the house, belongings, and children following the husband's death. Custom obligates his brother to marry the widow and engage in intercourse with her as a form of cleansing. Often, working with these women involves helping her with decision analysis for how she wants to manage the situation with her in-laws, conceptualized as a dispute. The therapeutic process includes providing psychoeducation about her rights and helping her consider family members who hold power and can help her negotiate with her in-laws. If these means are unsuccessful, then seeking legal assistance may be an option. The dispute is typically handled first, especially if legal services need to be involved, before grief is addressed. Even in cases where in-laws do not acquire widows' belongings, women have significant life stressors in supporting children and meeting their basic needs. These newfound life stressors are conceptualized as life transitions.

For the dispute problem area, it has been helpful to look at marriages in the Mozambique context. Disputes and disagreement between couples are common. Mozambique is, for the most part, a patriarchal culture, and women are expected to be deferential to their husbands. Those women may not see it as possible to communicate directly with their husbands to resolve a disagreement. We have found it necessary to invite the male partner for consultation to work with the couple together. Given high rates of intimate partner violence in the country, we have received a NIMH-funded mentored training grant to adapt IPC to work with couples to reduce violence and improve women's mental health (Dr. Jennifer Mootz is principal investigator, Dr. Palmira dos Santos is sub-award principal investigator, and Saida Khan is the lead trainer and supervisor).

The same strategies are used to address life transitions and loneliness; the latter is less frequently seen as a problem area. Given high rates of HIV in the country, common transitions occur after losing a family member (losing a spouse or parent[s]). Children or women may need to take financial responsibility for the household or move into households where many other family members are living (aunts, uncles, grandparents, cousins). Disputes can easily occur in these settings and are related to the life transition of a changing family structure and/or housing. IPC strategies in this context help patients accept the new condition of their life and identify people who can help and note how they can help (*quem e como*, "who and how").

COVID-19

When COVID-19 started, the National Health Service provided psychological support for patients and family members who tested positive for COVID-19. A national phone line was initiated. Patients were asked screening questions from a brief mental wellness tool developed in Mozambique.[13] Those who screened positive for a CMD received IPC by phone. Saida Khan and Paulino Feliciano led an online, 2-week training for 15 mental health specialists to provide IPC by phone.

IMPLEMENTATION CHALLENGES

We have experienced some challenges in scale-up and implementation. For supervision, challenges in network connectivity limited our ability to supervise trainees in large groups. Supervision groups were formed with 2 or 3 people, which required increased human resources and time to carry out supervision. Given the distance between clinics, especially in rural areas, in-person supervision was also not feasible.

IMPLEMENTATION FACILITATORS

Interpersonal counseling is a simple therapy to learn and apply and addresses many everyday issues and life events that are relevant for Mozambicans. Positive organizational dynamics (e.g., engagement qualities of leadership) of the research team also facilitated scale-up. Having active and dynamic coordinators and research assistants improved the interaction between trainers and trainees. We created checklists of the session objectives to support trainees before the app was developed.

CASE EXAMPLE

In this case, M. L., 43, separated, lived in her mother's house with her 5 children and nephews whose ages ranged from 12 to 22 years old. She was a domestic worker in someone's home. Her initial consultation was to gynecology, where she presented with severe stomach pain (gastritis) and pain in her uterus, left leg, and neck. She reported having had difficulty sleeping for more than 2 months. The patient was followed in gynecology for 1 year, and all tests were negative. A consultation was also made to the orthopedics department, where M. L.'s tests were also negative.

SESSION ONE

The therapist conducted the PHQ-9. M. L. had a score of 17, indicating moderately severe depression. M. L.'s primary symptoms were insomnia, neck pain and other body aches, gastritis, headaches, sadness (frequent crying), difficulty concentrating, fear, and shame. The therapist gave feedback about the results of the PHQ-9 to the patient and assigned the sick role. The therapist then explained the relationship between symptoms and life events. The therapist conducted the Interpersonal Inventory to understand M. L.'s sources of support and distress. The inventory showed that M. L. considered 2 older siblings and a son as sources of support. Those who caused M. L. more distress were her ex-husband, mother, mother-in-law, and 2 of her children (a 17-year-old daughter who had a baby and another daughter in her early 20s who was not attending school or working).

Through conducting the timeline, the therapist learned that M. L.'s husband had gone to South Africa for mining work when their third child was born. At first, even though their relationship was not very good, he still provided some money for her and the children and came home once a year for vacation. He was sexually coercive during his visits and demanded sexual intercourse without contraception. M. L. felt she could not refuse him because of his financial support. After the fourth child was born, their relationship worsened. He stopped coming home and sending money. When her husband left, M. L. and her 5 children, who had been living in her in-laws' home, were forced by her in-laws to move out. M. L. moved into her parents' home for 3 months, but it was difficult to stay there with her 5 children. She had many disagreements with her mother, who called her a failure, blamed her for being abandoned by her husband, and repeatedly told M. L. that she had achieved nothing in life. M. L. proceeded to rent a place where she could stay with her children and experienced a lot of financial difficulties trying to pay her rent and support her children. M. L. shared: "I feel very overloaded with children, food, school, and other expenses. There is a lot of pressure at work, too."

The therapist identified dispute or life changes as possible problem areas. The patient elected to work with the life changes area to focus on the difficulty she was having living alone with her children, being both their father and mother, and her challenges supporting them with education and basic needs, such as food. The patient explained that she felt a lot of pressure because none of her children worked. The two oldest daughters had children, who also depended on her. Sometimes she mentioned that she would sleep where she worked because she could not afford both a bus fare home and food for her children, and she had to choose one or the other. M. L. expressed a desire for the husbands of the eldest daughters to secure a source of income to help support her. She noted she could talk with her children about her health problems and her difficulty in providing support and paying her children's school bills. She said: "I'm going to try to open up to them, because I've never talked to them about it. They only know that I'm sick. They don't know that I suffer at night because of thinking, and that I don't go home because I don't have money."

SESSION TWO

The therapist began by summarizing the first session and then conducted the PHQ-9, which showed a score of 10, indicating moderate depression. M. L. reported still having some difficulty sleeping. The pain in her belly and neck had reduced, but the pain in her leg and uterus continued. She was able to talk to the 3 older children about her financial worries. The children cried and said they didn't know she was going through all this because she always showed herself to be strong. They said they were going to look for a job, and that one of their brothers would try to help. The son was willing, and the mother talked to his boss for him to work in her company to do laundry and go to school at night. M. L.'s plan for the week was to spend time with a friend from church and try to talk with her mother because the dispute with her mother was bothering her.

SESSION THREE

M.L.'s PHQ-9 score dropped to 6, indicating mild depression. She reported that her symptoms had improved. Sleep and gastritis improved a lot, and she had no neck pain. She said she didn't overthink anymore, and that her stomach hurt less. Her mood improved, and the work became a little lighter. Her presentation improved a lot. She came with her hair done and a nice outfit, which was not the case in the two previous sessions. She still experienced some pain in her uterus and leg. She said she went to visit her mother with her friend, and it was good, although she still felt her mother was a little aggressive toward her. Her daughters

continued to look for work and wait for their uncle to lend them the money so
they could start a business. Her son was working in the mistress's laundry, and
sometimes he slept with his mother in the back house. M. L. planned to go to
church with a friend and continue helping her daughters look for work, while
waiting for financial assistance from her brothers to help her daughters start a
business.

SESSION FOUR

In Session 4, M. L.'s PHQ-9 score was 4, below the cutoff for mild depression. She
came to the session with her daughters. M. L. spoke briefly about her somatic pains
and shared: "I can only thank you here, because my headaches and stomachaches
and other pains that I used to feel no longer feel. Sometimes my head hurts a little,
but I don't feel like before. Now I can sleep. I wake up very early, but I can sleep.
The only thing that still bothers me is the pain in the uterus." M. L. discussed how
it felt to know that she could count on her daughters, and that her son was already
working. She explained: "I always thought that my obligation was for my children
to study and have a home. If they couldn't, it was because sometimes I didn't have
the money for them to enroll. So now they go to night school. They've lost many
years without studying. But I realize that they are big, and the doctor says that
I can't blame myself for that. But I feel like I failed as a mother, and as they practi-
cally didn't have a father, I suffer a lot for that. My children have always lived from
charity of others. They ate what was left over. When I started to work, it got better.
But even so, my salary is not enough, but I can manage. I raised my children with
a lot of suffering. I accept everything we are talking about here, but I don't want
my daughters to be domestic servants like me." The therapist worked with M. L. to
discuss her feelings about termination. M. L. was very calm and said that with
everything she learned in the sessions and with the help of her brothers, boss, and
children, she was going to make it.

SESSION FIVE

One month after the termination session, the therapist saw M. L. for a follow-up
session. Her PHQ-9 score remained a 4, and she continued to be below the cutoff
threshold for depression. She reported almost a total improvement in symptoms.
Her sleep had improved a lot, and she had better socialization. She noted being
in a better mood and having improved communication with her children, with
whom she could discuss issues of lack of money. She felt good about being able
to share these difficulties with her daughters. Her older brother committed to
helping her daughters with some money at the end of the month so that they
could start a business. M. L. shared: "My brother helps me a lot. All these years it
was thanks to him that I managed to feed my children. The problem now is how
to know what business we can do. Because the money he is going to give us is not

much, and we have to try to see what we can do to earn it and not ask him again. But I'm happy. I don't get upset all the time. I don't even care when my mother talks. One day she'll understand everything." The only remaining symptom was that M. L. continued to have some pain in her uterus. The therapist planned to refer her for another gynecology consultation.

THE FUTURE

In Maputo city, IPC continues to be scaled up for all mental health professionals (around 54 professionals in 25 health units). Plans are to continue to scale-up IPC at the national level. We aim to train nonspecialized professionals in the National Health System at the main entrance doors of health units, in chronic disease consultations, and given that Mozambique has a high number of HIV cases, in specialty HIV care clinics. Learning IPC has given greater confidence to providers, specialized and nonspecialized, who continue to be encouraged with the many success stories observed with facilitation of IPC.

REFERENCES

1. GBD 2019 Mental Disorders Collaborators. Global, regional, and national burden of 12 mental disorders in 204 countries and territories, 1990–2019: a systematic analysis for the Global Burden of Disease Study 2019. *Lancet Psychiatry*. 2022;9(2):137–150.
2. Patel V, Maj M, Flisher AJ, et al. Reducing the treatment gap for mental disorders: a WPA survey. *World Psychiatry*. 2010;9(3):169–176.
3. United Nations Development Programme. *Human Development Report 2020*. United Nations Development Programme; 2020.
4. Audet CM, Wainberg ML, Oquendo MA, et al. Depression among female heads-of-household in rural Mozambique: a cross-sectional population-based survey. *J Affect Disord*. 2018;227:48–55.
5. Vos T, Flaxman AD, Naghavi M, et al. Years lived with disability (YLDs) for 1160 sequelae of 289 diseases and injuries 1990–2010: a systematic analysis for the Global Burden of Disease Study 2010. *Lancet*. 2012;380(9859):2163–2196.
6. World Bank. *Mozambique Overview: Development News, Research, Data*. World Bank; 2022.
7. Schwitters A, Lederer P, Zilversmit L, et al. Barriers to health care in rural Mozambique: a rapid ethnographic assessment of planned mobile health clinics for ART. *Global Health Sci Pract*. 2015;3(1):109–116.
8. Dos Santos PF, Wainberg ML, Caldas-de-Almeida JM, Saraceno B, Mari JD. Overview of the mental health system in Mozambique: addressing the treatment gap with a task-shifting strategy in primary care. *Int J Ment Health Syst*. 2016;10:1–9.
9. Murray LK, Skavenski S, Bass J, et al. Implementing evidence-based mental health care in low-resource settings: a focus on safety planning procedures. *J Cogn Psychother*. 2014;28(3):168–185.

10. Matsuzaka C, de Mello MF, Clougherty K, et al. Supervision Skype calls Brazil-Mozambique-USA. In International Society for Interpersonal Psychotherapy. 2019.
11. Weissman M, Verdeli H. *Interpersonal Counseling for Primary Care*. 2018.
12. Weissman MM, Hankerson SH, Scorza P, et al. *Interpersonal Counseling for Primary Care and Community Health Workers–Tablet Version*. 2019.
13. Lovero KL, Basaraba C, Khan S, et al. Brief screening tool for stepped-care management of mental and substance use disorders. *Psychiatric Serv*. 2021;72(8):891–897.

Interpersonal Psychotherapy Group in Senegal

First Steps and Future Plans

SALAHEDDINE ZIADEH, CHARLOTTE BERNARD,
IBRAHIMA NDIAYE, AND MOUSSA SEYDI ■

BACKGROUND

Senegal, the "gateway to Africa," is an ethnically and ecologically diverse sub-Saharan country on the western side of the continent.[1] Its capital, Dakar, houses many of the country's medical and research facilities, including the Fann National University Hospital Center (FNUHC), home to the oldest psychiatric department in the country and the site of our work. It was there, in 2019, and in the context of a research project by the West Africa International Epidemiological Databases to Evaluate AIDS that interpersonal psychotherapy (IPT) was first introduced to Senegal to treat depression in people living with HIV (PLHIV).

Depression is the most common psychiatric disorder[2] in sub-Saharan Africa (SSA) and is highly prevalent[3] among PLHIV on antiretroviral therapy (ART). It has been associated with suboptimal HIV treatment outcomes (i.e., decreased adherence to ART, rapid progression to AIDS stage, and slow increase in CD4 count)[4-6] and negative consequences for quality of life.[2] Yet, depression remains underdiagnosed and undertreated in SSA.[2,6,7] Also, a large mental health care gap continues to be observed in resource-limited countries,[8] such as Senegal (e.g., shortage in mental health specialists[8]), where only 46 psychiatrists provided care in 2018 according to the Ministry of Health and Social Action.[9] Most services were in Dakar, to the detriment of other areas. Accessibility and affordability of care are further limited with the exclusion of mental health from primary health

Salaheddine Ziadeh, Charlotte Bernard, Ibrahima Ndiaye, and Moussa Seydi, *Interpersonal Psychotherapy Group in Senegal*
In: *Interpersonal Psychotherapy*. Edited by: Myrna M. Weissman and Jennifer J. Mootz, Oxford University Press.
© Oxford University Press 2024. DOI: 10.1093/oso/9780197652084.003.0021

care, compelling patients to seek alternate ways of healing in traditional and religious practices.[9]

In the face of resource scarcity, the World Health Organization (WHO) recommends "task shifting"—a practice that involves the training of nonspecialists to provide mental health care under the guidance of specialists.[10,11] Further, it recommends group interpersonal therapy (IPT-G) to treat depression in low- and middle-income countries. However, the acceptability and feasibility of IPT-G was never evaluated in Senegal, let alone with a task-shifting approach. Thus, the present authors sought to test it out, with PLHIV as target population.

The project, conducted jointly by the psychiatry and outpatient departments at FNUHC, involved the IPT-G training of hospital staff (i.e., 4 social and community workers). Participating PLHIV were predominantly middle-aged women (50%) and men who had been screened for depression with the Patient Health Questionnaire-9 (PHQ-9) by the referring doctor on the project, with confirmatory diagnosis by a psychiatrist for any score of 5 or greater. Some were recently diagnosed with HIV, whereas others had been living with HIV for years. Exclusion criteria included hospitalization or medical emergency; diagnosis with a psychiatric illness other than depression; vision or hearing impairment that would seriously hinder group interaction; and imminent suicide risk. None of the participants were prescribed antidepressants at time of diagnosis, during, or following IPT-G implementation, in neither the training phase nor the study phase of the project, which involved 13 groups over the span of 2 years.

GENERAL IPT ADAPTATIONS

Interpersonal psychotherapy adaptation centered on treatment modality, protocol, language, and training. Context and population informed the choice of modality and protocol. Previous work with PLHIV in Uganda had shown group IPT-G to be effective in treating depression[12,13] and the group modality lined up with Senegal's collectivistic culture. The adoption of a brief 8-session IPT-G protocol developed by WHO placed less burden on patients and the resource-strapped system. IPT's multiphasic structure (i.e., pregroup, initial, middle, termination) was preserved. However, groups were limited to same-sex members (including facilitators) in line with Senegalese norms and previous practice. Also, the age range was extended within groups, given the shortage in patients needed to form similar-age groups.

Following authorization by WHO, the treatment manual was translated from English to French,[14] Senegal's official language. This was critical for Senegalese staff who were French educated, though they belonged to the Wolof ethnic majority and often spoke Wolof with hospital patients. The use of Wolof arguably enhanced cultural relevance. Yet, it potentially challenged staff-patient communication around key terms in the manual, including signs and symptoms of depression. For this reason, these terms were discussed with staff psychiatrists for accurate use in Wolof throughout the training. The expression *naxaru xol* (literally, "loss of taste for doing things" in Wolof) was chosen to refer to depression.

Training nonspecialists in the context of task shifting also informed IPT adaptation in terms of implementation. Given the scarcity of mental health specialists, and in line of recommendations by WHO on task shifting, 3 social workers and 1 community health worker were tasked with group facilitation, though they had no prior experience with therapy. Budgetary constraints and previous experimentation with individual IPT confirmed IPT-G as the modality of choice, largely because of its cost-effectiveness.

ADAPTATIONS TO TRAINING AND SUPERVISION

Training in IPT-G was undertaken in the context of a feasibility and acceptability study.[15,16] The plan consisted of a 5-day intensive training followed by 6–8 months of supervised practice. The primary objective was to build competency in IPT-G so that its effectiveness could be tested. The benchmark was successful facilitation of 2 patient groups (6 patients each). By design, the first IPT group was led by 2 trainees; the second, by 1. Cofacilitation was intended to reduce the work burden of the trainees and enable them to assist one another in their first group. Two additional incentives helped cement this model: (1) parsimony (e.g., fewer patients needed) and (2) operational cost reduction. Feedback from trainees supported the usefulness of this training model.

Group facilitators were paired to form 2 supervision groups led by an IPT master trainer (S. Z.) from the United States. Trainees who cofacilitated the same group were supervised together. Supervision consisted of weekly online sessions (90 minutes each) conducted in French. On completion of their first group, trainees went on to facilitate a second group, this time by themselves. In this round, supervision was provided per IPT group, and each facilitator received a full hour of weekly supervision.

Contextual limitations called for additional adaptation. First, case identification to form groups depended on diagnostic confirmation by busy psychiatrists. This meant (1) longer wait time for patients to join a group and for facilitators to start training and (2) longer study duration. Therefore, group size was limited to 6. Second, work demands on trainees in the context of task shifting called for schedule flexibility with supervision to ensure attendance. On a more global level, the COVID-19 pandemic that hit Senegal in the study phase brought all group and supervision activities to a halt, thus forcing a reality of its own and raising a global question about how IPT-G can work in similar conditions.

A retrospective examination of adaptation, in the context of training, identified some areas for improvement. For one, the WHO manual (used in training) could be better adapted to the local context with Senegalese case examples and minor revisions to IPT strategies. Here, follow some illustrations in the context of grief, dispute, and transition.

In classic grief work, tears are expected and perhaps encouraged as patients "mourn their loss." However, in predominantly Muslim Senegal (95%), the approach needed to be adapted since crying in this context produces "burning tears that hurt the deceased." Praying for the beloved would be more appropriate. The same goes for items used to facilitate grieving. Jewelry and clothes, inherited or gifted, are more laden with significance in Senegalese culture than photographs. And, given cultural expectations to speak well of the dead, caution is advised when helping patients "reconstruct" their relationship with the dead person. The focus should be on validating the loss and honoring the memory of the deceased.

In the area of "disputes," the collectivistic and hierarchical nature of Senegalese society lends itself nicely to mediation as a primary strategy for resolving conflict. People traditionally live with their extended family in dwellings governed by social hierarchy and specific expectations, such as "centrality of family" and "filial duty." Polygamy, widely practiced in Senegal, adds some complexity to marital relationships and often requires some change in patient expectation or a "give-to-receive" approach. Role disputes can generally be resolved with the help of a respected elder (e.g., uncle; imam).

As regards role transitions, IPT-G strategies seem straightforward and appropriate for the Senegalese context overall. Nonetheless, specific challenges need to be addressed when working with PLHIV. These include stigma and poor understanding of the condition. Patients avoid help lest they be discovered. Therefore, offering IPT-G in a setting associated with HIV (i.e., infectious diseases treatment facility) was not ideal for our PLHIV participants. Yet, there were no viable alternatives at the time.

While relocation wasn't feasible, forming same-sex groups was. Participants were informed their groups would be entirely composed of same-sex PHLIV. Sharing one's HIV status is difficult enough in Senegalese society and more so with the opposite sex. PLHIV live with their "secret" for years, not only due to stigma but also because they perceive it as a condition that cannot be helped. Deep social isolation and despair ensue. Therefore, in training IPT-G providers, special attention was given to education about HIV, hope instillation, and breaking social isolation.

The IPT techniques of role play, communication analysis, and decision analysis were well received by our trainees. The same was true of group facilitation skills and IPT-G-specific techniques, such as "harnessing the power of the group" and the "interpersonal lab."[17] Trainees were especially moved by the power of the group (e.g., sharing experiences and supporting one another, which resonated nicely with local culture).

IMPLEMENTATION CHALLENGES

Challenges to IPT-G implementation were primarily organizational in nature and nonspecific to the intervention itself. They included patient identification, service integration, and treatment accessibility. The IPT-G feasibility and acceptability study required a confirmed diagnosis of depression for participation. This had two implications. It increased the burden on psychiatrists and restricted the pool of PLHIV to those with diagnosable depression. Given the stigmatization of mental health and HIV in Senegal, case identification thus became more problematic. Further, IPT service integration into a preexisting operational system increased work demands on staff tasked with implementation, in not only amount but also coordination. Adverse consequences such as worker dissatisfaction, burnout, and attrition constituted a potential threat.

Other challenges involved service recipients and were mainly associated with treatment burden and accessibility. Though the adoption of an 8-session treatment protocol significantly reduced the intervention's burden, some patients still voiced concern over weekly attendance. For a couple, it was employment with a changing schedule; for a few, stigma; for most, transportation. Participants got a flat fare from the IPT-G program, but those who lived far found it insufficient.

A different form of patient accessibility pertained to Senegal's ethnic and linguistic diversity. It had to do with language spoken in session. Group facilitators routinely spoke Wolof, which is widely spoken in Senegal as *lingua Franca*; however, in a couple of groups, participants had to intermittently use French or another local language to keep a nonfluent ethnic minority member in the loop. This is quite normal in polylinguistic Senegal and may indicate group cohesiveness. Nonetheless, the point is raised in the interest of broader inclusion and accessibility.

To address the above challenges, we propose that future training include providers from diverse backgrounds and more trainees to counter attrition. Further, shifting focus from a diagnosis-based to a symptom-based identification process would enable more depressed PLHIV to be included and decrease the system's dependence on psychiatrists. Also, because depressed PLHIV carry a double stigma that makes them difficult to identify and treat, awareness-raising and destigmatizing education campaigns targeting HIV and mental illness would be in order.

IMPLEMENTATION FACILITATORS

Group IPT was well implemented overall.[15,16] At the organizational level, direct support by the department head (M. S.) secured the resources needed for running groups; supervisory oversight and team management (C. B.) smoothed operational activities. Service delivery was optimized with ongoing competence building through training and clinical supervision (S. Z.). Despite hard work time pressure, group facilitators enjoyed several satisfiers, including professional growth and opportunity for achievement. They were enthusiastically engaged in training and practiced professionally. Their social work background and related interpersonal competencies helped them implement IPT-G with no prior therapy experience.

Contextually, IPT-G implementation benefited from cultural relevance. All group facilitators were Senegalese and observed cultural norms in their practice.

Punctuality was encouraged but not strictly enforced. Members who came on time completed their PHQ-9 and chatted while waiting for the rest to arrive. On average, groups began within 30 minutes of scheduled time. Similarly, it was normal for group members to exchange phone numbers, socialize, and support one another outside of group. Following termination, members stayed in touch. Many continued to meet, months after their group ended.

Some IPT-G features contributed to its successful implementation. The group modality resonated well with the collectivistic nature of Senegalese society, with its relational and storytelling culture. In effect, focused discussions with facilitators identified experience sharing as a primary strength of IPT-G. Group processes and techniques proved potent and made sense to Senegalese participants. Further, the very constitution of PLHIV groups was helpful, inasmuch as it broke individual isolation and accessed support.

FUTURE PLANS AND RECOMMENDATIONS

The IPT-G feasibility and acceptability study laid the grounds for future work in Senegal. One future direction is upscaling service delivery. The country's health settings are adequate in number but not in distribution. Most are concentrated in Dakar, making them less accessible to out-of-area patients.[18] Further, given the study's geographic bounds (limiting its generalizability), program replication in a less centralized context seems warranted. In this vein, two facilities outside the capital will be used to evaluate IPT-G in different contexts of care.

The upcoming project wouldn't be possible without trained personnel. To this end, our IPT-G providers in Dakar are presently cosupervising new providers following a training-of-trainers model. The plan is to create a self-sustaining training system—perhaps in collaboration with the national School of Social Work, where IPT-G would be studied. Such a move would considerably facilitate the dissemination of interpersonal therapy in Senegal and beyond.

Additional future plans include (1) systemic screening at health facilities to help with case identification; (2) a stepped-care model with newly diagnosed PLHIV, with interpersonal counseling as a first step; (3) use of specific nonclinical indicators of improvement (e.g., social and economic impact) to broaden treatment outcome assessment; and (4) application of IPT to more disorders (e.g., anxiety, distress, and trauma).

In terms of recommendations, context and organization stand out. IPT-G implementation requires more than good training. And, though supervision can increase trainee satisfaction, it cannot resolve organizational and contextual issues. Systemic support (e.g., by leadership) is primary and should be accompanied by procedural and structural reform. Personnel management, critical to service sustainability (e.g., staff retention) and quality, may be optimized with improved "conditions of service" (e.g., professional advancement). Therefore, we recommend systemic integration for successful implementation. As regards patients, PLHIV may especially benefit from health education outreach programs targeting depression and HIV. In the era of COVID-19, we also need alternate forms of service delivery (e.g., online; satellite service units).

CASE EXAMPLE

Amadou was a 53-year-old man who returned with his family to his native Senegal from Mali following a serious decline in his wife's health. Traditional healers told him that his wife had been "marabouted by family members." Hospital medical tests, on the other hand, showed Amadou's family (except 2 of his 5 children) to be HIV+, information he kept to himself.

Amadou's wife eventually died, following a long hospitalization, leaving him with 3 young children, all seropositive. Depression set in, as he grieved the death of "the woman he loved so enormously" and felt trapped with his HIV+ secret and hospital bills. Leaving Mali had left him with no income, and, with his wife gone, he was at loss about "how to care for his young children." In the intake session, he reported deep sadness, depressed mood, and disturbed sleep and was visibly upset and overwhelmed.

In group, Amadou was no longer alone. He opened up and shared his experience with loss and HIV. As he successfully grieved, he began to engage socially, build friendships, and take steps to get medical care for himself and his children. In the sixth session, he took the leap to share his HIV status with his eldest son. This opened a major support pathway for Amadou. It brought him closer with his son, who, in turn, stood by him and helped with child care. By the termination session, Amadou was gainfully employed, capably caring for himself and children, and depression free (PHQ-9 = 2).

The above case illustrates a typical PLHIV case, with "role transition" as primary problem area exacerbated by stigma. It also showcases other challenges PLHIV face, such as loss of loved ones and HIV care burden. The following discussion nuances the case in a Senegalese context.

Amadou's case reflects a characteristic feature in PLHIV presentation: multiple problem areas. This, combined with the brevity of an 8-session treatment protocol, dictates prioritization. In Amadou's case, grief seemed a good place to start inasmuch as he couldn't get past the death of the woman he loved so much. Strategies for grief were straightforward, except for a minor adaptation in the context of Amadou's faith (i.e., Islam): honoring his wife's memory through prayer (vs. shedding tears), remembrance, and being a good father. The group supported Amadou's efforts to draw on his faith—which valued steadfastness and patience in the face of hardship and gave meaning to his "trials," thus enabling him to work through grief.

Absent from Amadou's case, the problem area of "dispute" was nonetheless present in numerous PLHIV cases seen in Senegal (along with "transition"). Some were HIV related (e.g., being shunned by family due to HIV), but others occurred in different contexts, such as preferential treatment in polygamous marriages. In Amadou's case, an interpersonal dispute could have erupted in the context of the "curse" placed on his wife by members of his own family. Arguably, it didn't because none were specifically identified.

With his wife passing, Amadou was catapulted into a double role transition as widow and PLHIV. Without a spouse by his side, he became the sole caretaker of three seropositive children. Jobless, he couldn't afford medical care or sustenance. Social stigma stood between him and others, including his adult children, further deepening his loneliness and isolation. The group, however, proved a powerful antidote in both support and composition. Knowing that all members were PLHIV, Amadou related well and found it easier to share. This practice would subsequently prove useful in reaching out to the adult son. Given the centrality of the family in Senegalese culture, Amadou's talk with his son was critical to his recovery. It not only reduced his isolation and got him help, but also "put him together" in terms of collective identity.

PUBLICATIONS

Since its introduction to Senegal in March 2019, IPT-G has incrementally shown promise. The first results of the project are to be published in 2 articles (in preparation) that focus on quantitative and qualitative findings, respectively. Preliminary results were presented in 3 congresses, in the form of 1 oral presentation[19] and 3 posters.[15,16,20] Related publications include the French translation of the treatment manual, available online through the WHO web page.[14]

REFERENCES

1. Camara C, Clark A, Hargreaves JD et al. Senegal: References & Edit History. https://www.britannica.com/place/Senegal. "Senegal". Encyclopedia Britannica, 3 November 2023. Accessed November 5, 2022. (Last Updated: Oct 7, 2023).
2. Abas M, Ali GC, Nakimuli-Mpungu E, Chibanda D. Depression in people living with HIV in sub-Saharan Africa: time to act. *Trop Med Int Health*. 2014;19(12):1392–1396.
3. Bernard C, Font H, Diallo Z, et al. Prevalence and factors associated with severe depressive symptoms in older West African people living with HIV. *BMC Psychiatry*. 2020;20(1):442.
4. Memiah P, Shumba C, Etienne-Mesubi M, et al. The effect of depressive symptoms and CD4 count on adherence to highly active antiretroviral therapy in sub-Saharan Africa. *J Int Assoc Provid AIDS Care*. 2014;13(4):346–352.
5. Wroe EB, Hedt-Gauthier BL, Franke MF, Nsanzimana S, Turinimana JB, Drobac P. Depression and patterns of self-reported adherence to antiretroviral therapy in Rwanda. *Int J STD AIDS*. 2015;26(4):257–261.
6. Berhe H, Bayray A. A: prevalence of depression and associated factors among people living with HIV/AIDS in Tigray, North Ethiopia: a cross sectional hospital based study. *Int J Pharm Sci Res*. 2013;4(2):765–775.

7. Parcesepe AM, Mugglin C, Nalugoda F, et al. Screening and management of mental health and substance use disorders in HIV treatment settings in low- and middle-income countries within the global IeDEA consortium. *J Int AIDS Soc.* 2018;21(3):e25101.

8. World Health Organization. *mhGAP Mental Health Gap Action Programme: Scaling Up Care for Mental, Neurological and Substance Use Disorders.* World Health Organization; 2010. https://iris.who.int/bitstream/handle/10665/43809/978924 1596206_eng.pdf?sequence=1. Accessed November 5, 2022.

9. Petit V. Mental health: an underestimated development issue. in Y. Charbit (ed.), *Population and Development Issues.* ISTE-Wiley; 2022:157–181. https://www.iste.co.uk/book.php?id=1877. Accessed November 5, 2022.

10. Lancet Global Mental Health Group, Chisholm D, Flisher AJ, et al. Scale up services for mental disorders: a call for action. *Lancet Lond Engl.* 2007;370(9594):1241–1252.

11. World Health Organization. *Task Shifting: Rational Redistribution of Tasks Among Health Workforce Teams: Global Recommendations and Guidelines.* Geneva: WHO; 2008.

12. Verdeli H, Clougherty K, Bolton P, et al. Adapting group interpersonal psycho-therapy for a developing country: experience in rural Uganda. *World Psychiatry.* 2003;2(2):114.

13. Weissman MM, Markowitz JC, Klerman GL. *The Guide to Interpersonal Psychotherapy.* Oxford University Press. 2018.

14. World Health Organization. Group Interpersonal Therapy (IPT) for Depression. 2020. https://iris.who.int/bitstream/handle/10665/250219/WHO-MSD-MER-16.4-eng.pdf?sequence=1. Accessed November 5, 2022.

15. Bernard C, Ziadeh S, Tine JM, et al. Acceptabilité et faisabilité de la thérapie interpersonnelle dans la prise en charge de la dépression chez des personnes vivant avec le VIH au Sénégal. Eleventh Conférence Internationale Francophone VIH/Hépatites/Santé sexuelle–AfraVIH. Marseille, France; April 6–9, 2022.

16. Bernard C, Font H, Mané I, et al. Management of depression in people living with HIV in Senegal: acceptability and feasibility of group interpersonal therapy. AIDS Conference. Montréal, Canada; July 29 to August 1, 2022.

17. Wilfley DE, Mackenzie KR, Welch R, Ayres V, Weissman MM. *Interpersonal Psychotherapy for Group.* Basic Books; 2000.

18. United States Agency for International Development. 2017b. Senegal Conflict Vulnerability Assessment: Final Report. https://www.usaid.gov/sites/default/files/documents/1860/20180213_Senegal_CVA_Report_External.pdf. Accessed November 5, 2022.

19. Bernard C, Ziadeh S, Seydi M. Group interpersonal therapy to treat depres-sion in people living with HIV: Senegal first appraisal. International Congress of Psychology. Prague, Czech Republic; July 19–24, 2020.

20. Bernard C, Ziadeh S, Tine JM, et al. Thérapie interpersonnelle et prise en charge de la dépression chez des personnes vivant avec le VIH: une expérience sénégalaise. Tenth Conférence Internationale Francophone VIH/Hépatites/Santé sexuelle—AfraVIH; 2020.

21

Interpersonal Psychotherapy Group

A Scalable Solution to the Depression Epidemic in Zambia and Uganda

SEAN MAYBERRY ∎

STRONGMINDS

According to the Lancet Commission on global mental health and sustainable development, despite substantial research advances showing what can be done to prevent and treat mental disorders and to promote mental health, translation into real-world effects has been painfully slow. The global burden of disease attributable to mental disorders has risen in all countries in the context of major demographic, environmental, and sociopolitical transitions. Only 0.3% of global healthcare aid is directed toward mental health in low- and middle-income countries.[1]

The global development community is beginning to embrace good mental health as the foundation of thriving individuals, families, and societies. The World Health Organization (WHO) now recognizes that mental health is linked to each of the 17 Sustainable Development Goals (SDGs). The SDGs[2] are a collection of interlinked global goals, developed in 2015 by the United Nations General Assembly, which were designed to create a better and more sustainable future for all. Each specific goal is set to be achieved by 2030.

StrongMinds is a social enterprise and nongovernmental organization (NGO) that treats African women and adolescents suffering from depression, one of the most neglected health and development problems in Africa. According to WHO, an estimated 322 million people suffer from depressive disorders globally,[3] with the number of depression sufferers expected to increase, especially in lower income countries. Depressive disorders are the leading cause of disability globally,[3]

Sean Mayberry, *Interpersonal Psychotherapy Group* In: *Interpersonal Psychotherapy*. Edited by: Myrna M. Weissman and Jennifer J. Mootz, Oxford University Press. © Oxford University Press 2024. DOI: 10.1093/oso/9780197652084.003.0022 and women and girls are affected at 1.5x the rate of men and boys.[1] At its worst, depression can lead to suicide, the fourth leading cause of death among 15- to 19-year-olds worldwide.[4]

When a woman is depressed, she is less productive, has a lower income, and has poorer physical health. If she is a mother, we see the negative impact extends to her entire family. Research shows that children of depressed mothers are more likely to have poor health, struggle in or miss school, and suffer from depression themselves.

Depression impairs an individual's ability to focus and concentrate. People with depression may be less able to respond to health initiatives or livelihood trainings, rendering these programs less effective. Depression is not just a health problem; it is a development problem. This is StrongMinds' theory of change, and it is also encapsulated in the WHO 2022 World Mental Health Report[2]—that we cannot achieve the SDGs without prioritizing mental health.

THE MENTAL HEALTH TREATMENT GAP

No one can thrive without good mental health; yet, governments in low-income countries typically devote less than 1% of healthcare spending to mental health.[5] The mental health treatment gap for Africans has grown wider as a result of the COVID pandemic. Africa has 1.3 qualified mental health professional for every 100,000 individuals. By contrast, in Europe, there are 45.5 per 100,000.[6] More than 75% of people with depression in low- and middle-income countries have no access to effective treatment.[7] To address the growing mental health epidemic, we need a cost-effective, scalable, and evidence-based solution.

THE ORIGINS OF STRONGMINDS

My awareness of the issue took hold during my 10 years living and working in Africa implementing HIV/AIDS and malaria programs. During that time, I noticed that there was often a percentage of people—perhaps one in five—who did not respond to our behavior change interventions, even when the changes were small and the benefits life saving. It seemed that the effort required, no matter how seemingly small, was simply too much for some people. Having witnessed the impact of depression on people in my own life—how it sapped strength and motivation and impaired focus—I wondered if perhaps something similar was at play among the people I was trying to help. Were undiagnosed, untreated mental health disorders holding back development efforts in Africa?

In 2013, I came across the findings of a randomized controlled trial in Uganda from 2002 that had remarkable success in treating depression with group inter-personal psychotherapy (IPT-G). The study, by researchers from Johns Hopkins University (JHU) and Columbia University used lay community workers with only a high school education. The IPT-G intervention was simple, cost-effective, and highly scalable.

I founded StrongMinds that same year, with the mission of scaling access to mental health services for women in Africa using the IPT-G approach, relying on lay community health workers that we would train to facilitate IPT-G sessions. Each facilitator receives 2 weeks of training and ongoing supervision by mental health professionals. Since each facilitator is a community member, they are well -received by the depressed clients.

A DATA-DRIVEN APPROACH

We started running pilot IPT-G groups in Kampala, Uganda, in 2014—the site of the original JHU study—where we would try to replicate the results of the JHU study among low-income and marginalized women. Our first cohort consisted of 500 women who were experiencing depression, as indicated by their Patient Health Questionnaire-9 (PHQ-9) scores. Initial IPT-G sessions ran for 16 weeks, and we measured the results by administering the PHQ-9 at baseline, midline, and end of the sessions and then again at 18 and 24 months posttreatment. The results were overwhelmingly positive, with more than two-thirds of the women remaining depression free well beyond the conclusion of formal therapy groups. After therapy, clients reported improvements in their economic and social lives.

A MODEL BUILT FOR SCALE

StrongMinds now serves tens of thousands of individuals with depression each year throughout Uganda and Zambia. StrongMinds therapy is always free for participants, delivered in local languages, and led by lay facilitators who are trained in the IPT-G curriculum and supervised by StrongMinds staff and qualified partners. Our therapy groups consist of 10–14 individuals and meet over a period of 8 weeks for 60–90 minutes. As of this writing in 2023, we have treated over 230,000 individuals with depression. On average, 80% of our clients are free of depression by the conclusion of therapy, and the results are sustained 6 months later.

INNOVATION AND LEARNING TO REACH
NEW POPULATIONS

While the IPT-G model is the core of our program, constant innovation is required to reach new populations under ever-evolving conditions. Our clients typically subsist on less than $2 per day and have little formal education. Our therapy groups take place in communities through songs and with visual aids developed by our local staff, always in collaboration with local leaders. People who exhibit moderate-to-severe depression are invited to join a therapy group, which begins with an initial 1:1 private consultation with a facilitator. Should we need them, we also have tools and systems in place to identify and refer clients at risk of suicide or self-harm and for child protection.

Figure 21.1 shows how individuals would access our mental health chatbot, Amani.

Figure 21.2 shows the scale we use to help clients identify their current burdens/ challenges.

Figure 21.3 shows a visual method of assessing grief.

In 2017, we began training former clients to run their own therapy groups as peer facilitators, drawing on their lived experiences of depression and recovery. This effort allowed us to further embed mental health knowledge and resources

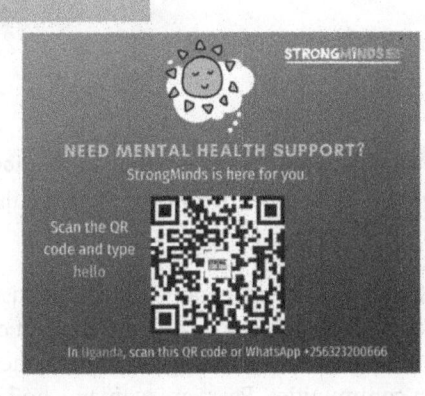

Figure 21.1 Chatbot tool.
CREDIT: StrongMinds grew from the conviction of Sean Mayberry, the author of this chapter.

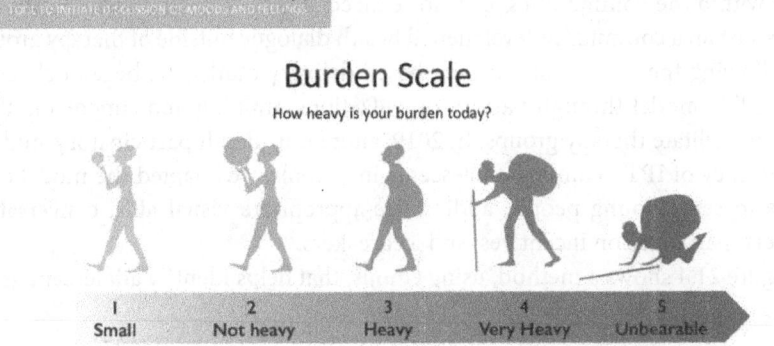

Figure 21.2 Tool to initiate discussion of moods and feelings: Burden Scale.
CREDIT: StrongMinds grew from the conviction of Sean Mayberry, the author of this chapter.

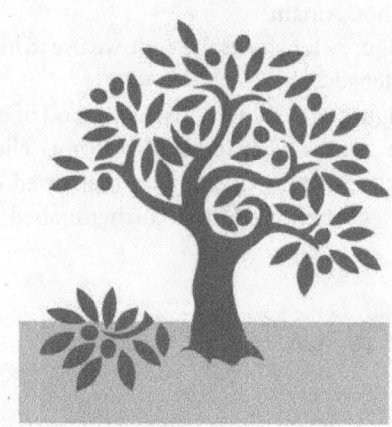

Figure 21.3 Tool to initiate discussion of grief and loss: Branches Tool.
CREDIT: StrongMinds grew from the conviction of Sean Mayberry, the author of this chapter.

within communities. This makes our therapy model self-sustaining, by removing the stigma around depression and normalizing the concept of mental health. Our peer facilitators are identified by the StrongMinds staff members who lead initial therapy groups in communities. Peers are women who have shown a remarkable recovery from depression through IPT-G and who have also—within their groups—demonstrated exceptional empathy and support for others. Peers are very receptive to training because they have already been through the program, so they have a frame of reference for the teachings, and they have firsthand experience of the beneficial outcomes. We see that peers are very successful at leading groups because they are already known to the community and trusted. Their public presence within the communities leads to reduced stigma around mental health and helps sustain a community-level mental health dialogue outside of therapy groups.

Following the success of our peer-based delivery model, we began delivering our IPT-G model through partner organizations, training and supporting their staff to facilitate therapy groups. In 2019, after an in-depth participatory study of the efficacy of IPT-G among adolescents in schools, we adapted the model once more to serve young people, adding age-appropriate visual aids, conversation starters, participation incentives, and icebreakers.

Figure 21.4 shows a method, using emojis, that helps identify adolescent grief.

ADAPTATION DUE TO COVID-19

The COVID-19 pandemic served as a catalyst for rapid innovation and growth. In the immediate days and weeks following the initial outbreak, StrongMinds surveyed 12,000 former clients by phone to understand the impact on the women

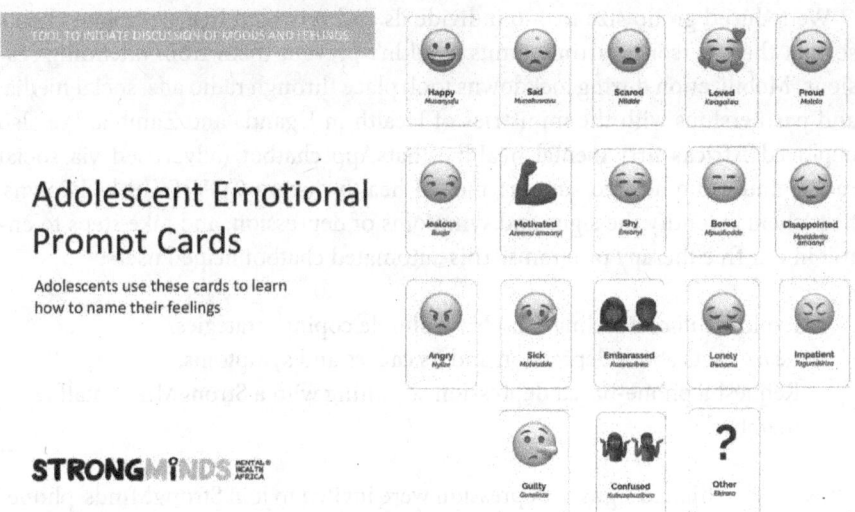

Figure 21.4 Tool to initiate discussion of moods and feelings: Adolescent Emotional Prompt Cards.
CREDIT: StrongMinds grew from the conviction of Sean Mayberry, the author of this chapter.

we had treated for depression. The number of participants who answered the phone call, consented, and completed the survey was 12,681. This survey was possible because we had a roster of staff who were unable to deliver therapy due to lockdowns and were working from home. We put their skills to use to conduct this survey, which ultimately helped us transition to our teletherapy offering a couple months later. We learned that lockdowns were causing intense distress, and that our services were needed more than ever. But we also learned that these women—all of whom had already been through IPT-G—had retained the skills they had learned in their groups, and that this had had a bolstering effect on their ability to remain resilient during the lockdown crisis.

Unable to run therapy groups in person, StrongMinds staff worked quickly to adapt the IPT-G model for phone-based delivery. Our staff were trained to ensure clients were in a safe place during calls, to read emotional cues through voices rather than faces, and to deploy various techniques to effectively facilitate phone-based group discussions. The trainings were given by our in-house clinician to mental health facilitators over several interactive Zoom sessions. As an example, facilitators in this training were reminded that—for in-person groups—they can observe posture, eye contact, hygiene, body language, and more in a client to assess her well-being. So even if someone doesn't speak much in group, the facilitator can observe them. On the phone, this isn't possible, so facilitators were coached to ask more open-ended questions of each individual and to avoid yes/no questions. For example, instead of, "Did you sleep well tonight?" you ask, "Betty, how was your sleep last night?" Then you ask another member to react to or comment on what Betty said.

We reduced group size to 4–6 individuals and provided free airtime to clients so that their personal airtime limits wouldn't prevent them from attending sessions. Mobilization during lockdowns took place through radio ads, social media, and partnerships with the ministries of Health in Uganda and Zambia. We also deployed Africa's first mental health WhatsApp chatbot (advertised via social media and radio ads) to support mental health during COVID-19 lockdowns, help clients identify the signs and symptoms of depression, and take steps to enroll in our free therapy programs. This automated chatbot helped users:

- Explore difficult feelings and learn simple coping strategies.
- Learn facts about depression and its causes and symptoms.
- Request a phone-based depression screening with a StrongMinds staff member.

Those who exhibited signs of depression were invited to join StrongMinds' phone-based group teletherapy group. Ultimately, we treated 11,390 individuals in 2020 through this teletherapy innovation, with PHQ-9 score changes on par with those we see with in-person group scores taken at baseline, midline, and end. As far as we know, this is the first instance of teletherapy IPT-G serving Africa. A portion of our clients reported that teletherapy was a preferable delivery method to in-person therapy, affording them flexibility, anonymity, and a welcome opportunity to learn from people with similar experiences outside of their immediate community. Teletherapy is not appropriate for all, however, and is especially difficult in areas with poor networks or for people with shared phones or limited access and privacy. For those who prefer it, we continue to offer teletherapy options to our clients, even now that in-person groups have resumed.

INTEGRATING DEPRESSION TREATMENT WITHIN THE GOVERNMENT IN UGANDA

In the wake of the pandemic, we are seeing a surge in mental health interest among NGOs and governments, who are turning to us for technical support and capacity building. We are now working with the Ministry of Education in Uganda to train teachers in schools to deliver IPT-G to their students. Anecdotal evidence suggests that this innovation is not only alleviating depression symptoms among students, but also keeping at-risk students in school, improving academic performance, and enhancing social connections. Numerous teachers have also asked to participate in IPT-G themselves to address their depression symptoms. We hope this leads to lower burnout rates and improved retention and job satisfaction among these educators.

In Uganda, we are also training village health technicians—who provide village-level healthcare outreach on behalf of the Ministry of Health—to provide IPT-G in the communities they serve. This has helped us treat depression in tens of thousands of people we would not otherwise have been able to reach.

The manualized nature of the IPT-G curriculum—combined with our toolkit of training and technical support—has kept results consistent for our clients through these various delivery methods. Our adaptations and enhancements of the IPT-G model include extensive guidance from quality assurance, monitoring, evaluation, and learning. This guidance is the result of StrongMinds' years of accumulated experience testing, learning, and iterating on these processes.

SUSTAINED RESULTS FOR HUMAN WELL-BEING

No one can thrive without a foundation of good mental health. StrongMinds surveyed clients to understand the impact of depression recovery on other aspects of their lives. Of those surveyed, 16% reported working more days, 13% reported that their families ate more meals, 30% reported that their children attended more school, and 28% reported an increased sense of social support.[1] These results align with existing research illustrating the extensive benefits of depression treatment for health and adherence to medication, economic productivity, and children's health and development. Furthermore, we estimate that for every 1 woman who recovers from depression, 4 household members feel the benefits, meaning that our programs have ultimately improved the well-being of some 700,000 people to date.

The benefits of the StrongMinds IPT-G model have been externally validated by organizations such as Founder's Pledge, Inciting Altruism, and Happier Lives Institute as one of the most cost-effective ways to improve human well-being in Africa. The organization has also been covered by publications such as *Psychology Today, The World Economic Forum, Forbes, Devex,* and *Psychiatric News.*[8] IPT-G has now become a World Health Organization-recommended first-line intervention for depression.[9]

REFERENCES

1. Liese BH, Gribble RS, Wickremsinhe MN. International funding for mental health: a review of the last decade. *Int Health.* 2019;11(5):361 369.
2. World Health Organization. WHO world mental health report: transforming mental health for all. 2022. https://www.who.int/publications/i/item/9789240049 338. Accessed June 18, 2022.
3. World Health Organization. *Depression and Other Common Mental Disorders: Global Health Estimates.* World Health Organization; 2017:8.
4. World Health Organization. Adolescent mental health fact sheet. November 17, 2021. Accessed July 2022. https://www.who.int/news-room/fact-sheets/detail/ado lescent-mental-health
5. World Health Organization. *Mental health atlas.* 2021.72. https://iris.who.int/bitstr eam/handle/10665/345946/9789240036703-eng.pdf?sequence=1. Accessed June 18, 2022.
6. World Health Organization. Depressive disorder (depression). https://www.who. int/news-room/fact-sheets/detail/depression. Accessed June 18, 2022.

7. StrongMinds. 2019 Q4 report. 2019. https://strongminds.org/wp-content/uploads/2020/03/SM-Q4-report-8.5x11_03.12.20.pdf

8. StrongMinds. Media, awards, and validation. https://strongminds.org/media-awards-and-validation/?swcfpc=1. Accessed June 18, 2022.

9. World Health Organization. Group interpersonal therapy (IPT) for depression. 2016. https://iris.who.int/bitstream/handle/10665/250219/WHO-MSD-MER-16.4-eng.pdf?sequence=1. Accessed June 18, 2022.

PART V

Interpersonal Psychotherapy in Asia

22

Interpersonal Psychotherapy in Mainland China

The Rapidly Growing Practice

WANHONG ZHENG, WEIHUI LI, YANLI LUO, MANLI HUANG, XIA SUN, AND XIAOYI ZHOU ∎

China is one of the largest countries in the world. Its current population is over 1.4 billion and comprises about 18% of the world's population. The World Health Organization (WHO) estimates that 54 million people in China suffer from depression, and about 41 million suffer from anxiety disorders (WHO, n.d.).[1] One recent major change in mental health care in China has been that psychotherapy is now recognized as a scientific and effective method of treatment, as reflected in the new law's specification of psychotherapy as an integral part of medical care that should be provided at medical facilities across levels of care.[2]

Interpersonal psychotherapy (IPT) is particularly well suited to China for several reasons. First, it focuses on interpersonal relationships, which are especially important in Chinese culture. Confucianism, the dominant cultural belief system in China for thousands of years, strongly emphasizes the interdependence of individuals through social connections. Unlike in Western countries, interpersonal relationships in China rely heavily on networks of trust and mutual obligation operating across personal, familial, and societal levels. These relationships have such a huge impact on everyday life in China that they affect an individual's ability to get things done. In daily clinical practice in China, it was common to see patients whose mental health problems were triggered by malfunctioning *guanxi*, or personal connections, relationships, and social networks. Second, mental health has been a primary focus of ongoing improvements in the healthcare system in China. In Shanghai and Hangzhou, where new health-related

Wanhong Zheng, Weihui Li, Yanli Luo, Manli Huang, Xia Sun, and Xiaoyi Zhou, *Interpersonal Psychotherapy in Mainland China*
In: *Interpersonal Psychotherapy*. Edited by: Myrna M. Weissman and Jennifer J. Mootz, Oxford University Press.
© Oxford University Press 2024. DOI: 10.1093/oso/9780197652084.003.0023

policies encourage the practice of evidence-based psychotherapy, local mental health facilities have received tremendous support for training practitioners and implementing mental health programs. Finally, the rapid economic development in many areas of China has led to improvement in people's quality of life. Consequently, the demand for mental health services has increased significantly. Evidence shows that, as the pace of life in China has increased, so has the incidence of mental health problems.[3] Although previous surveys have shown low rates of treatment-seeking among individuals with mental disorders in China,[4,5] we have noted recent improvements in mental health literacy and an increase in the number of Chinese people willing to seek professional help when needed. This anecdotal evidence is consistent with evidence from recent studies.[6,7]

Following an organized series of lectures, workshops, and case supervisions over the past 4 years, IPT practice in mainland China has been on the increase.[8] We estimate that by early 2022, as a result of this solid foundation of training, there were more than 2500 clinicians equipped with the basic skills necessary to integrate IPT into their practice, including psychiatrists, nonpsychiatry physicians, nurses, psychologists, and certified therapists.

While Chinese therapists are delivering IPT services all over the country, most of the training and practice has taken place in the coastal and central parts of China, particularly in Shanghai, Zhejiang, and Hunan. Patients are seen in both inpatient and outpatient settings, through either individual or group sessions, in person, online, or blended. The target population is primarily those with depression, anxiety, somatoform disorder, adjustment disorder, and bipolar disorder, and they vary in age from adolescent to geriatric. Individual IPT treatment routinely comprises weekly sessions over 8–20 weeks, with each session lasting 50–60 minutes. IPT group treatment generally included 8–12 weekly sessions, with each session lasting 90 minutes.

To better address the needs of patients and maintain alignment with Chinese cultural values, our pioneering Chinese IPT therapists have made some adaptations to practice. For individual IPT, examples of these adaptations include the following:

1. Shortening the course of IPT (8 sessions or fewer) with flexibility regarding frequency. Many Chinese therapists preferred brief interpersonal psychotherapy brief (IPT-B). For one thing, there have been too few psychotherapists to meet the ever-increasing demand for services. Providing a shortened course of treatment is one practical way to address this shortage. Also, in a country developing as rapidly as China is, most patients want to resolve their problems in a relatively short time and quickly return to their normal lives. Many must go back to work or study as soon as possible and therefore prefer short-term IPT. Finally, as IPT is currently still not covered by government or commercial insurance in many provinces, financial cost is a big concern for most Chinese patients. A short, efficient, and focused course of therapy is more affordable. In some cases, weekly sessions can be

changed to biweekly to accommodate patients' concerns with regard to time and financial cost. Therapists have noticed no difference in treatment outcome with the reduction in the number of sessions.

2. Involving families at an appropriate time to improve treatment efficacy. In our experience using IPT with Chinese patients, many have had interpersonal conflicts with family members. This may also be true for patients in Western countries, but Chinese culture is particularly family oriented. In traditional Confucianism, obedience and devotion to parents and elder family members form the basis of moral conduct and social harmony. The extreme shame a Chinese patient can experience because of conflict with family members over failure to meet their unreasonable expectations (e.g., admission to a prestigious university) cannot be resolved without the understanding and cooperation of those family members.

3. Initially focusing on one problem area and, when permitted, extending sessions for additional problem area(s). Chinese people have intricate interpersonal relationships. Whether at home or in the extended family, community, workplace, or school, guanxi has a significant effect on their lives. Daily, each Chinese person must fulfill multiple social roles and can encounter interpersonal problems with each. This is more salient for mental health patients. It is not uncommon to see an individual patient dealing with several problem areas at once. Therefore, when practicing IPT in China, we had to spend more time exploring the problem areas that were most urgent and choose one to focus on initially. If needed, after the first set of sessions was complete, we strongly encouraged patients to continue therapy to address other problem areas.

For group IPT, examples of these adaptations include these:

1. Incorporation of the social media app WeChat for connection and support. For most Chinese people, WeChat is a ubiquitous all-in-one app that can be used to communicate with everybody from family members to old classmates. People shop and pay bills, coordinate with coworkers, and swap stories through WeChat. IPT therapists in Shanghai took advantage of the app's ubiquity and used it to boost group participation and interaction. This innovation was extremely helpful during times in the COVID-19 pandemic when face-to-face meetings were restricted. While Zhumu, a videoconferencing tool similar to Zoom, was used for conducting therapy groups, therapists also established a WeChat group right after the first session to facilitate communication between group members between sessions. Group members agreed to a set of rules to govern use of the group chat, and the IPT therapist managed the group through the eighth session. After that, the therapist would rename the group and switch group management to a volunteer group member. The therapist would finally leave the group 3 months after transferring

management to a group member. Involvement in the WeChat group was mandatory for all group members through the initial sessions because the therapist would immediately post important therapy-related group messages for all group members after sessions. Participation beyond the initial 8 weeks was voluntary but highly encouraged. Therapists felt WeChat made it much easier to instill a sense of participation and friendship in the group. It also provided a convenient way for group members to submit therapy practice homework between sessions.

2. Incorporation of photos into group sessions. As smartphones with cameras have also become ubiquitous, we added photos as a treatment element of group sessions. Members were encouraged to share pictures of life events, moments that evoked strong emotions, or anything else that might be useful for group discussion.

3. Focusing on treatment goals instead of current symptoms or distress. We noticed that in some patients with moderate-to-severe anxiety, talking too much about current symptoms could worsen the condition. Rather, we found that instilling hope through focusing on treatment goals was the most effective approach.

4. Use of subgroups to focus on particular issues. Subgroups of 2 or 3 members with similar symptoms could be helpful in certain circumstances, especially for those with severe anxiety. The subgroups could easily be created in Zhumu videoconferencing, where a member could be in both a subgroup and the larger group at the same time. For those who were initially uncomfortable with the large-group setting, a subgroup could serve as a transition to moving into full participation with the larger group.

5. Use of traditional ways to encourage interactions during each group session. For example, *jiguchuanhua* ("beating the drum and passing the flower") is a traditional Chinese game played by a group of people sitting in a circle. When the drum sounds, the players start to pass the flower. When the drum stops without warning, the player who currently has the flower in their hands must do something, such as sharing feelings, singing a song, or telling a story. This game engenders a sense of community and proved to be a lot of fun for Chinese IPT group members.

The experiences over these initial years of IPT practice in China have indicated its acceptability among patients, families, and practitioners. However, as with any other treatment option, there have been challenges in implementing IPT in China. First, we are still at the initial phase of IPT development in China. Only a small number of the growing cadre of therapists in the country have received IPT training. Many have voiced uncertainty about its suitability for Chinese patients. Clinical evidence on treatment outcomes in the Chinese population is not yet robust enough to convince practitioners who have these concerns, which hinders broader implementation in daily practice. Second, the career path for professional development in IPT practice is unclear. People are waiting for a formal certification system that will recognize training and help with securing work. Third, not many experienced bilingual IPT therapists are available who can provide advanced training or case supervision to Chinese speakers who want to learn IPT. Fourth, as with any psychotherapy in China, counseling is not currently covered by health insurance in most provinces. We believe that it is only through increasing the practice of IPT in China that we can prove its efficacy and advocate for its inclusion in the future healthcare plans. Finally, given the philosophical, traditional, and societal differences between Oriental and Western cultures, solid evidence of the practicality and efficacy of IPT in the Chinese population must be demonstrated. Clinical trials are thus needed, including the testing of adaptations of IPT practice to achieve cultural congruency with Chinese patients. Though this task is complicated and will take time, it is particularly important. The new generation of IPT therapists in China must be cognizant of the cultural needs of their patients when using an IPT framework and techniques that were initially developed for a Western cultural context. Future IPT training and case supervision must continue to emphasize this need for adaptation.

The following case example both demonstrates the applicability of IPT to the challenges of a typical Chinese family and highlights the importance of adapting IPT to meet the cultural needs of patients in China.

CASE EXAMPLE

Mary was a 40-year-old female working in a midlevel management position in a business financed by foreign investment. Her husband had a stable job working for the government. They had a 12-year-old daughter who was in the 6th grade. About 5 months before entering therapy, Mary started a new work project that required a lot of overtime. She routinely had to use her weekends for work instead of being with family. She presented to the clinic with complaints of increased sadness, decreased energy level, poor concentration, and diminished interest in activities. Her score on the Hamilton Depression Rating Scale (HAMD-17) assessment was 20. A psychiatrist diagnosed her with major depressive disorder, prescribed citalopram, and recommended therapy. Mary agreed to try "a brief therapy" and started weekly 50-minute IPT sessions.

In the initial phase of treatment, the therapist reviewed Mary's symptoms and assigned her the "sick role." A brief psychoeducational intervention helped her understand the severity and nature of her symptoms. Mary identified her relationships with her husband and daughter as her most significant ones, followed by those with her sister and parents in her interpersonal inventory. She admitted that her recent busy work schedule had estranged her from her husband and daughter. She also recalled the sharp exchanges between her and her husband when she expressed her concern and lack of readiness for a second child. Her husband has always wanted a second child, but Mary was very worried about pregnancy in older age and the potential that it would affect her job performance and further career development. Neither Mary nor her husband, themselves, had siblings because of China's long-term family-planning policy. Having more than 1 child in a family is a dream but is, in practice, quite unfamiliar to them. In addition, Mary and her husband have always disagreed over their daughter's education. While her husband prefers to grant their daughter more autonomy and opportunities for self-teaching of skills, Mary believes a teenager should always be taught what to do because of their immaturity.

It was thus not difficult for Mary and her therapist to agree on focusing on the problem area of role dispute. They determined treatment goals to be gaining further understanding of the disputes between her and her husband, improving the marital relationship through communication modification and gaining additional interpersonal support. The therapist then focused on helping Mary analyze the stages of disputes, identify faulty condemnations, and explore options for making changes. Mary noted that the trigger for the current dispute was their daughter's declining school performance. Due to her busy work schedule, Mary had not paid much attention recently to their daughter's schoolwork. The couple had been arguing more and more about how to better support their daughter and improve her school performance. Her husband had also accused her of being "controlling" and "hard to reason with" as a mother. The therapist helped Mary recognize her feelings and learn to normalize and validate them. Through communication analysis and role playing, Mary practiced how to control her anger, speak out about her own needs, and negotiate using reasonable compromise. She also formed a plan to reestablish connections with and gain psychosocial support from other people in her inventory, such as her sister and an old classmate. By the end of the 10-week course of treatment, Mary felt significant improvement in her depressive symptoms, her relationship with her husband had improved, and her HAMD-17 score had fallen to 2, indicating remission. Mary reported that her life had returned to normal. She was now capable of balancing family life and a busy work schedule. The therapy was terminated successfully.

As the case example above demonstrates, rapid economic growth and an increase in the pace of daily life have led to increasing mental health problems in China and a corresponding increase in the demand for a brief, highly effective, and focused psychotherapy modality such as IPT. With more and more attention being paid to mental health, the Chinese government has offered new mental health policies to support psychotherapy training and practice in the country. The increasing number of successful IPT lectures and workshops over the past 4 years is one result of these changes in demand and policy. In 2021, the International Society of Interpersonal Psychotherapy Chinese chapter (IPT China) was established. Within 2 months, IPT China started the first group supervision for Chinese IPT practitioners. In August 2021, a group of first-generation Chinese IPT therapists successfully published *Interpersonal Psychotherapy for Depression: Theory and Case Practice*,[9] the first Chinese-language book on IPT and a milestone in the development of IPT in China. The book uses many clinical examples to describe how to stage IPT and choose problem areas in clinical encounters with Chinese patients, therefore providing practical guidance for any Chinese clinician who wants to use IPT in their clinical practice.

The time for IPT practice in China has arrived. IPT China has several plans to promote the growth of this modality in the country. First, the organization will continue to expand IPT education and training, with a focus on training Chinese-speaking trainers who can then train others. For those who have already received training, IPT China is developing a model to combine domestic and international expertise to provide supervision and a path for professional development. Within each province, the organization plans to strengthen training of clinicians in community hospitals and continue to offer IPT workshops as part of annual provincial psychiatric conferences. Second, IPT China will encourage adaptation of IPT by exploring and improving the practice of IPT in the context of Chinese culture. Third, the organization will seek to expand involvement in IPT China to encourage participation and support more local training activities. IPT China will also continue to encourage committee members to practice IPT in different settings and modalities, including group therapy and therapy for specific populations. Finally, the organization will promote IPT-related clinical research, facilitate collaborations among regional hospitals and clinics, and collect evidence on treatment outcomes to pave the way for widespread IPT practice in China.

REFERENCES

1. World Health Organization. Mental health. Accessed April 11, 2022. https://www.who.int/china/health-topics/mental-health
2. Chen HH, Phillips MR, Cheng H, et al. Mental Health Law of the People's Republic of China (English translation with annotations): translated and annotated version of China's new mental health law. *Shanghai Arch Psychiatry*. 2012;24(6):305.
3. Que J, Lu L, Shi L. Development and challenges of mental health in China. *Gen Psychiatry*. 2019;32(1):e100053.
4. Shen YC, Zhang MY, Huang YQ, et al. Twelve-month prevalence, severity, and unmet need for treatment of mental disorders in metropolitan China. *Psychol Med*. 2006;36(2):257–267.
5. Wang PS, Aguilar-Gaxiola S, Alonso J, et al. Use of mental health services for anxicty, mood, and substance disorders in 17 countries in the WHO world mental health surveys. *Lancet*. 2007;370(9590):841–850.
6. Liu F, Zhou N, Cao H, et al. Chinese college freshmen's mental health problems and their subsequent help-seeking behaviors: a cohort design (2005–2011). *PLoS One*. 2017;12(10):e0185531.
7. Shi W, Hall BJ. Help-seeking preferences among Chinese college students exposed to a natural disaster: a person-centered approach. *Eur J Psychotraumatol*. 2020;11(1):1761621.
8. Zheng W, Liu X, Chandran DN, et al. Interpersonal psychotherapy knowledge dissemination in China. *Heart Mind*. 2021;5(4):144.
9. Huang ML, Xu Y, Chung PY, et al. *Interpersonal Psychotherapy for Depression: Theory and Case Practice*. Zhejiang Science and Technology Publishing House; 2021.

23

Interpersonal Psychotherapy in Hong Kong

JOSEPH PUI-YIN CHUNG ∎

Interpersonal psychotherapy (IPT) was first introduced to Hong Kong in 2007 by Dr. John Markowitz. He was invited by the psychologists in government hospitals to conduct an introductory workshop. At that time, IPT was almost unheard of by mental health professionals in Hong Kong. Most therapists in those days practiced cognitive behavioral therapy, and some practiced psychodynamic psychotherapy. In the ensuing 15 years, IPT had been slowly disseminated throughout Hong Kong, but not without obstacles. Now, it has become a well-recognized psychological treatment among mental health professionals in this modern city located in the southern part of China.

Hong Kong is a metropolitan city in Southeast Asia. It has a population of 7 million, of which 92% are Chinese. Hong Kong was a British colony from 1841 to 1997 and reunited with China on July 1, 1997. As a result, many people in Hong Kong, especially the younger generation, are bilingual, and they were influenced by traditional Chinese as well as Western cultures. Thus, implementation of a psychological treatment developed in the Western culture may be easier in Hong Kong compared to other parts of China, but still requires some cultural adaptations. The healthcare system in Hong Kong is influenced by the British medical system and well developed. Cognitive behavioral therapy is routinely used in mental health service, but dissemination of other forms of psychotherapies, including IPT, is often limited by the lack of clinical training and supervisions.[1]

When IPT was first introduced to Hong Kong, there was skepticism about its effectiveness. Some therapists were unsure if a therapy that focused exclusively on improving interpersonal relationships and social support, without addressing the cognitive distortions, would work. They also doubted if the techniques used in IPT were too simple to result in meaningful clinical changes. Other therapists

Joseph Pui-yin Chung, *Interpersonal Psychotherapy in Hong Kong* In: *Interpersonal Psychotherapy.*
Edited by: Myrna M. Weissman and Jennifer J. Mootz, Oxford University Press. © Oxford University Press 2024.
DOI: 10.1093/oso/9780197652084.003.0024

worried that a short-term therapy not addressing the complex psychodynamic background of patients would not result in sustainable improvement in maladaptive interpersonal patterns and behaviors, and hence the depressive mood would return.[2] Because of the unfamiliarity about the theories behind this newly introduced therapy, therapists did not realize the powerful role of relationships in alleviating mood symptoms in depression,[3] and the value of a structured psychological treatment[4] in addition to the techniques in facilitating changes to improve health outcomes. The fact that IPT was an evidence-based treatment helped dispel many doubts about its effectiveness,[5] but it was the sequential training workshops in 2010, 2011, 2014, 2016, and 2018 by Drs. Michael O'Hara, Scott Stuart, and Betsy Bledsoe that answered questions from therapists new to IPT and prepared a fertile soil for IPT dissemination and implementation in Hong Kong.

In 2014, there was only 1 trained IPT local supervisor in Hong Kong. Clinical supervision by overseas experts was challenging because of the lack of suitable English-speaking patients for training as 92% of the Hong Kong population were Chinese. IPT not adapted to the local culture made it less effective,[6] and it created further obstacles to training by the sole reliance on nonlocal trainers and supervisors. Supporting local change agents who were capable of a high level of effort by the international community, cultural adaptations, formation of a peer-to-peer network, developing local training materials and videos, organizing local workshops, and publishing local case reports[7] all helped the process of local dissemination. Around 2012, IPT became one of the psychological treatments psychiatric residents in Hong Kong could choose to receive training in to fulfill the requirement for residency training. Such a system change enhanced residents' motivation to receive training in IPT, and it also facilitated IPT dissemination in Hong Kong. Another important factor that affected dissemination was certification. Certification is important in Asia, especially among Chinese, where people pride themselves in hard work to achieve recognition in their respective field. IPT certification, although not required for a licensed mental health professional in Hong Kong to practice IPT, is a recognition to the skill of a therapist, and it gives therapists motivation to receive training. In 2021, the International Society of Interpersonal Psychotherapy launched its certification system for therapists, supervisors, and trainers, and it was helpful to facilitate IPT dissemination in Hong Kong and in Asia by providing a systematic pathway for therapists to be trained and to receive recognition by the international community of IPT.

Cultural adaptation is another important step in the dissemination and implementation of IPT in a non-Western society like Hong Kong. Psychotherapy studies among Chinese have shown that treatments not adapted to the local culture were significantly less effective than adapted treatments.[8] The ways Chinese express their emotions, negotiate conflicts, and seek social support are different from their Western counterparts. Chinese tend to express their emotions indirectly and may be less comfortable talking about difficult emotions.[9] When conducting IPT in Chinese, it is important to spend more time to help patients identify their emotions so they can link their mood to changes in interpersonal relationships. Therapists also need to provide a sense of security for Chinese patients to express difficult emotions and adapt to their pace by offering support and encouragement instead of rushing them through the therapy agenda. This is especially true when working with patients who have grief and loss. The Chinese cultural value of filial piety affects the way patients express their feelings about the loss of a family member. Sometimes, Chinese patients may feel guilty about not spending enough time with a family member with terminal illness before he or she dies or not doing enough to prevent sickness or death. Such feelings may be difficult to express. Some are not willing to talk about negative feelings toward a deceased family member to avoid being seen as disrespectful to the dead (e.g., not talking about the stress in looking after an irritable relative with cancer who passed away). Such feelings and emotions need to be sensitively explored in the therapy sessions to help patients mourn their loss.

Chinese society has a clear relationship hierarchy.[10] The relationship hierarchy affects the handling of interpersonal disputes in workplace and in family, between subordinates and supervisors, and between younger and older members of a family. A typical example occurs in the treatment of adolescent depression, in which parents often expect unquestioned obedience from the adolescent and consider the adolescent as a problem to be fixed[6] instead of seeing the struggles the adolescent is experiencing related to depression. This is often complicated by the cultural expectation Chinese parents have for their children to succeed academically, creating a high-pressure environment that makes communication difficult. A typical example is a parent who keeps asking a depressed child to work harder in school. The child thinks the parent only cares about his academic result instead of caring about him, but the parent thinks caring about his academic result in a competitive society is caring about him. Very often therapists need to involve parents in treatment sessions to help both the parent and the adolescent to understand each other's expectations, and to observe and coach their communication, for the therapy to be successful.[6] Communication analysis and role play of IPT will be very useful in such scenarios, to help both the parent and the child to understand the expectations behind communication and role play how to talk in a way that the child feels being understood and the parent feels being respected.

The core structure, the 4 interpersonal foci and the IPT techniques, can be used in Chinese patients with few modifications. In randomized controlled trials of IPT conducted among Chinese, the basic structure was the same, and the treatments were found to be efficacious.[11,12] It is the cultural sensitivities that matters. In Chinese, family support is very important, and it is often the first source of interpersonal support the therapist should explore with patients in IPT sessions. In a case report of IPT for postnatal anxiety disorder, the therapist focused on improving communication between the patient and her husband. With improvement of the family relationship, the patient could expand her social network and adapt to the role transition of being a mother on her own,[7] and anxiety symptoms were reduced. In Chinese elderly patients, children can be an important support both emotionally and financially.[9] A survey among psychiatric nurses in Hong Kong about their cultural framework of interpersonal relationships and social support found that improving interpersonal relationships to improve mood in IPT was relevant to their culture. However, they considered maintaining family cohesion as more important than resolving disputes and viewed parental control over adolescents as culturally appropriate. They also considered it difficult to openly negotiate an interpersonal conflict at the workplace because of workplace hierarchy.[2] These attitudes illustrate cultural adaptations therapists might need to be aware of when conducting IPT among Chinese. Below are two case examples for illustration.

CASE EXAMPLES

Case example 23.1

Ms. A was a 30-year-old mother with a 2-month-old newborn son. She suffered from postnatal depression because of interpersonal disputes with her mother-in-law, who visited the couple daily and often criticized Ms. A over her child care methods. Ms. A's husband was the only child in his family, and he avoided mediating the conflict between his wife and his mother. He considered speaking up to his mother as disrespectful and contradicted filial piety. He also worried that not letting his mother visit her grandson daily would rupture family cohesion. He asked Ms. A to tolerate his mother, which worsened Ms. A's depression. The therapist coached Ms. A to be assertive with her mother-in-law in the middle phase of IPT, but Ms. A was not able to do so, probably because she also saw assertiveness as being disrespectful to a senior member of the family. Finally, the therapist's supervisor suggested the therapist involve Ms. A's husband in the session to understand his need to maintain family cohesion and coached him to talk with his mother about being less critical toward his wife to maintain family harmony. With the couple working together on the goal of fostering family harmony, interpersonal relationships in the family improved, conflicts were reduced, and Ms. A's depression score was reduced.

This case example highlighted how the Chinese cultural value of filial piety affects the way members in a family see interpersonal disputes.

Case example 23.2

Mr. B was a 70-year-old elderly man suffering from complicated grief and depression. His wife died 1 year ago from cancer, and Mr. B had been depressed since then. His depression did not improve despite psychopharmacotherapy treatment for 6 months. He had a 30-year-old daughter who tried to support him, but he did not want to be an emotional burden to her. In IPT, the therapist helped him mourn his loss, and his mood improved. Subsequently, the therapist used several therapy sessions to help the patient connect with his daughter. It was only after he improved communication with his daughter and re-invited her into his life that the depressive symptoms completely resolved. It was not necessary to explore other social supports before symptoms improved.

This case example highlights the importance of family support in Chinese culture. It is especially true for Chinese elderly experiencing grief and loss.[9] When facilitating mourning, because of the close family ties in Chinese culture, we found it is important to give patients enough time to talk about the relationship with the deceased family member, especially the positive aspects, such as how they met or the good times they spent together, before discussing the circumstances of death and exploring negative emotions.

The Chinese chapter of the International Society of Interpersonal Psychotherapy was established in 2021. With this platform, collaborations among Hong Kong and Chinese professionals who use IPT became possible. Research and exchange of experiences enabled therapists to better understand how to deliver IPT among Chinese. With the support from the International Society of Interpersonal Psychotherapy in certification, more IPT therapists, supervisors, and trainers are being trained, and dissemination has become more widespread in Hong Kong and in the rest of China. In the future, we expect greater participation of Chinese trainers and supervisors in the global IPT community to foster collaborations and disseminate and implement widely in the Chinese population that makes up one-fifth of the population of the world.

REFERENCES

1. Wong OL, Ma JLC. Development of family therapy in Hong Kong. *Contemp Fam Ther.* 2013;5:244–256.
2. Chung JPY, Bledsoe B. IPT trainings and dissemination in Hong Kong and the cultural specific considerations in conducting IPT among Hong Kong Chinese patients. Paper presented at the 8th Conference of the International Society of Interpersonal Psychotherapy (ISIPT); 2019; Budapest, Hungary. https://interpe rsonalpsychotherapy.org/wp-content/uploads/2019/11/ISIPT-AGENDA_web-1.pdf. Accessed November 2, 2022.
3. Sullivan HS. *The Interpersonal Theory of Psychiatry.* Norton; 1953.
4. Psychotherapy for Major Depressive Disorder and Generalized Anxiety Disorder: A Health Technology Assessment. Health Quality Ontario. *Ont Health Technol Assess Ser.* 2017;17(15):1–167.
5. Klerman GL, DiMascio A, Weissman M, Prusoff B, Paykel ES. Treatment of depression by drugs and psychotherapy. *Am J Psychiatry.* 1974;131:186–191.
6. Stuart S, Pereira XV, Chung JP. Transcultural adaptation of IPT in Asia. *Asia Pac Psychiatry.* 2021;13(1):e12439.
7. Chung JPY. Interpersonal psychotherapy for postnatal anxiety disorder. *East Asian Arch Psychiatry.* 2015;25:88–94.
8. Ng TK, Wong DF. The efficacy of cognitive behavioral therapy for Chinese people: a meta-analysis. *Aust N Z J Psychiatry.* 2018;52(7):620–637.
9. Xu H, Koszycki D. Interpersonal psychotherapy for late-life depression and its potential application in China. *Neuropsychiatr Disord Treat.* 2020;16:1919–1928.

10. Li MG, Duan C, Ding BK. Psychotherapy integration in modern China. *J Psychother Pract Res*. 1994;3(4):277–283.

11. Jiang, RF, Tong HQ, Delucchi KL. Interpersonal psychotherapy versus treatment as usual for PTSD and depression among Sichuan earthquake survivors: a randomized clinical trial. *Confl Health*. 2014;8:14.

12. Tang TC, Jou SH, Ko CH. Randomized study of school-based intensive interpersonal psychotherapy for depressed adolescents with suicidal risk and parasuicide behaviors. *Psychiatry Clin Neurosci*. 2009;63(4):463–470.

24

Interpersonal Psychotherapy in Japan

HIROKO MIZUSHIMA ■

BACKGROUND

Surrounded by the Pacific Ocean and the Sea of Japan, Japan is an island country with a beautiful seasonal landscape, unique traditional architecture, and culture. The population of Japan is about 120 million (48% male), about 30% are over 65 years old, and it is considered an aging society. Interpersonal psychotherapy (IPT) was introduced in Japan in 1997 when Dr. Hiroko Mizushima and colleagues at Keio University published the Japanese translation of the first manual *Interpersonal Psychotherapy of Depression.*"[1] As a young psychiatrist specializing in eating disorders and mood disorders, Dr. Mizushima sought guidance from Drs. Weissman and Markowitz and other authorities in the United States. She actively introduced IPT into her clinical practice and disseminated it in Japan.

She energetically introduced IPT in academic conferences, wrote review articles about IPT in Japanese mental health journals, translated English manuals, and wrote easy books for laypeople consisting of psychoeducation and adaptation of IPT of each disorder.[2–8] The self-help books have sold more than 10,000 copies each. IPT is well known and popular among Japanese users. In 2007, Dr. Mizushima founded an IPT study group (currently IPT-JAPAN) and started training and disseminating IPT in Japan. The study session is divided into an introductory course given every 3 months and a monthly group supervision course. About 2 times a year, workshops focused on role playing take place. The introductory course is an 8-hour course that strictly adheres to the ideas and basic approaches of IPT by Drs. Klerman and Weissman. To make it a practical workshop, Dr. Mizushima introduces her real cases using video and verbatim script.[9]

Hiroko Mizushima, *Interpersonal Psychotherapy in Japan* In: *Interpersonal Psychotherapy.* Edited by: Myrna M. Weissman and Jennifer J. Mootz, Oxford University Press. © Oxford University Press 2024. DOI: 10.1093/oso/9780197652084.003.0025

The group supervision course is by case study. As of May 2022, there were 924 professionals who had participated in the introductory course. COVID-19 has slowed the increase in the numbers. All mental health professionals now know the IPT name, even if they have not received training in IPT.

Currently, IPT is widely used to treat depression, eating disorders, post-traumatic stress disorder, bipolar disorder, and more. Like the United States, it extends from adult outpatients to adolescents, couples, and patients with coexisting physical illnesses. It is also attracting attention as a powerful treatment for perinatal mental health. After establishing the IPT study group, Dr. Mizushima built the Japan chapter of the International Society of Interpersonal Psychotherapy (ISIPT), appointing several young experts from all over the country as board members and inviting core leaders in Japan's mental health as the board advisers. Currently, 8 members of the board with Dr. Mizushima as a president oversee dissemination, education, training, and research of IPT.

ADAPTATIONS OF IPT

The following adaptations to IPT have been made:

1. Many young people in Japan live with their parents even in their 20s. This tendency is increased in young people with mental illness. Therefore, we are actively introducing IPT for adolescents to these patients in their 20s and treating them with their parents. We find that the understanding and assistance of their parents is essential to the young person's progress.
2. In Japan, bullying has become a major social problem. Many patients have been bullied in the past. When treating these patients, 12 to 16 treatment sessions are often insufficient because of the complex trauma. Even after treatment ends, we continue to recontract another 12 to 16 sessions.
3. There are many cases in which autistic spectrum disorders and attention deficit hyperactivity disorder coexisted with the main complaint of mental illness. In such cases, in addition to psychoeducation for mental illnesses, it is necessary to conduct the psychoeducation of developmental characteristics and establish careful treatment alliances in the early stages. We are trying to double the number of early stage sessions for these patients.
4. In Japan, peer pressure at home, in the workplace, in communities, and in schools is problematic. We are required to follow not only explicit but also implicit rules to avoid disturbing the group's harmony. Especially since some Japanese family systems remain, we sometimes meet patients who live without saying what they want to say, prioritizing family harmony over their feelings. As a result, inadequate verbal communication often leads to increased role disputes and psychiatric

symptoms. Therefore, therapists need to carefully follow IPT treatment procedures to help patients learn effective verbal communication and resolve role disputes.

Finally, the stigma of mental illness persists in Japanese society. Psychoeducation for mental illness is sometimes rejected by not only patients but also their families. Working to deepen the understanding of mental illness in society will be a significant issue for us in the future.

There are few trainers or supervisors certified by ISIPT in Japan. Many Japanese do not speak or understand English and are reluctant to receive training in English abroad. Therefore, several Japanese senior therapists are currently applying for supervisors certified by ISIPT based on what they have learned at IPT-JAPAN and the biennial IPT workshops. As the next step, we plan to start creating a system for training therapists and supervisors in Japan using the group supervision course of IPT-JAPAN.

BARRIERS AND FACILITATORS OF IMPLEMENTATION

One of the barriers to implementing IPT is that the National Health Insurance Plan does not cover IPT. As a result, patients who wish to receive IPT must pay the total cost of medical treatment (30% payment if covered by the National Health Insurance Plan). Therefore, patients and providers (e.g., therapists in hospitals and clinics that provide National Health Insurance treatment) may hesitate to use IPT. This situation also deters the dissemination of IPT. In addition, if the therapists are not medical doctors, they are not officially permitted to perform medical procedures such as diagnosis and treatments, so a physician's direction is required. At least under the direction of medical doctors familiar with IPT, there is an opportunity for those who are not to conduct IPT.

On the other hand, we have established a system in which each of our board members nationwide serves as a consultant for the region for which they are responsible. We expect that they will contribute to the increase of IPT therapists and the dissemination of IPT by serving as a guide for beginners and specialists in each region who want to learn IPT in the future.

FUTURE PLANS

We aim to make IPT-JAPAN an official academic society, which can give points to maintain professional qualifications. The COVID-19 pandemic has postponed this plan, but we will resume after the pandemic has converged. At the conference of the new academic society, we will invite clinicians/researchers active in ISIPT to give lectures or hold workshops so that the content will be suitable for the Japan chapter of ISIPT.

CASE EXAMPLE

Ms. A, a woman in her 30s, came to the clinic with the chief complaint of binge eating and self-induced vomiting. She also had a depressed mood and lack of energy. She had been married for 4 years and had a 2-year-old child. She had worked as a caregiver in a nursing home but had left soon after becoming pregnant. Because her child had a congenital disease and required full-time care, she chose not to work after the birth and focused on housework and child care.

Her husband, a dentist, had been physically weak as a child, and his mother was quite overinvolved. Since she lived in the western part of Japan, which was far away from her son in Tokyo, her daily interference was done over the phone. That was already stressful enough for Ms. A, but when she visited Tokyo once during Ms. A's pregnancy, she criticized her: "You are feeding this stuff to my son!" Ms. A's husband didn't take her side, which hurt her. After that incident, Ms. A. began to feel depressed and to binge eat and vomit.

At the time of initial presentation, she met the *Diagnostic and Statistical Manual of Mental Disorders, Fourth Edition (DSM-IV)* criteria of major depressive disorder and bulimia nervosa. She also was increasingly consuming alcohol and just missed meeting criteria for alcohol abuse. She noted that binge eating and drinking were done to relieve her stress.

> I don't take my mother-in-law's phone calls any longer; I don't see her, so I'm not under any direct stress. But I feel guilty and also, I can't forgive my husband for taking my mother-in-law's side when she did something terrible to me. Also, I don't like my husband behaving like a 'medical professional.' When I talk to him about my child's illness, he only talks about medical data as a dentist, not as my husband. I don't feel like talking to him about anything. I don't want to divorce him because I must raise my child. It will work if we keep living separately in our house.

When the therapist recommended IPT as an effective treatment for both depression and an eating disorder, she said that she would like to get better, but did not want to undergo treatment to improve her relationship with her husband. When the therapist asked her if she was confident enough to raise a child in her current condition, she said she said she wanted to be healthy both physically and mentally for the sake of her child.

The therapist said: "IPT is a treatment for your depression and eating disorder, which will improve your relationships. The relationship with your husband may be one of the treatment focuses, but it is not the main objective." The patient agreed to focus on the disputes with her husband, which were at the impasse stage.

Although there were number of life events, such as the birth of a child with a congenital disease, the change from a full-time job to a stay-at-home mom, and the relationship with an overinvolved mother-in-law, the patient's current feelings of distrust toward her husband were the center of her stress. She decided to choose role disputes with her husband rather than transitions as a problem area.

During treatment, repeated communication analysis about disputes with her husband revealed that the nuances that Ms. A's thought she conveyed were not conveyed at all. It also became clear that Ms. A's expectation that her husband should lead the conversation if he were loving was unrealistic. It is also become clear that her husband was very vulnerable to blame. By discussing and implementing a communication style in which Ms. A leads the conversation and does not blame her husband, the couple's relationship improved significantly, and there were occasions when Ms. A thanked her husband. In addition, the couple was able to decide on a policy of not involving the overinvolved mother-in-law, with her husband acing as a liaison and only the husband returning to their home region for visits, when necessary.

Treatment was terminated at 16 sessions, and both depression and eating disorder were in remission, as confirmed by symptom scores. Drinking was also no longer a problem. At the 1-year follow-up, this state was maintained, and the couple expressed satisfaction with their relationship.

REFERENCES

1. Klerman GL, Weissman MM, Rounsaville BJ, et al. *Interpersonal Psychotherapy of Depression*. Basic Books; 1984. (Japanese version translated by H. Mizushima, M. Shimada, & Y. Ono. Iwasaki Academic Publisher; 1997.)
2. Mizushima H. *Series of Self-Help Books for Patients and Families of Depression, Bipolar Disorder, PTSD, Dysthymic Disorder, Social Anxiety Disorder, and IPT for Couples*. Sogensha; 2009–2011.
3. Mufson L, Dorta KP, Moreu D, Weissman MM. *Interpersonal Psychotherapy for Depressed Adolescents*. 2nd ed. Guilford Publication; 2004. (Japanese version translated by F. Suzuki and supervised by T. Nagata. Sogensha; 2016.)
4. Weissman MM, Markowitz JC, Klerman GL. *Comprehensive Guide to Interpersonal Psychotherapy*. Basic Books; 2000. (Japanese version was translated by Hiroko Mizushima. Iwasaki Academic Publisher, 2000).
5. Weissman MM, Markowitz JC, Klerman GL. *Clinician's Quick Guide to Interpersonal Psychotherapy*. Oxford University Press; 2007. (Japanese version translated by H. Mizushima. Sogensha; 2007.)
6. Wilfley DE, MacKenzie KR, Welch RR, Ayres VE, Weissman MM. *Interpersonal Psychotherapy for Group*. Basic Books; 2000. (Japanese version translated by H. Mizushima. Sogensha; 2006.)
7. Frank E. *Treating Bipolar Disorder: A Clinician's Guide to Interpersonal and Social Rhythm Therapy*. Guilford Press; 2005. (Japanese version translated by Y. Abe, K. Oga, & T. Shimoyama. Seiwa Shoten Publishers; 2016.)
8. Markowitz JC. *Interpersonal Psychotherapy for Posttraumatic Stress Disorder*. Oxford University Press; 2017. (Japanese version translated by T. Nakamori and supervised by H. Mizushima. Sogensha; 2019.)
9. Mizushima H. Efficacy study of interpersonal psychotherapy on Japanese bulimia nervosa women [in Japanese]. Health Labor Sciences Research Grant; 2010:76–82.

25

Interpersonal Psychotherapy for Refugees in Malaysia

XAVIER V. PEREIRA AND SHARUNA VERGHIS ■

INTRODUCTION

As cities in the developing world become destinations for about two-thirds of displaced people globally,[1] the Greater Kuala Lumpur area and other cities in Malaysia now host about 182,960 refugees and asylum seekers registered with the United Nations High Commissioner for Refugees (UNHCR).[2] However, owing to the lack of a legal and administrative framework for asylum and refugee protection, refugeehood in Malaysia is protracted and precarious related to ongoing vulnerability to arrest, whipping, detention, poor and abusive work conditions, extortion by local gangs, and xenophobia.[3–5] Healthcare access is fraught with economic barriers and the risk of arrest at public hospitals. Thus, premigration experiences of violence and loss and postmigration psychosocial impacts of fear, helplessness, and loss continue to be exacerbated during asylum.

HUMAN RIGHTS AND REFUGEE MENTAL HEALTH

Alongside discourses on civil and political rights, the ascendancy of trauma and post-traumatic stress disorder (PTSD) concepts since the 1970s provided a scientific framework to examine and assess the consequences of human rights violations experienced by refugees.[6] The Victorian Foundation for Survivors of Torture Trauma Recovery Framework[7] and the Adaptation and Development after Persecution and Trauma (ADAPT) model[8] are examples of conceptual frameworks that incorporate human rights violations in mental health interventions for refugees fleeing abusive and repressive contexts. Both models

Xavier V. Pereira and Sharuna Verghis, *Interpersonal Psychotherapy for Refugees in Malaysia* In: *Interpersonal Psychotherapy.* Edited by: Myrna M. Weissman and Jennifer J. Mootz, Oxford University Press. © Oxford University Press 2024. DOI: 10.1093/oso/9780197652084.003.0026 pay attention to the role of culture in understanding the experience of trauma and facilitating recovery. Similarly, the Mental Health and Psychosocial Support (MHPSS) interventional framework of the Inter-Agency Standing Committee (2007)[9] also recognized the psychological sequelae of human rights violations experienced by refugee populations and aims to address the infringements of rights via multilayer supports and services that seek to enhance safety, protection, and mental well-being for displaced people.

In tandem with these developments, the emerging salience of the right to health in the 1990s and 2000s focused on the neglected healthcare needs of disadvantaged populations like refugees and asylum seekers. Considering the suitability of interpersonal psychotherapy (IPT) for refugees,[10-12] expanding access to mental health interventions such as IPT with other psychotherapies would be an instrumental part of a right to health approach to recovery for refugees. Further, specialized mental health interventions like psychotherapy, including IPT, are included in the topmost layer of the MHPSS pyramid, which focuses on specialized services, with the other three layers in descending order being focused nonspecialized support, community and family supports, and basic services and security.[9]

HEALTH EQUITY INITIATIVES

Against this background, Health Equity Initiatives (HEI) is a nonprofit, nongovernmental organization in the Greater Kuala Lumpur area that provides mental health services using the MHPSS approach to address the mental health challenges of refugees and asylum seekers. HEI currently provides mental health services to around 350 patients from Afghanistan, Myanmar, Sri Lanka, Pakistan, and others, including Somalia, Sudan, Yemen, and Iraq. These patients have been diagnosed with mood disorders, anxiety disorders, psychotic disorders, trauma and stress-related disorders, somatic symptoms disorders, substance-related disorders, neurodevelopmental and neurocognitive disorders, and others. In its management of refugees with mental health challenges, HEI has found that it is critical to address the psychosocial needs of refugees before proceeding to use psychological and behavioral therapies, aligning with the literature highlighting the importance of psychosocial support in treatment adherence related to common mental health disorders, symptom reduction, and improved social functioning.[13-15] Thus, an adaptation of IPT for refugees should include addressing the psychosocial needs of these refugees before proceeding to apply IPT for depression and PTSD.

CASE STUDIES OF REFUGEES WHO HAVE RECEIVED IPT

The case studies in this chapter have been selected from those who received IPT in HEI's mental health services.

Case study 25.1

Ms. M. K., a young woman from a West Asian country, sought treatment at HEI. She was diagnosed as having moderate major depressive disorder, moderate generalized anxiety disorder, and PTSD according to validated psychometric measures and the clinical criteria of the *Diagnostic and Statistical Manual of Mental Disorders, Fifth Edition* (DSM-5).[16]

She, her mother, and her elder sister had fled her home country for Malaysia because of threats from her maternal uncle. Her uncle wanted to forcibly marry her widowed mother and her elder sister to men of his choice. He physically and verbally abused M. K.'s mother. The civil war in her home country had begun in early 2015. M. K. heard and felt bombs exploding close to the house, which terrified her. It became unsafe to venture out of her home. Water and electricity supply was often disrupted. M. K., her mother, and her sister fled home with a day's notice. They had to take 3 flights before arriving in Malaysia. M. K. said that they were very nervous because they feared that her uncle might catch up with them.

Against this background, arriving in Malaysia was a relief for them. They felt safe and enjoyed good amenities. They initially had challenges transitioning to Malaysia. They lived in cramped living quarters, all 3 living in a rented room. They had financial challenges, and M. K. had difficulty resuming school. These challenges were addressed over a period of time. M. K. received a scholarship to a private school. All 3 are currently working. This has allowed them to rent a 3-bedroom apartment. They have rented 1 room to another refugee and are thus able to defray some of the rental expense. At HEI, she has been prescribed an antidepressant and a benzodiazepine. When she did not improve, IPT was offered to her.

The IPT problem areas identified for Ms. M. K. were *interpersonal conflict* with her uncle, who was threatening her, and *grief and loss* on the death of her maternal grandmother in her home country. Her Interpersonal Inventory revealed that her support was from her mother, her sister, two friends who had been her classmates in school, and the patient manager of HEI. M. K.'s attachment style was ascertained to be anxious-avoidant.

The interpersonal threat from MK's uncle, who threatened to kill all 3 women, was addressed individually with M. K. and in a joint session with M. K.'s mother. It was concluded that it was unlikely that M. K.'s uncle would be able to carry out his threat in Malaysia. This reassured M. K. and reduced her anxiety.

The death of her grandmother in her home country filled M. K. with guilt and self-blame. She felt that her grandmother was harassed by her uncle because of her, and that this constant harassment had contributed to her grandmother's death. The complicated grief she was experiencing was addressed utilizing an adaptation of faith and religion. She found that being a Muslim helped address the grief she was experiencing. Reading verses from the Quran and praying to God assisted her in coping with the loss of her grandmother. During therapy, her faith helped her conclude that her grandmother was in heaven and thus was in a better place. She also cherished her grandmother, who was always nice, kind, and generous and was always there for her and protected her from her uncle. Thus, M. K. firmly believed her grandmother deserved to be in heaven. Talking about her grandmother in the light of faith reduced her psychological pain and feelings of loss, guilt, and self-blame. M. K. added that this was the first time she had talked about her grandmother's death in detail and the loss she had experienced. The therapy sessions made her grandmother's death "real" because she previously felt that her grandmother's death was "unreal" as she could not view her grandmother's remains.

At the end of 8 sessions of IPT, M. K.'s depression was minimal and anxiety was mild. The gains that she had made in IPT were that she was able to express her thoughts and feelings without being judged, she was able to reduce self-blame related to her grandmother's death, her mood had improved, and she was able to function independently and with greater self-competence. Monthly maintenance IPT sessions were agreed on.

Case study 25.2

K. Y. was a married lady in her 40s displaced from a neighboring Southeast Asian country. She sought help from HEI for anxiety and depression. She was diagnosed to have moderate depression and mild anxiety according to *DSM-5*, clinical criteria, and validated psychometric measures. K. Y. had fled her home country in Southeast Asia because of threats to her life and well-being. There was a civil war between the national armed forces and the local resistance army in her home state. She was smuggled over land. The migration journey was fraught with much difficulty and danger. She was relieved when she reached Malaysia safely.

The IPT problem areas identified in her were *difficult transitions* and *complicated grief.*

She had arrived in Malaysia in 2008, about 13 years ago, and she was yet to be resettled in a third country. She had watched her friends, who had arrived in Malaysia after her, be resettled. This had affected her mood, and she lacked hope that she would be relocated. She had lost her mother in Malaysia. She had provided care for her mother but felt that she could have done more. Thus, she felt guilty and blamed herself.

The transition to living in Malaysia as a refugee was initially suitable for her but became increasingly difficult as time passed. She said that her freedom was suppressed, and she lived with the constant fear that she might be arrested and detained by the Malaysian police. She said that she was treated like an illegal migrant and was not allowed to open a bank account, and this troubled her because she could not keep money in the bank for safekeeping.

Her interpersonal inventory revealed that although she shared a close relationship with her spouse, her primary sources of support were her sister and two friends, who she felt understood her better as women. Her attachment style was discussed. She had secure attachment in her close relationships and was anxious-avoidant in other relationships.

During the therapy sessions, she identified two timelines resulting in transitions. The first was when she arrived in Malaysia in March 2008, and the second was when the restrictions resulting from the COVID-19 pandemic were implemented in March 2020. On inquiry, she said that this episode of depression was attributed to the March 2020 transition, but the issues of the earlier change continued to bear heavily on her.

Her responsibility to implement COVID control strategies of masking and physical distancing at the workplace brought criticism and resistance from peers. Moreover, transitioning to online modes of work exacerbated the pressure of resource constraints brought about by the need for connectivity and devices. She said that her passion for her work had decreased during this period.

She would also avoid attending farewell parties for her community members who were being resettled because of unpleasant thoughts and emotions that were stirred in her to remind her that she was yet to receive news of resettlement. She added that the therapy sessions had allowed her to discuss these issues openly and without being judged. This helped her feel better.

The technique utilized to address her transitions was identifying the two timelines and discussing the changes in each transition. The positives of these transitions were emphasized: a safer environment in Malaysia, the opportunity to do meaningful work to serve others, and the support from her sister, friends, and ethnic community. She also resorted to her faith in God and rationalized that the consequences of the transitions were God's will for her.

K. Y. also wanted to discuss the grief that she was experiencing at the loss of her mother. She acknowledged the loss of her mother, a family and community leader who gradually became dependent on others. The family and community had lost a kind and generous person. Most of her family and community members respected and loved her mother. She felt guilty that she could not do more for her mother and should have spent more time with her. She was relieved that her mother's passing was peaceful. She said she also felt relieved that no one blamed her for her mother's death. Her family and community members said it was her mother's "time to go." She also received support from her community to transport her mother's remains to her home village for burial.

In the next session, we continued to discuss her grief. She acknowledged the loss of her mother. She said that even though her mother had passed away, she felt her mother was still with her. Staying in the same room reminded her of her mother. Sometimes she would talk to her mother as if her mother was still with her. She used to feel lonely and was able to fill her loneliness with work and the presence of her colleagues and students.

She held a faith perspective on her mother's death. She believed her mother had returned to God. This belief consoled her. The structure of the IPT sessions for K. Y. was 2 initial sessions, 7 middle sessions, and 1 terminal session. Monthly maintenance sessions were agreed on at the end of the tenth session.

In the final session, we reviewed her gains in therapy. The gains were the opportunity to talk openly about her transitions and her grief in a safe and non-judgmental space, and she was also able to avail of support within the extended therapeutic relationship (therapist and HEI patient manager) and outside of therapy (her sister and her two colleagues). At the end of 10 sessions, she had psychometric scores indicating mild depression and minimal anxiety.

DISCUSSION

Despite IPT being effective for the refugees in Case Study 25.1 and Case Study 25.2, it is challenging to do IPT with refugees who have experienced multiple traumatic experiences, sexual- and gender-based violence (SGBV), and severe ongoing stressors. IPT is relevant for treating refugees with depression because it can address problem areas typical of refugees.[17] Some of the problem areas distinct for refugees and the following adaptations are discussed here.

The migration journey

In our work with refugees, our initial assessment includes exploring the refugee's migration journey. Entry into Malaysia is by air, sea, or land. The migration experiences over sea and land are often stressful, traumatic, and fraught with difficulties and adversities. Asylum seekers from Myanmar are often smuggled into Malaysia via Thailand by land. Rohingya refugees are known to have traveled a treacherous journey by sea.[18] Arrest and detention can occur in a transit country like Thailand or Indonesia, and this experience can be very stressful and traumatic, resulting in depression, anxiety, and PTSD. Thus, an adaptation of IPT for refugees who live in Malaysia would need to address the migration journey.

Transitions

The migration from the country of origin to a transit country like Malaysia is a significant transition because of multiple transit journeys. In the past, Afghan asylum seekers of Hazara ethnicity would initially migrate to Iran because of similarities in language and religion. They then would migrate to Malaysia directly or via Indonesia. Afghan refugees are also known to arrive in Malaysia via India.

Refugees find living in Malaysia difficult. Although Kuala Lumpur has a UNHCR office, Malaysia is not a signatory of the 1951 Refugee Convention or its 1967 Protocol. This limits opportunities for work for adult refugees and education for children.

The most common role transition for married refugee men is the difficulty or inability to provide for the family. Refugees are not allowed to work formally;

thus, much stress is experienced because of a lack of steady income to support themselves and their families. This also poses a challenge for refugees who are single mothers. They need to be gainfully employed to provide for their families. Teenagers and young adults have limited access to formal education and thus cannot enter tertiary educational institutions. This becomes a stressor for not only the young adult but also the parents of these young people.

Safety and security become an issue in this transition to living in Malaysia. Since the Malaysian government does not recognize refugee status, a refugee in Malaysia is under constant threat of arrest and detention by the Malaysian police and Malaysian immigration. This precarity of refugee life in Malaysia was exacerbated during COVID-19 when they lost jobs, experienced housing and food insecurity, and had to endure ongoing mobility restrictions and lockdowns.[19] The psychosocial needs that arise as a result of forced migration, and thus the transition of migration, must be addressed as an adaptation of IPT for refugees.

Grief and loss

Refugees suffer much loss. They often lose everything they possess when they are forcibly displaced. The loss of loved ones is also a common experience for refugees. Afghan Hazara refugees have witnessed the murder of relatives. Myanmar refugees have experienced losing their family members at the hands of military personnel. Sri Lankan Tamil refugees have experienced the disappearance of family members.

Complicated grief is a common experience for refugees. The inability to be at the dying relative's side, attend the dead relative's funeral, or bury the deceased relative contribute to complicated grief. Our experience doing IPT with refugees shows that discussing the loss of loved ones in a safe and nonjudgmental environment contributes to healing.

Interpersonal disputes/conflicts

Some refugees experience family conflicts in their home country and face threats to their lives and well-being. There are refugee women who are forced to marry a man of the family's choice. Some Afghan and Yemeni women refugees have fled their home country because they disagree with this spouse choice. This becomes an issue of family honor, and these women are threatened with death.

Domestic violence is also prevalent among refugees. Some refugee men abuse their partners or spouses physically and verbally. SGBV is commonplace in not only families of refugees but also their ethnic communities. Conflict with the government and the Army has been the experience of ethnic Kachin, Shan, and Rohingya in Myanmar. It used to be an issue for Sri Lankan Tamil refugees until 2015. The most severe interpersonal trauma experienced by refugees includes abuse and torture in detention. It is very challenging to treat these victims of abuse and torture, including trying to treat them with IPT.

Trust and the therapeutic relationship

Many refugees have difficulty trusting others. The therapeutic relationship in IPT allows the refugee patient to build trust again. The refugees who have undergone IPT have listed a confidential, trusting, and nonjudgmental therapeutic environment as one of their favorable experiences in therapy. This allows healing to take place in the therapeutic relationship. The therapeutic relationship is also a relationship that contributes to more secure attachment styles for the refugee patient.

Adaptations of faith, religion, and religious community support in treating refugees with IPT

Many of the refugees in Malaysia are people who profess faith in God and are affiliated with a particular religion. Many are also persecuted because of the faith they profess. In treating refugee patients with IPT, some patients include God in the Interpersonal Inventory. Many refugees have been waiting for years to be resettled, and hope can be eroded. Trusting in God helps instill hope. It has been found that the faith communities provide social and material support for refugees, especially Christians and Muslims. Shared prayer and communitarian sharing from religious books have been used as adaptations in IPT treatment of refugees and the local population who profess faith in God and belong to a religious community.[20]

CONCLUSION: ADAPTATIONS AND TRAINING—IPT FOR DISPLACED PEOPLE

Adaptations of IPT for the refugee population are not new. The adaptations and training of Verdeli et al., who implemented group IPT for depressed youth in internally displaced people camps in Northern Uganda, were groundbreaking in addressing a specific refugee population in Uganda.[21] In collaboration with Schultz et al., Verdeli and colleagues also developed an adapted stepped-care brief IPT intervention for psychologically distressed women displaced by conflict in Bogota, Columbia.[22] Susan Meffert and associates successfully carried out a randomized pilot trial of IPT for Sudanese refugees in Cairo, Egypt.[11]

The case studies in this chapter, based in an Asian upper-middle income country, add to the existing work of adapting IPT for refugee populations in a different geographical and refugee protection context and demonstrate the suitability and fruitfulness of IPT for this population. However, as the context of flight, asylum, and durable solutions vary across the globe, the adaptation of IPT for this population would require context specificity.

REFERENCES

1. United Nations High Commissioner for Refugees (UNHCR). Global trends. Forced displacement in 2018: United Nations High Commissioner for Refugees. 2021. https://www.unhcr.org/62a9d1494/global-trends-report-2021. Accessed July 7, 2022.

2. United Nations High Commissioner for Refugees (UNHCR). Figures at a glance in Malaysia Kuala Lumpur. 2022. https://www.unhcr.org/en-my/figures-at-a-glance-in-malaysia.html. Accessed July 7, 2022.

3. Hoffstaedter G, Missbach A. Facilitating irregular migration into Malaysia and from Indonesia: illicit markets, endemic corruption and symbolic attempts to overcome impunity. *Public Anthropologist.* 2021;3(1):8–31.

4. Nungsari M, Flanders S, Chuah H-Y. Poverty and precarious employment: the case of Rohingya refugee construction workers in Peninsular Malaysia. *Hum Soc Sci Commun.* 2020;7(1):120.

5. Togoo R, Ismail F. Security dilemma of Rohingya refugees in Malaysia. *Open J Polit Sci.* 2021;11:12–20.

6. Steel Z, Steel CR, Silove D. Human rights and the trauma model: genuine partners or uneasy allies? *J Trauma Stress.* 2009;22(5):358–365.

7. Kaplan I. *Rebuilding Shattered Lives: Integrated Trauma Recovery for People of Refugee Background.* 2nd ed. Victorian Foundation for Survivors of Torture (Foundation House); 2020.

8. Silove DM. The ADAPT model: a conceptual framework for mental health and psychosocial programming in post conflict settings. *Intervention.* 2013;11:237–248.

9. Inter-Agency Standing Committee. *IASC Guidelines on Mental Health and Psychosocial Support in Emergency Settings.* IASC; 2007. https://interagencyst andingcommittee.org/system/files/2020-11/IASC%20Guidelines%20on%20Men tal%20Health%20and%20Psychosocial%20Support%20in%20Emergency%20Setti ngs%20%28English%29.pdf. Accessed July 7, 2022.

10. Bolton P, Bass J, Neugebauer R, et al. Group interpersonal psychotherapy for depression in rural Uganda: a randomized controlled trial. *JAMA.* 2003;289(23):3117–3124.

11. Meffert SM, Abdo AO, Alla OAA, et al. A pilot randomized controlled trial of interpersonal psychotherapy for Sudanese refugees in Cairo, Egypt. *Psychol Trauma.* 2014;6(3):240–249.

12. Murray KE, Davidson GR, Schweitzer RD. Review of refugee mental health interventions following resettlement: best practices and recommendations. *Am J Orthopsychiatry.* 2010;80(4):576–585.

13. Depp CA, Moore DJ, Patterson TL, Lebowitz BD, Jeste DV. Psychosocial interventions and medication adherence in bipolar disorder. *Dialogues Clin Neurosci.* 2008;10(2):239–250.

14. Tarrier N, Bobes J. The importance of psychosocial interventions and patient involvement in the treatment of schizophrenia. *Int J Psychiatry Clin Pract.* 2000;4(1):35–51.

15. Kohrt BA, Song SJ. Who benefits from psychosocial support interventions in humanitarian settings? *Lancet Glob Health.* 2018;6(4):e354–e356.

16. American Psychiatric Association. *Diagnostic and Statistical Manual of Mental Disorders.* 5th ed. American Psychiatric Association; 2013.

17. Pereira X, Yong A. Interpersonal psychotherapy for depressed refugees. Poster presentation at: 6th ISIPT Conference; 2013; London.

18. Pereira X, Verghis S, Cheng KH, Ahmed AB, Nagiah S, Fernandez L. Mental health of Rohingya refugees and asylum seekers: case studies from Malaysia. *Intervention.* 2019;17(2):181–186.

19. Verghis S, Pereira X, Kumar AG, Koh A, Singh-Lim A. COVID-19 and refugees in Malaysia: an NGO response. *Intervention.* 2020;19(1):15–20.

20. Stuart S, Pereira XV, Chung JP-Y. Transcultural adaptation of interpersonal psychotherapy in Asia. *Asia-Pacific Psychiatry.* 2021;13(1):e12439.

21. Verdeli H, Clougherty K, Onyango G, et al. Group interpersonal psychotherapy for depressed youth in IDP camps in Northern Uganda: adaptation and training. *Child Adolesc Psychiatr Clin N Am.* 2008;17(3):605–624.

22. Shultz JM, Verdeli H, Gómez Ceballos Á, et al. A pilot study of a stepped-care brief intervention to help psychologically-distressed women displaced by conflict in Bogotá, Colombia. *Glob Ment Health (Camb).* 2019;6:e28.

26

Group Interpersonal Psychotherapy for Adolescents in Nepal

INDIRA PRADHAN, KELLY ROSE-CLARKE, HELEN VERDELI, AND PRAGYA SHRESTHA ∎

THE NEPALI CONTEXT

Nepal is a South Asian lower middle-income country with a population of over 30 million.[1] Owing to 10 years of government-Maoist conflict (1996–2006), 2 devastating earthquakes (2015), and annual flooding and landslides, the need for mental health care is significant and largely unmet. Transcultural Psychosocial Organization Nepal has been working for the past 17 years to try to fill this gap in mental health care.[2] Our recent work has focused on adolescent mental health because of the opportunity to alleviate suffering in these formative years and prevent morbidity later in their lives.

In collaboration with King's College London and Columbia University, we adapted and tested the feasibility of delivering interpersonal therapy (IPT) to adolescents with depression in Nepal. We used the World Health Organization *Group IPT Manual* as a starting point because it was designed for nonspecialist health workers in low-resource settings such as Nepal.[3] We adapted the manual based on evidence from formative research (25 qualitative interviews with boys and girls aged 13–18 with depression; 4 focus group discussions with adolescents, 4 with parents/caregivers, and 2 with teachers; 6 interviews with community health workers; and one interview with a representative from a local nongovernmental organization, a total of 126 participants). We also received feedback from IPT trainers, facilitators, participants, and a youth mental health advisory board.

Indira Pradhan, Kelly Rose-Clarke, Helen Verdeli, and Pragya Shrestha, *Group Interpersonal Psychotherapy for Adolescents in Nepal* In: *Interpersonal Psychotherapy.* Edited by: Myrna M. Weissman and Jennifer J. Mootz, Oxford University Press.
© Oxford University Press 2024. DOI: 10.1093/oso/9780197652084.003.0027

Our study site was Sindhupalchowk, a remote mountainous district of 300,000 people. Agriculture is the main source of income, along with remittances from labor migrants. More than half the population is Hindu (59.0%); 38% are Buddhist. Society is stratified according to caste/ethnic group: Brahman (10.3%), Newar (11.1%), and Chhetri (18.2%) are the most privileged, followed by Tamang (34.3%) and the least privileged Dalit groups (7.4%).[4] Some 95% of children are enrolled in primary school, but enrollment in upper secondary education (43%) drops substantially as adolescents marry and take up paid work.[5]

NEEDS OF ADAPTATIONS IN IPT FOR ADOLESCENTS IN NEPAL

The adaptation was guided by the ecological validity framework,[6] and we made adaptations related to the following domains: *context* (the intervention environment), *persons* (the therapeutic relationship), *treatment goals*, *methods* (how goals are achieved), *concepts* (cultural and contextual concepts of treatment), *language*, *metaphors* (symbols and sayings), *content* (cultural knowledge), and *developmental stage*.[6] We tested the feasibility of the intervention among 62 adolescents aged 13–19. Examples of adaptations in each domain of the framework are provided below.

Methods

Our intervention comprised 2 individual pregroup and 12 group meetings. In the first pregroup meeting, the group facilitator met with the adolescent to explore the history of depression and key relationships, identify the problem area, and link it to the adolescent's depressive symptoms. The second pregroup meeting involved parents and aimed to mobilize family support. We extended the overall number of sessions from 8 to 12 because adolescents did not feel comfortable opening up until the fourth session. Group meetings were held weekly for around 90 minutes during school lunch break, free periods, or before or after school.

Context

We integrated IPT into the education system because community members explicitly mentioned that they would only trust an intervention if it was delivered through schools. We ran separate groups for girls and boys because adolescents said they would be embarrassed to talk in front of the other gender.

Persons

We recruited nurses to facilitate IPT because of a government policy to employ a nurse in each secondary school. Adolescents told us they wanted a facilitator of the same gender, but most nurses in Nepal are female. We therefore recruited male facilitators from the local community.

Goals

In the manual, we clarified the aims of each phase of group sessions.

Concepts

We moved away from the concept of the "sick role" toward a "recovery role" (i.e., shifting from "I cannot do anything because of my sickness" to "I can do things despite my sickness").

Adolescents had difficulty expressing their emotions, so we introduced a game called inside/outside feelings (*Bhitri-Bahiri Bhawana*), where each group member drew a face showing their true inner feelings and another showing the feelings they project to others (Figure 26.1). The cultural expectation in Nepal is for the children to show a happy face. This technique helped the teens differentiate the public display of their affect from their internal states.

Facilitators struggled to understand social isolation as a problem area, so we provided locally relevant examples, such as adolescents from the Dalit caste or a minority religion being socially excluded by their peers. It helped the facilitators to understand the nature of isolation whether it is because of social structure or the rest of the problem area. It was helpful to find the resources to reduce the symptoms and case management.

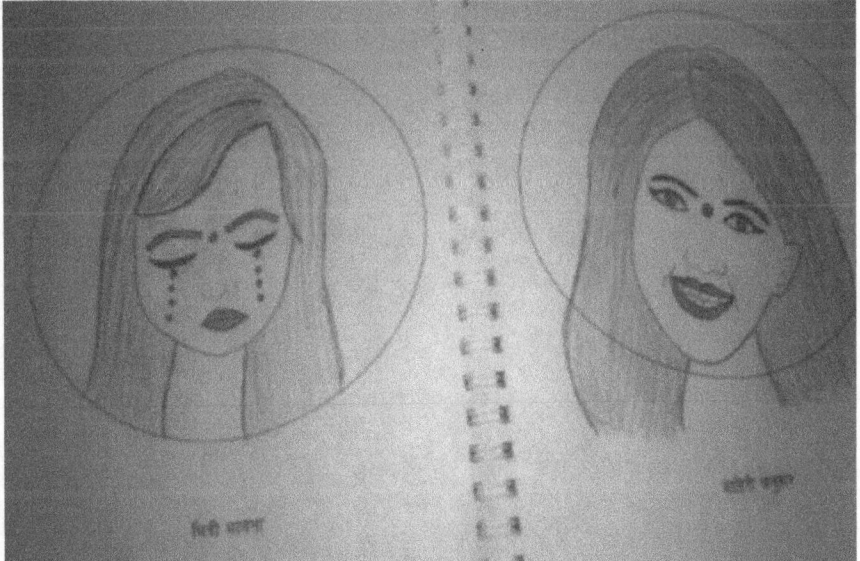

Figure 26.1 Inside/outside feelings.
CREDIT: Copyright of TPO Nepal in the sketch. Received permission to publish this picture.

Language

Informed by our formative research and Nepali ethnopsychological literature,[7,8] we used the term *manko samasya* (meaning "heart-mind problem") to refer to mental health problems, and *udas-chinta* ("sadness-worry") to refer specifically to depression as one type of heart-mind problem.

Metaphors and content

We added content to the manual to make it more relevant to the lives of local people. For example, we described how depression "gets in the way of working on the farm" and makes it difficult "to do your household work." Adolescents participating in our formative work told us the intervention had to be fun, so we included games and activities. Each session started with the activity "Share a talent" (*Prativa Dekhaune Kriyakalap*), where members of the group took turns telling jokes and stories, dancing, or singing.

Developmental stage

Adolescents were given a "friend diary" (*Saathi Dainiki*) (Figure 26.2) and asked to bring it to each session. The diary was a place for adolescents to record their progress and write helpful information and advice, dates of the sessions, and

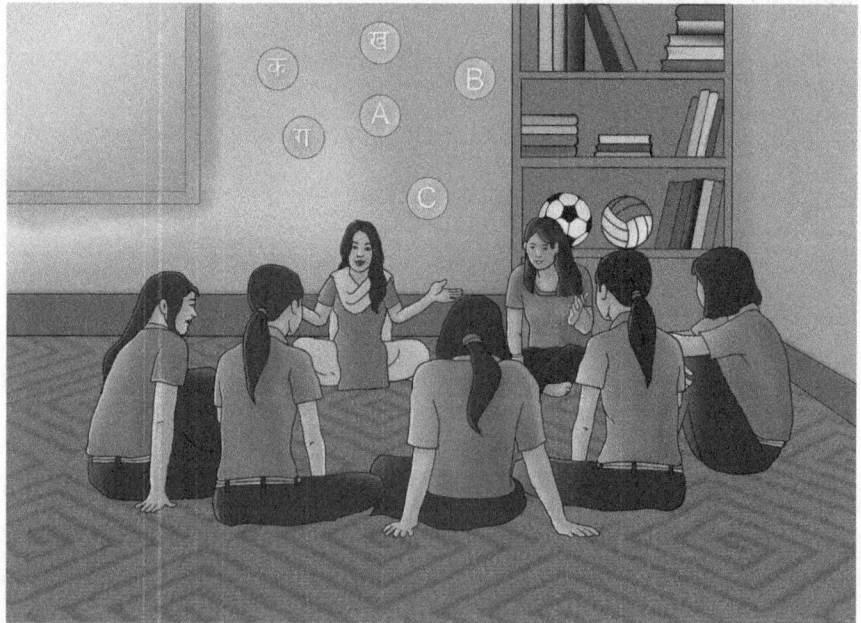

Figure 26.2 Friend diary.
CREDIT: Copyright of TPO Nepal in the sketch. Received permission to publish this picture.

contact details of local health and social organizations. We provided pens and stickers and encouraged adolescents to be creative and personalize their diaries.

TRAINING AND SUPERVISION RELATED TO THE INTERVENTION

Training supervisors

Prior to our study, there were no IPT supervisors in Nepal. Led by master trainers Dr. Helen Verdeli and Ms. Kathleen Clougherty, supervisor training comprised an 8-hour virtual workshop on the theory behind IPT and 4 days of in-person training to build knowledge and skills. A knowledge test was administered the week after the training (a passing grade was 75%). After the training workshop, the supervisors facilitated IPT with individuals and groups and received supervision by master trainers to build their confidence and experience.

Training facilitators

We trained 9 individuals (3 male and 6 female), none of whom had experience in mental health treatment. Three were nurses, and the others were from the local community with a high school education. First, facilitators completed a 10-day curriculum to build their knowledge about mental health problems, communication and group management skills, confidence working with family and managing child protection issues (e.g., domestic and gender-based violence, and suicide), and case management. Next, facilitators attended a didactic training workshop using the IPT manual, completed an IPT knowledge test, and practiced IPT with a small group of adolescents. In these practice groups, facilitators learned how to apply their IPT knowledge and skills and built confidence using basic helping skills. The size of the group was limited to around 4 adolescents, so facilitators could focus on practicing IPT rather than group management skills.

Before and after training, supervisors assessed facilitator competency with the ENhancing Assessment of Common Therapeutic factors (ENACT) rating scale, the Working with children—Assessment of Competencies Tool (WeACT),[9,10] and standardized lists of session-specific IPT tasks. Based on these assessments, we selected the best 6 facilitators (3 females and 3 males) from the 9 individuals we had trained. These facilitators demonstrated a good ability to work in teams and proactive behavior and skills in social engagement, which were felt to be key ingredients for facilitating groups.

Supervising facilitators

Facilitators required support to apply IPT knowledge and skills and initially found it difficult to understand participants' needs and help them find the way to recovery. Supervisors engaged facilitators in a process of review and reflection through various supervision activities: (1) group supervision where facilitators participated together to share, learn, and practice new skills; (2) distance individual weekly supervision (via phone and Skype or Viber) with each facilitator, focusing on challenges facilitators had faced during sessions; (3) on-site supervision to observe the group process, assess and feedback on facilitators' competency, and provide on-the-spot feedback and support; and (4) peer supervision where facilitators encouraged and supported each other, validated their IPT skills, and brainstormed ideas. Supervisors were based in Kathmandu and regularly traveled to the study site. Supervisors received weekly remote supervision from master trainers.

Facilitators were distressed by some of the cases they were managing, especially those involving suicidality and parental abuse. We therefore integrated psychosocial support for facilitators into the supervision activities. We encouraged facilitators to be creative and draw on their own local cultural knowledge to understand adolescents' problems and identify potential solutions.

MAJOR BARRIERS AND FACILITATORS OF IMPLEMENTATION

Involving caregivers

In the formative research, adolescents told us that parents would be reluctant to allow them to attend groups because the parents perceived household chores, paid work, and studying to be adolescents' priorities. While adolescents told us that they did not want to formally involve their parents in IPT groups, they advised us to meet with parents to explain the intervention and obtain their permission. In pregroup session 2, facilitators therefore visited adolescents' homes to speak with the adolescent and their family. This was felt to be an effective way to build rapport, learn more about the adolescent, and mobilize family support.

Stigma

In the community, we encountered discrimination against people with mental health problems, who were referred to as *Pagal* ("crazy"), *Saiko* ("psycho"), and "mental." In the intervention, we mitigated stigma in several ways. We used the idiom of distress *manko samasya* because this is a socially acceptable condition and reason for seeking treatment. Supervisors and facilitators ran orientation sessions in schools for teachers and students and worked closely with school leads. IPT was conceptualized as training in interpersonal skills, rather than a psychological therapy. Facilitators emphasized the potential functional benefits of IPT to parents, teachers, and adolescents, including improvements in family relations and engagement in school. A group-based delivery approach enabled adolescents to form close-knit peer groups that supported individuals in and out of IPT meetings. Facilitators emphasized and explained the importance of confidentiality to adolescents and their parents. Confidentiality was also a key topic in facilitator training. Meetings took place in quiet, private rooms in schools where adolescents felt comfortable and safe. The intervention embodied a rights-based approach where facilitators ensured each adolescent was listened to and valued and made to feel comfortable and able to share and trust other group members.

Managing child protection issues and suicidality

We looked for mental health (trained health professionals) and child protection services (shelters, nongovernmental organizations) in the study setting, but they were limited. We therefore developed safety protocols for facilitators to ensure appropriate, feasible, and timely support that engaged clinical supervisors, a psychosocial counselor (employed through the project and based in the study location), and family members, teachers, and friends as required.

Effects of the COVID-19 pandemic

Lockdown restrictions in early 2020 put a stop to face-to-face group meetings. This forced us to test the feasibility of individual phone-based meetings in sessions 9 to 11. These meetings were surprisingly well accepted by adolescents, especially among those who were too shy to share in earlier group meetings. Research is therefore needed to further explore the feasibility of a hybrid delivery model.

Scheduling meetings

In Sindhupalchowk, adolescents often walk for more than an hour to reach school. Due to concerns about safety, girls were reluctant to travel without their friends, especially in the evening, so it was difficult for them to attend IPT meetings after school. During school time, lessons were prioritized, and adolescents had limited free time. We therefore organized meetings according to the group members' needs. Most meetings were held in the morning before school, some were during the day, and a few were on Friday afternoons when school finishes at lunchtime.

FUTURE PLANS AND RECOMMENDATIONS

We have secured funding to evaluate our intervention through a randomized controlled trial where we will explore the overall effects of IPT on depression, as well as mediators and moderators. Informed by data from the feasibility study that showed that improvements in adolescent mental health happened early in the intervention, and that attendance dropped off in later meetings, we intend to reduce the number of group meetings to 9 or 10. The trial will help to consolidate IPT capacity in Nepal by training additional trainers and facilitators, refining manual and training materials, and raising the profile of IPT with a view to integrating techniques and skills into existing national mental health training programs.

Based on our experience, key recommendations for future work in Nepal are as follows:

1. A standardized IPT trainer's manual and supervision model to promote consistency and quality delivery.
2. A separate counseling provision for parents with mental health problems—adolescent depression was often linked to parental mental health in our study, but there were no local services for parents.
3. School-based psychoeducation to mitigate stigma or discrimination toward adolescents with mental health problems.

CASE EXAMPLE

The following case study illustrates how group IPT was used to address grief in an adolescent boy with depression. Details have been removed or changed to ensure participant anonymity.

Orientation and pre-group phase

X lives with his father, mother and grandmother. He attends the local school. In the first pregroup meeting, X shared his manko samasya with the facilitator. He felt lonely after his sister died in the 2015 earthquake. In the days following her death, X had felt extreme sadness, helplessness, and guilt that he had survived the earthquake, but his sister had not. He planned to die by suicide but convinced himself that this was not a good way to be reunited with his sister. A year later, X had a dispute that led to him being excluded from his friendship group. He felt lonely and struggled to concentrate on his studies. He attempted suicide by hanging himself, but his mother found him and stopped him. Over the following 2 years, he increasingly isolated himself from friends and family. His attendance at school dropped, and his grades suffered. He mostly spent his time alone at home, using his father's phone to watch videos.

After listening to his story, the facilitator explained to X that many of the feelings he was experiencing were a normal part of the grieving process and gave him hope that things would get better. The facilitator encouraged X to share memories of his sister and to think about what he would like to change moving forward. X wished to reduce the extent to which grief impacted his daily life. The facilitator helped him to plan to manage his suicidal thoughts and to identify key supportive people such as his mother and a cousin who lived locally.

In pregroup meeting 2, the facilitator met X and his mother to clarify the aims and potential benefits of IPT and to obtain consent and support from the family.

Initial and middle group phases

X joined a group with other boys from his school. The facilitator began the first meeting by outlining the aims of IPT, introducing each of the adolescents, and reminding them about the need to respect each other, and the importance of maintaining confidentiality outside meetings. The facilitator encouraged X to talk to the group about his sister and the problems he was facing with his friends. Group members made suggestions to help with his schoolwork, including studying in a group and taking regular study breaks for relaxation.

The facilitator helped X to mourn his sister. X wrote a poem about her and read it to group members, who praised his talent and effort. They suggested other ways he might safely express his grief, such as singing and sharing his sorrow with his family. After the fourth meeting, X's mood started to improve, which he attributed to the new ways he had learned to cope with his sister's death. In later meetings, the facilitator encouraged him to use interpersonal skills to improve his loneliness, build confidence at school and in his studies, and improve relationships with his relatives.

Termination phase

In the last meeting, the facilitator reviewed group members' individual progress. X identified possible warning signs that could indicate his mood was worsening, and he worked with the facilitator to develop a plan to manage this. His future goal was to strengthen the friendships he had made with other group members so that they could continue to support each other. He no longer felt disturbed by grief and was able to focus on his studies. He had no suicidal ideation and felt ready to make new friends.

REFERENCES

1. Chaulagain TR. Population and households characteristics. *Cent Bur Stat*. 2021:7–8.
2. Introduction—TPO Nepal. https://www.tponepal.org/indroduction/. Accessed October 6, 2022.
3. World Health Organization. *Group Interpersonal Therapy (IPT) for Depression*. World Health Organization; 2016. http://apps.who.int/iris/bitstream/handle/10665/250219/WHO-MSD-MER-16.4-eng.pdf;jsessionid=713E2FF0ECC3B042136E1C3F33910A75?sequence=1. Accessed October 6, 2022.
4. National Statistics Office. *National Population and Housing Census 2011 (National Report)*. Government of Nepal; 2012.

5. Relief Web. *Sindhupalchok Gender Profile*. UN Women. Published online 2016. https://reliefweb.int/report/nepal/sindhupalchok-gender-profile-august-2016. Accessed October 6, 2022.

6. Rose-Clarke K, Pradhan I, Shrestha P, et al. Culturally and developmentally adapting group interpersonal therapy for adolescents with depression in rural Nepal. *BMC Psychol*. 2020;8(1):1–15.

7. Kohrt BA, Maharjan SM, Timsina D, Griffith JL. Applying Nepali ethnopsychology to psychotherapy for the treatment of mental illness and prevention of suicide among bhutanese refugees. *Ann Anthropol Pract*. 2012;36(1):88–112.

8. Pylayeva-Gupta Y, Kelsey C, Ho MV, Lee J-A. KCM 基因的改变NIH Public Access. *Bone*. 2012;23(1):1–7.

9. Kohrt BA, Jordans MJD, Rai S, et al. Therapist competence in global mental health: Development of the ENhancing Assessment of Common Therapeutic factors (ENACT) rating scale. *Behav Res Ther*. 2015;69:11–21.

10. Jordans MJ, Coetzee A, Steen HF, et al. Assessment of service provider competency for child and adolescent psychological treatments and psychosocial services in global mental health: evaluation of feasibility and reliability of the WeACT tool in Gaza, Palestine. *Global Ment Health*. 2021;8:e7.

These are in Nepali. Our publications, describing this work, translation of the IPT manual in Nepali Language.

Rose-Clarke K, Hassan E, Prakash BK, et al. A cross-cultural interpersonal model of adolescent depression: a qualitative study in rural Nepal. *Soc Sci Med*. 2021;270:113623.

Rose-Clarke K, Pradhan I, Shrestha P, et al. Culturally and developmentally adapting group interpersonal therapy for adolescents with depression in rural Nepal. *BMC Psychology*. 2020;8(1):1–5.

The IPT manual has been translated in Nepali, and the back translation in English is completed. Contact the chapter authors for more information.

Interpersonal Psychotherapy in Europe

27

Interpersonal Psychotherapy in Finland

ROSLYN LAW AND KLAUS RANTA ∎

INTERPERSONAL PSYCHOTHERAPY

In 1996, interpersonal psychotherapy (IPT) dissemination began in Mikkeli, Finland, when secondary care clinicians, working with adults with depression in psychiatric outpatient clinics, embarked on peer-supported learning and supervision. This self-guided practice reflected the demand to meet the needs of a growing number of people with depression seen in these services and led to a clinical research project helmed by Professor Hannu Koponen.[1] IPT dissemination was further advanced through a series of training events delivered by John Markowitz between 2000 and 2014 and hosted by Finland's University of Turku and Professor Hasse Karlsson.[2] Over time, graduates of these trainings established the Finnish Association for Psychodynamic and Interpersonal Psychotherapy (DIPY), and, since 2008, they have run IPT training for up to 500 participants with the support of national and international IPT experts. IPT has been disseminated to several Finnish provinces, mainly in Southern and Central Finland, and secondary-level psychiatric outpa tient clinics.[3] DIPY now oversees training standards and Finnish registration of IPT supervisors and trainers. Both qualifications require completion of an IPT supervisor course and a degree-level psychotherapy license. DIPY has developed a curriculum and training program for Finnish IPT supervisors, soon to be launched.

INTERPERSONAL COUNSELING

Interpersonal counseling was introduced into adult primary care services with a randomized controlled trial (RCT) comparing IPC in primary care to IPT in

Roslyn Law and Klaus Ranta, *Interpersonal Psychotherapy in Finland* In: *Interpersonal Psychotherapy.*
Edited by: Myrna M. Weissman and Jennifer J. Mootz, Oxford University Press. © Oxford University Press 2024.
DOI: 10.1093/oso/9780197652084.003.0028

secondary care.[4] The study was conducted across 5 municipal primary care units in Savonlinna by Finnish psychologist and psychotherapy trainer Dr. Jarmo Kontunen (J. K.), who already had played a key role in the introduction of IPT in Finland.[1] The short IPC intervention (6 + 1 sessions) was delivered by primary care nurses and social workers and targeted those with mild-to-moderate depression. IPC and IPT produced comparable results, with approximately 60% of participants achieving recovery, in their respective clinical settings. An adaptation for adults with depression following myocardial infarction has been developed in Turku University Central Hospital.[5]

INTERPERSONAL PSYCHOTHERAPY FOR ADOLESCENTS

Interpersonal psychotherapy for adolescents (IPT-A) was initially introduced to Finland around 2010, following a workshop by its developer, Dr. Laura Mufson. Subsequent IPT-A training, delivered by DIPY for secondary care services in university hospitals, was integrated into IPT training. Access to IPT-A remained limited until 2015 despite the high demands on secondary care psychiatric services for adolescents with depression. However, one such training event, delivered at Helsinki University in 2011, was attended by 3 clinicians who would go on to act as supervisors on projects focused on implementing IPC for adolescents (IPC-A) in secondary schools in the capital area of Finland and that within a few years would extend across all of Finland.

INTERPERSONAL COUNSELING FOR ADOLESCENTS

A state-funded initiative to build a national model for dissemination and implementation of brief, evidence-based treatments for adolescent depression in primary care began in Helsinki University Hospital (HUH) in 2016. This program targeted a wide range of professionals working in schools, mental health services, and social services. It was led by Dr. Klaus Ranta, with Dr. Roslyn Law from the Anna Freud Center, United Kingdom, acting as the main interpersonal counseling for adolescents (IPC-A) trainer. The pilot program in the city of Espoo ran in parallel with a research trial on the feasibility and effectiveness of IPC-A in primary-level services.[6,7]

This dissemination and implementation initiative increased demand for early interventions for young people at risk of developing mental health difficulties. Capacity for training and dissemination of IPC-A was extended by training supervisors working in secondary-level services across the country. An annual program of IPT-A supervisor and IPC-A practitioner trainings, coordinated by HUH and conducted by Dr. Law, followed. These trainings were attended by staff from secondary services and primary services, respectively, from several healthcare districts between 2018 and 2019. The dissemination plan was adopted by the

Finnish government in 2020 and used as the basis for a nationally funded program, based in schools and primary care, for improving adolescent mental health across Finland.[6] Twenty hospital districts and 5 university hospital districts embarked on the complex task of targeted training and dissemination of evidenced-based interventions for adolescents, including IPC-A, to establish mental health interventions in their respective primary care services. As part of this nationwide program, Dr. Tarja Koskinen from Kuopio University Hospital conducted the first IPC-A trainings across the country, reaching over 700 participants in 1 year. By 2022, almost 1700 IPC-A counselors had been trained through this cumulative effort.[6,7]

MODEL AND ADAPTATIONS

Interpersonal psychotherapy

Interpersonal psychotherapy training focuses on the original 12- to 16-session model.[8] Experienced mental health and social care professionals, mostly working in psychiatric outpatient clinics, attend 3 to 5 training days. Finnish practitioners then attend approximately 24 hours of monthly group supervision over 1 year. The small-group supervision covers casework on 2 cases, with additional telephone support as required. Audio or video recordings of clinical sessions are reviewed by supervisors between meetings and on completion of the casework. The therapists and supervisors independently rate the casework using an IPT adherence and competence scale and reflect on the therapeutic process. The result of this review forms the basis of the fifth closing day of the training seminars.

Interpersonal counseling for adolescents

One aim of the government-funded pilot project in 2016–2018 was to review and identify adolescent mental health interventions that would be feasible for use in the school health and welfare services. This process included reviewing research evidence and prior Finnish development programs for adolescents' mental health and their outcomes; analysis of the functioning of the mental service system for adolescents; and analysis of mental health work in primary-level services. HUH, the city of Espoo, and the Finnish Institute for Health and Welfare collaborated on this project. In discussions, the primary care service leaders and the project lead from HUH estimated the mental health work that was feasible to offer in schools, that is, time and resources available, and the type of work and length of intervention that could be implemented in the school services.

One of the innovations in the subsequent workshops lay in training school psychologists, social workers, and nurses, inexperienced in offering mental health interventions, to help young people with mild depressive symptoms directly and at an early stage. Given the high demands, poor service-level co-ordination, and absence of evidence-based interventions that characterized the Finnish school health care at the time, the brief and highly scripted IPC-A model was considered the most viable treatment option to pilot. IPT-A-trained professionals from HUH were recruited to supervise the IPC-A trainees. Secondary-level professional support and supervision were considered key in maintaining the interventions.

The Espoo feasibility study arranged by HUH was used to pilot IPC-A in secondary schools for 13- to 16-year-olds. It aimed to demonstrate the poten-tial benefits of school-based early intervention and to inform national policy. Until that point, evidence-based mental health interventions were not available in schools, with young people being directed to an overstretched secondary care system with long waiting lists.

The IPC-A training was delivered to therapists in the intervention group of the study in 2016 and to therapists from the control group in 2017. Training took place over 3 days with simultaneous translation. Experienced IPT-A practitioners attended the training, facilitated small-group exercises in Finnish, and provided posttraining supervision on one case for each participant. In 2018, these IPT-A practitioners and nascent IPC-A supervisors attended the first IPT-A/IPC-A supervisor training with Dr. Law. In subsequent years, IPC-A trainees were encouraged to complete at least 2 cases with 12 months of monthly supervision to consolidate skills more robustly.

Jarmo Kontunen's experience of using IPC and Dr. Law's expertise in the de-velopmental adaptations necessary to use IPT-informed approaches with young people and their parents or caregivers were combined in training the school work-force. This collaboration greatly benefited from parallel work on using IPC with young people in the United Kingdom by Paul Wilkinson, who generously shared his practice manual.[9] In 2016, Dr. Risto Heikkinen translated Wilkonson's IPC-A manual into Finnish, adding developmentally appropriate descriptions of the IPT focal areas. The standard IPC framework was retained in this training, with 3 phases of work, a mixed focus on prevention and early intervention for mild de-pression, and 4 focal areas. Scripts were modified to be developmentally relevant and accessible, and resource materials were in multimedia formats to enhance en-gagement. Where possible, parental involvement, through psychoeducation and/ or joint sessions, was encouraged to consolidate learning and encourage between-session support.

The relational approach was easily adopted by Finnish trainees, but the active focus on skills development, through decision analysis, communication analysis and role play proved more challenging.[10] This reluctance was identified in the pilot study, and more support and attention were given to these features in sub-sequent practitioner and supervisor trainings to encourage use of the full range of strategies. Increased confidence and willingness to use these strategies were reported by participants in later trainings, and these strategies were deliberately encouraged in supervision groups.

BARRIERS AND FACILITATORS OF IMPLEMENTATION

Implementation barriers

Implementation of IPT-A and IPC-A has been markedly different from implementation of IPT for adults in Finland. This reflects systemic differences in the structure of service and the sharp increase in demand for treatment for adolescents, the limits of which were a cause of national concern. The fragmented structure of adolescent primary care services and lack of personnel and time allocated to mental health work in these services have been the most significant legislative, structural, and ideological barriers for implementation.

The legislative barrier arose from Finnish law that limits welfare service professionals in primary-level education (i.e., comprehensive schools up to age 15 or 16) to providing mainly preventive work or generic support to young people. Clinical treatment is not part of school health and welfare services until secondary-level education (i.e., in high schools and vocational schools from age 16). The HUH dissemination model was built on the assumption that IPT-A-trained secondary care professionals would supervise IPC-A in primary care services. In practice, this required clinicians with limited posttraining experience in practicing IPT-A to supervise a shortened model (IPC-A) they had not used and had no opportunity to gain expertise in. This proved to be more challenging and anxiety provoking than originally anticipated. Additionally, novice supervisors were forced to use materials provided in a second language. Translating materials fell behind implementation because for most of the time those driving dissemination were doing so alongside demanding "day jobs" and without additional time or funding. Most IPC-A supervisors were also trying to add this activity to already busy jobs and consequently had very little scope for taking on more time-consuming supervision activities, such as recurrent constructive corrective feedback to support active learning and deliberate practice.[11] Demand for training consistently outstripped capacity for robust supervision. This was particularly evident when the central funding in the national program from 2020 on was distributed via the provinces with very different resources and service structures. Many areas did not perceive the need for supervision when the workforce was faced with many competing demands, which made it very difficult to confidently evaluate the competence and adherence of IPC-A being delivered post-training.

Implementation facilitators

Finnish implementation of IPT has focused on well-established outpatient units in secondary psychiatric services in several areas. Early adopters included Mikkeli in South-Eastern Finland and Turku in the Turku University Central Hospital District in Southwest Finland. Thereafter, IPT has spread into other hospital district regions in Southern Finland, Capital, Central Finland, and in Northern Finland. With further training programs after 2010, dissemination to secondary services followed, partially concurrent with clinical research projects arranged in Turku, in the Helsinki region and Jyväskylä.[1-3] Clinical and academic collaborations have facilitated dissemination financially and by working through established networks.

International collaboration throughout the planning and delivery of IPT, IPT-A, and IPC-A workshops and making use of a tried-and-tested training approaches has enhanced efficiency and impact. Adopting a competency-based framework and corresponding training requirements clearly set out parameters and training structures for therapists and supervisors. Existing materials have been generously shared with openness to the necessity of changes and adaptations to suit the local context and culture.

Regarding IPC-A, support from local healthcare administrators and state funding for a pilot project allowed disseminators to progress on a small scale and created the foundation of all training from 2016 to 2020. In 2020, in part responding to high demand for IPC-A from potential providers, government targeted funds on adolescent mental health, specifically training, helped dissemination and implementation of brief interventions for depression and anxiety in primary care services. In accordance with a plan designed in collaboration with HUH, the Ministry of Social Affairs and Health also funded the creation of regional teams for disseminating evidence-based interventions.[6]

In 2021, IPC-A training pivoted significantly to become a 16-hour online self-study course followed by a 1-day implementation workshop. The midterm progress report on the National Future Health and Social Services Centres programme, published by the Finnish National Institute for Health and Welfare, recorded 1507 IPC-A counsellors and 68 IPC-A supervisors had completed training by March 2023. In 2022–2023, 145 IPC-A counsellors commenced training through the web -based training provided by the Hospital District of Helsinki and Uusimaa.[12] Based on clinical experience, supervision on at least 2 cases post training is recommended to consolidate skills and support sustained practice. In 2022, three IPC-A supervisors completed a 2-year train-the-trainer program delivered remotely by Dr. Law to support Finnish innovation and sustainability.

FUTURE PLANS AND RECOMMENDATIONS

Collaborating with academic colleagues where possible is encouraged, including conducting pilot trials and assessing outcomes to inform economic planning. In pursuit of this aim, the improving mental well-being as a means of increasing inclusion of young people consortium (IMAGINE), with the support of the Anna Freud Center, has secure funding to conduct an evaluation of the cost-effectiveness of the ongoing national implementation and dissemination of IPC-A and provide structure and tools for future implementations. Additionally, the University of Tampere has funded a collaboration on training and research infrastructure with the Anna Freud Center to introduce clinical training for master's-level psychology students for the first time, focusing on IPT-A Skills Training (IPT-AST). Dr. Law will provide training and supervision to Tampere University teaching staff, collaborators, and students with the aim of establishing self-sustaining provision. This model of training will be the subject of a research collaboration between the 2 centers to evaluate the feasibility of using top-level psychotherapy training to extend the scope of current psychology training. Above all, collaborate, be patient and be resilient.

IPC-A CASE EXAMPLE

This case example is drawn from group supervision for novice IPC-A school counselors. The group is facilitated by an IPT-A-trained psychologist working in an adolescent psychiatric outpatient clinic, and IPC-A is provided by an IPC-A-trained school nurse.

Helena was a 14-year-old girl referred by her mother, who attended a presentation about IPC-A given by the school counselor at a parent-teacher meeting. Helena's mother noticed her daughter had become increasingly withdrawn at home. She spends a lot of time in her room, cries easily, and her grades have started to drop. Helen's parents divorced when she was 11, and her mother would like her daughter to spend more time with her father, who has moved away and rarely reaches out to his daughter. Helena used to meet up with her friends more often, but now rarely goes out and has begun to feel left out, which increases her loneliness and sadness.

Providing a psychological intervention is new to the school nurse, and she brings details of the referral to the group to discuss the potential for IPC-A to be of benefit to Helena. Criteria for offering IPC-A are reviewed, and, based on early indicators of depression and the interpersonal themes surrounding their onset, it is agreed that an assessment will be booked. The school nurse attends supervision once a month, with the option of contacting the primary supervisor by telephone between meetings if necessary, so feels under some pressure to conduct this new intervention independently and welcomes the group support.

Following a screening session and first IPC-A meeting, the school nurse returns to the group and shares more background details and asks them to help her to think about the most useful focal area to use in her work with Helena. The group is asked to consider 2 options, 1 listening for themes of role transition and the other for role dispute.

Following her parents' divorce, Helena describes a deterioration in her relationship with her father. She is angry with him for moving away and feels he has no time or interest in her after meeting a new partner. She is disappointed that the father rarely calls or asks how she is doing. She would like to spend more time with him but feels it should be his job as a parent to reach out to her. She has lost confidence in herself following her father's departure and finds it hard being around her friends. Helena is upset when her friends talk about their parents, even when they complain about them, but hasn't told them how she feels. It felt easier to avoid their company and the possibility of feeling upset at first, but now Helena fears they have forgotten about her, and she feels even more alone.

Following discussion, the supervision group suggests both focal areas could be useful but on balance recommend role transition. It is agreed that this should be discussed openly with Helena to ensure this is a shared decision-making process. This also prompts a wider discussion in the group about how strictly the IPC-A counselor needs to follow the manual. Those in the group are used to adopting a person-centered approach, following the young person's needs as they arise, and are all adjusting to a manualized approach. Some group members express concern about deviating too much from the manual and forgetting key parts of the intervention, while others worry that they will miss some important themes the young person brings to the session if they follow the manual too closely. The group helps each other consider how a manualized approach can be personalized for each young person and the relevance of communication and emotionally focused work across all focal areas.

The importance of an open and collaborative process of formulating the problem with the young person is highlighted when Helena expressed a preference for using the role disputes approach to improve communication with her father rather than adjusting to his absence. Helena and her IPC-A counselor agree that directly involving her father in at least 1 session may be helpful in supporting direct and constructive communication.

The IPC-A counselor is anxious about conducting a joint session and takes this concern to the supervision group for support and guidance. The supervisor suggests the group could role play conducting a joint session in small groups. A cultural barrier to IPC-A dissemination becomes apparent at this point, with the Finnish participants expressing anxiety and reluctance to engage in role play, something that was also highlighted in the initial trial of IPC-A in Finland.[7-10] The group members describe feeling silly, awkward, and fake acting out the proposed session. The supervisor uses this response as a learning opportunity and invites the group to consider the advantages and disadvantages of practicing. This not only invites more thought about avoided features of the approach but also models taking a decision analysis approach to the kind of reluctance that the counselors may encounter in session. A compromise is reached, and the IPC-A counselor participates in the role play as Helena and the supervisor as the IPC-A counselor, with the others observing and making notes, which they share with the participating counselor. The group is also reminded of prerecorded role play demonstration available in their course materials.

The IPC-A counselor's confidence is boosted by the role play experience, and she successfully navigates the session with Helena and her father. When the intervention is complete, a good outcome is reported. Helena's symptoms on the Patient Health Questionnaire-9 have decreased from 15 (moderate range) to 5 (healthy range), and she rated satisfaction with the approach at 9/10. Helena said she had gained more insight into her relationship with her father, and the atmosphere at home with her mum felt more relaxed. Helena was pleased that she had talked about her feelings to her father at the joint appointment. She discovered that her father hadn't realized she wanted him to reach out to her more. He reminded her that when he moved he told her that she could, "come over anytime," and explained that he thought Helena hadn't wanted to visit him or keep in touch.

At 1-month follow up, Helena says that she is still doing well, and her relationship with her father continues to improve. She has been visiting him regularly, and he has started calling her to check in on how she's doing. This has boosted her confidence, and she has begun seeing her friends more regularly and is enjoying her time with them. Helena described feeling significantly less lonely at the end of the intervention.

ACKNOWLEDGMENT

Special thanks to Heidi Martelin, Kristiina Mämmi, Mari Hintikka, and Maikku Lenkkeri for sharing clinical experience in the case report.

REFERENCES

1. Löyttynen AM, Koponen H, Kontunen J, Lehtonen J, Marttunen M. Introducing interpersonal psychotherapy (IPT) to psychiatric outpatient care: early experiences in training therapists and treating depressed outpatients. *Psychiatria Fennica*. 2008;36:78–84.
2. Karlsson H, Säteri U, Markowitz JC. Interpersonal psychotherapy for Finnish community patients with moderate to severe major depression and comorbidities: a pilot feasibility study. *Nord J Psychiatry*. 2011;65(6):427–432.
3. Saloheimo HP, Markowitz J, Saloheimo TH, et al. Psychotherapy effectiveness for major depression: a randomized trial in a Finnish community. *BMC Psychiatry*. 2016;16(1):1–9.
4. Kontunen J, Timonen M, Muotka J, Liukkonen T. Is interpersonal counselling (IPC) sufficient treatment for depression in primary care patients? A pilot study comparing IPC and interpersonal psychotherapy (IPT). *J Affect Disord*. 2016;189:89–93.
5. Oranta O, Luutonen S, Salokangas RK, Vahlberg T, Leino-Kilpi H. The outcomes of interpersonal counselling on depressive symptoms and distress after myocardial infarction. *Nord J Psychiatry*. 2010;64(2):78–86.
6. Linnaranta O, Ranta K, Marttunen M, et al. A national implementation of interpersonal counselling, adolescent version (IPC-A) in Finland. *Psychiatria Fennica*. 2022;53:24–35.
7. Parhiala P, Ranta K, Gergov V, et al. Interpersonal counseling in the treatment of adolescent depression: a randomized controlled effectiveness and feasibility study in school health and welfare services. *School Ment Health*. 2020;12:265–283.
8. Klerman GL, Weissman MM, Rounsaville B, Chevron ES. *Interpersonal Psychotherapy for Depression*. Basic Books; 1984.

9. Wilkinson PO, Cestaro V, Pinchen I. Pilot mixed-methods evaluation of interpersonal counselling for young people with depressive symptoms in non-specialist services. *BMJ Ment Health.* 2018;21(4):134–138.

10. Ranta K, Parhiala P, Law R, Marttunen M. Treating adolescent depression in multiprofessional school services with IPC-A: implementation results from the national pilot trial. *Psychiatria Fennica.* 2022;53:36–55.

11. Rousmaniere T, Goodyear RK, Miller SD, Wampold BE, eds. *The Cycle of Excellence: Using Deliberate Practice to Improve Supervision and Training.* John Wiley & Sons; 2017.

12. Koivisto J, Muurinen H. Tulevaisuuden sosiaali- ja terveyskeskus -ohjelman hyötytavoitteiden toteutumisen kansallinen seuranta ja arviointi. Kevät 2023. THL Työpaperi 29/2023. National Institute for Health and Welfare: Helsinki, 2023. Report in Finnish. https://www.julkari.fi/bitstream/handle/10024/146851/TY%c3%962023_029_%20final%20s.pdf?sequence=4&isAllowed=y. Accessed September 25, 2023.

28

Interpersonal Psychotherapy in Germany

EVA-LOTTA BRAKEMEIER ■

Interpersonal psychotherapy (IPT) was founded in Germany in the early 1990s and has since established itself in Germany, which is the outstanding achievement of Elisabeth Schramm of the Department of Psychiatry and Psychotherapy at Freiburg University Medical Center. This chapter illustrates the implementation and dissemination of IPT in Germany referring to three important steps.

THE GERMAN IPT MANUAL

An important first step in this process was the publication of the first German book on IPT in 1996, which Elisabeth Schramm edited, including the translation of the original IPT treatment manual by Klerman, Weissman, Rounsaville, and Chevron. In the fourth edition, published in 2019, Elisabeth Schramm and her author team described the numerous modifications of the approach for other forms of disorders, settings, and time frames that had been studied and applied in recent years.[1] In addition, the fifth focus "work stress" was also introduced.

IPT ASSOCIATIONS IN GERMANY

The second important step was the foundation of the *Arbeitsgemeinschaft Wissenschaftliche Psychotherapie* (AWP) in Freiburg in 1998 by Martin Bohus and Elisabeth Schramm, inspired by the upswing that structured, evidence-based therapeutic concepts had gained in the United States at that time. The aim was to make empirically proven therapeutic approaches known in German-speaking

Eva-Lotta Brakemeier, *Interpersonal Psychotherapy in Germany* In: *Interpersonal Psychotherapy.*
Edited by: Myrna M. Weissman and Jennifer J. Mootz, Oxford University Press. © Oxford University Press 2024.
DOI: 10.1093/oso/9780197652084.003.0029

countries. It started with dialectical behavioral therapy (DBT) for borderline personality disorder by Linehan and with IPT by Klerman and Weissman. For organizational reasons, the AWP now splits into the AWP-Freiburg (DBT and trauma
therapy) and the AWP-Depression (IPT and in cognitive behavioral analysis
system of psychotherapy [CBASP]). In 2015, the association *Deutsche Gesellschaft
für Interpersonelle Psychotherapie* (DG-IPT; German Society for Interpersonal
Psychotherapy) emerged from AWP-Depression, which is dedicated to the dissemination of IPT as a method and the networking of practitioners. The DG-IPT
currently counts 130 members. The board members of the association meet regularly under the leadership of the president, Elisabeth Schramm, in order to disseminate IPT in Germany in a systematic and high-quality manner to practitioners
and patients. In addition, there is also a scientific advisory board, whose members
include, among others, Prof. Mathias Berger as medical director emeritus of the
Department of Psychiatry and Psychotherapy at the University Hospital Freiburg.
The DG-IPT home page informs all interested parties about current developments
and news concerning IPT. In addition, the IPTalk is announced there, which is
very well accepted (see https://www.dg-ipt.de).

TRAINING IN IPT IN GERMANY

Training in IPT in Germany—as the third step—is stimulated in particular by
the DG-IPT. The DG-IPT presents the certification criteria for IPT therapists,
supervisors, trainers, and clinics on its home page along with the criteria
used for the US National Institutes of Mental Health Treatment of Depression
Collaborative Research Program. For example, therapists who seek certification
in IPT should

1. be a psychologist or medical doctor with completed psychotherapy
   training or advanced training;
2. have basic knowledge in the treatment of depressive patients (at least
   1 year of active treatment);
3. read the treatment manual[1];
4. complete an extensive training program (including at least 24 didactic
   units, 10 supervision units, and the fulfillment of the formal adherence
   criteria).

The IPT workshops and trainings are organized by the DG-IPT or universities
and private training centers. Within the framework of the state-funded project Competence Center Psychotherapy at the Medical Faculties of Baden-
Württemberg, a 2.5-day German-speaking webinar on IPT was created. The
webinar can be held simultaneously in a seminar room setting at different locations
that are in contact with each other via videoconference. Alternative forms of
use (e.g., playback on one's own PC) are also possible. The webinar consists of

recorded lecture units, therapy demonstration videos, small-group exercises with online support, and discussion rounds via videoconference. Through this webinar, clinics and therapists can be trained in IPT at different locations without having to travel to another place with large investments of time and money. Through the video technology, it is still possible to practice the IPT techniques under coaching and to discuss difficulties and problems in the implementation afterward in the discussion rounds. In addition, there are also IPT video sequences on a DVD, which are often used for teaching at universities and other institutes to familiarize students with IPT.[2]

ADAPTATIONS OF IPT

IPT for specific age groups

In 2022, the first German IPT manual for older people suffering from depression in an inpatient setting was published by Petra Dykierek, Elisa Scheller, and Elisabeth Schramm. The manual describes IPT-Late Life as individual and group therapy.[3] IPT-Late Life has a clear psychosocial-interpersonal focus and is particularly suited to address the lived realities of older people with experiences of loss, loneliness, and serious life changes.

Regarding IPT in adolescents (IPT-A), in January 2018 an article on IPT-A in an inpatient setting was published in the journal for psychiatry, psychotherapy, and psychosomatics *PSYCH up2date*.[4] In the article, the basic principles, procedures, and modifications specifically for the inpatient treatment of depressed adolescents were presented. The IPT-A manual of Laura Mufson is being translated in German and is in press. Both modifications are mostly applied in specialized wards in different hospitals.

IPT IN SPECIAL SETTINGS AND FOR SPECIFIC PROBLEMS

IPT inpatient program

The possibility that patients suffering from severe depression are treated for several weeks as inpatients with intensive psychotherapy concepts (in combination with medication) is certainly specific for German-speaking countries. Inpatient treatment with IPT is described in detail in an IPT casebook.[5] In the early 2000s, Elisabeth Schramm and Matthias Berger developed IPT as an inpatient multidisciplinary concept, implemented it in a university clinic, and evaluated it in a randomized controlled trial (see Schramm et al., 2007, for the main publication).[6] Since then, many hospitals have introduced IPT as an inpatient treatment program.

IPT group treatment

In 2022, the second edition of the updated manual *Interpersonal Psychotherapy in Group*,[7] describing how therapists can use IPT in group settings, was published. It introduces the role of the group leader and explains session by session which content can be conveyed. With this training program, psychotherapists can learn the IPT group method relatively quickly. IPT groups have become widespread in German-speaking countries, mainly in inpatient contexts.

IPT integrated in Internet- and mobile-based interventions

For relatives and significant others of depressed individuals, the "Family Coach Depression" was developed as a freely available online program under the leadership of Elisabeth Schramm and her research group based on interventions from IPT. The self-help online program (https://depression.aok.de) offers participants information and instructions on how to support their depressive relatives, improve the relationship, and protect themselves from overload. A study is currently underway with family members of people with depressive illnesses to determine whether the Family Coach has advantages with individualized guidance per mail support over automated guidance and over psychoeducational material.

In the CADY (Conversational Agent to Treat Depression in Young People, https://psychologie.uni-greifswald.de/cady/) research project led by Florian Kuhlmeier, Stefan Lüttke, and Eva-Lotta Brakemeier, a chatbot is being developed to support young people (13 to 21 years old) suffering from depression. The chatbot CADY regularly asks how the user is doing and offers therapeutic exercises based on content from cognitive behavioral therapy (CBT) and IPT. The project started in June 2021, and the CADY app is expected to be ready in early 2023. CADY is primarily intended for young people who are waiting for a therapy place or who do not want traditional therapy. There is another Internet-based project that integrates the IPT (eHELP-MV). As this was developed in the context of the COVID-19 pandemic, it is described under COVID.

IPT for work-stress-related depressive disorders

Since more and more depressive patients complain about depressive and burnout symptoms associated with intense work stress and because work stress belongs to the most common triggers of depressive disorders, the working group of Elisabeth Schramm has conceptualized a fifth IPT focus on stress in the work role, which directly refers to changes and/or conflicts in the work environment.[8] The best investigated psychosocial work stressors include increased job demands in connection with low control possibilities and lack of gratification, interpersonal conflicts, role stress, and social isolation or lack of support. Thus, this problem area focuses on not only specific communication in the workplace (e.g., in conflicts, bullying); on stressful, involuntary changes (e.g., change of boss, change of work position); and social role stress (e.g., colleague and supervisor role in one person), but also the reduction of external stressful working conditions. In the first studies, the work stress program proved to be an effective method for treating work-related depressive disorders.[1] However, further studies are needed to evaluate the efficacy of this newly designed problem area.

IPT IN THE CONTEXT OF CRISES

All global crises directly affect the interpersonal context. Crises are role transitions; conflicts are usually a trigger or are consequences of crises; changes in the social network can cause loneliness and isolation; and deaths trigger grief, which can be long lasting or complicated. IPT, which has been proven as an effective short-term therapy and as a preventive intervention, is therefore particularly suited for short-term and specific support to people affected by crises. Projects from Germany in the context of crises are briefly outlined below.

Berlin model project in the context of the refugee crisis of 2015

Due to the high number of refugees with mental disorders who sought protection in Berlin in the refugee crisis of 2015, the Interpersonal Integrative Pilot Project for Refugees (IIPPR) was initiated.[9] This short-term intercultural psychotherapy program aimed for a timely treatment of mental problems, while supporting the integration of the refugees into the working and social world. Thus, the project was funded by the Federal Ministry of Labour and Social Affairs. The psychotherapy program was based on a modified version of IPT (10 sessions of interpreter-assisted individual therapy), supplemented by z sessions of social counselling, among others. The intercultural program is described in detail in an unpublished manual (Brakemeier et al., 2015). Within the scope of an open study, feasibility and outcome were examined by quantitative and qualitative analyses.[10] A total of 37 patients, mainly from Syria, participated in the IIPPR. The most frequent diagnoses were depression (70.2%) and post-traumatic stress disorder (43.2%). The dropout rate was 24.3%, while 85.5% of patients who completed the program rated the project as "good" or "very good." The initially high mental distress decreased, while the quality of life significantly improved with medium effect sizes. A helpful cooperation with job centers was successfully established. Qualitative interviews also made it possible to explore the importance of language for psychotherapeutic work and multilingualism in intercultural interpreter-assisted IPT. The experience of foreignness, which the different languages convey a moment of (relative) exclusion to those involved in the treatment process, could be identified in the sense of not only role transition as the central theme of psychotherapy with refugees but also an opportunity for therapeutic progress.[11]

Vorpommern model project in the context of the war against Ukraine in 2022

Based on the promising results of the IIPPR, in 2022, in the context of the war on the Ukrainians and the renewed large-scale refugee movement, I launched another IPT-based intercultural project in Western Pomerania. This support project of the initiative "Together for Mental Health," initially carried out in cooperation with the Psychosocial Center for Asylum Seekers and Migrants in Western Pomerania based on voluntary commitment, aims to help people of all ages who are psychologically stressed or traumatized by the war in Ukraine (especially those seeking protection in Western Pomerania). The project offers free and interpreter-supported counseling sessions directly in community shelters, at the Center for Psychological Psychotherapy at the University of Greifswald, or in therapeutic practices in Mecklenburg-Western Pomerania. Virtual counseling via telehealth is also possible. If indicated, short-term psychotherapy is initiated. In addition, an open digital group is offered weekly for people living in Germany who have been burdened by war and who would like to be involved proactively. These psychological support services are based, among other methods, on IPT. The intercultural program is described in detail in a manual (Brakemeier & Harder, 2022, unpublished). So far, more than 100 counseling sessions have been conducted, and the strategies from the IPT area of role transition have emerged as particularly helpful. Thanks to financial support from the Bosch Foundation, the project can now be implemented in a more sustainable and professional way, led by Eva-Lotta Brakemeier, Florian Harder, and Anna-Lena Zietlow (https://psychologie.uni-greifswald.de/gemeinsam/beratung/).

In these two intercultural projects, it is important that adjustments are made in training and supervision. In particular, the culture-specific characteristics of certain interpersonal issues should be addressed in workshops in order to achieve intercultural sensitivity among all participants. For example, the way of dealing with mourning and death sometimes differs considerably in different cultures. In some Islamic conceptions, for example, mourning is forbidden because the belief is that God has commanded death. In addition, interpreters should receive a brief introduction to IPT and be sensitized to specific topics. Interpreters often originate from the same countries as the patients. Many have themselves experienced traumatic events in their lives (like war and flight) or, because of the cultural similarities, may be particularly affected by the events that the patients describe in therapy. For example, it would be inappropriate if an interpreter began to cry uncontrollably in therapy or even left the therapy room. Thus, it is important to offer continuous supervision to not only the therapists, but also the interpreters to help them address any of their own concerns and suffering. The therapists should also take a short time before and after the therapy to talk with the interpreters without the patients present. In this setting, the intercultural content of the therapy or the feelings triggered about the therapy can be discussed. The interpreters can also explain to the therapist certain terms that may be unclear or draw attention to cultural differences.

Psychological help in the context of the COVID-19 pandemic 2020

In the context of the COVID-19 pandemic, an increase in mental health problems in the general population and an increased need for psychotherapeutic support for people with preexisting mental health problems and disorders was observed in Europe.[12-14] Therefore, low-threshold prevention and intervention measures are urgently needed to provide rapid help to those with mental distress to counteract an increase in mental disorders and to minimize the overload of the existing psychotherapeutic and psychiatric care systems. At the same time, these measures should reduce the risk of infection with the COVID-19 virus and be compliant with the applicable security measures, which is why digital offerings appear to be particularly suitable.

Loneliness increased by 20%–30% during the pandemic,[15] and IPT's focus on the interpersonal context and helping people regain emotional support makes it particularly suitable as a preventive or therapeutic intervention. With the onset of the pandemic in the first and second wave, I conducted digital IPT training for therapists to present these helpful strategies. In addition, together with a working group, we created videos and worksheets for those who were living under COVID-19 restrictions (https://psychologie.uni-greifswald.de/43051/lehrstue hle-ii/klinische-psychologie-und-psychotherapie/corona-pandemie/psychologis che-unterstuetzung-im-umgang-mit-der-corona-pandemie/). These short video clips are intended as a self-help tool to help people cope better with the pandemic-associated stressors. One video, "Well-being and Positive Living Despite the Corona Pandemic," introduces the problem area of role transition and presents helpful strategies. People can ask themselves, for example: "What roles do I take on in life? What has changed within my roles as a result of the pandemic? Have I lost roles temporarily? Have new roles been added?" In addition, the following questions were added: "How can I compensate for losses? How can I use what has remained the same in such a way that it leads to more well-being? How can these experiences positively influence my life in the long term?" Two other videos present helpful strategies for dealing with conflicts that can occur more frequently, especially in domestic isolation. The Kiesler circumplex model was also included here, which complements the IPT strategies well. Especially in the problem area of conflicts, the Kiesler circle helps to analyze how the partners influence each other (e.g., dominant behavior triggers submissive reactions, hostile behavior leads to hostile reactions, friendly behavior triggers friendliness) and through which behavioral changes in the "negotiation phase" solutions can be brought about. In the problem area of isolation/loneliness, the interpersonal circumplex model also shows ways to get out of the isolation/distance. In addition, the Kiesler circle is helpful for role plays (see also Guhn et al., 2019).[16]

Our project eHELP-MV is considered as self-help in the pandemic and is a modularized, online-based therapy for people with psychological stress in Mecklenburg-Western Pomerania (https://psychologie.uni-greifswald.de/43051/ lehrstuehle-ii/klinische-psychologie-und-psychotherapie/nadja-hagewiesche/ praxisbasierte-forschung/ehelp-mv-1/). It pursues the goals of developing, implementing, and scientifically evaluating a guided 4-week digital self-help intervention in order to be able to offer it in the long term to those affected throughout Mecklenburg-Western Pomerania. After inclusion in the study, patients with mental disorders who are on the waiting list for outpatient psychotherapy will participate in 1 of the 5 developed digital self-help interventions, whereby each intervention contains symptom-reducing strategies as well as practical exercises from evidence-based psychotherapy methods. One of the modules is based on IPT. Implementation is supported by trained e-coaches and digital applications to increase ease of use and effectiveness. To tailor the self-help intervention to the individual needs of patients, we will investigate in a second phase whether algorithm-based personalization increases the effects of self-help to a meaningful extent. This project is funded by the Mecklenburg-Vorpommern State Funding Institute as part of the "Health and Prevention" program.

Finally, we made an effort to draw attention to the IPT model through media, social media, and the Internet (e.g., an article about IPT in a general population magazine covering topics in psychology, brain research, and medicine).[17]

BARRIERS AND FACILITATORS OF IMPLEMENTATION

Concerning implementation and dissemination, the DG-IPT website currently lists around 130 therapists from Germany, Switzerland, and Austria who are certified in IPT. In addition, there are 19 clinics in German-speaking countries (including 4 in Switzerland) listed that offer IPT on certified wards. Apart from the certified therapists and wards, IPT is of course also used in Germany by other therapists who are not certified.

Experiences with the projects in the context of crises showed that the IPT concept and its elements are gratefully accepted by not only therapists but also interpreters and other volunteers and can be used quickly after a short training. IPT is also popular with young students in psychotherapy courses at universities, when it is taught. Many theses by students were completed in the respective refugee projects. However, such projects including the involvement of students and therapists as well as the inclusion in the teaching at universities are the exceptions in Germany. It is necessary to further stimulate, evaluate, and disseminate such projects in the future.

The main reason why IPT is not spreading faster is due to the fact that IPT in outpatient psychotherapy is not reimbursed since it is not classified as a guideline procedure (*Richtlinienverfahren*). In Germany, only CBT, psychoanalysis/

psychodynamic, or systemic therapy are reimbursed by the public health insurance. Currently, IPT is only approved as a method in the treatment of depression in the context of the above-mentioned approaches. To be clear, IPT is reimbursed only when the method is integrated into a CBT, psychoanalysis/psychodynamic, or systemic therapy. An application to the Federal Joint Committee for consideration of IPT as a guideline procedure is currently being processed.

FUTURE PLANS AND RECOMMENDATIONS

Due to the new "psychotherapists law" that was passed in 2019 and included the new *Approbationsordnung* ("licensing regulations"), Germany is currently in a phase of transition as the education and training of psychotherapists is being re-formed. This holds many opportunities especially for psychotherapy research and methods like IPT. In this law, it is stated that scientifically evaluated and approved methods of psychotherapy must be taught. Since IPT is approved as an evidence-based method for the treatment of depression, it can also be increasingly integrated into education at the university master's programs and training. However, efforts should be made to ensure that the range of indications for IPT is also expanded in accordance with the available studies. The current scientific debate and focus in the Society on Psychotherapy Research on the so-called personalized psychotherapy (i.e., the adaptation of psychotherapy methods and techniques to the individual patient and progress in psychotherapy)[18] is also increasingly finding its way into Germany. Thus, together with Wolfgang Lutz (University of Trier) and other colleagues, I founded an interest group "Evidence-Based Personalized Psychotherapy" within the framework of the German Society of Psychology. In this context I also would like to ensure that IPT research is intensified (see, e.g., Huibers et al., 2015).[19] Whether called modular psychotherapy, process-oriented psychotherapy, or personalized psychotherapy, IPT should be an important component or ingredient in the repertoire of psychotherapy methods.

In the future, it will be necessary to deal more intensively with the important psychotherapy research question: "What works for whom?" This is especially helpful in determining which patient benefits from which psychotherapy method in which setting and in which phase of treatment. It is hoped that IPT will play an essential role here, and not only in Germany. Finally, IPT as a practice-oriented therapy can help to narrow the gap between research and practice contributing to the relevant paradigm of a practice research network,[20] which should now consistently move to the center of research.

CASE EXAMPLE

To conclude, I would like to illustrate how, in two counseling sessions with a Ukrainian boy and his mother seeking protection in Mecklenburg-Western

Pomerania, IPT strategies were helpfully applied in the problem area of role transition.

A 12-year-old Ukrainian boy and his mother took up the offer of a counseling session in the context of the support project. Both had arrived at the shared accommodation only a few days prior. The mother reported that she was very worried about her son because he was withdrawn, spoke little, and had sleeping problems. The boy said that he missed his father and his friends and was afraid of the war. After an empathic validation of these feelings in the context of the war and the flight, the therapist explained the role transition in which they both found themselves. The boy indicated his transition as from a relatively happy and care-free boy in Ukraine to a refugee without a father and friends who is full of fear.

Together, they listed all that he had lost and took the time and offered support to cry and mourn. Then, the therapist asked the question about what still remained the same despite the war and flight. Here, the boy recognized that besides the supportive relationship with his mother, he had also kept all his skills and hobbies, especially his artistic abilities and his love for art and music. The boy vividly told how much he liked drawing, and that he had been playing the saxophone for 3 years. Then he became sad when he reported that he could not take his saxophone with him when fleeing. However, he planned to make music with his community in the refugee home. In addition, he intended to make friends with other children from the home and also village. Specifically, he planned to participate in the painting group that women from the village organized for the children from Ukraine. Finally, they even briefly discussed what possibilities or challenges could arise in the context of this serious crisis. He said that he had the feeling that he would grow up faster and also become more mature, which might not be such a bad thing. In conclusion, the boy was able to resolve the transition to pursue his hobbies with others more intensively and to establish more contacts with children of the same age. The therapist managed to find a volunteer who wanted to give a used saxophone to the boy. During the second session, the therapist was able to give him this saxophone as a present, and the boy and his mother seemed overjoyed.

This short case study illustrates how, by applying the strategies from the area of role transition, a young boy could be helped. The pragmatic approach of providing help directly through the saxophone corresponds to the idea of IPT. Even independent of the saxophone, the boy already seemed to be coping much better. It was especially nice that this boy was able to play in a jazz orchestra at his new German school and was thus able to pursue his hobby in relationship with other children and to make new friends more easily. Thus, IPT could unfold the beneficial effect.

ACKNOWLEDGMENT

I would like to thank Elisabeth Schramm as the IPT expert of Germany for her careful review of this book chapter.

REFERENCES

1. Schramm E, Mack S, Thiel N, Jenkner C, Elsaesser M, Fangmeier T. Interpersonal psychotherapy vs. treatment as usual for major depression related to work stress: a pilot randomized controlled study. *Frontiers in Psychiatry*. 2020;11:193.

2. Brakemeier EL, Jacobi F. *Verhaltenstherapie in der Praxis*. Beltz Video-Learning. Beltz; 2017. (Herausgeberwerk)

3. Dykierek P, Scheller E, Schramm E,.eds. *Interpersonelle Psychotherapie im Alter (IPT-Late Life)*. Kohlhammer Verlag; 2021.

4. Von Lucadou A, Schramm E. Interpersonelle Psychotherapie bei affektiven Störungen. *PSYCH up2date*. 2018;12(1):39–54.

5. Schramm E. IPT for inpatient depression. In Weissman MM, Markowitz J, eds. *Casebook of Interpersonal Psychotherapy*. Oxford University Press; 2012:393–410.

6. Schramm E, van Calker D, Dykierek P, et al. An intensive treatment program of interpersonal psychotherapy plus pharmacotherapy for depressed inpatients: acute and long-term results. *Am J Psychiatry*. 2007;164(5):768–777.

7. Schramm E, Thiel N, Zehender, N. (überarbeitete und erweiterte Auflage). *Interpersonelle Psychotherapie in der Gruppe. Das Therapiemanual*. Schattauer Verlag; 2022.

8. Schramm E, Berger M. Interpersonal psychotherapy for work-related stress depressive disorders. *Nervenarzt*. 2013;84:813–822.

9. Brakemeier EL, Rump S, Spies J, Schouler-Ocak M. Interpersonelles integratives Modellprojekt für Flüchtlinge mit psychischen Störungen (IIMPF): Ein interkulturelles Kurzzeit-Hilfsprogramm für Flüchtlinge mit psychischen Störungen zur Unterstützung und Förderung der Integration in die Arbeits-und Sozialwelt. *Rep Psychol*. 2015;11(12):442–443.

10. Brakemeier EL, Zimmermann J, Erz E, et al. Interpersonelles Integratives Modellprojekt für Geflüchtete mit psychischen Störungen. *Psychotherapeut*. 2017;62:322–332.

11. Storck T, Brakemeier EL. Sprache und Fremdheit in der interkulturellen dolmetschergestützten Psychotherapie. *Psychotherapeut*. 2017;62(4):291–298.

12. Gilan D, Röthke N, Blessin M, et al. Psychomorbidity, Resilience, and exacerbating and protective factors during the SARS-CoV-2 pandemic: a systematic literature review and results from the German COSMO-PANEL. *Dtsch Arzteblatt Int*. 2020;117(38):625–630.

13. Luo M, Guo L, Yu M, Jiang W, Wang H. The psychological and mental impact of coronavirus disease 2019 (COVID-19) on medical staff and general public—a systematic review and meta-analysis. *Psychiatry Res*. 2020;291:113190.

14. Wirkner J, Christiansen H, Knaevelsrud C, et al. Mental health in times of the COVID-19 pandemic. *European Psychol*. 2022;26(4):310–322.

15. Buecker S, Horstmann KT. Loneliness and social isolation during the COVID-19 pandemic. *Eur Psychol*. 2021;26:272–284.

16. Guhn A, Köhler S, Brakemeier EL. *Kiesler-Kreis-Training: Manual zur Behandlung interpersoneller Probleme: mit E-Book inside und Arbeitsmaterial*. Beltz; 2019.

17. Leu M, Brakemeier EL. *Beziehungen im Fokus: Interpersonelle Therapie*. Gehirn & Geist; 2021.

18. Brakemeier EL, Herpertz SC. Innovative Psychotherapieforschung: auf dem Weg zu einer evidenz-und prozessbasierten individualisierten und modularen Psychotherapie. *Der Nervenarzt.* 2019;10(11):e0140771.

19. Huibers MJ, Cohen ZD, Lemmens LH, et al. Predicting optimal outcomes in cognitive therapy or interpersonal psychotherapy for depressed individuals using the personalized advantage index approach. *PloS One.* 2015;10(11):e0140771.

20. Herzog P, Kaiser T, Brakemeier EL. Praxisorientierte Forschung in der Psychotherapie. *Z Klin Psychol Psychother.* 2022;51(2):127–148.

29

Interpersonal Psychotherapy in Hungary

ADRIENNE STAUDER AND MÁRTA NOVÁK ∎

The story of interpersonal psychotherapy (IPT) in Hungary started with a grant of the British Know How Fund to the Hungarian government. Márta Novák, as a resident in psychiatry, was involved in their project Implementing Evidence-Based Medicine into the Hungarian Health Care System. She was particularly interested in evidence-based mental health and, as she reviewed the literature, realized that IPT was completely unknown in Hungary. This was somewhat surprising since Hungary is well known for its strong history of various psychotherapies, including psychoanalysis and cognitive behavioral therapy (CBT).

Marta became interested in bringing IPT to Hungary and contacted Dr. Myrna Weissman, the developer of IPT. She was very supportive and recommended inviting Dr. John Markowitz to present IPT in Budapest. Sponsored by the Austrian American Foundation, he gave a full-day IPT workshop in English in Budapest at the National Institute of Mental Health and Neurology for about 100 participants (psychiatrists, psychologists, and psychotherapists) in November 2001. Subsequently, Márta Novák and her colleague László Lajtai had an opportunity to attend a 4-day IPT workshop in Edinburgh, United Kingdom, organized and presented by Dr. Roslyn Law. The opportunity to become more deeply involved in IPT came to Marta during her fellowship at the University of Toronto in 2003, when she was supervised for her IPT training by Dr. Paula Ravitz. While Marta accepted a position at the University of Toronto, she continued with a cross-appointment at the Institute of Behavioral Sciences, Semmelweis University, Budapest, Hungary, and organized three 1-day workshops in IPT together with Dr. Ferenc Túry in cooperation with the Family Therapy Association.

Adrienne Stauder and Márta Novák, *Interpersonal Psychotherapy in Hungary* In: *Interpersonal Psychotherapy*. Edited by: Myrna M. Weissman and Jennifer J. Mootz, Oxford University Press. © Oxford University Press 2024. DOI: 10.1093/oso/9780197652084.003.0030

This is where Dr. Adrienne Stauder (psychiatrist and psychotherapist) became interested in IPT and subsequently completed a clinical fellowship at the Mount Sinai Hospital and University of Toronto to be trained in IPT under the supervision of Dr. Paula Ravitz during the 2012–2013 academic year.

Starting in 2014, we together began to provide yearly Continuing Medical Education (CME)–accredited 1-day IPT workshops at the Institute of Behavioral Sciences, Semmelweis University. On average, 10 to 20 participants attend these workshops. The workshop has been announced on the Hungarian website, and we reached out to professional contacts, but we had lack of resources for more extensive marketing of the course. Most of the participants at the workshop are senior psychotherapists (mostly psychoanalysts and CBT therapists). They usually become quite interested in IPT, and we have engaged in discussions comparing various methods of psychotherapy.

In addition, we seized opportunities such as the annual conference of the Hungarian Psychiatric Association to offer shorter introductory workshops or symposia to introduce IPT. We were honored to host in Budapest the Biannual Meeting of the Society of Interpersonal Psychotherapy (ISIPT) in 2019, which facilitated the introduction of the outstanding international IPT faculty to our Hungarian colleagues. Another step to raise awareness of IPT as an evidence-based psychotherapeutic approach is its presentation as part of graduate and post-graduate training. A 90-minute lecture "Basics of Interpersonal Psychotherapy" has been included in the 4-year residency of clinical psychologists since 2019. A 90-minute lecture "Interpersonal Counseling" has been part of the curriculum of the Behavioral Medicine and Psychosomatics elective course for medical students since 2020. Also, there is a chapter on IPT in the course book of the Introduction to Psychotherapy required course for senior medical students at Semmelweis University. Over the years, we had a number of opportunities to give shorter presentations to interested healthcare professionals at various local workgroup meetings, such as the Williams Lifeskills Facilitator workgroup supervision meeting. Some of in attendance attended the full-day workshop after this.

CURRENT DEVELOPMENTS

About 160 professionals completed the basic 1-day workshop, and there was a clear interest expressed by many of them to continue the training and to start IPT therapy with supervision. However, there is not enough trained staff and personal capacity locally available to provide regular supervision. Language is an important barrier to the involvement of experienced colleagues from other parts of the world. However, during the COVID pandemic, many colleagues became comfortable with online work, so this experience opens new opportunities for online supervision. We are also implementing some IPT techniques and the interpersonal counseling (IPC) concept in the framework of the Student Counseling Service at Semmelweis University.

POSSIBILITIES FOR FURTHER DEVELOPMENT

As we have mentioned, currently the main obstacle of IPT development is the lack of human resources, especially the lack of trained, committed supervisors. It might be relevant to know that there are very high expectations toward trainings in a psychotherapeutic method. There are a number of well-established therapies (psychodynamic, CBT) and currently in-development psychotherapy schools (schema therapy, mindfulness) offering long, strict (and often expensive) training programs.

PSYCHOTHERAPY TRAINING IN HUNGARY

Being a psychotherapist requires a university diploma and completion of a psychotherapy specialization exam. Therefore, officially, IPT can be practiced as a psychotherapy only by professionals having obtained such a specialization. Psychotherapy is a second specialization in Hungary based on a 46- to 78-month basic training that must be in either adult or child psychiatry, clinical and mental health psychology, or other medical specialty. Specialization in psychotherapy necessities 24 to 36 months of additional training and at least 150 hours of therapy in individual or group settings. The specialty training can be provided by 1 of the 16 accredited psychotherapy associations in Hungary, all members of the Hungarian Council of Psychotherapy. Professionals with university degrees in other helping professions can provide mental health interventions, which qualify as counseling but cannot be called psychotherapy.

FUTURE DIRECTIONS

Considering the above professional context, we believe we can aim to

1. Increase the psychotherapeutic competencies of certified psychotherapists by teaching them IPT;
2. Provide psychotherapy skills to psychiatrists and psychologists working by teaching them IPT;
3. Increase the counseling competencies of other mental health specialists not eligible for providing psychotherapy by teaching them IPC; and
4. Organize supervision and peer supervision groups.

How can we disseminate IPT in Hungary?

1. General education: Raise awareness that IPT is an evidence-based psychotherapy;
2. Professional education: Continue to offer lectures or short introductory workshops where professionals can learn about the basic concept of IPT

as a CME workshop (e.g., training in psychology, mental health–related conferences);

3. Other opportunities: Offer workshops at conferences where the participants get a theoretical overview and practice IPT techniques;
4. Training in IPT: Provide advanced workshops preparing professionals to provide IPT or IPC;
5. Supervision: Provide regular group supervision (most feasible online);
6. IPT manuals: Translate into Hungarian for a helpful resource; and
7. International IPT trainings: Advertise among mental health professionals who speak English (e.g., ISIPT-accredited courses).

DIFFICULTIES AND LIMITATIONS

We continue to face certain challenges, for example, lack of financial and professional resources. These include IPT trainers, dedicated time available and financial barriers.

FURTHER PLANS

We hope to facilitate the translation of IPT books into Hungarian and organize group supervision for those who are ready to start IPT after completing our workshop. We would like to present a case where IPT tools and techniques have been applied at the Student Counseling Service of Semmelweis University. The service is provided by the colleagues of the Institute of Behavioral Sciences.

CASE EXAMPLE

All students studying at the various faculties of the university can get an appointment for 1 to 5 sessions of counseling. If a longer psychotherapeutic treatment is needed, they are referred to the Outpatient Clinic of the institute. Besides Hungarian students, counseling is also available for international students in German or in English.

Most students present with symptoms of stress-related somatic symptoms or mood and anxiety symptoms. The onset of their symptoms often can be related to interpersonal conflicts that they have a hard time managing because of the lack of a support network related to the move to the university from another place or from another country. Their relationships with parents, siblings, and other family members and old friends necessarily change. Living alone (or with strangers) for first time in their lives poses new challenges. In addition, international students, coming mostly from Germany, the Scandinavian countries, Middle East, Asia, or Africa, often feel isolated and alienated in a very different cultural environment and not understanding the local language.

Most often the focus of the counseling in our service can be conceptualized along the IPT problem areas of role transitions and role conflicts, occasionally grief. We have found the Interpersonal Inventory a useful tool to explore these issues. It is also an invaluable tool to identify potential new resources of social support and also explore old ones in a deeper way. Communication analysis, brainstorming, and role plays are also useful techniques to understand conflicts and to improve the ways of sharing emotions and expressing needs.

To illustrate the implementation of this IPC-informed intervention, we briefly present the case of Maria, a third-year pharmacy student. She came from a small Hungarian town and shared a flat with 2 other students. She performed well at the university and also worked part-time. She described her parents as rather isolated, not very good communicators, and as carrying a grudge toward their closest relatives. She had several friends and a new supportive partner. Her current source of stress, which impacted her mood and sleep, was that her new flatmate has been messy and not contributing to the household chores. She became upset and anxious and felt that she was unable to bring up these issues with her.

The exploration revealed her long-standing pattern of conflict-avoidant behavior, which often left her frustrated, feeling used, upset, sad, and helpless, not only with the flatmate, but also at her workplace and with her parents. The focus of the intervention was identifying and formulating her needs and communicating them assertively. Brainstorming during the second session resulted in a plan on how she could discuss the rules regarding the household chores, instead of doing everything herself or expecting each other to do something. She came to the next session in a bright mood and pleased because she found an opportunity to raise the issue, and the flatmates agreed on a household system that seemed to function in a satisfactory way. In the third session, her difficulties setting limits for the unrealistic expectations of her boss and her parents were discussed, and Maria enjoyed role playing what and how she would communicate with them. At the fourth session, the counseling was concluded by reviewing her progress and planning ahead. Maria expressed that she felt more able to communicate her needs assertively, which resulted in the significant decrease of her stress level and improvement of her mood and her self-esteem.

REFERENCES

1. Lajtai L. Az interperszonális pszichoterápia bemutatása (Introduction to interpersonal psychotherapy). *Pszichoterápia. XI. évf.* 2002;199–207.
2. Miller MD, Frank E, Cornes C, et al. Applying interpersonal psychotherapy to bereavement-related depression following loss of a spouse in late life. *J Psychother Pract Res*. 1994;3(2):149–162. (Translated to Hungarian by L. Benczúr & J. Pilling. 1999. Interperszonális pszichoterápia alkalmazása a gyásszal összefüggő depresszióban házastársukat elveszített időseknél. Kharon, Spring–Summer online. https://kharon.hu/docu/1999-tavasz-nyar_mark-interperszonalis.pdf.) Accessed January 31, 2023.

3. Lajtai L, Unoka Zs. Az interperszonális pszichoterápia. In Unoka Z, Purebl G, Túry F, Bitter I, eds. *Pszichoterápia az orvosi gyakorlatban* [*Psychotherapy in medical practice*]. Semmelweis Kiadó; 2011:108–110.

4. Zalai D, Novák M. Interperszonális pszichoterápia evészavarokban. In Túry F, Pászthy B eds. *Az evészavarok terápiájának aktuális kérdései* [*Interpersonal Psychotherapy in Eating Disorders*]. Semmelweis Kiadó; 2011:60–66.

30

Interpersonal Psychotherapy in Italy

SILVIO BELLINO AND PAOLA BOZZATELLO ∎

BACKGROUND

The arrival of interpersonal psychotherapy (IPT) in Italy can be traced to the 1980s and was promoted by the cooperation between Klerman[1] and Giovanbattista Cassano of the University of Pisa. The IPT manual was translated into Italian by Giuseppe Berti Ceroni in 1989. However, for a real spread of this therapy in Italy, we had to wait until the mid-1990s, when the first IPT workshops, training courses, and seminars by IPT experts from the United States (John Markowitz and Ellen Frank) were organized in several Italian cities.[2-4]

A decade later, in 1999, Filippo Bogetto and Silvio Bellino of the University of Turin wrote a chapter on IPT for the second edition of the Italian *Treatise of Psychiatry* published by the Italian Society of Psychopathology. In the same years, Andrea Pergami and Luigi Grassi, in collaboration with John Markowitz (1999), published the Italian monograph on IPT in the treatment of depressive symptoms among patients with HIV: *La psicoterapia interpersonale (IPT). Il trattamento psicologico della depressione nell'infezione da HIV.*[5,6]

The first trial of IPT in Italy was conducted in 2001 and was the result of the collaboration between the investigators of the University of Pittsburgh coordinated by Ellen Frank and those of the University of Pisa directed by Giovanni Battista Cassano. The study "Depression: The Search for Treatment Relevant Phenotypes" was aimed at identifying demographic, biological, and psychopathological mediators and moderators of treatment response with psychotherapy, antidepressant, or their combination.[7]

The emergence of IPT in Italy was promoted by a partnership of several Italian clinical centers (the Universities of Turin, Bologna, Pavia, Varese, Perugia, Bari,

Silvio Bellino and Paola Bozzatello, *Interpersonal Psychotherapy in Italy* In: *Interpersonal Psychotherapy.*
Edited by: Myrna M. Weissman and Jennifer J. Mootz, Oxford University Press. © Oxford University Press 2024.
DOI: 10.1093/oso/9780197652084.003.0031

and Foggia and the Departments of Mental Health of Cagliari and Modena) that produced a multicenter, randomized, controlled trial on the efficacy of interpersonal counseling (IPC; a brief, structured psychological intervention derived from IPT) in comparison with pharmacotherapy (administering selective serotonin re-uptake inhibitors, SSRIs) in mild-to-moderate major depression. A second step of this study aimed to investigate the efficacy of augmentation with SSRI or IPC in depressed patients who did not respond to monotherapy.[6,8] Over the years, IPT, originally conceived for treatment of major depression, has been applied to other psychiatric disorders because of their frequent and often predominant interpersonal dimension: dysthymia, bipolar disorder, substance abuse, post-traumatic stress disorder, social phobia, panic disorder, eating disorders, and borderline personality disorder (BPD). In addition, IPT has been proposed in contexts of liaison psychiatry and in particular populations of patients (i.e., women after breast reconstructive surgery).

Understandably, the progressive broadening of applications of IPT for other disorders with heterogeneous clinical characteristics required adaptations of the traditional format to address the needs of new diagnostic targets.[9] In the most common applications (i.e., in depressive and anxiety disorders), the clinical population predominantly consisted of female subjects both for the higher prevalence of depression and anxiety in female gender and for the greater willingness of women to be engaged in psychotherapy. Adult subjects between 30 and 50 years of age were most common, although this therapy can be delivered with good effects also to adolescents and has been performed in older patients.

In Italy, in the years 2004–2005, the research group of the University of Turin carried out clinical trials in patients with major depression and comorbid BPD and then in BPD patients with no other concomitant disorders. In the first studies, we used the traditional format of IPT for depression. Then we adopted the adaptation of IPT to BPD proposed by John Markowitz in the United States (IPT-BPD). The recent application of IPT to treat BPD saw a change in the characteristics of patients. People with BPD treated with adapted IPT were mainly younger adults and, in an increasing proportion of cases, adolescents. Over the years, we felt the need to make some changes to the model of IPT-BPD designed by Markowitz. The main changes of our revision (IPT-BPD-R) consisted in extending the duration to 10 months (40 sessions), adding a maintenance phase of 8 months (1 session per month), offering an intervention of IPC to cohabiting family members and supervising therapists.

In addition, at the University of Turin, an IPT group (IPT-G) is underway for patients with BPD who are receiving individual IPT. It is a 4-month intervention with 1 session per week with 6 patients in each group. It should be emphasized that IPT has been implemented and developed in Italy mainly in the University Centers of Tuscany, Turin, Bologna, and Padua. This approach has been favorable for research and proposal of new intervention strategies, but it entailed some limits in terms of spread of IPT in general clinical practice.

Training of IPT in Italy

The training of therapists strictly adheres to the official guidelines of the International Society of Interpersonal Psychotherapy. IPT of major depression was administered to Italian patients according to the model described in Klerman's manual. First- and second-level courses have been conducted in recent years in the Centers of Turin and Tuscany and at the National Congresses of the Italian Society of Psychopathology. Advanced courses are in the program. Regarding the adaptation of IPT to BPD, training has begun at the Center for Personality Disorders of Turin and supervision of therapists in training is offered. Moreover, an IPT course has been activated at the School of Specialization in Psychiatry of the University of Turin.

RANDOMIZED CONTROLLED TRIALS

At the University of Turin, 7 clinical trials[10-16] and 1 brain imaging study[17] were carried out to evaluate the efficacy of IPT in BPD with or without major depression in comorbidity. In addition, we participated in 2 multicenter genetic studies on IPC for major depression.

Clinical trials

To begin studying the efficacy of this new proposal of psychotherapy, we performed initial trials in samples of patients with major depression and BPD who received a combination of IPT with medications. The first investigation[9] aimed to compare combined therapy (IPT + fluoxetine) with pharmacotherapy alone (fluoxetine 20–40 mg/day) for 24 weeks in 39 people receiving outpatient care who had concomitant major depression and BPD. The two treatments had no differences in terms of responder rates and improvement of anxiety and global symptoms, but the combination of IPT and fluoxetine produced a greater effect on depressive symptoms, subjective perception of quality of life, and interpersonal relationships. The following study[10] compared the efficacy of 2 combined therapies for 24 weeks: IPT + fluoxetine (20–40 mg/day) and cognitive therapy (CT) + fluoxetine (20–40 mg/day) in a sample of 35 people receiving outpatient care who had major depression and BPD. The 2 treatments were not different for the rate of responders, improvement in global symptoms, and socio-occupational functioning. CT was found superior in improving anxiety symptoms and subjective psychological functioning, while IPT was more efficacious in improvement of subjective perception of social and relational functioning (an elective target of this psychotherapy).

The adaptation of IPT to BPD proposed by Markowitz (IPT-BPD) was tested in our center in patients with BPD without other concomitant psychiatric disorders.[11]

We compared the efficacy of combined therapy (IPT-BPD + fluoxetine 20–40 mg/day) to pharmacotherapy alone (fluoxetine 20–40 mg/day) for 32 weeks in 55 outpatients with BPD. Combined therapy showed better results in improving anxiety symptoms, subjective perception of quality of life, and symptom domains of interpersonal relations, impulsiveness, and affective instability (according to the items of the Borderline Personality Disorder Severity Index [BPDSI]). Most of these advantages were confirmed after a follow-up study.[13] Forty-four patients who completed the 32-week trial underwent 24 months of follow-up. The addition of IPT-BPD to medication produced greater effects on BPD symptoms (impulsivity and interpersonal relationships) and quality of life (perception of psychological and social functioning) that endured after termination of psychotherapy until the end of follow-up. In the subgroup of 27 patients allocated to combined therapy with IPT-BPD and fluoxetine in the 32-week efficacy study (2010), clinical factors that predicted response to combined therapy were investigated. Patients with more severe BPD psychopathology and with a higher severity of fear of abandonment, affective instability, and identity disturbance had a better chance to improve with a combination of modified IPT and antidepressant.

The more recent investigation of ours[16] is a pilot study designed to assess the efficacy of IPT-BPD-R (our revised model of Maerkowitz's IPT-BPD)[18] as a single treatment with 43 patients with BPD for 10 months. Results for patients receiving IPT-BPD-R were compared with a control group of BPD patients on a waiting list plus clinical management. Results showed differences between groups in favor of psychotherapy in terms of reduction of severity of general psychopathology, improvement of social and occupational functioning, decrease of global BPD symptoms and improvements in interpersonal relationships, impulsivity, and identity. It is noticeable to observe that we did not find any differences between groups for self-harm and aggressive behaviors. The dropout rate was rather low in all our investigations (20% or less), and none of the patients that completed our studies fulfilled diagnostic criteria for BPD at endpoint, although they still presented a subthreshold number of BPD traits.

Genetic and brain imaging studies

We participated in 2 multicenter studies in Turin designed to explore the potential effects on outcome of pharmacological and psychological interventions induced by gene variants controlling the serotonin pathway in patients with major depressive disorder (MDD).[19,20] In the first randomized controlled trial,[19] 160 patients with depression were randomized to receive either IPC or antidepressants. IPC resulted in an effective psychological intervention with the same effects of antidepressants in mild-to-moderate MDD. Concerning the effects of polymorphisms related to the serotonin system, results were negative in both treatment groups. The second trial[20] aimed to evaluate a possible different effect of gene variants on response to pharmacotherapy and IPC. One hundred and thirty-seven patients with MDD were randomly assigned to the 2 groups, and 5 gene variants were analyzed.

Results suggested that the allele rs8076005 in the SLC6A4 gene produced a different effect: It was significantly associated with response rate to antidepressants, while in the IPC group only a nonsignificant trend was obtained. While these initial findings are stimulating, they need replication.

Based on the results of a first study of functional magnetic resonance imaging (fMRI) performed to assess differences in brain functioning between BPD patients and healthy subjects during an autobiographical memory reenactment task, we designed a second fMRI study in order to examine changes of brain activity during the same task in patients with BPD who received IPT-BPD-R compared with patients in waiting list and clinical management.[17] Forty-three patients with a diagnosis of BPD were randomly assigned to the 2 groups for 10 months. Both groups underwent pre- and posttreatment fMRI. Findings of this study indicated that positive therapeutic effects produced by IPT-BPD-R in BPD patients were reflected in the functional changes of specific brain areas registered with fMRI. Areas that showed modulation of their activity after psychotherapy were the right temporoparietal junction and the right anterior cingulate cortex, both involved in mentalization processes fundamental for BPD psychopathology. The results obtained in genetic and fMRI studies of patients receiving IPT are initial, but show promising findings. They deserve to be replicated in large samples.

CASE EXAMPLE

E. is a 38-year-old man. He had been a songwriter, but at the beginning of psychotherapy did not have a job. He lived with his parents but had a conflictual relationship with both. He had a sister who lived independently and was a point of reference for him. E. had previous hospitalizations in a psychiatric setting for benzodiazepine and alcohol abuse. He came to our observation with a diagnosis of MDD. During the first psychiatric visits, he complained of a persistent feeling of dejection and loss of hope. He had been living in a condition of interpersonal isolation and often argued with parents. During the following visits, other aspects of E. emerged. A pattern of emotional instability, poor control of impulsiveness, constant feelings of emptiness and boredom, and turbulent and unstable relationships was observed. These symptoms had been present since late adolescence. E. showed up dressed in black clothes, had long hair and lots of tattoos and piercings, and looked like a rock singer.

E. was evaluated with standardized instruments (Structured Clinical Interview for DSM-5 Personality Disorders and Millon Clinical Multiaxial Inventory-III), which confirmed the clinical assessment. He received the diagnosis of BPD. Before beginning treatment with IPT-BPD-R, he completed the assessment with other evaluation tools specific for his diagnosis: The BPDSI, an instrument to measure specific BPD symptoms, and the Hamilton Depression Rating Scale (HDRS). E. obtained a score of 55 on the BPDSI (medium-high severity of BPD symptoms) and 15 on the HDRS (mild depressive symptoms).

Acute phase of psychotherapy (sessions 1–22)

In the initial sessions, the IPT therapist shared with the patient the diagnosis and attributed the "sick role." E. reported a difficult situation at home because his mother was depressed and his father didn't seem to understand the suffering of the mother or E. E. had an attitude of comprehension toward his mother, while he often quarreled with his father. His parents had controlling behaviors. They treated E. like an adolescent, hindering his autonomy. He experienced these parental behaviors with discomfort, but at the same time was dependent on them for financial support and making decisions about his future.

On the interpersonal inventory, E. had few meaningful relationships outside of family members. The positive relationships were with his sister and niece. He had 2 friends who were part of the band he used to play with, but he hadn't met them in years.

He had recently ended a 2-year romantic relationship with L. In this relationship, he required care because he was "sick," and, when he no longer felt cared for, he decided to break up with L. In the first sessions, the therapist shared the choice of the interpersonal problem area on which to work in the coming months of therapy. The therapist proposed to E. the possibility of role transition: "You feel excessively submissive to your parents' supervision. You feel anxious about their warnings, which are often recurrent in your thoughts. You should consider that you can maintain a relationship with your parents even if you set boundaries in your relationship, without feeling guilty about it. You could try to empower yourself by moving from the role of a child dependent on his parents to that of an adult capable of taking responsibility and making decisions about his own life." E. gladly accepted this interpersonal area.

During the sessions, feelings of anger emerged toward the parents for the lack of trust they showed him (in relation to his past dysfunctional conducts), and at the same time, E. expressed feelings of guilt for not having met their expectations. He had difficulties putting himself in the shoes of others, in particular his father, whom he perceived as authoritarian and insensitive to his psychological discomfort. In this initial phase of therapy, the therapist established a therapeutic alliance with E., assigned him the role of patient, discussed with him the diagnosis and the symptoms that created the highest degree of discomfort in him (also providing elements of psychoeducation). The main difficulties in this phase derived from E.'s tendency to assume that he knew the motivations of others actions and words without needing open communication. A major communication problem in the family was a tendency to make others understand one's emotional states without expressing them directly.

Techniques adopted in this phase were encouragement of affect, empathic participation of the therapist, clarification, and organization of contents. E. generally respected the rules of the setting and rarely missed a session. So, the therapist decided to continue the intervention with the continuation phase. At the end of the acute phase, E. showed an improvement of depressive symptoms with a decrease in HDRS score to 7 (remission of depression).

Continuation phase (sessions 23–42)

Conflicts with family members emerged even more clearly during the continuation phase. E. looked for an alternative to cohabitation with parents in the family home, but they did not agree with this decision. E., on one hand, wanted to leave their home but, on the other hand, was afraid of no longer receiving parental support. In addition, he did not feel that his efforts to gain independence were acknowledged.

During the therapeutic sessions, E. capably reflected on the possibility of living alone without breaking the relationship with his parents and feeling guilty for having "disobeyed" them. He considered the opportunity of helping them with daily activities at a distance (e.g., offering to go shopping, paying bills online for them, and accompanying his grandmother to medical visits). E. moved to a new home in another city. In the first few weeks, there were episodes of crisis (related to loneliness and a sense of emptiness), during which E. asked his father to come and take him back to his parents' house.

Over time, he succeeded in staying in his new home even during critical episodes. He also learned to express his disagreement with his parents not through outbursts of anger, but waiting for when he felt more relaxed.

Physical separation from his family allowed E.'s symptoms to improve quickly. He contacted his 2 friends and began to hang out with them again in moments of leisure. He abandoned the role of "rock star" to take on a more authentic role as an adult man almost 40 years old. He attended computer training courses and began a real search for a job. Romantic relationships were still problematic. He struggled to separate himself from the idealized image of his last girlfriend and undertook noncommittal and casual relationships.

The conclusion phase was particularly difficult with this patient. A maintenance phase of 6 monthly sessions was necessary. In addition, 6 sessions of IPC were offered to his parents. At the end of therapy, E. no longer fulfilled diagnostic criteria for BPD. The BPDSI score had decreased to 24 (mild BPD symptoms), and the HDRS remained below the threshold of 7. After IPT-BPD-R discontinuation, a follow-up of 24 months with monthly visits began and was currently underway. Techniques that had been used in the continuation phase were confrontation and observation (a more explorative intervention) in addition to other techniques already used during the acute phase. Changes of the IPT model were not necessary to deal with cultural differences in Italy.

REFERENCES

1. Klerman GL, Dimascio A, Weissman M, Prusoff B, Paykel ES. Treatment of depression by drugs and psychotherapy. *Am J Psychiatry.* 1974;131(2):186–191.
2. Beck AT, Rush AJ, Shaw BF, Emery G. *Cognitive Therapy of Depression.* Guilford Press; 1979.
3. Klerman GL, Weissman MM, Rounsaville BJ, Chevron ES. *Interpersonal Psychotherapy of Depression.* Basic Books; 1984.

4. Weissman MM. Interpersonal psychotherapy: history and future. *Am J Psychother.* 2020;73(1):3–7.

5. Menchetti M, Bortolotti B, Rucci P, et al. Depression in primary care: interpersonal counseling vs. selective serotonin reuptake inhibitors. The DEPICS Study. A multicenter randomized controlled trial. Rationale and design. *BMC Psychiatry.* 2010;10:97.

6. Magnani M, Sasdelli A, Bellino S, et al. Treating depression: what patients want; findings from a randomized controlled trial in primary care. *Psychosomatics.* 2016;57(6):616–623.

7. Ellen F. Depression: The Search for Treatment-Relevant Phenotypes. *University of Pittsburgh.* Pittsburgh, United States. 2003. https://grantome.com/grant/NIH/R01-MH065376-01A1. Accessed April 26, 2022.

8. Pergami A, Grassi L, Markowitz JC. *La psicoterapia interpersonale (IPT). Il trattamento psicologico della depressione nell'infezione da HIV.* Franco Angeli; 1999.

9. Pancheri P, Cassano GB. *Trattato Italiano di Psichiatria.* Masson; 1999.

10. Bellino S, Zizza M, Rinaldi C, Bogetto F. Combined treatment of major depression in patients with borderline personality disorder: a comparison with pharmacotherapy. *Can J Psychiatry.* 2006;51(7):453–460.

11. Bellino S, Zizza M, Rinaldi C, Bogetto F. Combined therapy of major depression with concomitant borderline personality disorder: comparison of interpersonal and cognitive psychotherapy. *Cana J Psychiatry.* 2007;52(11):718–725.

12. Bellino S, Rinaldi C, Bogetto F. Adaptation of interpersonal psychotherapy to borderline personality disorder: a comparison of combined therapy and single pharmacotherapy. *Can J Psychiatry.* 2010;55(2):74–81.

13. Bellino S, Bozzatello P. Interpersonal psychotherapy adapted for borderline personality disorder (IPT-BPD): a review of available data and a proposal of revision. *J Psychol Psychother.* 2015;5(6):1–5.

14. Bellino S, Bozzatello P, Bogetto F. Combined treatment of borderline personality disorder with interpersonal psychotherapy and pharmacotherapy: predictors of response. *Psychiatry Res.* 2015;226(1):284–288.

15. Bozzatello P, Bellino S. Combined therapy with interpersonal psychotherapy adapted for borderline personality disorder: a two-years follow-up. *Psychiatry Res.* 2016;240:151–156.

16. Bozzatello P, Bellino S. Interpersonal psychotherapy as a single treatment for borderline personality disorder: a pilot randomized-controlled study. *Front Psychiatry.* 2020;11:578910.

17. Bozzatello P, Morese R, Valentini MC, Rocca P, Bellino S. How interpersonal psychotherapy changes the brain: a study of fMRI in borderline personality disorder. *J Clin Psychiatry.* 2021;83(1):21.

18. Markowitz JC, Skodol AE, Bleiberg K. Interpersonal psychotherapy for borderline personality disorder: possible mechanisms of change. *J Clin Psychol.* 2006;62(4):431–444.

19. Serretti A, Fabbri C, Pellegrini S, et al. No effect of serotoninergic gene variants on response to interpersonal counseling and antidepressants in major depression. *Psychiatry Investig.* 2013;10(2):180–189.

20. Matsumoto Y, Fabbri C, Pellegrini S, et al. Serotonin transporter gene: a new polymorphism may affect response to antidepressant treatments in major depressive disorder. *Mol Diagn Ther.* 2014;18(5):567–577.

Interpersonal Psychotherapy
in the Netherlands

FRENK PEETERS, KOSSE JONKER, AND MARC BLOM ■

Interpersonal psychotherapy (IPT) was first introduced in the Netherlands during a 2-day workshop by John Markowitz in 1994. Participation in this workshop was by invitation only, resulting in a small but dedicated group of clinicians and researchers that received some initial familiarity with this approach. The emphasis of the workshop was mostly on IPT for depression, which was in line with its primary indication and the majority of the data on its efficacy in those years.

When looking back, it is clear that this workshop inspired most attendees to start practicing IPT, which, over the years, resulted in a nationwide implementation of IPT in selected clinical settings, the availability of postdoctoral courses for therapists interested in learning IPT, the publication of a first Dutch introductory book on IPT, the foundation of the Dutch Society for Interpersonal Therapy, and initiatives for clinical studies and adaptations. We address these developments consecutively below and close with an outlook on the future of IPT in the Netherlands.

IMPLEMENTATION

Implementation of IPT in the Netherlands went relatively smoothly. The Netherlands is one of the smaller countries in Europe, with a little over 17 million inhabitants with a rather homogeneous demographic population that was from the outset comparable to the population in the United States. No specific adaptations to the mental health system were therefore needed. The inclusion of IPT for depression as one of first-line psychotherapeutic treatments in the national guideline greatly supported further acceptance and implementation of IPT.

Frenk Peeters, Kosse Jonker, and Marc Blom, *Interpersonal Psychotherapy in the Netherlands* In: *Interpersonal Psychotherapy.* Edited by: Myrna M. Weissman and Jennifer J. Mootz, Oxford University Press. © Oxford University Press 2024. DOI: 10.1093/oso/9780197652084.003.0032

In recent decades, the population composition has changed, with immigration from many parts of the world creating a more multicultural society, creating some challenges for mental health services. Luckily, IPT has been shown to be effective in various cultures and parts of the world. In line with this, an early study into the effectiveness of IPT for depression in the Netherlands found that patients from ethnic minority groups benefited equally from IPT, but that there was a higher dropout rate (45.9% vs. 24.4%) in this group.[1] An important conclusion of the study was that therapists in this patient group should focus on improving compliance. Some small adaptations to the initial protocol were made to improve uptake with minority groups. These adaptations were published in Dutch.[2]

INSTRUCTIONS IN IPT

To stimulate implementation of IPT in daily practice, basic 3-day introductory courses were offered in different parts of the country in the curricula of postdoctoral training institutions for psychologists, psychotherapists, and to some extent psychiatrists. Over the years, we estimate that around 300 of these courses were given, which yields a total of over 4000 mental health professionals trained in IPT in the Netherlands. The courses were supported by the publication in 1997 of the first Dutch textbook on IPT.[3] This book was updated and extended in 2011 and is to date being used as a basic textbook for IPT in the Netherlands.[2]

THE DUTCH SOCIETY FOR INTERPERSONAL THERAPY

The initiatives outlined above stimulated the founding of the Dutch Society for Interpersonal Therapy in 2008, with a stable number of around 70 members, among which there are 10 supervisors. The society's major goal is to transfer IPT knowledge and experience in the Netherlands. The society is involved in the organization of IPT courses and certification of therapists, supervisors, and trainers. Additionally, over the years some national conferences were organized with national and international speakers. In 2011, the fourth International Society of Interpersonal Psychotherapy (ISIPT) conference on IPT was held in Amsterdam with over 200 participants from all over the world.

CLINICAL RESEARCH

Some early adopters of IPT were also the first to initiate clinical studies in the Netherlands in IPT for depression, and at a later stage were involved in the studies of adaptations in content, delivery, and clinical populations. Marc Blom and Kosse Jonker conducted a study that examined the effectiveness of IPT for depression. They reported equal effectiveness of IPT and IPT combined with antidepressant medication but more effectiveness of these interventions when compared with medication alone.[4] Higher baseline severity and longer duration of the index episode predicted less clinical improvement. The presence of personality factors was not related to short-term outcomes.[5]

These findings were partially replicated and extended in both a pragmatic trial and an randomized controlled trial in which IPT and cognitive behavioral therapy (CBT) were compared head to head.[6,7] IPT was found to be as effective as CBT, most interestingly also after a 2-year follow-up providing strong support for an enduring effect of short-term IPT without additional maintenance sessions.[8,9] The widespread implementation of IPT for depression also enabled a nationwide 4-arm study in which the timing of IPT and CBT were altered in a design with twice-weekly sessions in comparison to once-weekly sessions for both conditions while keeping the total number of sessions equal in all 4 arms.[10] Patients who received twice-weekly sessions showed a statistically significant larger decrease in depressive symptoms, lower dropout rates, and an increased rate of clinical response when compared with those who received weekly sessions. These in-depth studies also provided knowledge on processes and mechanisms of change in both IPT and CBT for depression.[11–16] Finally, with the use of state-of-the-art statistical approaches, preliminary prediction and moderation models were developed and tested.[17–20]

Over the years, studies into adaptations in other formats and patient groups were carried out. Dina Snippe developed and published a depression treatment protocol for providing IPT in a group format.[21] Pilot data suggested significant improvement of depressive symptomatology and well-being. Anneke van Schaik reported that IPT (10 sessions) for elderly patients with depression in general practice was more effective than general practitioners' care as usual (CAU).[22] IPT in this context appeared to be an attractive treatment modality for patients, general practitioners, as well as therapists from mental health organizations,[23] but was not more cost-effective than CAU.[24] More recently, Sjoertje Vos published one of the few papers on IPT for panic disorder with agoraphobia in comparison to CBT.[25] IPT appeared less efficacious than CBT for this indication.

Finally, Tara Donker examined the effectiveness of short (4-week), Internet-delivered, self-guided IPT and CBT. She found both interventions equally effective in reducing depressive symptoms but reported high dropout rates and low participant satisfaction.[26,27]

THE FUTURE OF IPT IN THE NETHERLANDS

Interpersonal psychotherapy has set foot in the Netherlands as one of the first-line psychotherapeutic treatments for depression. Its introduction has also stimulated clinical research, mainly in the field of depression. The application of IPT for the treatment of post-traumatic stress disorder has gained interest and recently resulted in a Dutch translation of John Markowitz's book on this subject.[28]

Some concerns for the future are, however, warranted. As can also be witnessed during the ISIPT conferences, IPT seems to have little appeal for younger professionals; this is certainly the case in the Netherlands. Founded in the 1980s of the last century and introduced in the Netherlands in 1994, IPT never became a significant mainstay in the Netherlands. Most of the same therapists who started to use IPT 30 years ago are still the main protagonists, and only a very small number of young therapists are active in delivering and teaching IPT. It has a minor and often no role in most curricula of training programs for (future) mental health professionals. Although through the years many courses were given (it is the longest-running single course in the postdoctoral training program in Amsterdam), only a small number of those trained continued practicing IPT. As a rule of thumb, IPT seems to survive in clinical settings, where it is being practiced by 3 or more therapists; apparently, a minimal critical mass is needed for continued application in daily clinical practice. A further hindrance to more widespread implementation into standard practice is, like in many Western countries, the dominance of CBT in our country. CBT is taught at all the major universities and postdoctoral programs. There is a huge amount of comparatively well-funded research at universities, and the Society of Behavioral and Cognitive Therapy is by far the largest of the psychotherapy associations with over 9000 members nationwide.

As Markowitz et al.[29] pointed out, psychotherapy is an important and often ignored treatment for treatment-resistant depression, which is typically seen in the secondary and tertiary care settings in which most IPT therapists in the Netherlands work. However, it remains unclear to what extent and in what format IPT is a good treatment for these difficult-to-treat patients. Future work should incorporate theoretical reflections on possible adaptations that need to be followed by empirical clinical testing for this clinically important patient population.

In the meantime, courses in IPT will still be held with an emphasis on supervision to ingrain IPT into the standard of care in mental health organizations. Despite the limited implementation of IPT following training, attendees rate these courses as excellent and helpful. It is our understanding that although the full protocol is not always implemented, the theoretical approach of IPT with important aspects and techniques, such as the interpersonal focus and communication analysis, are used frequently for the well-being of patients.

REFERENCES

1. Blom MB, Hoek HW, Spinhoven P, Hoencamp E, Judith Haffmans PM, van Dyck R. Treatment of depression in patients from ethnic minority groups in the Netherlands. *Transcult Psychiatry*. 2010;47(3):473–490.
2. Blom M, Peeters F, Jonker K, eds. *Leerboek Interpersoonlijke Psychotherapie*. Bohn Stafleu van Loghum; 2011.
3. Blom M, Kerver M, Nolen W, eds. *Inleiding in de interpersoonlijke psychotherapie*. Bohn Stafleu Van Loghum; 1997.
4. Blom MB, Jonker K, Dusseldorp E, et al. Combination treatment for acute depression is superior only when psychotherapy is added to medication. *Psychother Psychosom*. 2007;76(5):289–297.

5. Blom MB, Spinhoven P, Hoffman T, et al. Severity and duration of depression, not personality factors, predict short term outcome in the treatment of major depression. *J Affect Disord*. 2007;104(1-3):119–126.

6. Peeters F, Huibers M, Roelofs J, et al. The clinical effectiveness of evidence-based interventions for depression: a pragmatic trial in routine practice. *J Affect Disord*. 2013;145(3):349–355.

7. Lemmens LH, Arntz A, Peeters FP, Hollon SD, Roefs A, Huibers MJ. Clinical effectiveness of cognitive therapy v. interpersonal psychotherapy for depression: results of a randomized controlled trial. *Psychol Med*. 2015;45(10):2095–2110.

8. Lemmens LH, Van Bronswijk SC, Peeters F, Arntz A, Hollon SD, Huibers MJ. Long-term outcomes of acute treatment with cognitive therapy v. interpersonal psychotherapy for adult depression: follow-up of a randomized controlled trial. *Psychol Med*. 2019;49(3):465–473.

9. Bruijniks SJ, Lemmens LH, Hollon SD, et al. The effects of once-versus twice-weekly sessions on psychotherapy outcomes in depressed patients. *Br J Psychiatry*. 2020;216(4):222–230.

10. Bruijniks SJ, DeRubeis RJ, Lemmens LH, Peeters FP, Cuijpers P, Huibers MJ. The relation between therapy quality, therapy processes and outcomes and identifying for whom therapy quality matters in CBT and IPT for depression. *Behav Res Ther*. 2021;139:103815.

11. Bruijniks SJ, Meeter M, Lemmens LH, Peeters F, Cuijpers P, Huibers MJ. Temporal and specific pathways of change in cognitive behavioral therapy (CBT) and interpersonal psychotherapy (IPT) for depression. *Behav Res Ther*. 2022;151:104010.

12. Bruijniks SJ, Meeter M, Lemmens L, et al. Mechanistic pathways of change in twice weekly versus once weekly sessions of psychotherapy for depression. *Behav Res Therapy*. 2022;151:104038.

13. Lemmens LH, Galindo-Garre F, Arntz A, et al. Exploring mechanisms of change in cognitive therapy and interpersonal psychotherapy for adult depression. *Behav Res Ther*. 2017;94:81–92.

14. Lemmens LH, van Bronswijk SC, Peeters FP, et al. Interpersonal psychotherapy versus cognitive therapy for depression: how they work, how long, and for whom—key findings from an RCT. *Am J Psychother*. 2020;73(1):8–14.

15. Lemmens LH, DeRubeis RJ, Arntz A, Peeters FP, Huibers MJ. Sudden gains in cognitive therapy and interpersonal psychotherapy for adult depression. *Behav Res Ther*. 2016;77:170–176.

16. Bruijniks SJ, van Bronswijk SC, DeRubeis RJ, Delgadillo J, Cuijpers P, Huibers MJ. Individual differences in response to once versus twice weekly sessions of CBT and IPT for depression. *J Consult Clin Psychol*. 2022;90(1):5–17.

17. Van Bronswijk SC, Bruijniks SJ, Lorenzo-Luaces L, et al. Cross-trial prediction in psychotherapy: external validation of the Personalized Advantage Index using machine learning in two Dutch randomized trials comparing CBT versus IPT for depression. *Psychother Res*. 2021;31(1):78–91.

18. van Bronswijk SC, DeRubeis RJ, Lemmens LH, et al. Precision medicine for long-term depression outcomes using the Personalized Advantage Index approach: cognitive therapy or interpersonal psychotherapy? *Psychol Med*. 2021;51(2):279–289.

19. van Bronswijk SC, Lemmens LH, Keefe JR, Huibers MJ, DeRubeis RJ, Peeters FP. A prognostic index for long-term outcome after successful acute phase cognitive

therapy and interpersonal psychotherapy for major depressive disorder. *Depression Anxiety.* 2019;36(3):252–261.

20. Snippe D. *Interpersoonlijke psychotherapie in een ambulante groep.* Bohn Stafleu van Loghum; 2009.

21. Van Schaik A, Van Marwijk H, Adèr H, et al. Interpersonal psychotherapy for elderly patients in primary care. *Am J Geriatr Psychiatry.* 2006;14(9):777–786.

22. Van Schaik DJ, Van Marwijk HW, Beekman AT, De Haan M, Van Dyck R. Interpersonal psychotherapy (IPT) for late-life depression in general practice: uptake and satisfaction by patients, therapists and physicians. *BMC Fam Pract.* 2007;8(1):1–7.

23. Bosmans JE, Van Schaik DJ, Heymans MW, Van Marwijk HW, Van Hout HP, De Bruijne MC. Cost-effectiveness of interpersonal psychotherapy for elderly primary care patients with major depression. *Int J Technol Assess Health Care.* 2007;23(4):480–487.

24. Van Schaik DJ, Van Marwijk HW, Beekman AT, De Haan M, Van Dyck R. Interpersonal psychotherapy (IPT) for late-life depression in general practice: uptake and satisfaction by patients, therapists and physicians. *BMC Fam Pract.* 2007;8(1):1–7.

25. Vos SP, Huibers MJ, Diels L, Arntz A. A randomized clinical trial of cognitive behavioral therapy and interpersonal psychotherapy for panic disorder with agoraphobia. *Psychol Med.* 2012;42(12):2661–2672.

26. Donker T, Batterham PJ, Warmerdam L, et al. Predictors and moderators of response to Internet-delivered interpersonal psychotherapy and cognitive behavior therapy for depression. *J Affect Disord.* 2013;151(1):343–351.

27. Donker T, Bennett K, Bennett A, et al. Internet-delivered interpersonal psychotherapy versus Internet-delivered cognitive behavioral therapy for adults with depressive symptoms: randomized controlled noninferiority trial. *J Med Internet Res.* 2013;15(5):e82.

28. Markowitz J. *Interpersonal Psychotherapy for Posttraumatic Stress Disorder.* Oxford University Press; 2016.

29. Markowitz JC, Wright JH, Peeters F, Thase ME, Kocsis JH, Sudak DM. The neglected role of psychotherapy for treatment-resistant depression. *Am J Psychiatry.* 2022;179(2):90–93.

32

Internet-Delivered Interpersonal Psychotherapy (i-IPT) in the Netherlands

ELS DOZEMAN, TARA DONKER, AMRAH Y. SCHOTANUS, AND ANNEKE VAN SCHAIK ∎

BACKGROUND

The Netherlands is a country in the northwestern part of Europe. In 2021, about 17 million residents lived in an area of 41.583 square kilometers, which makes the Netherlands one of the most densely populated countries in Europe. The lifetime prevalence of depression in the Netherlands is 20%, and the 12-month prevalence is 5.2% in the general population.[1]

The general practitioner (GP) is the gatekeeper of the healthcare system. Patients who need professional help for depression will visit their GP first. Treatment is delivered in a stepped-care format: general care or primary mental health care, if possible, and secondary (specialized) mental health care, if necessary. Specialized mental health care offers treatment to patients with more complex depression, when first-step interventions such as psychoeducation, lifestyle advice, and (online) self-help have not been effective.[2] In specialized mental health care, psychotherapy for depression mainly consists of cognitive behavioral therapy (CBT) and, to a lesser extent, interpersonal psychotherapy (IPT), but these psychotherapies are difficult to access due to long waiting lists caused by a short supply of mental health care professionals.[3,4] Internet-delivered formats may help to reduce waiting lists given less therapist time is needed. Moreover, these formats have other advantages that are discussed below. In the Netherlands, Internet-delivered CBT is widely available and reimbursed by insurance companies. As IPT is a good

Els Dozeman, Tara Donker, Amrah Y. Schotanus, and Anneke van Schaik, *Internet-Delivered Interpersonal Psychotherapy (i-IPT) in the Netherlands* In: *Interpersonal Psychotherapy*. Edited by: Myrna M. Weissman and Jennifer J. Mootz, Oxford University Press. © Oxford University Press 2024. DOI: 10.1093/oso/9780197652084.003.0033 alternative to CBT, Internet-delivered IPT (i-IPT) may serve as an additive treatment option for depression in primary and secondary care. This chapter describes an Internet-delivered version of IPT our team has developed.

INTERNET-DELIVERED TREATMENT FOR DEPRESSION

Over the past 2 decades, Internet-delivered therapy programs have been designed to improve access to healthcare. Unrestricted by time and place, electronic health (eHealth) may provide personalized treatment, increase patient empowerment, and contribute to accessible and affordable treatment.[5] Especially for depression, electronic interventions have been well researched and successfully launched. They have fewer and lower thresholds, have less intense treatment characteristics, and are cost-effective.[6] These Internet-delivered treatments are almost exclusively CBT based, while IPT may fit some patients and therapists better.[7]

i-IPT

i-IPT was modeled after the brief 6-session version of IPT, interpersonal counseling (IPC), which was developed by Klerman and Weissman for primary care settings.[8] Therefore, i-IPT consists of 6 online sessions and follows the structure of IPC. It was studied in an unguided (self-help) format by Donker et al. in Australia in 2013.[9] Between 2015 and 2019, the authors of this chapter (Vrije Universiteit and GGZ in Geest Mental Health Care, Amsterdam), in collaboration with Dr. Myrna Weissman, translated and adapted this first version of i-IPT for use in primary and specialized mental health care in the Netherlands. It can be offered in a guided format, with email support from therapists, or in a blended format. In the blended format, 6 online sessions and 6 to 10 face-to-face sessions with a therapist are delivered in an integrated treatment approach. Face-to-face sessions are alternated with online sessions. In specialized mental health care in the Netherlands, blended formats of CBT are increasingly being used and found to be effective in specialized mental health care.[10] It seems to fit better than guided formats for patients who have more complex depression and need more therapist support. Adding a human component to enable the development of a therapeutic alliance was found to be associated with higher motivation to initiate and sustain engagement in blended care.[11]

In i-IPT, the basic principles of IPT, the structure of the treatment, and the various techniques that may be used to improve interpersonal functioning are explained in the online sessions and combined with various writing exercises. In the online sessions, case examples are provided to help patients cope with their problems by identifying with the problems and solutions of others. In i-IPT, patients are empowered to actively participate in the treatment. For example, in regular IPT, the therapist suggests a treatment focus at the end of the initial phase. However, in i-IPT, patients learn about the different foci in sessions 1 and 2 and are asked to describe in online exercises what focus they think will fit best their problems.

After every online session, the therapist gives written feedback. In the face-to-face sessions, the therapist may use regular IPT strategies and techniques to elaborate on the online exercises and to guide patients through the different phases of IPT. If needed, extra face-to-face sessions may be added. Table 32.1 shows the content of each online session.

Every online session begins with the Patient Health Questionnaire-9, a self-administered mood questionnaire to monitor depressive symptoms. Patients are asked to reflect on changes in the scores, so they learn to link interpersonal problems to mood changes. The first session further includes general information and psychoeducation about depression. The second online session focuses on triaging to 2 of the 4 problem areas. The third, fourth, and fifth online sessions are different for every problem area. In the treatment phase, one can only access the sessions that are part of the problem area that was chosen. In the sixth online session, the therapy is evaluated through written exercises in which patients are asked to reflect on the helpful elements of the therapy and on how they have learned to master their problems. Also, they are asked to fill out a relapse prevention plan. In the closing face-to-face session with the therapist, the exercises and relapse prevention plan are discussed and elaborated when necessary.

Each online focus has its own type of exercises. The focus of grief is elaborated with writing sessions about the grief experiences. In the first online exercise, the patient is asked to describe the relation with the loved one. It is suggested to describe how they first met, what the positive and negative aspects of the

Table 32.1 OVERVIEW OF THE ONLINE I-IPT SESSIONS

Session	Content
1	Psychoeducation on depression. IPT rationale. Linking important life events to depression using a timeline.
2	Choosing a problem area with the help of case vignettes, questions, and a sociogram: grief/disputes/role transition/loneliness.
3–5 Complicated grief	Psychoeducation on depression and the process of grief, building new social networks and social support.
3–5 Role dispute	Exploring the dispute and work on communication patterns.
3–5 Role transition	Psychoeducation about depression and role transitions. Revalidating the old and the new role, adapting to a new role.
3–5 Loneliness	Psychoeducation on depression and social isolation. Working on social skills and creating a social network.
6	Recapitulation of the lessons learned, making a relapse prevention plan.

relationship were, and what kind of person the loved one was. In another exercise, the patient is asked to describe the circumstances of the sickness and death of the loved one, what they felt, with whom they shared their emotions, and who was supportive. In the online sessions on role dispute, patients are first asked to describe the role dispute, with whom, what kind of disputes, how they feel. In another exercise, they are asked to describe the expectations of themselves and the other person. Later, they are given information about different phases of a dispute and different communication styles. They are asked to watch video fragments of people arguing with each other and, in the accompanying online exercise, comment on what they have seen in the video. By working through the session, they become aware of different phases in a role dispute and learn about helpful and nonhelpful interaction styles, such as reading other people's minds or not sharing thoughts or emotions. As a next step, they are asked to describe what communication styles they recognize and to describe a recent dispute in their own life. Finally, they learn how to communicate their needs, wishes, and expectations through exercises. In the sessions on role transitions, online writing exercises on the old and the new roles have to be worked through. The feelings on the old and new roles are explored, and the patient writes about the positive and negative elements of the old and new roles. In the next sessions, the patient makes a plan on how to adjust to the new situation. The sessions of the fourth focus, loneliness, provides patients with examples and exercises on social behavior. Information is given about possible social activities by referring to informative websites. Internet IPT is programmed on a specific e-health platform, Minddistrict. See Figure 32.1 for a visual example. It may serve as an example that can be used to build i-IPT on other platforms.

Training in i-IPT

To train therapists in i-IPT, we developed an in-person workshop (at 2 days, 2.5 hours per day). The trained therapists were both experienced and inexperienced IPT therapists and had different backgrounds (psychologists, psychiatrists in training, and nurse specialists). The first session focused on IPT in general, and the second session was on how to work with i-IPT in a guided or blended format. A treatment manual for therapists was made available in which the content and aim of each session were described. Also, various examples of online feedback were included. The training is shorter in time than the traditional IPT training. This seems feasible as, aside from the detailed manual, the online IPT sessions support not only the patient, but also the therapist to adhere to the IPT structure and strategies from the moment they started i-IPT with one or more patients. Therapists attended supervision sessions with a certified IPT supervisor 1 hour every 2 weeks over a period of 4 months. In the blended protocol, alternating biweekly face-to-face sessions and written sessions is recommended. However, the frequency of face-to-face sessions versus online feedback can be adjusted according to the patient's needs. For example, more severe depression and

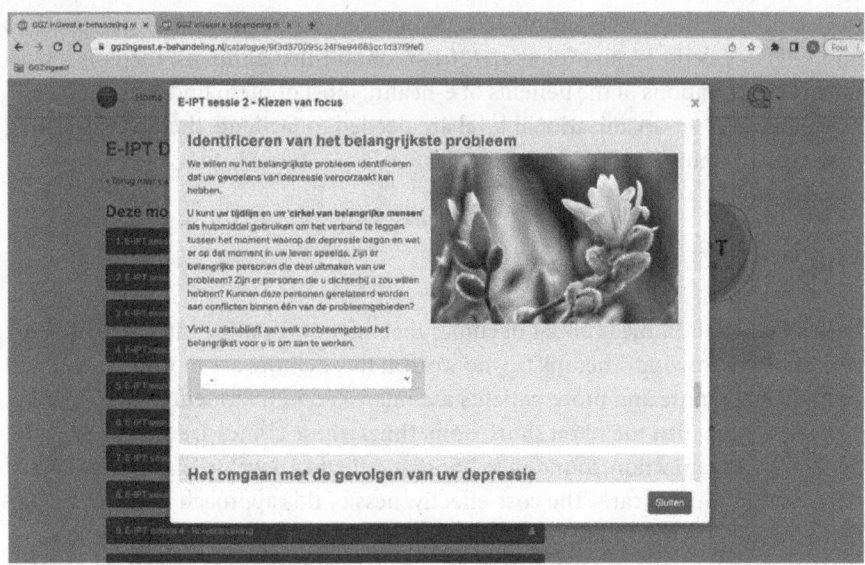

Figure 32.1 Screenshot of Internet-delivered IPT, session 2: choice of focus (in Dutch). Translation: Identifying the main problem. We now want to identify the main problem that may have caused your feelings of depression. You can use your timeline and your "circle of important people" to help you make the connection between when the depression started and what was going on in your life at that time. Are there important people who are part of your problem? Are there people you would like to have closer to you? Can these people be related to conflicts within one of the problem areas? Please tick which problem area is most important for you to work on. (There is a drop-down menu in the text box showing the 4 problem areas.)

accompanying motivational problems may be reasons to increase the frequency of the face-to-face sessions for extra motivation and support. The number of face-to-face sessions may vary from 6 to 10. In the face-to-face sessions, the exercises are further explored and elaborated, for example, through use of role plays.

IMPLEMENTATION

We conducted a pilot study in both primary care (guided format) and specialized mental health care (blended format). However, since the number of sessions reimbursed in primary care is limited, we suggested offering i-IPT in a guided format. Yet, the therapists from our primary care clinics did not perceive a guided intervention without face-to-face contact as acceptable. In contrast, in secondary care, it was not difficult to find therapists who were enthusiastic to work with i-IPT in a blended format. Thus, we conducted a pilot study on blended i-IPT in specialized mental health care. Based on the promising preliminary results regarding patient satisfaction and adherence, the blended IPT intervention has been made available for other therapists.[12] However, availability has not automatically led to the use of the online intervention. In a qualitative study on therapists' perspectives on i-CBT for depression, Mol et al. (2019)[13] found that although therapists have positive expectations of the benefits of e-health, most of them find it hard to use.[12] More efforts at an organizational level are needed to facilitate therapists learning to work with Internet-delivered therapies.

THE FUTURE

In the Netherlands, the number of clinics that offer only online Internet-delivered treatments is growing. Therapists who work at these clinics are motivated and well trained. Also, more and more patients are interested in treatment at these clinics, because waiting lists are often short. Sometimes, these clinics are part of a mental health care organization, founded to boost and further develop Internet-delivered treatment in routine care. The cost-effectiveness of this approach needs to be further studied.

REFERENCES

1. Trimbos. *Depressie in Nederland: Feiten en cijfers*. Geraadpleegd op. 2022. https://www.trimbos.nl/kennis/cijfers/ depressie. Accessed June 3, 2022.
2. Spijker J, Meeuwissen JAC, Aalbers S, et al. De zorgstandaard Depressieve stoornissen [The care standard "Depressive disorders"]. *Tijdschr Psychiatr*. 2019;61(2):112–120.
3. Donker T, Kleiboer A. Innovative technology based interventions for psychological treatment of common mental disorders. *J Clin Med*. 2020;9(10):3075.
4. Fairburn CG, Patel V. The impact of digital technology on psychological treatments and their dissemination. *Behav Res Ther*. 2017;88:19–25.
5. Donker T, Cornelisz I, Van Klaveren C, et al. Effectiveness of self-guided app-based virtual reality cognitive behavior therapy for acrophobia: a randomized clinical trial. *JAMA Psychiatry*. 2019;76(7):682–690.
6. Cuijpers P, Noma H, Karyotaki E, Cipriani A, Furukawa TA. Effectiveness and acceptability of cognitive behavior therapy delivery formats in adults with depression: a network meta-analysis. *JAMA Psychiatry*. 2019;76(7):700–707.
7. Lemmens LH, van Bronswijk SC, Peeters FP, et al. Interpersonal psychotherapy versus cognitive therapy for depression: how they work, how long, and for whom—key findings from an RCT. *Am J Psychother*. 2020;73(1):8–14.
8. Weissman MM, Hankerson SH, Scorza P, et al. Interpersonal counseling (IPC) for depression in primary care. *Am J Psychother*. 2014;68(4):359–383.
9. Donker T, Bennett K, Bennett A, et al. Internet-delivered interpersonal psychotherapy versus Internet-delivered cognitive behavioral therapy for adults with depressive symptoms: randomized controlled noninferiority trial. *J Med Internet Res*. 2013;15(5):e82.
10. Kooistra LC, Wiersma JE, Ruwaard J, et al. Cost and effectiveness of blended versus standard cognitive behavioral therapy for outpatients with depression in routine

specialized mental health care: pilot randomized controlled trial. *J Med Internet Res*. 2019;21(10):e14261.

11. Lungu A, Jun JJ, Azarmanesh O, Leykin Y, Chen CE. Blended care-cognitive behavioral therapy for depression and anxiety in real-world settings: pragmatic retrospective study. *J Med Internet Res*. 2020;22(7):e18723.

12. van Schaik DJ, Schotanus AY, Dozeman E, Huibers MJ, Cuijpers P, Donker T. Pilot study of blended-format interpersonal psychotherapy for major depressive disorder. *Am J Psychother*. 2023;76(2):69–74.

13. Mol M, van Genugten C, Dozeman E, et al. Why uptake of blended Internet-based interventions for depression is challenging: a qualitative study on therapists' Perspectives. *J Clin Med*. 2019;9(1):91.

33

Interpersonal Psychotherapy in Different Populations in Scotland

PATRICIA GRAHAM AND LINDA IRVINE FITZPATRICK ∎

Responsibility for the National Health Services in Scotland resides with the Scottish government, which makes the decisions regarding policy and resourcing. The 4 nations of the United Kingdom each operate independently of each other in terms of healthcare and therefore have a different set of priorities and models of delivery. In Scotland, there has been an active delivery of interpersonal psychotherapy (IPT) since 1998, when the first Scottish IPT randomized controlled trial (RCT) of IPT versus cognitive behavioral therapy (CBT) was conducted in primary care.[1] IPT in Scotland has developed from initially having a charitable status as an entity, into 1 of the 4 nations linking directly with IPT-UK in terms of an overarching training pathway. There have been many different adaptations and applications of IPT that have been piloted and tested in Scotland, all of them drawing on the essential elements of IPT, which are described as follows:

1. **Medical model**: "You are a person with an illness, distress, symptoms, which we recognize."
2. **Sick/recovery role**: "Take care of yourself; who can help?"
3. **Interpersonal inventory/network**: "Who is in your life?"
4. **Symptoms** specifically linked to the onset of the problem: "Grief, interpersonal dispute, transition, loneliness."
5. **Target** symptom reduction and improved social functioning, not personality.
6. **Time** limits are specified.

Patricia Graham and Linda Irvine Fitzpatrick, *Interpersonal Psychotherapy in Different Populations in Scotland* In: *Interpersonal Psychotherapy*. Edited by: Myrna M. Weissman and Jennifer J. Mootz, Oxford University Press. © Oxford University Press 2024. DOI: 10.1093/oso/9780197652084.003.0034

This chapter focuses on the following:

1. Features of IPT for population mental health in Scotland
2. Delivery of IPT for a specific *population* in Scotland
3. An adaptation of IPT within a specific *setting* in Scotland.

POPULATION MENTAL HEALTH: FEATURES OF IPT FOR POPULATION MENTAL HEALTH IN SCOTLAND

Thrive Edinburgh is the capital city's mental health and well-being strategy,[2] an ambitious 10-year framework that focuses on addressing the social determinants of health through intersectoral collaborations and partnerships. The strategy is underpinned by shared values of kindness, respect, and love and focuses on 4 objectives:

1. Identifying and addressing root causes of poor mental health
2. Building resilience and opportunities for people to flourish
3. Providing treatment that is easy to access and makes a difference
4. Focusing on those who are at greatest risk of mental illness

All of our work in Edinburgh is geared around relationships as mediators of stress that buffer hardship[3] and support a cohesive community.[4,5] Relational systems of friendship, kinship, and formal and informal associations build a sense of belonging,[6-9] and a sense of belonging leads to a society with a shared sense of morality and common purpose, social control, social order, and social interactions.[4,10-14] Developing healthy relationships with others and developing positive social networks fosters self-esteem and improves well-being.[9,13] Communities, whether geographical, identity, or of interest, with high levels of social capital are indicated by norms of trust, reciprocity, and participation[15-17] and have advantages for mental health.[18-20]

The worldwide COVID-19 pandemic has given us a deeper understanding and new insights into the different ways that people live and make use of places and spaces.[21,22] If we are to thrive, we need access to spaces that engage our senses to enjoy causal and meaningful social connections, to be included in the life of our city.[23] The recent experiences of social distancing have accelerated the development of the Thrive Line in Edinburgh.[2]

The Thrive Line: Edinburgh

The Thrive Line is a way to connect places and spaces across the city that help to promote and improve mental health and well-being. This may include public or private services such as parks, museums, libraries, gyms, and community centers. A 1-hour awareness-raising course has been developed for employees and volunteers who work in these settings in recognition that the initial inter-action can determine whether a person leaves, stays, or returns to that setting. The awareness session provides participants with an opportunity to increase their understanding of interpersonal relationships and how they may impact their well-being, understand how places and spaces can impact mental health, and gain in-sight into how an interpersonal approach and communication can impact how everyone experiences places and spaces. The session is underpinned by the prin-ciples of attachment theory and understanding the importance of interpersonal communication and how this relates to places. This is demonstrated by drawing participants' attention to how verbal and nonverbal communication can affect how people feel or view themselves in relation to the world and, in turn, how people experience others and spaces they encounter. An interpersonal circle, a simple version of the Interpersonal Inventory, is then used to illustrate connec-tivity. Following the awareness session, the place becomes part of the Thrive Line and added to the visual, which depicts physical assets across the city, staffed by people with awareness of the importance of attachment and interpersonal com-munication styles to establish places where people can thrive.

DELIVERY OF IPT FOR THE VETERAN COMMUNITY

As of 2019, there were an estimated 240,000 veterans living in Scotland.[24] The broader veterans' community living in Scotland, including family members and dependents, has been estimated to make up 10% of Scotland's population.[25] This figure is forecast to fall to around 6% of Scotland's population by the year 2030, and the demographics of Scotland's veterans are increasingly made up of older adults.[26] Adapting and catering to the changing needs of veterans and the broader veteran community is therefore an important consideration for Scottish health services.

Veterans First Point (V1P) Scotland aims to address the needs of Scotland's veterans through provision of a veteran-designed service that acknowledges the unique profile and needs of veterans as a group. Basing V1P Scotland on an ethos of accessibility, coordination, and credibility aims to deliver a service in line with both the expressed needs of Scotland's veterans and the evidence base on how best to engage veterans with mental health services.[27] V1P Scotland's overarching aim is to deliver a credible service through employment of experienced veteran peer support workers and clinicians who are highly trained and experienced in working with veterans. Previous research based in the V1P Lothian service found that veteran peer support workers provided a positive first impression to service users due to their credibility, which is associated with their military connections.[28]

V1P Scotland ensures credibility of clinicians by ensuring that they are highly trained in a range of evidence-based interventions[29] and experienced in working with veterans so that they can provide the best possible care for them. Psychological therapists working in V1P Scotland were all trained in IPT for Veterans[30] through a 5-day experiential workshop-based training. The V1P Scotland peer sup-port workers were also trained in the use of interpersonal counseling (IPC), an intervention that has been found to be effective in the treatment of mild-to-moderate depression and deemed as an appropriate intervention for service users at assessment.[31] IPT for Veterans[30] is the same model as the original model of IPT[32] but delivered specifically to a veteran population. A significant addition is the inclusion of *motivational enhancement* to promote initial and ongoing engagement of veterans in IPT, who are often unfamiliar with evidence-based psychotherapies.

Once discharged from psychological therapy, veterans remain registered with the service with easy access to peer support and drop-in groups to re-engage with the service as needed. This stepped-care model aims to retain engagement with veterans and supports accessibility through re-engagement with clinical support when appropriate.

ADAPTATION OF IPT FOR THE EMERGENCY DEPARTMENT

Interpersonal psychotherapy was adapted for those who presented to an emergency department in Scotland, United Kingdom, in crisis, specifically for those who had attempted suicide. IPT-Acute Crisis (IPT-AC) aims to reduce distress and decrease the risk of self-harm and suicide by providing the intervention as soon as possible after presentation. It aims to improve help seeking from the individual's natural network, develop problem-solving skills, and assist appropriate access to other services. The 4 sessions focus on the following:

1. The reduction and normalization of distress
2. The acceptance of painful affect
3. Problem-solving (clarifying and naming the problem and making sense of it)
4. Understanding who is there for the patient (using the Interpersonal Inventory)
5. Enhancement of interpersonal relationships (including appropriate help seeking from services)
6. Agreement on goals and ways to work on them
7. Preparing for future problems (including signposting to further help or support)

Tann et al.[33] profiled patients who had received IPT-AC as part of the pilot testing to form a descriptive characterization of the cohort, document their engagement, and provide an overview of the outcomes at 6 months after IPT-AC. The authors described a high completion rate (71.3%). A large percentage (59.1%) of patients required no further follow-up from mental health services at 6 months. The results of the pilot study will inform the IPT-AC proof of concept to aid refinement of patient selection. The next stage of the feasibility of IPT-AC will be to conduct an RCT to determine the effectiveness of IPT-AC against an alternative intervention.

IPT for adolescents with acute crisis

Catalan et al.[34] have described their acute crisis adaptation for adolescents as the Ultra-Brief Crisis IPT-A Based Intervention for Suicidal Children and Adolescents (IPT-A-SCI). In their pilot study, they described suicidal behaviors in adolescence as a major public health concern with the worldwide rise in self-injurious behaviors among adolescents. Their intervention was formed based on brief and focused interventions that were found to be effective among suicidal adults, using an adaptation of interpersonal psychotherapy for adolescents. As in the adult version, the intervention has 4 main objectives:

1. A focused treatment for reducing suicide risk
2. A short and immediate response
3. A treatment plan built based on understanding the emotional distress and interpersonal aspects underlying suicidal behavior
4. Generation of hope among adolescents and their parents

The intervention includes intensive 5-weekly sessions, followed by 3 months of email follow-up. Preliminary results of their pilot study of 26 adolescents indicated meaningful trends for both suicidal ideation and depression outcome measures. Significant interaction was found concerning suicidal ideation but not for depression. The authors reported the same as IPT-AC for adults in that the treatment appeared to be safe, feasible, and acceptable, and initial results showed promising trends to support further study. The approach will form part of a planned RCT to test feasibility and how it compares to an alternative crisis psychological intervention.

The Scottish government is currently reviewing its approach to mental health and well-being to develop approaches that will further accelerate whole-system change for more resilient communities and a sustainable health and social care system that focuses on improving population health and tackling inequalities through preventive and proactive care.[35] We believe the features and adaptations of IPT have a key role to play and will continue to advocate and create opportunities for growth and innovation.

REFERENCES

1. Power MJ, Freeman C. A randomized controlled trial of IPT versus CBT in primary care: with some cautionary notes about handling missing values in clinical trials. *Clin Psychol Psychother*. 2012;19(2):159–169.
2. Irvine FL, Campbell P, Gall E, Young C. Thrive Edinburgh—a 10 year road. Edinburgh Health and Social Care Partnership. 2019. Accessed April 4, 2022. https://assets.website-files.com/5e9c71b09aae7e6c3cb9b761/5edfaa100da830a dbece7969_Edinburgh%20Thrive%20Strategy%20Roadmap.pdf
3. Hernandez R, Bassett SM, Boughton SW, Schuette SA, Shiu EW, Moskowitz JT. Psychological well-being and physical health: associations, mechanisms, and future directions. *Emot Rev*. 2018;10(1):18–29.

4. Holt-Lunstad J, Smith TB, Baker M, Harris T, Stephenson D. Loneliness and social isolation as risk factors for mortality: a meta-analytic review. *Perspect Psychol Sci.* 2015;10(2):227–237.

5. Ham C, Alderwick H. *Place Based Systems of Care; a Way Forward for the NHS in England.* King's Fund; 2015.

6. McAdam, DP. The psychology of life stories. *Rev Gen Psychol.* 2001;5(2):100–122.

7. Joseph Rowntree Foundation. *Resilience and the Recession in Six Deprived Communities: Preparing for Worse to Come?* Joseph Rowntree Foundation; 2010.

8. Kallathil J. *Recovery and Resilience: African, African-Caribbean and South Asian Women's Narratives of Recovering From Mental Distress.* Mental Health Foundation; 2011.

9. Mental Health Foundation. *Relationships in the 21st Century: The Forgotten Foundation of Mental Health and Wellbeing.* Mental Health Foundation; 2016. Accessed January 4, 2022. www.mentalhealth.org.uk/publications/relationships-21st-century-forgotten-foundation-mental-health-and-wellbeing

10. Cohen S. Social relationships and health. *Am Psychol.* 2004;59(8):676.

11. Whitehead M, Dahlgren G. Concepts and principles for tackling social inequities in health: levelling up part 1. World Health Organization: Studies on social and economic determinants of population health. 2006;2:460–474.

12. Jetten J, Haslam C, Haslam SA. *The Social Cure: Identity, Health and Well-Being.* Psychology Press; 2012.

13. Cruwys T, Dingle GA, Haslam C, Haslam SA, Jetten J, Morton TA. Social group memberships protect against future depression, alleviate depression symptoms and prevent depression relapse. *Soc Sci Med.* 2013;98:179–186.

14. Hassan Z. *The Social Labs Revolution: A New Approach to Solving Our Most Complex Challenges.* Berrett-Koehler; 2014.

15 Bourdieu P. The forms of capital. In Richardson JG, ed. *Handbook of Theory and Research for the Sociology of Capital.* Greenwood Press; 1986:241–258.

16. Putnam RD. *Bowling Alone.* Simon and Schuster; 2000.

17. Hancock L, Mooney G, Neal S. Crisis social policy and the resilience of the concept of community. *Crit Soc Policy.* 2012;32(3):343–364.

18 Laub JH, Sampson RJ. Understanding desistance from crime. *Crime Justice.* 2001;28:1–69.

19. Morgan A, Ziglio E. Revitalising the evidence base for public health: an assets model. *Promot Educ.* 2007;14(2 suppl):17–22.

20 Maruna S. Strengths-based approaches to reentry: extra mileage toward rcintegration and destigmatization. *Jpn J Sociol Criminol.* 2009;34:58–80.

21. Whittle N. *The 15 Minute City; Global Change Through Local Living.* Luathe Press; 2021.

22. Roe J, McCay L. *Restorative Cities—Urban Design for Mental Health and Wellbeing.* Bloomsbury Visual Arts; 2021.

23. Keyes CLM. The mental health continuum: from languishing to flourishing in life. *J Health Soc Behav.* 2002;43(2):207–222.

24. Scottish Veterans Commissioner. Veterans' health and wellbeing: a distinctive Scottish approach. 2018. Accessed May 2, 2022. https://www.gov.scot/publications/veterans-health-wellbeing-distinctive-scottish-approach/

25. Poppy Scotland. Health and welfare of the ex-service community in Scotland. 2014. Accessed April 6, 2022. https://www.ageuk.org.uk/globalassets/age-scotland/documents/veterans-project/poppyscotland-household-survey-research-2014.pdf

26. Ashworth J, Hudson M, Malam S. A UK household survey of the ex-service community. Royal British Legion; 2014. Accessed April 5, 2022. https://storage.rblcdn.co.uk/sitefinity/docs/default-source/campaigns-policy-and-research/rbl_household_survey_report.pdf?sfvrsn=5bcbae4f_4

27. Fitzpatrick LI, McArdle A, Gall E, Abraham L. *An Evaluation of Veterans First Point Scotland: Scotland's Specialist Mental Health Service for Veterans.* 2020.

28. Weir B, Cunningham M, Abraham L, Allanson-Oddy C. Military veteran engagement with mental health and well-being services: a qualitative study of the role of the peer support worker. *J Ment Health.* 2018;28(6):647–653.

29. NHS Scotland. The Matrix: a guide to delivering evidence-based psychological therapies in Scotland. 2015. Accessed October 1, 2022. https://www.nes.scot.nhs.uk/our-work/matrix-a-guide-to-delivering-evidence-based-psychological-therapies-in-scotland/.

30. Clougherty KF, Hinrichsen GA, Steele JL, et al. *Therapist Guide to Interpersonal Psychotherapy for Depression in Veterans.* US Department of Veterans Affairs; 2014.

31. Weissman MM, Hankerson SH, Scorza P, et al. Interpersonal counseling (IPC) for depression in primary care. *Am J Psychother.* 2014;68(4):359–383.

32. Weissman MM, Markowitz JC, Klerman GL. *The Guide to Interpersonal Psychotherapy.* Oxford University Press; 2018.

33. Lin T. Profiling the interpersonal psychotherapy acute crisis (Scotland) cohort: suicidality and risk factors. Poster presented at: International Society of Interpersonal Psychotherapy Conference; November 2019; Budapest, Hungary.

34. Catalan HL, Frenk LM, Spigelman AE, et al. Ultra-brief crisis IPT-A based intervention for suicidal children and adolescents (IPT-A-SCI) pilot study results. *Front Psychiatry.* 2020;11:553422.

35. Scottish Government. Scottish government's COVID 19, Scotland's Strategic Framework update. 2022. Accessed April 18, 2022. https://www.gov.scot/publications/coronavirus-covid-19-scotlands-strategic-framework-update-february-2022/#:~:text=Coronavirus%20(COVID%2D19)%3A%20Scotland's%20Strategic%20Framework%20update%20%2D%20February%202022,-Published%2022%20February&text=This%20update%20of%20the%20Strategic,calmer%20phase%20of%20the%20pandemic

34

Interpersonal Psychotherapy in Ukraine

ROSLYN LAW, VITALII KLYMCHUK, AND
VIKTORIIA GORBUNOVA ■

CONTEXT AND BACKGROUND

Ukraine is an eastern European country prominent in the minds of people around the world, more so now than at any other time in its existence. A humanitarian crisis has faced its population in 2022 and continuing in 2023. Over 6.5 million people have been forced to leave their country, and a further 5 million have been displaced within its borders, an urgent reminder of the need for mental health care and psychosocial interventions in the relief and recovery work of the present and future.[1] The journey toward disseminating interpersonal psychotherapy (IPT) across Ukraine did not begin in such circumstances. However, even in mid-2018, when the first emails were exchanged, it was a country of more than 43 million people who were already 5 years into a conflict with an aggressive neighbor, forcing change, conflict, and loss on sections of its population.

Mental health services in Ukraine have traditionally been centralized and provided by psychiatrists and psychologists in outpatient psychiatric clinics of large mental health facilities. Approximately 20% of those who need support receive it in these public services. Additional access, available mostly in large cities, has been provided by a large multidisciplinary private sector, offering multiple psychotherapeutic modalities and reflecting varying levels of professional education. As there is no legislative regulation of psychotherapeutic practice in Ukraine, commitment to ethical practice and to evidence-based interventions has been mostly a matter of a professional's personal conscience.

Roslyn Law, Vitalii Klymchuk, and Viktoriia Gorbunova, *Interpersonal Psychotherapy in Ukraine* In: *Interpersonal Psychotherapy.* Edited by: Myrna M. Weissman and Jennifer J. Mootz, Oxford University Press. © Oxford University Press 2024. DOI: 10.1093/oso/9780197652084.003.0035

The process of IPT dissemination began as it has in many places around the world, with 2 people having a conversation. Networks build networks, and within 5 days we had been introduced and a conversation that was to run for several years started. This chapter describes the intentions, progress, and future objectives arising from those exchanges.

Vitalii Klymchuk (V. K.), professor of psychology and mental health expert for the Ukrainian Ministry of Health next describes his ambitious vision of IPT in Ukraine and the steps necessary to achieve it.

THE VISION

The vision is to bring IPT to Ukraine in accordance with international standards and establish the IPT institute in Ukraine.

THE STEPS

1. Provide training in IPT for a multidisciplinary group of 20–30 Ukrainian mental health professionals, including psychologists, psychotherapists, and psychiatrists;
2. Establish an institute for IPT in Ukraine;
3. Promote IPT through written material, videos, practice handbooks, and translation of existing manuals that will be used as a foundation for additional IPT training courses; and
4. Conduct IPT-focused research in Ukraine.

The first round of training would focus on IPT for working-age adults, and subsequent waves would move on to models adapted for children and adolescents. Those professionals educated in this first IPT wave were expected to be experienced psychologists and psychiatrists, working in public and private sectors.

TRAINING PROCESS

Step 1, bringing an external expert in IPT to Ukraine to deliver in-person training, encountered the predictable hurdles and delays inherent in dissemination:

- aligning diaries for planning and delivery—seemingly simple but not to be underestimated;
- the financial burden for a low- and middle-income country recruiting support from a wealthier economy;
- adapting accreditation standards to reflect an emerging rather than established IPT workforce; and
- navigating language barriers in supervision.

In the months of discussion that followed, we considered alternative models of dissemination to address these challenges:

- a small number of clinicians traveling to the United Kingdom to attend an established course with a view to being fast-tracked through training to deliver first language courses in Ukraine on completion;
- delivering training to a larger group, 50–60 clinicians, to generate income and interest that would be used to support more targeted training.

After several months of discussion, reduced fees were approved, primary objectives were agreed on, and training dates were confirmed for April 2020, which proved to be just one of the highly fateful decisions to befall this process. The intention was to raise awareness of IPT through a large-scale training. Supervised practice was not yet financially or logistically within reach, and consequently the number of participants that could attend was not limited to a corresponding supervision capacity. V. K. complemented this awareness-raising exercise by speaking about IPT at a psychotherapy conference in Ukraine and generating promotional material to encourage interest in colleagues (http://iptukraine.mh-solutions.pro/).

However, as the impact of COVID became clear in early 2020, the plan for this face-to-face event was reluctantly postponed. In its place, and to sustain interest, an online introduction to IPT was conducted by Roslyn Law (R. L.) in April 2020, attended by 25 participants who had been registered to attend the original event. Attention was also turned to translating materials for use by Ukrainian clinicians, and V. K. was introduced to Little Brown Books Publishers and given permission to translate R. L.'s books. Energy was initially invested in rescheduling the face-to-face teaching, but as the delay imposed by a global pandemic extended, learning forced by lockdown allowed us to pivot to remotely delivered training. Three days of practitioner training were delivered during November and December 2020 for 30 trained clinicians working with adults and children. Training materials were provided in advance to allow information to be reproduced in Ukraine and help participants to process the information at a manageable pace. Simultaneous translation was also provided to facilitate participation. Feedback was positive and enthusiastic, but highlighted the need for more in-depth and practice-based training to build confidence in adopting this new way of working. Supervision and more attuned personalized guidance were training needs expressed by almost all trainees, reflecting the need for combined training and supervision of deliberate and feedback-based practice as a foundation for sustainable dissemination.[2]

Following completion of this step, and in response to the feedback and enthusiasm for further guidance, we tried to find Ukrainian-speaking supervisors in the International Society of Interpersonal Psychotherapy (ISIPT) community to support future dissemination, but unfortunately none was identified. Drawing on our own and others' experience, alternative models were also considered:

- Focus on peer-to-peer learning
- Translated transcripts of clinical practice for supervision

- English-speaking Ukrainian therapists work with English-speaking clients
- Simultaneous translation of supervision of first-language therapy

In order not to lose momentum, peer-to-peer learning was adopted as a first step, and R. L. shared resources that could be used in this context. During the next year, the Ukrainian group of trainees created a community of practice. Those who attended the training were invited to join the discussions and attend monthly meetings. Each meeting consisted of shared learning about new theory or review of the material from the training, prepared by one of the participants, and a case review, presented by others.

In parallel with this work, ISIPT was developing a framework for regional chapters, and V. K. had a meeting with the ISIPT then-President Oguz Omay to discuss chapter-related options. Two pathways are under consideration—either establishing the Ukrainian chapter with the support of the National Psychological Association of Ukraine or creating a separate Ukrainian IPT nongovernmental organization. The idea of a Ukrainian chapter has not yet become a reality, but the idea is still in place and waiting for the implementation.

CURRENT CONTEXT AND PLANS FOR THE FUTURE

On February 24, 2022, life for our Ukrainian colleagues was irrevocably changed. Despite being displaced within his own country, V. K. and his colleagues remain committed to pursuing the objective of disseminating IPT and to extend the options for psychological care available to his community now and when they rebuild. Communities are scattered across continents, experiencing unimaginable transitions, cross-border conflicts in families as well as between nations, and they have been subjected to tragic, brutal loss.

In the face of all this, how can we keep going?

- We write this and remain in each other's minds.
- We will work on generating high-quality materials for use when Ukrainian communities begin the work of rebuilding.
- Four Ukrainian clinicians were sponsored by Myrna Weissman, the Anna Freud Center, and Teachers College of the University of Columbia to attend the 2022 Global Mental Health IPT Summer Institute, focusing on working with populations exposed to severe adversities and trauma and provided training in group IPT. R. L. and the attendees formed a peer supervision group to review and learn from initial group practice.
- Knowing we are stronger together, V. K. will work in collaboration with the ISIPT Dissemination Committee to introduce 250 displaced Ukrainian clinicians who are living in our international communities to ISIPT and IPT national group members. Our Ukrainian colleagues will be invited to accessible IPT activity in their host environments,

supporting their IPT learning and helping us to move at pace when they return home and begin to rebuild.
- We will ground our work on empirically supported principles in the aftermath of humanitarian crises.[3]
  o Promote a sense of safety
  o Promote calming
  o Promote a sense of self- and collective efficacy
  o Promote connectedness
  o Promote hope

REFERENCES

1. Shi W, Navario P, Hall BJ. Prioritising mental health and psychosocial services in relief and recovery efforts in Ukraine. *Lancet Psychiatry*. 2022;9(6):e27.
2. Rousmaniere T, Goodyear RK, Miller SD, et al. *The Cycle of Excellence: Using Deliberate Practice to Improve Supervision and Training*. John Wiley & Sons; 2017.
3. Hobfoll SE, Watson P, Bell CC, et al. Five essential elements of immediate and mid-term mass trauma intervention: empirical evidence. *Psychiatry*. 2007;70(4):283–315.

Guided Self-Help Interpersonal Psychotherapy in the United Kingdom

ROSLYN LAW ■

INTRODUCTION

Guided self-help, in the form of bibliotherapy, has been widely used to treat mild-to-moderate or subthreshold depressive symptoms, as either a sole or supplementary intervention. Individuals work through a structured book, either independently or with supportive guidance. Multiple studies have shown that bibliotherapy, reflecting a range of therapeutic approaches, is cost-effective, facilitates positive change, and improves self-management and resilience.[1] Self-help resources may be accessed directly or through coordinated reading schemes that aim to make selected self-help materials more readily available to the public, such as the Reading Well Books on Prescription scheme.

Self-help materials have been a relatively late addition to the interpersonal psychotherapy (IPT) library of publications. Service-user focused IPT materials have primarily been developed as supplementary resources, and to date none have been the subject of empirical evaluation of clinical outcomes. The current selection occupies a position somewhere between stand-alone interventions and supplementary resources used prior to or alongside traditional IPT. Four publications are discussed in this chapter, 3 focus on IPT for adults and 1 on IPT for adolescents (IPT-A) experiencing depression.

The first self-help style guide to be published was *Mastering Depression Through Interpersonal Psychotherapy—Patient Workbook* and the accompanying *Mastering Depression Through Interpersonal Psychotherapy: Monitoring Forms*

Roslyn Law, *Guided Self-Help Interpersonal Psychotherapy in the United Kingdom* In: *Interpersonal Psychotherapy*. Edited by: Myrna M. Weissman and Jennifer J. Mootz, Oxford University Press. © Oxford University Press 2024. DOI: 10.1093/oso/9780197652084.003.0036

(Treatments That Work).[2,3] This short workbook and the monitoring forms provide psychoeducation about depression and IPT and primes the reader to consider questions they may be asked if they engage in IPT with a trained therapist. The focus is on describing the IPT process and objectives of each phase of the work and tracking outcomes with relevant monitoring forms. Brief case examples are provided to illustrate the focal areas and the ways in which IPT may help in each context. This is available in paperback and as an e-book.

Defeating Depression: How to Use the People in Your Life to Open the Door to Recovery[4] provides a complete guide to IPT that could be used either independently or with a therapist. The book was commissioned following IPT's inclusion in Improving Access to Psychological Therapies (IAPT), the framework for primary care services for common mental health problems across England. *Defeating Depression* explains IPT, provides psychoeducation on depression, explains the importance of understanding the interpersonal narrative that gives context to this experience, and walks the reader through the whole IPT process step by step. From the outset, the reader is encouraged to recruit a backup team with whom to tackle depression as a collective effort. The therapist may be part of the team as can members of the reader's personal network. Multiple exercises that reflect IPT interventions are described and illustrated in brief, as are chapter-long case examples. The book is available in paperback and as an e-book and has been approved for translation in Estonian and Ukrainian but these have not yet been published.

When IPT for adolescents with depression (IPT-A) was added to the Children and Young People's IAPT (CYP IAPT) program in England, *Defeating Teenage Depression—Getting There Together*[5] was published. This was initially commissioned as an update on the 2013 publication described above, but recognizing the omissions that can result when interventions for adolescents are reduced to "downward adaptations of adult treatments or upward adaptations of child treatments,"[6] the book was completely rewritten for an adolescent audience. A group of young people with experience of mental health difficulties were enlisted as first editors on this publication. The IPT-A self-help guide includes additional chapters on adolescent brain development and the resulting interpersonal and conceptual implications, developmentally relevant case examples, and information for parents and caregivers. Online resources are referenced, and clinical materials are available to download.[4] This publication is available in paperback and as an e-book.

The most recent IPT self-help book is *Feeling Better: Beat Depression and Improve Your Relationships With Interpersonal Psychotherapy.*[7] This resource guides the adult reader through the IPT process step by step, with the authors acting as coaches along the way with upbeat encouragement and multiple personal examples. This publication has additional sections throughout that specifically target men experiencing depression and is available as a paperback, e-book, and as n audiobook. In 2021, a Russian translation was published.[8]

ADAPTATIONS IN A SELF-HELP FORMAT

Each of the published IPT self-help books follows the standard models of IPT or IPT-A. The period over which they will be read is determined by the reader, although the recommendation is to work through the sections on a week-by-week basis, as with face-to-face work. The language in each of the publications is simplified and less academic than in the professional manuals. The aim is to make clinical concepts accessible and easy to follow with a clinician or alone. Multiple case examples are provided to illustrate each step of the process, and detailed exercises are described to guide the individual. Readers are encouraged to use the questions to prime discussions in therapy or with their support networks.

BARRIERS TO IMPLEMENTATION

One central challenge of writing a self-help book for IPT is that the approach is interpersonal and not intended to be used in isolation. Each of the publications has addressed this issue in a slightly different way. Weissman[2,3] prepares the reader for therapeutic work that will be completed with a therapist. Law[4,5] explicitly encourages the reader to recruit a team with whom to work through the book and includes the possibility that the book will be used in the context of ongoing therapy. Stulberg and Frey[7] give the authors prominent voices throughout, acting as coaches during the process.

As written resources with few translations to additional languages, the current self-help resources are primarily of benefit to literate, English-speaking populations. The most recent publication,[7] which is available as an audiobook, is a partial exception. Text-to-speech features of some e-reader devices and apps now allow written publications to be read aloud, which goes some way to improving access.

The existing resources all originated in Western contexts, which is reflected in most of the clinical examples. The limited range of culturally diverse case examples, including limited or no consideration of gender identity, sexuality, physical ability, and neurodivergence, is likely to limit the relevance and nuance for communities that are not sufficiently represented.

FACTORS ASSISTING DISSEMINATION

Having each of the publications available electronically has increased their accessibility and privacy of use, allowing people to carry them on their phone or tablet rather than being limited to a hard copy. The *Defeating Depression* book also provides online copies of many of the worksheets and prompts that can be freely downloaded from the "Overcoming" website.[4] Some of the publications have been adopted as training texts on IPT practitioner and supervisor courses in the United Kingdom, including Northern Ireland; United States; Sweden; Canada; Philippines; and Finland. Consequently, they have been widely used by trainers and supervisors to inform and guide novice trainees as they learn IPT and IPT-A. Additionally, they are often used by qualified therapists offering additional resources during and after therapy and occasionally as guidance for family members supporting the person in depression (see Table 35.1). *Defeating Depression*[4] is included in the Reading Well bibliotherapy program,[9] making it freely available in every library in England and Wales. This is funded by the Department for Digital, Culture, Media, and Sport of the UK government. Reading Well books, which reflect interventions included in the National Institute for Health and Care Excellence (NICE) guidelines,[10] are recommended for selection by independent health experts and people with lived experience of the conditions covered. Over 2.6 million Reading Well books have been borrowed from public libraries in England and Wales.

Defeating Teenage Depression was highly recommended by the British Medical Association (BMA) British Medical Awards book prize for Popular Medicine. The BMA Medical Book Awards 2017 Review stated:

> The book's main strength has to be its appeal to a wide range of clinical and non-clinical readers. It is topical, clinically sound and empowering. It is engaging and therapeutic—a positive book which guides the reader to reflect on experiences and thought processes and enable them to seek change and shape the thinking process. It is a well-written therapeutic text which could have a positive impact on many. It could empower teachers, clinicians, parents and most importantly the teens themselves to problem solve and understand the depth of emotion and behaviours that shape their mental health. It is also a valuable tool for those who do not present to a GP or teacher but wish for support or help. This book challenges any reader to evaluate thinking patterns and reflect. This is an informative thought-provoking read which every reader will take something positive from.[11]

HOW ARE SELF-HELP MATERIALS USED BY IPT CLINICIANS?

Members of International Society of Interpersonal Psychotherapy (ISIPT) and Interpersonal Psychotherapy UK (IPTUK) were surveyed to ask about their knowledge and use of the IPT self-help materials that are available. Seventy-five responses were received from the United Kingdom (72%), North America (11%), Europe (7%), Australia and NZ (5%), and Israel (1%). It is not possible to determine if the response rate reflects differences in use of self-help materials internationally or a bias of response from the author's regional network.

Eighty-five percent of responders had used at least 1 self-help resource to inform their own learning and practice, and 16% reported using 2 or more of

Table 35.1 Qualitative descriptions of use of IPT self-help materials

Training resource	Resources in session
"Use [Feeling Better] when training clinicians to do IPT therapy." "We have asked students to refer to *Defeating Depression* and how to use the people in their life to open the door to recovery. This book is so easy for students to follow and we often discuss aspects of the book and integrate sections into our training sessions." "I like both these publications and recommend them for trainee therapists as they break down the content and rationale for session in a meaningful way" "Ros Law's self-help books are useful support for trainees trying to think about how to translate IPT theoretical concepts into patient friendly language and so I often give trainees chapters to read as part of their own learning."	"The self-help book is amazingly accessible and helpful in normalising the language we use in sessions." "In-depth helpful explanations of the main strategies, e.g., timeline, IPI, all 4 focal areas and examples contribute to my planning of sessions and explanations to patients. I also use the appendices as handouts, e.g., info for family and ending." "I find it helps the client to have a greater understanding of what we do in sessions."
Learning resource "Good analogies and explanations to simplify complex ideas and helpful case studies to visualise aspects of IPT in practice whilst training." "I find them useful if I'm looking to refresh my knowledge and skills in delivering the model and also when I want to think about how to approach client sessions or say things in a different way." "It has helped a lot to understand in a clear and practical way some theory I was not very confident about."	**Resource between sessions** "Using the self-help resource outside of therapy is a useful parallel to the therapy process, particularly in IPT-A when used by parents and carers, as it engages significant others and proactively supports the network to help." "It's very helpful to underscore IPT model between sessions and assists with homework practice. Treatment is more efficient." "They have been a supportive backbone and sometimes reference point for both myself and the client. For the client, I have found that when we have perhaps met for a review 3–6 months after end of treatment, they have reported that the books consolidated their understanding."

Feedback from individuals in therapy

"I knew nothing about IPT so, pleased to say I wouldn't be where I am today without the help of *Defeating Depression*. All easy to read and explained in understandable and workable chapters. I feel that if I can get through depression with this wonderful aid, then anyone can."

Table 35.2 USE OF SELF-HELP MATERIALS

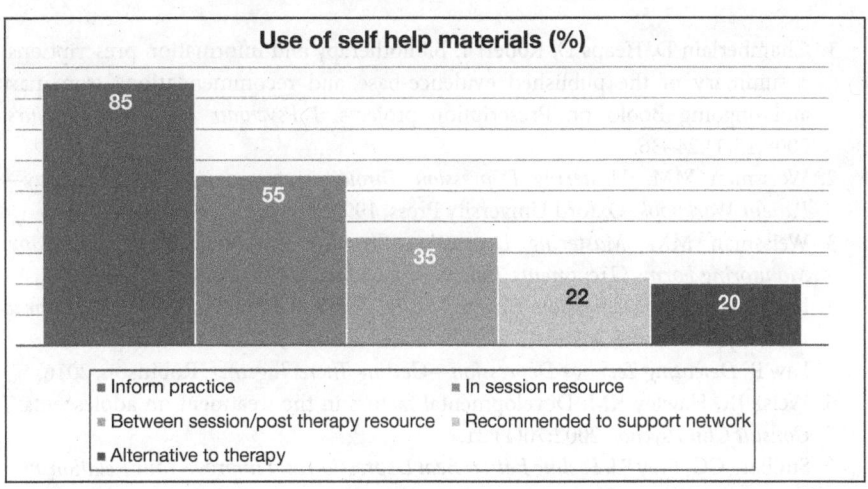

the available resources. The country of origin was highly correlated with re-ported use, with limited crossover of North American and UK texts beyond their local regions. More than half of responders (55%) used at least 1 self-help resource in session with clients. Almost half (47%) supplemented work in session with targeted use of self-help resources between sessions or following the end of therapy as part of a maintenance plan. Twenty-nine percent additionally encouraged their clients' networks (e.g., family members, parents) to use at least 1 of the self-help resources to guide their understanding and involvement between session and following completion of therapy. More than a quarter of responders (27%) recommended at least 1 self-help resource as an alternative to face-to-face therapy (see Table 35.2).

RECOMMENDATIONS

Future editions and new publications should carefully consider the length of the resource to ensure they fall within the capacity of a depressed population with concentration and memory difficulties. Existing and future resources should be available across multiple formats and specifically targeted at social media platforms to increase ease of access. The ISIPT Dissemination committee and Anna Freud Center have both adopted the production of short, freely available resources as a leading priority. Self-help resources adapted for different cultural groups and made available in multiple languages should be developed to increase equity of access and relevance. Researchers should examine the optimal use of self-help materials for different clinical populations. This could inform pathways of care and opportunities to sustain the impact of IPT as a time-limited intervention, delivered face to face or through guided support.

REFERENCES

1. Chamberlain D, Heaps D, Robert I. Bibliotherapy and information prescriptions: a summary of the published evidence-base and recommendations from past and ongoing Books on Prescription projects. *J Psychiatr Ment Health Nurs.* 2008;15(1):24–36.
2. Weissman MM. *Mastering Depression Through Interpersonal Psychotherapy— Patient Workbook.* Oxford University Press; 1995.
3. Weissman MM. *Mastering Depression Through Interpersonal Psychotherapy: Monitoring Forms (Treatments That Work).* Oxford University Press; 1995.
4. Law R. *Defeating Depression: How to Use the People in Your Life to Open the Door to Recovery.* Robinson; 2013.
5. Law R. *Defeating Teenage Depression—Getting There Together.* Robinson; 2016.
6. Weisz JR, Hawley KM. Developmental factors in the treatment on adolescents. *J Consult Clin Psychol.* 2002;70(1):21.
7. Stulberg CG, Frey RJ. *Feeling Better: Beat Depression and Improve Your Relationships With Interpersonal Psychotherapy.* New World Library; 2018.
8. Stulberg CG, Frey RJ, Maria Smirnova, Trans. *Мне лучше: Межличностная терапия против депрессии.* Transatlantic Literary Agency Inc. and Van Lear Agency LLC; 2021.
9. The Reading Agency. *Reading Well.* https://reading-well.org.uk/books/books-on-prescription/mental-health#self-help; 2023. Accessed September 17, 2023.
10. National Institute for Health and Care Excellence. *Depression in adults: treatment and management.* https://www.nice.org.uk/guidance/ng222/resources/depression-in-adults-treatment-and-management-pdf-66143832307909; 2023. Accessed September 17, 2023.
11. British Medical Association. *Medical Book Awards.* https://www.bma.org.uk/about-us/corporate-social-environmental-responsibility/bma-awards/medical-book-awards; 2023. Accessed September 17, 2023.

PART VII

Interpersonal Psychotherapy in the Middle East

Interpersonal Psychotherapy in the Middle East

36

Interpersonal Psychotherapy in Iran

NILOOFAR RAFIEI ALHOSAINI AND
HASAN REZAEI-JAMALOUEI ∎

INTRODUCTION

Epidemiological studies have found that the lifetime prevalence of depression in Iran is about 25%–35%[1-4] and approximately twice as prevalent in women compared to men.[5] Interpersonal psychotherapy (IPT) effectively treats major depressive disorder (MDD) and is well matched with Iranian culture, where interpersonal relations are important and people consider themselves part of a family and a community before they see themselves as individuals. Iranian culture values relationships, especially family ties.

To understand the extent of the dissemination of IPT across Iran and learn of adaptations made for the Iranian cultural context, we conducted searches in 6 bibliographical databases (google scholar, SID, Magiran, Sivilica, Irandoc, and Adineh book) by searching "interpersonal psychotherapy" in Persian "روان درمانی بین فردی". Of the 59 examined abstracts (37 after removal of duplicate records), 20 full-text articles[6-25] were retrieved for further consideration (see Table 36.1).

Generally, these included trials were published after 2007 (around 2 articles published per year). The 20 studies included a total of 583 participants (226 in IPT conditions, 44 in the IPT plus usual care condition, 1 in the IPT for adolescents [IPT-A] condition, 3 in the family-based IPT [FB-IPT] condition, 38 in the cognitive behavioral therapy [CBT] condition, 43 in the usual care condition, 204 in the wait list control condition, and 24 lost to attrition.

Iran is subdivided into 31 provinces. Sixty percent ($n = 12$) of trials took place in the capital city of Tehran, 2 in Lorestan Province, 2 in Mazandaran Province, 2 in Karaj Province, 1 in Razavi Khorasan Province, and 1 study was reported in

Niloofar Rafiei Alhosaini and Hasan Rezaei-Jamalouei, *Interpersonal Psychotherapy in Iran* In: *Interpersonal Psychotherapy*. Edited by: Myrna M. Weissman and Jennifer J. Mootz, Oxford University Press. © Oxford University Press 2024. DOI: 10.1093/oso/9780197652084.003.0037

Table 36.1 FULL-TEXT JOURNAL ARTICLES

	Study authors reference number	IPT type[a]	Diagnosis[b]	Target group	Study interventions (N)[c]	Format[d]	Sessions	Outcome measures[b]	Method	City
1	Moradi et al.[6]	O	Dysthymia	Female	IPT-A (N = 1)	IND + TEL (between sessions)	12 (1x weekly)	BDI	Case study	Tehran
2	Abbaspour et al.[7]	O	Major depression symptoms	Male and their mother	FB-IPT (N = 3)	IND (Client + parents)	14 (2x weekly)	MAQ	Single-case experimental design	Tehran
3	Rouzbahani et al.[8]	A	Generalized anxiety	Female	IPT (N = 15); WL (N = 15)	GRP	8	BAI, FTAS-20	Pre-test, posttest	Tehran
4	Mohammadi[9]	A	Dyslexia	Students	IPT (N = 15); WL (N = 16)	GRP	8	BAI, FTAS-20	Pretest, posttest	Karaj
5	Ahmadi Sabzevari et al.[10]	O	Major depression symptoms	Female	IPT (N = 15); WL (N = 15)	GRP	8	TPT, BAI	—	Lorestan
6	Gholamrezaei et al.[11]	O	Eating disorder symptoms	Female students	IPT (N = 16 + 2 dropout); WL (N = 18)	GRP	14 (2x weekly)	BDI-II, Reef	Pretest, posttest	Lorestan
7	Pouyan et al.[12]	A	Postpartum depression	Female	IPT + UC (N = 44 + 2 dropout); UC (N = 43 + 3 dropout)	IND (N = 2, 60 min) + TEL (N = 1)	3	EAT-26, CIA-V3	Pretest, posttest	Karaj

#	Author		Condition	Population	Groups		Sessions	Measures	Design	Location
8	Bodaghi et al.[13]	A	Social anxiety disorder	College students	IPT (N = 9 + 1 dropout); WL (N = 10)	GRP	10	LSAS, EEQ	Pretest, posttest	Razavi Khorasan
9	Gharadaghi et al.[14]	A	Marital satisfaction	Female	IPT (N = 12); CBT (N = 12); WL (N = 12)	GRP	8	ENRICH	Pretest, posttest	Tehran
10	Tarkhan.[15]	O	Marital dissatisfaction	Female	IPT (N = 15); WL (N = 15)	GRP	10 (1x/2x weekly)	Bell, Shiring	Pretest, posttest	Mazandaran
11	Shoja'Kazemi & Momenijavid.[16]	A	Infidelity	Female	IPT (N = 8 + 2 dropout); WL (N = 8 + 2 dropout)	GRP	8	Vaughan, MR-AI	Pretest, posttest	Tehran
12	Momeni Javid et al.[17]	A	Marital betrayals	Female	IPT (N = 8); WL (N = 8)	GRP	20 (2x weekly)	Vaughan, MR-AI	Pretest, posttest	Tehran
13	Morteza[18]	O	Low psychological well-being and life quality	Female	IPT (N = 15); WL (N = 15)	GRP	10	WHOQOL-BREF, RSPWB	Pretest, posttest	Mazandaran
14	Alizadehfard et al.[19]	A	Social anxiety	University students	IPT (N = 20); WL (N = 20)	GRP	12	SPIN, RMET	Pretest, posttest	Tehran

(continued)

Table 36.1 Continued

Study authors reference number	IPT type[a]	Diagnosis[b]	Target group	Study interventions (N)[c]	Format[d]	Sessions	Outcome measures[b]	Method	City
15	Tavoli et al.[20]	Social anxiety disorder	Students	IPT (N = 16 + 4 dropout); CBT (N = 14 + 6 dropout)	GRP	12 (1x weekly)	FAQ, SPIN, BFNE-II	Pretest, posttest	Tehran
16	Asl Soleimani et al.[21]	Social anxiety disorder	Students	IPT (N = 12); WL (N = 12)	IND (N = 1) + GRP (N = 12)	13	SPIN, CERQ, PEPQ	Pretest, posttest	Tehran
17	Danekar et al.[22]	Major depression symptoms	Female students	IPT (N = 13); WL (N = 13)	GRP	12	BDI, DLQ	Pretest, posttest	Tehran
18	Zemestani et al.[23]	Major depression symptoms	Male	IPT (N = 10 + 2 dropout); WL (N = 12)	GRP	12	BDI	—	Tehran
19	Shafiea Abadi et al.[24]	Nonclinical depression	Female	IPT (N = 12); CBT (N = 12)	GRP	8	BDI	—	Tehran
20	Qaderi Bagajan et al.[25]	Resilience	Female	IPT (N = 15); WL (N = 15)	GRP	12	CD_RSC	Pretest, posttest	Kurdistan

[a] A = acute treatment using an adapted manual; O = acute treatment using original manual.

[b]DSM: *Diagnostic and Statistical Manual*; BDI: Beck Depression Inventory; QIDA: Questionnaire about Interpersonal Difficulties for Adolescents; MAQ: Mood Affect Questionnaire; BAI: Beck Anxiety Inventory; FTAS-20: Farsi version of the Toronto Alexithymia Assessment Test; TPT: Topnotch Placement Test; Reef: Reef psychological well-Being questionnaire; EAT: Eating Attitudes Test; CIA: Clinical Impairment Assessment Questionnaire; EPDS: Edinburgh Postnatal Depression Scale; PSS:NICU: Parental Stressor Scale: Neonatal Intensive Care Unit; LSAS: Liebowitz Social Anxiety Scale- self-report; EEQ: King & Emmons, Emotional Expression Questionnaire; ENRICH: ENRICH

Marital Satisfaction Scale; Bell: Bell's Affective, social adjustment questionnaire; Shiring: Shiring's assertiveness questionnaire; Vaughan: Vaughan questionnaire of evaluation of infidelity; MR-AI: marital-relations author-inventory; WHOQOL-BREF: The World Health Organization Quality of Life; RSPWB: Reef Psychological Well-Being Scale; SPIN: Connor AR Inventory; RMET: Reading the Mind in the Eye Test, Baron-Cohen; FAQ: Focus of Attention Questionnaire; BFNE-II: Brief Fear of Negative Evaluation Scale revised version; CERQ: Garnefski Cognitive Emotion Regulation Questionnaire; PEPQ: Post Event Processing Questionnaire; DLQ: Dehshiri loneliness questionnaire; CD_RSC: Connor and Davidson's 2003 resilience scale questionnaire

[c]TPT-A: Interpersonal Psychotherapy for Adolescents; FB-IPT: family-based interpersonal psychotherapy; CBT = cognitive-behavioral therapy; COCT = coping-oriented couples therapy; IPT = interpersonal psychotherapy; PHA = pharmacotherapy; PLA = placebo; UC = usual care; WL = waiting list.

[d]GRP = Group treatment; IND = individual treatment; TEL = telephone treatment.

Kurdistan Province. Forty percent ($n = 7$) of trials targeted depressive symptoms ($n = 4$ MDD; $n = 1$ dysthymia; $n = 1$ postpartum depression; and $n = 1$ nonclinical depression); 1 targeted eating disorders, 4 aimed to improve social anxiety disorders, 1 addressed generalized anxiety disorder, 1 was adapted for dyslexia, and the remaining 6 focused on other mental health problems and psychological variables.

Interpersonal psychotherapy appeared to be effective in reducing depression[7,10,22-23]; nonclinical depression[24]; postpartum depression[12]; dysthymia[6]; anxiety[6,8]; social anxiety (performance anxiety, performance avoidance, and situational avoidance)[13,19-21]; alexithymia[8]; and eating disorder symptoms (dieting, bulimia, and oral control).[11] Three trials compared IPT with CBT but found no significant differences between the 2.[14,20,24]

CULTURAL ADAPTATION

These studies showed that adaptations of IPT retained its basic structure.[6-26] However, it may be unacceptable to directly ask about some subjects and issues in questionnaires. Areas to assess carefully relate to sexual relationships, having a friend of the opposite sex, and substance/alcohol misuse or addiction. Providers usually ask about these areas after establishing a strong therapeutic alliance.[27-32]

Sometimes there is conflict within families about expectations and rules. Alhosaini et al.[26] mentioned that respecting parents, elders, and individuals with a higher rank or status is highly valued in Iran. It is only acceptable or permissible to disagree and "respectfully" be assertive. Therefore, resolving disagreements with elders in the context of the IPT role dispute problem area might be challenging. While families often encourage their children to be independent and plan for their future, they also expect their children to consult with them and consider their rules and suggestions when making life choices.

To address this cultural value, we have found in our own work[26] that IPT therapists can use a social role transition (rather than dispute) problem area focus. This focus helps clients learn how to navigate being adult children and modify how they manage difficult interpersonal relationships and conflicts with parents, elders, or others with a higher social status. Clients usually start by resolving their problems respectfully (no matter what or how severe the stage of the dispute is) and renegotiate based on understanding the problem(s) and finding new ways to communicate about the problem. Iranian culture does not accept dissolution of a relationship with parents.[33-35] If strategies for renegotiation are unsuccessful, adult children must still be respectful[34-35] and focus on a role transition problem area to give up the old role and develop skills to adapt to their new role.[26,28] The research work in Iran is quite active, and a new trial with depressed women was recently published.[36]

CASE EXAMPLE

Maryam is a 45-year-old homemaker who is the mother of 2 adult sons, Ali and Ahmad. Her life collapsed when her 23-year-old son Ali died by suicide. Maryam and Ali were close, but they had suffered some rockiness over his engagement, about which they disagreed. They finally settled on finding another partner who matched better with Ali and his family (e.g., same family ranking/position, religion, and no prior romantic relationships). Ali had long suffered from dysthymia, and it resulted in poor relationships with his parents and friends. Nevertheless, Ali and Maryam were looking forward to enjoying their lives now. Maryam, in her usual way, handled everything and made homemade dishes to make money and carried on as the backbone of the family. A couple of months later, when Maryam thought everything was fine, Ali unexpectedly died by suicide in his room.

Since Ali's death, Maryam has been unable to sleep. She lost interest in celebrating events and visiting her family and believed that everyone was gossiping about Ali. She thought that when people passed her in the street, they started talking about what had happened and how much she should have been shattered. She was also angry at and in conflict with her parents. She stopped going out or visiting anyone. Convinced that she had an underlying medical problem, she consulted with doctors and started taking several kinds of medications, but nothing changed. She gained weight, felt exhausted, and became unable to work as usual.

In the initial sessions, she was diagnosed with dysthymia. The therapist inquired about what had been going on in Maryam's life when her symptoms began. Although it had been 8 years since Ali's death, she still visited his gravesite 2 to 3 times weekly and cried like his death was yesterday. Her Beck Depression Inventory-II (BDI-II) revealed a score of 39, which is in the severely depressed range.

Her son's death became the focus of attention. The therapist focused on the narrative; the sudden, unforeseen, painful, and stigmatized circumstances of his death; their close relationship; and her immediate resumption of activities to avoid mourning. It was also clear that Maryam's symptoms worsened around the anniversary of Ali's death and when her younger son asked for her for blessing for an engagement.

Therapy progressed with a detailed discussion of the life she and Ali had together. Sessions covered the details of her daily activities, especially those she used to do with Ali, his role in the family, and how his loss felt to her. Over time, she began to visit Ali's room and look at the picture albums. She went to the gravesite less often and started morning workouts. She also started reconnecting with Ahmad and spent more time talking with him about their feelings about Ali. They also started to talk more about Ahmad's future and preferences.

Meanwhile, the dispute with her parents worsened, and she lost her relationship with them. Her parents had become strict about her relationship with family and friends and her work. They also had sharp tongues and blamed and made her feel guilty for Ali's death, which caused her to lose control and start fighting, shouting, and crying and not visiting her parents' home for months. The conflict with her parents thus became a temporary focus of attention for a few sessions. Although she attempted to resolve disagreements respectfully with them (e.g., bringing up the conflict while her parents were in good spirits and trying to solve the conflict calmly) in the context of the dispute problem area, she also had to use a social role transition conceptualization to understand and modify this difficult interpersonal relationship. She wanted to be connected with them, so she decided to talk with them about that. She convinced her parents that she is an adult who can protect herself and handle her relationships and roles. She also tried to work in a suitable and safe environment to follow their expectations. She additionally tried to improve her relationship with her husband and mobilize social support by talking with others about things she could not bring up with her parents. In the final sessions, Maryam's BDI-II score was in the normal range. She was planning for her youngest son's engagement celebration with her husband, friends, and parents.

FUTURE DIRECTIONS

Authors in our search have suggested conducting research with larger sample sizes, increasing the duration of follow-up assessment time points, examining IPT in children and adolescents, considering the effect of IPT across genders, and employing fidelity measures to ensure quality of IPT delivery. Although only a few trials have been conducted in Iran, our review of IPT studies showed that there is a lack of certified trainers, supervisors, and translated books and articles. Inviting therapists certified by the International Society of Interpersonal Psychotherapy to Iran to conduct trainings would help further disseminate IPT. Additionally, educating Iranian students can be useful. More work that focuses on cultural adaptation about focal areas in Iranian society is needed.

REFERENCES

1. Weissman M, Markowitz J, Klerman GL. *The Guide to Interpersonal Psychotherapy*. Oxford University Press; 2018.
2. Montazeri A, Mousavi SJ, Omidvari S, Tavousi M, Hashemi A, Rostami T. Depression in Iran; a systematic review of the literature (2000–2010). *Payesh*. 2013;12(6):567–594.
3. Khajeh Nasiri F. A study of depression prevalence of nurses and its effective factors in Tehran Emam Khomeini Hospital. *Tehran University Medical Journal Publications*. 2000;58(1):10–14.
4. Hashemi Mohammadabad N, Zadehbagheri Gh, Ghafarian Shirazi HR. A survey on some etiologic factors related to depression among university students in yasuj. *J Med Res*. 2003;2(1):19–27.
5. Albert PR. Why is depression more prevalent in women? *J Psychiatry Neurosci*. 2015;40(4):219–221.

6. Moradi AR, Shokri O, Daneshvar PZ. The effect of interpersonal psychotherapy on depression treatment of adolescents: A case study. *Res Psychol Health*. 2007;1(3):5–28.

7. Abbaspour Z, Poursardar F, Koraei A, Khosravani Shayan M. The effectiveness of family-based interpersonal psychotherapy (FB-IPT) on depression symptoms in adolescents. *Fam Psychol*. 2016;2(2):67–78.

8. Rouzbahani F, Sozanian Kashani N, Eftekhari N. Interpersonal psychotherapy on anxiety and alexithymia in women with generalized anxiety. *MEJDS*. 2018;8(96):1–7.

9. Mohammadi V. The effectiveness of interpersonal psychotherapy on reducing anxiety and improving English reading skills in dyslexic students. *J Learn Disabil*. 2020;9(2):116–131.

10. Ahmadi Sabzevari F, Jalali MR. Effect of short-term group interpersonal psychotherapy on depression symptoms reduction and mental well-being in women prisoners. *Police Med*. 2017;6(3):207–212.

11. Gholamrezaei S, Honarmand MM, Zargar Y, Davoudi I, Bassaknejad S. The effect of interpersonal psychotherapy on eating disorder symptoms and the psychosocial performance of female students. *Journal of Psychological Achievements*. 2014;21(1):33–54.

12. Pouyan F, Akbari Kamrani M, Rahimzadeh M, Esmaelzadeh–Saeieh S. Education based on interpersonal psychotherapy on postpartum depression in mothers of infants admitted to neonatal intensive care unit. *AUMJ*. 2021;11(1):23–23.

13. Bodaghi S, Asghari ebrahimabad M, Mashhadi A. The effectiveness of brief interpersonal psychotherapy on social anxiety disorder and emotional expression in college students. *Res Clin Psychol Counsel*. 2020;9(2):5–17.

14. Gharadaghi A, Shafiabadi A, Hossein Rashidi B, Kiumars F, Esmaeili M. Comparing the effectiveness of cognitive behavioral therapy (CBT) and interpersonal psychotherapy (IPT) for pregnant women to increase marital satisfaction. *FCPJ*. 2015;4(4):583–605.

15. Tarkhan M. The effectiveness of group interpersonal therapy on affective, social adjustment and self-assertion of women with marital dissatisfaction. *J Psychol Stud*. 2016;12(3):123–140.

16. Shoja'Kazemi M, Momenijavid M. The effectiveness of interpersonal psychotherapy in repairing needs among women involved in infidelity. *Women's Studies Sociological and Psychological*. 2013;11(1):151–174.

17. Momeni Javid M, Shoaakazemi M, Pourshahriyari M. The effect of group counseling with an interpersonal approach on improvement of marital relationship of mothers who were hurt by marital betrayals. *J Psychol Stud*. 2015;11(2):87–114.

18. Morteza T. The effectiveness of short-term group interpersonal therapy on the psychological well-being and the life quality of addicted individuals' wives. *J Educ Psychol*. 2011;2(1):23–36.

19. Alizadehfard S, Rafezi Z, Tadris Tabrizi M. The effect of interpersonal therapy on social anxiety and theory of mind. *Knowledge & Research in Applied Psychology*. 2018;19(2):88–96.

20. Tavoli A, Allahyari A, Azadfallah P, fathiAshtiani A. Comparison of interpersonal therapy and cognitive behavior therapy for cognitive symptoms of social anxiety disorder. *Clinical Psychology and Personality*. 2021;11(42):23–50.

21. Asl Soleimani Z, Borjali A, Kiani Dehkordi M. Effectiveness of interpersonal psychotherapy on cognitive emotion regulation strategies and post event processing in girl students with social anxiety. *Q J Psychol Stud.* 2017;13(2):7–24.

22. Danekar M, Golchin N, Tarkhan M, Dehestani M. The effect of group interpersonal therapy on depression and loneliness in depressed girl students. *J Psychol Stud.* 2014;10(1):55–72.

23. Zemestani M, Sohrabi F, Borjali A. The effect of interference in group supportive psychotherapy by IPT method in reducing depressive symptoms of addicted patients. *Couns Cult Psychother.* 2012;2(8):17–30.

24. Shafiea Abadi A, Hussein Rasidi B, Farahbakhsh K, Ismaeili M, Garadagi A. Comparison of effectiveness of cognitive behavior therapy and interpersonal psychotherapy in decreasing non-clinical depression of pregnant women. *Modern Psychol Res.* 2014;8(31):117–139.

25. Qaderi Bagajan K, Yousefi N, Akbari S, Sadeghi R. Effectiveness of group interpersonal psychotherapy on increasing the resiliency of disabled children's mothers. *Socialworkmag.* 2019;8(3):12–19.

26. Rafiei Alhosaini N, Zarrin H, Rezaei-Jamalouei H. *The Effectiveness of Interpersonal Psychotherapy on Reducing Depression Signs and Increasing Quality of Life in Depressed Women Aged 20–50 Years in Isfahan.* MA thesis. Islamic Azad University; 2021.

27. Mahmoudian H, Dorahaki A. Factors effecting on the attitudes to boy and girl friendship relations before marriage. *Strategic Studies on Youth and Sports.* 2014;13(23):1–25.

28. Zarani F, Behzadpoor S, Babaeai Z. Analysis of the role of culture in psychopathology. *Rooyesh.* 2017;6(1):191–224.

29. Farzi S, Shamsaei F, Tapak L, Sadeghian E. Relationship between the stigma and the family performance of psychiatric patients. *Iran J Nurs Res.* 2020;14(6):1–8.

30. Heydari A, Meshkinyazd A, Soodmand PA. Mental illness stigma: a concept analysis. *Modern Care J.* 2014;11(3):218–228.

31. Damari B, Akrami F. Sexual health challenges in Iran and the strategies for its improvement. *IJPCP.* 2021;27(2):216–233.

32. Mohammadi J, Sobhani P. Stigma culture and abusers narratives of gradual acceptance of addict stigma. *Journal of Social Problems of Iran.* 2021;11(2):111–140.

33. Nazari Moqaddam J, Norouzi MH. The collectivist and cooperative identity of Iranians as viewed by travel writers. *National Studies Journal.* 2019;20(80):3–24.

34. Koutlaki, SA. *The Persian System of Politeness and the Concept of Face in Iranian Culture.* Doctoral thesis. University of Wales, College of Cardiff; 1997.

35. Ahi Andi M, Razzaghi M. The cultural of respect and successful aging; underlying approach for participatory-oriented lifestyle. *Journal of Visual and Applied Arts.* 2017;10(19):75–91.

36. Rafiei Alhosaini N, Zarrin H, Rezaei-Jamalouei H. Pilot randomized controlled trial of interpersonal psychotherapy for women with depression in Iran. *AmJ Psychother.* 2022;75(4):181–185.

37

Interpersonal Psychotherapy in Israel

ANAT BRUNSTEIN KLOMEK, YAEL LATZER, AND ROMI HERA ▪

INTRODUCTION

Interpersonal psychotherapy (IPT) was introduced in Israel at Ben Gurion University by Professor Josh Lipshitz, who developed IPT for anxiety disorders and initiated the Israeli IPT group, along with Dr. Alexandra Klein Rafaeli, Dr. Sharon Ben Rafael, and Professor Anat Brunstein Klomek. Later, Professor Yael Latzer and Mrs. Hila Argentaro joined the group. In the last 5 years, many scholars and psychotherapists joined the core leading group, which now includes 23 professionals. Many trainings were conducted as university courses, and the interpersonal counseling (IPC) manual was translated into Hebrew with permission from Dr. Myrna Weisman and Dr. Helena Verdeli.

In the last decade, IPT has been used frequently by therapists in Israel. Israel is a multicultural nation to which many have immigrated from a multitude of countries within an exceptionally brief period. Additionally, Israeli society includes many ethnic and religious groups and is anchored in ancient traditions yet poised at the apex of cutting-edge technology. Therefore, Israel presents a unique opportunity to study and present how the IPT framework enables patients and clinicians to overcome various cultural and religious differences.

The aim of the present chapter is to describe IPT in Israel. The first part of the chapter presents IPT in the Israeli education system and an adaptation of IPC for college students. The second part focuses on an IPT-based intervention for children and adolescents with specific learning disorders and attention deficit hyperactivity disorder (ADHD). The third part discusses IPT as part of the national suicide prevention program, while the fourth presents an adaptation of

Anat Brunstein Klomek, Yael Latzer, and Romi Hera, *Interpersonal Psychotherapy in Israel* In: *Interpersonal Psychotherapy*. Edited by: Myrna M. Weissman and Jennifer J. Mootz, Oxford University Press. © Oxford University Press 2024.
DOI: 10.1093/oso/9780197652084.003.0038

IPC for dieticians in Israel. The final section focuses on IPT for perinatal women. We then present two case examples illustrating some typical Israeli-oriented difficulties.

IPT IN THE ISRAELI EDUCATION SYSTEM

Interpersonal psychotherapy is part of the social-emotional learning (SEL) program called I Can Succeed (ICS), led by the Israeli Ministry of Education. ICS in Elementary Schools (ICS-ES) is the first SEL program based on IPT for adolescents (IPT-A).[1] The training followed a "whole-school" approach for SEL (Collaborative for Academic, Social, and Emotional Learning, CASEL). Initial training for all school staff at 5 schools included 30 hours of didactic and experiential training in ICS-ES theoretical background and contents. The school leadership team and all fourth-grade homeroom teachers met bimonthly with an ICS-ES leader for 2 hours of supervision. Supervision included reviewing the manual, solving implementation problems, sharing successes and challenges, and more. To measure fidelity, after each module teachers reported their implementation via a checklist questionnaire and interviews.

Teachers implemented the ICS intervention over 2 consecutive school years: 18 weeks in the first year and 15 weeks in the second. The ICS-ES lessons were 45 minutes. Modules are structured to support socioemotional skills in a "step-by-step" sequence and are designed to address interpersonal/social, emotional, and academic functioning in an integrative way. In the first year, modules included self-awareness and organizational skills. Second-year modules included self-regulation, interpersonal skills, and effective learning styles. Each module targets specific goals using active learning (e.g., role plays).

In the first ICS study, 419 fourth-grade students (204 girls and 215 boys, ages 9–10) were nonrandomly assigned to participate in ICS-ES ($n = 283$) or not participate in any SEL program (TAU; $n = 136$). At the end of the second year, analyses showed significant improvement in assertiveness and significant reductions in internalizing symptoms and bullying among the ICS-ES group. The groups did not differ in cooperation, responsibility, hyperactivity, empathy, self-control, and externalizing symptoms. In addition, academic achievements in their first language (Hebrew) significantly improved only among ICS-ES students, while there were no changes in their second language (English) achievements. In contrast, TAU students showed a decrease in their second-language achievements. Teachers reported overall high satisfaction with the training and implementation. These results suggest that ICS-ES is a feasible program for reducing internalizing symptoms and enhancing interpersonal skills and areas of academic functioning.

Interpersonal psychotherapy was further developed into an SEL program called I Can Succeed for Preschools, aiming to improve preschoolers' social/interpersonal, emotional, and academic skills.[2]

IPT IN ISRAELI UNIVERSITIES

Interpersonal psychotherapy has been implemented in many universities in Israel, such as schools for social work (Latzer), nutrition and behavior (Latzer), and psychology (Brunstein Klomek). An IPC adaptation, led by Dr. Alexandra Klein Rafaeli, was conducted among university students in Israel. The aim was to develop a brief, yet comprehensive, protocol for screening and intervening with distressed college students in 3–6 sessions. Individuals receiving IPC are initially assessed for symptoms of pathology and then encouraged to identify interpersonal problem areas that may contribute to their symptoms. Then, the IPC clinician works with the student to mobilize social support and rehearse effective communication strategies. Once the IPC protocol is completed, clinical decisions are made regarding clients' need for follow-up psychotherapy or alternative referrals.

Traditionally, counseling centers are not set up for research practice unless partnered with an academic department on the campus, but Israel has managed to bridge this gap. The local project has been modeled after pilot studies conducted in the United States[3] and Canada (internal review board approved, unpublished project with Paula Ravitz and the Wellness Center at University of Toronto) and related research.[4] Inspired by findings of Dennis Wilfley, the "train-the-trainer approach"[5] was adopted. A study at Tel Aviv University assessed the feasibility and acceptability of this project. These data have not yet been analyzed or published; however, hundreds of students have benefited from the pilot intervention. Recently, this inspired work has reached Ben Gurion University, where students can now receive IPT after intake. The first IPT group has been launched in collaboration with Dr. Colleen Conley.

IPT FOR CHILDREN AND ADOLESCENTS WITH SPECIFIC LEARNING DISORDERS AND ADHD

The first adaptation of IPT in Israel for children and adolescents diagnosed with specific learning disorders and ADHD was conducted at Schneider's Children Medical Center. This model describes the relationship between the child's learning disorder, emotional symptoms, and interpersonal functioning as a triangle. The protocol includes 13 sessions and 6 follow-ups. A preliminary study was conducted to assess the impact of the intervention model for adolescents with learning difficulties.[6] The intervention was given to adolescents ages 10–17. Findings revealed that by the end of the treatment, children showed improvement in attachment to mother, school avoidance, general anxiety, and social phobia. Overall, adolescents were satisfied with this intervention.

The Learning Disorders Clinic at Schneider Children's Medical Center currently has an integrated group based on IPT and cognitive behavior (CBT) for children and adolescents diagnosed with specific learning disorders and ADHD. Since COVID-19, the group has been conducted online and includes 13 sessions, 3 offline sessions, and 3 online parent meetings (last 2 in the initial, middle, and termination phases). The individual and parental sessions define the goals in the 3 areas of the IPT model: academic functioning, emotional, and interpersonal. Each cluster of sessions is dedicated to a specific skill acquisition, with many role plays during sessions and home experiments between sessions. The groups included the emotional and interpersonal techniques and skills from IPT-A. In addition, it included cognitive work from CBT- and learning disorder-specific organizational and learning strategies.

IPT AS PART OF THE NATIONAL SUICIDE PREVENTION PROGRAM

Interpersonal psychotherapy and IPT-A are both used as part of the national suicide prevention program; however, adaptations required flexibility in training and supervision. Three thousand school psychologists were trained through a few didactic trainings, which included about 600 school psychologists each. Later, supervisors received an additional 2 days of training, and each formed a supervision group. Groups met every other week for an hour and a half of supervision. In these meetings, cases were presented and discussed. The aim was to include supervision in the IPT framework when dealing with depression. The same groups included supervision of CBT for suicide prevention.[7] These groups were integrative in nature and aimed to teach clinicians to focus on reducing suicidal risk and depression as a significant risk factor.

IPC FOR NUTRITIONAL CONSULTATION BY DIETICIANS

Interpersonal psychotherapy in Israel is offered as a part of nutritional counseling implementation and aims to examine the pattern of the relationships affecting the eating behaviors. IPC is offered to the patient only if the nutritionist detects an association between mood changes, interpersonal relationships, and difficulties in eating behaviors. The implementation of this mechanism changed the emphasis of nutritional treatment and the methods of nutritional therapy. The nutritional focus of intervention includes the triangle demonstrating the correlation between interpersonal relationships, food behavior, and mood. In this IPC adaptation, emotional and interpersonal aspects are added to the nutritional assessment. For example, the consultation includes questions such as: "Do you eat differently around different people?" Additionally, mood evaluations are an integral part of nutritional therapy. Each questionnaire is reviewed twice, with the second time focusing on weight and body image. For example, "I do not feel sad" may be the answer when evaluating general mood. However, when incorporating weight and body image, the answer may be: "I am sad all the time." The Interpersonal Inventory is revised, aiming to identify the pattern of interpersonal relationships influencing a patient's mood, which may lead to disturbed eating habits. Future plans include training more nutritionists and studying the new protocol.

IPT FOR PERINATAL WOMEN IN ISRAEL

The Women's Mental Health Center at Tel Aviv Sourasky Medical Center was the first to offer IPT adapted for women in the perinatal period in Israel. Fieldwork in the women's center required a modified treatment manual to cater to women suffering from perinatal major depressive disorder (pMDD) and comorbid disorders. This IPT adaptation was first presented in a CBT conference[8] and later included in IPT workshops for perinatal mental health professionals. Interpersonal behavior psychotherapy (IBPT) leans on the conceptual framework of IPT with 2 major changes: an additional problem area (comorbid distress) and a reference to maladaptive behaviors and their influence on interpersonal factors. The IBPT formulation is based on a psychological, biological, behavioral, and social (PBBS) model of mental health.[9] The PBBS realms offer an understanding of the basis with which the woman arrives at the current crisis and the changes she experienced within each realm. These changes help us determine the appropriate problem area and provide a focus for interventions. The main goal of IBPT is to resolve the current crisis[10,11] by attending to behavioral and interpersonal patterns only when they interfere with the resolution of the current crisis. IBPT is considered when pMDD or perinatal difficulties are present along with a comorbid disorder that achieves best therapeutic gains by behavioral interventions.[11] Perinatal IPT and IBPT have been taught to clinicians in Israel since 2015. Recently, psychologists at Assuta Hospital were trained in this modality, and Clalit, the main medical insurance in Israel, integrated IPT into its perinatal services.

CASE EXAMPLES

The first case demonstrates interpersonal counseling therapy with a young Haredi (ultraorthodox) man with depression. The individual described below is a fictional character, representing common themes observed over time by Dr. Klein-Rafaeli.

Hillel is a 23-year-old male university student. He was born in Israel, grew up in a large Sephardi Haredi family, and was the first of his siblings to pursue a degree in higher education. Hillel was referred to the counseling center by a professor due to concerns about his emotional state after Hillel handed in a blank exam. At the initial intake, Hillel endorsed symptoms of moderate depression. He described a pattern of short-term relationships, both with friends and in trying to find someone he could imagine marrying. Hillel disclosed that he often felt socially awkward, like an "outsider."

The first session of the intervention included reviewing Hillel's symptoms of depression and social anxiety. The therapist provided psychoeducation and presented the "sick role." She noted that the feeling of "being an outsider" might abate if Hillel acquired interpersonal skills that would improve both his mood and interpersonal connections. In the closeness circle and the interpersonal inventory, Hillel did not include people besides his family, his rabbi, and his new roommates and wrote them in groups rather than individuals ("siblings," "roommates"). He noticed that there were no people he felt he could really turn to when in distress. The therapist shared the interpersonal deficits problem area formulation and ensured that Hillel both understood and agreed with it.

Throughout one of the middle sessions, Hillel and the therapist engaged in a communication analysis about an incident in which Hillel avoided voicing his opinion during a small-group assignment. They broke down the conversation to learn how Hillel had expressed himself, how he felt during the conversation, and how he might try to respond differently next time. Hillel was invited to role-play a similar future situation with the therapist; this time, the therapist challenged Hillel to say something early on in a small-group setting to "break the ice."

In the next session, Hillel reported that in another small-group session, he had been better able to tolerate his social anxiety and felt confident about trying to speak. He also reported he had spoken with his rabbi from home and said: "It helped so much to talk!" The therapist explained that it is common for people to isolate from those closest to them when their mood is low. She praised him for taking the initiative and expressed the importance of mobilizing social support when feeling depressed.

In the following session, Hillel's mood was lower, and he was less engaged than usual. He and the therapist discussed his week and noticed here were no other Haredi students in his program. In addition, he recalled a phone conversation with his mother in which he told her about his last arranged date; he could tell she was disappointed that the date wasn't more successful. At the end of this session, Hillel was encouraged to initiate another conversation with his mother, in which he would voice his feelings, the way he did in the session's role play.

In the termination phase, Hillel and his therapist reviewed his progress, noticing an improvement reflected in the self-report measures and linking this progress to specific events and efforts. Hillel reported that, overall, his mood improved, and he noted better understanding of the links between his moods and the life situations that affect them and found practicing communication skills empowering despite the cultural gap he was struggling with between the Western-oriented environment at the university and his traditional isolated "Haredi" house he came from. IPT succeeded to bridge this gap in a powerful way without putting him in a potential conflictual situation that may force him to choose between the two cultures.

The second case example is IPT with a young Christian-Arab-Israeli woman with depression. With the patient's consent, it is shared that changes were made to keep her privacy. It was clear that the IPT framework enables patients and clinicians to overcome various cultural and religious differences.

Ms. D., in her mid-20s, was born and raised in a Christian-Arab family living in a rural village in Israel, in which religion is part of everyday life. Ms. D. began therapy in a public clinic setting during a significant depressive episode in which she did not leave her room for a few days, drank large quantities of alcohol, and experienced suicidal ideation. At the intake, Ms. D. described growing up in a violent traditionally oriented environment with almost no rights for women. For a few years, she had been trying to get promoted at the company in which she works.

In the initial phase, her voice was soft, and she seemed to have very little energy, feeling as if she was not certain that she could trust the therapist. She was extremely harsh toward herself for not functioning at the level she expected, and so, the therapist proceeded to discuss the sick role. In the initial phase, the therapist and Ms. D. mapped the most significant people in her life, such as her parents, a good friend, and a sister. Out of these, it seemed that her sister and friend were great sources of support, and that the conflict with her father was the problem area (interpersonal disputes).

In the middle phase, they did a communication analysis about a fight with her father. Ms. D. shared that she rarely asks her father for anything, although she wished to ask him for financial support. They decided that she would try speaking to her uncle, which she did after a few weeks. Contrary to her expectations, Ms. D.'s father and uncle decided to help her financially. Following a discussion on additional sources of help, she reached out to a friend and an organization that assists with financial planning. Outside of the session, she decided to speak to another friend, engaging in positive social interactions throughout the week.

In the termination phase, Ms. D.'s depression was reduced, and they summarized the treatment and discussed ways in which she could apply the experiences and knowledge she gained to future situations. Although there were religious and cultural differences between Ms. D. and the therapist, IPT enabled them to focus on human interactions and relationships, a universal theme that connects everybody.

SUMMARY

Interpersonal psychotherapy in Israel has a few important adaptations, and it is growing. IPT in Israel can benefit people with a multitude of characteristics, cultures, religious backgrounds, and mental or emotional challenges. More local studies to examine its effectiveness are needed.

ACKNOWLEDGMENTS

We wish to thank Dr. Ika Weiss, Dr. Sharon Ben Rafael, Dr. Alexandra Klein-Rafaeli, Dr. Itay Rikon Beker, Nadia Grunstein-Cohen, Lilly Rosen, Sigalit Labunski, and Hila Argintaru for contributing parts of their work.

REFERENCES

1. Kopelman-Rubin D, Mufson L, Siegel A, Kats-Gold I, Weiss N, Brunstein-Klomek A. I can succeed, a new social emotional learning program for children based on interpersonal psychotherapy for adolescents. *Eur J Dev Psychol.* 2021;18(1):112–130.

2. Rafaeli AK, Bar-Kalifa E, Verdeli H, Miller L. Interpersonal counseling for college students: pilot feasibility and acceptability study. *Am J Psychother*. 2021;74(4):165–171.

3. Yamamoto A, Tsujimoto E, Taketani R, Tsujii N, Shirakawa O, Ono H. The effect of interpersonal counseling for subthreshold depression in undergraduates: an exploratory randomized controlled trial. *Depress Res Treat*. 2018;2018:4201897.

4. Fitzsimmons-Craft EE, Bohon C, Wilson GT, et al. Maintenance of training effects of two models for implementing evidence-based psychological treatment. *Psychiatr Serv*. 2021;72(12):1451–1454.

5. Brunstein-Klomek A, Kopelman-Rubin D, Apter A, Argintaru H, Mufson L. A pilot feasibility study of interpersonal psychotherapy in adolescents diagnosed with specific learning disorders, attention deficit hyperactive disorder, or both with depression and/or anxiety symptoms (IPT-ALD). *J Psychother Integr*. 2017;27(4):526.

6. Stanley B, Brown G, Brent DA, et al. Cognitive-behavioral therapy for suicide prevention (CBT-SP): treatment model, feasibility, and acceptability. *J Am Acad Child Adolesc Psychiatry*. 2009;48(10):1005–1013.

7. Ben-Rafael S. Integrating CBT and IPT for complicated perinatal disorders—a case study. Paper presented at: 45th Annual EABCT Congress; August 31–September 3, 2015; Jerusalem, Israel.

8. Ben-Rafael S. From interpersonal psychotherapy (IPT) to interpersonal behavior psycho therapy (IBPT) for comorbid perinatal disorders. In: Wenzel A, ed. *International Handbook of Perinatal Mental Health Disorders*. Routledge; 2022.

9. Anholt GE, Kalanthroff E. Do we need a cognitive theory for obsessive-compulsive disorder? *Clin Neuropsychiatry*. 2014;11(6):194–196.

10. Deacon BJ, Abramowitz JS. Cognitive and behavioral treatments for anxiety disorders: a review of meta-analytic findings. *J Clin Psychol*. 2004;60(4):429–441.

11. Lipsitz JD, Markowitz JC. Mechanisms of change in interpersonal therapy (IPT). *Clin Psychol Rev*. 2013;33(8):1134–1147.

Interpersonal Psychotherapy for Lebanese and Syrian Refugees in Lebanon

**HELEN VERDELI, KATHLEEN F. CLOUGHERTY,
SRISHTI SARDANA, CEMILE CEREN SÖNMEZ, AND
SANDRA PARDI MARADIAN ∎**

OVERVIEW

Lebanon is a small, middle-income country of 6.7 million, with a long history of war and political unrest. It hosts the highest number of refugees per capita worldwide, including 1.5 million registered Syrian refugees and 13,715 refugees of other nationalities.[1] The current context of collective stress and adversity in Lebanon is the culmination of more than 4 decades of continuous hardship and instability. The populations residing in Lebanon withstood a 15-year civil war (1975–1990); a series of bombings and assassinations from 2005 to 2021; the July 2006 war; the impact of the exodus of Syrian refugees (since 2011); the 2020 Beirut port blast[2]; and a spiraling economic crisis exacerbated by the COVID-19 pandemic (2019–present). The United Nations Office for the Coordinator of Humanitarian Affairs stated that 82% of the Lebanese population now lives in what is called multidimensional poverty.[1] The country is currently scoring the lowest minimum wage in the world, and there are immense shortages in basic need services and products, including medicine, fuel, electricity and water cuts.[3]

The chronicity and magnitude of adversities have placed millions of Lebanese at a high risk for depression and post-traumatic stress disorder (PTSD), creating a complex collective trauma.[4]

Helen Verdeli, Kathleen F. Clougherty, Srishti Sardana, Cemile Ceren Sönmez, and Sandra Pardi Maradian,
Interpersonal Psychotherapy for Lebanese and Syrian Refugees in Lebanon In: *Interpersonal Psychotherapy*.
Edited by: Myrna M. Weissman and Jennifer J. Mootz, Oxford University Press. © Oxford University Press 2024.
DOI: 10.1093/oso/9780197652084.003.0039

MENTAL HEALTH CARE CONTEXT IN LEBANON

Across Lebanon, the treatment gap is largely caused by the low availability of specialized mental health care resources and community-based mental health services.[5] Especially with the influx of displaced Syrians, local communities have been under unprecedented pressure to provide for the massive new and high-need population, overstretching resources and infrastructures already insufficient for the hosting communities. To address these needs, in 2015 the National Mental Health Program at the Ministry of Public Health (MoPH) of Lebanon, led by the psychiatrist Rabih El Chammay, initiated a 5-year mental health strategy (2015–2020), currently extended until 2030, to provide comprehensive, integrated, and responsive mental health services in community-based settings for vulnerable populations.[6] The strategy, which emphasizes human rights and evidence-based, community-centered services, is currently being implemented nationally. It aims to benefit both Lebanese and displaced populations, thus avoiding the creation of parallel systems.

In 2015, as part of the MoPH in collaboration with the Global Mental Health Lab (GMHLab) at Teachers College (TC), Columbia University, set the foundation for a sustainable national capacity-building in interpersonal psychotherapy (IPT) through the implementation of a series of trainings, with the aim of training psychologists working within the humanitarian response service system. Following consultations with Lebanese academic institutions, nongovernment organizations (NGOs), and mental health care practitioners and administrators, the MoPH became keen on adopting and endorsing IPT as the recommended evidence-based treatment for depression for the following reasons: IPT has been recommended as a first-line treatment for depression by the World Health Organization (WHO) *Mental Health Gap Action Program (mhGAP) Intervention Guide* for mental, neurological, and substance use disorders in nonspecialized health settings[7]; it has been adapted and tested with persons who have undergone severe adversities in a number of low- and middle-income countries (LMICs) in both community and primary care settings and is being disseminated globally by WHO (the digital version of the group IPT manual written by Verdeli, Clougherty, and Weissman has been copyrighted by WHO and translated in 8 languages.[8] Moreover, its focus on grief, life changes, disputes, and loneliness/social isolation were deemed to be particularly well aligned with the core mental health needs of both the displaced and host populations.

APPROACH AND ADAPTATION OF IPT ADOPTION
IN LEBANON

A training-of-trainers model was used in Lebanon, largely based on the "apprenticeship model" of psychotherapy training, initially articulated by Verdeli and Clougherty and adopted by other global mental health researchers.[9,10] This 3-tier cascade model involves coordination on 3 levels of training: *providers* with direct patient contact without prior exposure to IPT; *supervisors* with previous exposure to IPT; and master trainers with expertise in IPT.

The Lebanese IPT capacity-building project followed a competency-based training model that took place within a continuing education framework. It was implemented over 3 phases and funded by grants that the GMHLab team in collaboration with the MoPH received over the years. The team was systematically tracking provider and patient outcomes. Provider outcomes involved indicators of knowledge (IPT knowledge test); attitudes (attitudes toward evidence-based treatments, qualitative feedback on trainees' perceptions of the training); and skills (adherence to and competence in the IPT model). In addition, attendance at the training workshop and supervisions were tracked. Patient outcomes included depression scores and, in the last 2 phases, PTSD and generalized anxiety disorder scores. The patients were Lebanese and Syrian and were referred by NGOs and primary care staff or were self-referred in private practice. For all 3 phases, ethical approval was obtained by TC, Columbia University Institutional Review Board, in the United States and Saint Joseph University Institutional Review Board in Lebanon.

Phase I, in collaboration with the International Medical Corps and funded by the International Development Firm (2016–2017), explored the feasibility of training Lebanese providers in individual IPT. It started with a series of meetings of the GMHLab team with Dr. El Chammay's team from the MoPH, Lebanese academic institutions, the International Medical Corps and other NGOs. Selection criteria of the providers, informed by the discussions in these meetings, were drafted (Lebanese mental health care providers willing to make a 2-year commitment). The training consisted of a 4-day didactic workshop and a 2-day advanced workshop 6 months later (described below), during which proposed adaptations in IPT content and delivery were solidified. Predetermined competency criteria (passing the knowledge test at 75%, 100% attendance in the workshop, and meeting competency in 3 individual IPT cases). In addition, suicide risk assessment and safety planning adapted for contextual relevance were implemented. Provider and patient-level outcomes for all phases are described below.

Phase II, funded by the Grand Challenges Canada Transition-to-Scale grant mechanism (2018–2020) involved the training of a new and larger group of providers as well as supervisors selected by the previous trained providers. In the beginning of this phase, a group of representatives from the MoPH, academia, mental health professional associations, research institutions, and primary care providers and administrators and NGO providers met with the GMHLab. This time, a larger group of 62 candidates applied to be trained in IPT, indicating greater knowledge about and acceptance of IPT among the Lebanese mental health community. A didactic workshop on group IPT was conducted, for which the team followed the same criteria of competency milestones of phase I. For the training of supervisors, additional competency criteria were developed by the GMHLab team. The IPT master trainers (Verdeli and Clougherty) cosupervised the new group of supervisors as they in turn supervised new providers, as the master trainers progressively phased out.[11–13] For phase II, the national VA evidence-based psychotherapy dissemination and implementation model was followed, which tracked multilevel indicators (policy, provider, patient outcomes, local systems, and accountability mechanisms) of implementation and adoption in community clinics and primary care settings.[12,14]

For phase III, funded by the Economic and Social Research Council, UK Research and Innovation—R4HC MENA mechanism (2020–2022), a number of the supervisors were trained as trainers.[11,14] In this phase, following the newly established Order for Psychologists in Lebanon, a national initiative for the regulation of the practice was adopted, whereby only licensed clinical psychologists or psychiatrists were eligible for IPT training and certification. Therefore, the selection criteria for trainees in phase III included only licensed mental health professionals. There is increasing evidence on the importance of using a combination of active learning strategies, ongoing supervision, feedback, and coaching in sustaining skill acquisition and promoting adoption of newly learned treatments.[15] Thus, the training program was designed to start with a 4-day IPT didactic workshop where didactics were supplemented by video and live demonstrations, small- and large-group discussions, role plays, and feedback. Weekly 90-minute online supervision sessions were held in groups of 4 to 5 providers, a master trainer, and a supervisor. Approximately 6 months into training (when most providers completed their first or second clinical cases), a 2-day advanced IPT workshop is conducted, serving as both a refresher and collaborative learning platform where providers can hone their IPT skills and have more in-depth clinical discussions as a team. In this model, weekly supervision continues until all providers are deemed competent, dropped out, or withdrawn because they were deemed incompetent in IPT.

In addition to the manual, the IPT toolkit led by the first and second authors of this chapter also served as a guide for providers' ongoing self-evaluation and supervisors' discussion of the providers' progress with their assigned master trainer. Adaptations in both the content and delivery of IPT were implemented across the 3 phases in Lebanon, such as IPT application as a treatment-to-target intervention and its implementation within primary care as part of the collaborative care model. Predetermined criteria for patient-level improvement were defined as response (50% reduction in total baseline score) and/or remission (≤4) in depression scores as assessed on the Patient Health Questionnaire-9. Additional adaptations such as contextualized communication strategies and family engagement techniques are described elsewhere.[12]

RESULTS

Provider level

As part of the capacity-building work, from the series of trainings, we have 15 (phase I), 25 (phase II), 28 (phase III) providers; 9 (phase II) and 9 (phase III) supervisors; and 7 trainers (phase III). Of these, so far, 31 clinicians are certified by the International Society of Interpersonal Psychotherapy, with the rest planning for certification in the near future.

Patient level

Systematic tracking of patient-level outcomes was started at phase II. Eighty-eight accessed IPT, and 76 completed IPT, 3 were referred to higher care, and 9 were dropped due to relocation or lost to contact. Of the 88 that accessed, 72 patients (81.8%) met improvement criteria remission or response for depression, 1 patient (1.13%) was referred for higher care, and 3 patients (3.4%) were lost to contact or relocated. The tracking of patient outcomes continued in phase III, and data are being analyzed. Patients across phases II and III also reported significant reductions in PTSD and generalized anxiety symptoms, and these outcomes will be reported elsewhere.[12]

MAJOR BARRIERS AND FACILITATORS OF IMPLEMENTATION

During the IPT capacity-building work in Lebanon, the unending series of hardships and traumatic events had a deep impact on both patients and providers. Specifically, IPT providers who were enrolled in the training were themselves the survivors of several adversities and tragedies. However, the close collaboration with the GMHLab team over the years served as a contributing factor in establishing a nurturing environment and a nourishing network of support to provide stability, safety, and stimulation to the Lebanese community of IPT learners.

Finally, strained by the economic collapse in the country, some of the IPT-certified therapists in Lebanon have sought work opportunities in the gulf area, Europe, and the United States. Despite leaving the country, these therapists have continued offering their support to their home country through their active and close contribution throughout the different phases of the capacity-building work.

NEXT STEPS

Based on the IPT experience, the GMHLab and team and MoPH developed key recommendations for future work in Lebanon: The MoPH in collaboration with the GMHLab plans to link the capacity building of IPT to continuous mental health professional education in collaboration with the Ministry of Education. As a step forward, MoPH plans on integrating IPT within the curricula of postgraduate clinical psychology programs at different public and private universities. As such, these efforts in research and service capacity building through academic programs aim to serve as a canvas for the generation of local researchers and ensure sustained IPT training of future generations of clinical psychologists.

For strengthening the network and provision of continuing education to IPT practitioners of all levels, trained across the 3 phases, a digital, interactive platform—IPT Learning Collaborative—funded in phase III is currently under development. GMHLab is currently collaborating with University College London in a randomized controlled trial in both Lebanon and Kenya that aims at testing IPT for perinatal depression, through the provision of group IPT to the intervention arm of the study. Currently, several IPT therapists and supervisors are assisting the GMHLab in the dissemination of IPT in other regions worldwide, including in the Middle East/North Africa region, Africa, and Latin America.

ACKNOWLEDGMENT

This work was funded by the International Medical Corps, Economic and Social Research Council—UK Research and Innovation R4HC-MENA, and the Grand Challenges Canada.

REFERENCES

1. United Nations High Commissioner for Refugees (UNHCR). (2022). https://www. unhcr.org/news/stories/2022/1/61e6a6484.html. Accessed October 4, 2022.
2. El Hajj M. (). Prevalence and associated factors of post-traumatic stress disorder in Lebanon: a literature review. *Asian J Psychiatry*. 2021;63:102800.
3. United Nations Office for the Coordination of Humanitarian Affairs. Relief Web crisis figures data. 2021. https://data.humdata.org/dataset/0160cfdf-7dec-41a7-b0d2-8aa378f054d9. Accessed October 4, 2022.
4. Bosqui, T. The need to shift to a contextualized and collective mental health paradigm: learning from crisis-hit Lebanon. *Global Mental Health*. 2020;7:e26.
5. WHO-AIMS Lebanon. 2010. WHO-AIMS Report on Mental Health System in Lebanon. Microsoft Word—WHO-AIMS Lebanon Report October 2010 RM JM.doc. https://extranet.who.int/mindbank/item/1298. Accessed October 4, 2022.
6. Ministry of Public Health. *Strategic Plan of the Ministry of Public Health, 2015; 2016–2022*. 2015. Strategic Plan of the Ministry of Public Health 2016–2020 (Final Draft) (moph.gov.lb).
7. World Health Organization. mhGAP intervention guide for mental, neurological and substance use disorders in non-specialized health settings: mental health Gap Action Programme (mhGAP)—version 2.0. file:///Users/Jen_1/Downloads/9789241549790-eng.pdf. Accessed September 17, 2023.
8. *WHO Group Interpersonal Psychotherapy Manual*. Group Interpersonal Therapy (IPT) for Depression (who.int). 2016. file:///Users/Jen_1/Downloads/WHO-MSD-MER-16.4-eng.pdf
9. Verdeli H, Clougherty K, Bolton P, et al. Adapting group interpersonal psychotherapy for a developing country: experience in rural Uganda. *World Psychiatry*. 2003;2(2):114.

10. Murray L K, Dorsey S, Bolton P, et al. Building capacity in mental health interventions in low resource countries: an apprenticeship model for training local providers. *Int J Ment Health Syst.* 2011;5:1–12.

11. Verdeli H, Clougherty KF, Sardana S, et al. Interpersonal psychotherapy for healing in times of displacement and war in Lebanon: mental health capacity building and policy reform. Symposium presentation at: IPT for Persons Affected by the Syrian Crisis; November 9, 2019.

12. Verdeli H, Clougherty KF, Sardana S, et al. Multilevel evaluation of IPT adoption in Lebanon. In preparation. 2023. (Unpublished Manuscript).

13. Beidas RS, Kendall PC. Training therapists in evidence-based practice: a critical review of studies from a systems-contextual perspective. *Clin Psychol (New York).* 2010;17(1):1–30.

14. Karlin BE, Ruzek JI, Chard KM, et al. Dissemination of evidence-based psychological treatments for posttraumatic stress disorder in the Veterans Health Administration. *J Trauma Stress.* 2010;23(6):663–673.

15. Beidas, R. S., & Kendall, P. C. Training therapists in evidence-based practice: a critical review of studies from a systems-contextual perspective. *Clin Psychol (New York).* 2010;17(1):1–30.

PART VIII

Interpersonal Psychotherapy in Oceania

39

Interpersonal Psychotherapy in Australia

REBECCA E. REAY ■

Australia is the sixth largest country,[1] yet it is one of the most sparsely populated countries in the world, creating a unique set of challenges for access to mental health care. An equally significant feature of our modern society is the broad spectrum of cultures, including First Nations people, immigrants, refugees, and asylum seekers. Some of the mental health challenges we face include the high levels of psychological distress and high suicide rate among Aboriginal and Torres Strait Islander people.[2,3] People of migrant and refugee backgrounds are also at greater risk of mental health conditions due to trauma, racism, discrimination, loss of family ties, and unemployment. Young Australians are experiencing worse mental health outcomes and loneliness than they did prior to the COVID-19 pandemic.[4,5] Mental stress in parents also soared during COVID-19 due to job losses, economic uncertainty, role conflicts, and disrupted family and social networks.[6] Interpersonal psychotherapy (IPT) is a natural fit for addressing a range of mental health problems that resulted from the social upheaval and isolation caused by these life events. Australian academics and researchers have worked to translate the original IPT manuals, developing user-friendly clinician guides or manuals for a range of client groups and specific disorders, which are highlighted throughout this chapter.

IPT: EVOLVING AND EXPANDING

The pioneering work by Gerald Klerman, Myrna Weismann, and their colleagues[7] has had a significant impact on the field of psychotherapy. Australian clinicians were influenced by the strong empirical support of IPT for depression[8] and

Rebecca E. Reay, *Interpersonal Psychotherapy in Australia* In: *Interpersonal Psychotherapy*. Edited by: Myrna M. Weissman and Jennifer J. Mootz, Oxford University Press. © Oxford University Press 2024. DOI: 10.1093/oso/9780197652084.003.0040 other disorders. IPT emphasized the central role of interpersonal and social relationships within which mental health problems develop and are maintained. This paradigm shift spurred clinician interest in training, supervision, and certification in IPT. However, Australia is a large country and access to training and supervision opportunities has been challenging. Fortunately, training opportunities have expanded, partly due to the pandemic, with greater access to online training and accreditation bodies, such as the International Society of Interpersonal Psychotherapy and the IPT Institute in the United States. Australian clinicians have enthusiastically participated in introductory and advanced workshops, sharing their real-world clinical experiences during follow-up supervision. This interactive learning process contributed to the first IPT clinician's guide by Scott Stuart and Michael Robertson.[9] They encouraged therapists to combine their experience and clinical judgment with the framework of IPT to meet the needs of their clients. Examples include changes to the length of treatment, frequency of sessions, use of terminology, and greater flexibility with IPT techniques and strategies.

IPT FOR ADOLESCENTS AND YOUNG ADULTS

Pioneering research by Laura Mufson and colleagues demonstrated the efficacy and effectiveness of IPT with depressed adolescents aged 12–18 years.[10,11] Their seminal work provided therapists with a detailed, manualized approach to IPT with adolescents (IPT-A).[12] However, there were several major challenges to implementing IPT-A with our youth. Australian clinicians Robert McAlpine and Anthony Hillin gained extensive experience delivering and modifying the IPT-A model with youth from a diverse range of backgrounds. This included Indigenous; culturally and linguistically diverse; LGBTQIA (lesbian, gay, bisexual, transgender, queer/questioning, intersex, and asexual); homeless youth; and those in the criminal justice system. Their extensive clinical experiences provided the practice-based evidence that underpins their new book: *Interpersonal Psychotherapy for Adolescents: A Clinician's Guide.*[13]

Modifications to the original manual include extending the biopsychosocial model to incorporate cultural and spiritual dimensions in the assessment and treatment phases. This holistic model also includes (where appropriate) the domains of historical, political, and environmental factors. Historical factors include a client's experience of institutionalized and internalized oppression, including racism, homophobia, heterosexism, and sexism. Indigenous Australians view identity, culture, and connection to family, community, land, and sea as integral to their health and well-being.[14] Thus, the environmental domain can also encapsulate experiences of extreme weather events and concerns about the climate crisis. The authors underscore the importance of "access to country" and nature to promote well-being and greater resilience. Therapy sticking points related to culture can often be addressed by consulting Aboriginal Elders. Aboriginal mental health stakeholders have endorsed their holistic model, which explicitly acknowledges their issues of historical and current trauma, ongoing discrimination, and connection to country.

The extension of IPT-A to include young adults is also consistent with modern Australian youth mental health service models, which cater to individuals aged 12–25. Indeed, many young adults (>18 years) continue to grapple with role transitions, relationship issues, and developmental dynamics that are ideally addressed by the IPT-A framework. The clinician's guide underscores the importance of assessing the adolescent's attachment style to tailor treatment to help clients meet their attachment needs. LGBTQIA clients find the problem area of role transitions to be a helpful way to address significant changes in their life trajectory. The problem area of interpersonal gaps is preferred (rather than interpersonal deficits) as a less pejorative term for young people lacking confidence in communication or self-esteem. Other revisions include to the (third) consolidation phase of treatment, whereby continuation and maintenance are considered core components of therapy. Flexibility, rather than a prescribed number of sessions, is emphasized. The authors have also substantially expanded the range of IPT-A clinical tools and techniques, including the addition of mindfulness skills. Other IPT-A researchers have explored the mechanisms of therapeutic change in IPT for eating disorders (IPT-ED) in adolescents and young adults.[15] Their evidence-based theoretical model highlights the detrimental role of negative social evaluation on self-esteem and the engagement in eating disorder behaviors as a means of regulating emotions. IPT-ED treatment provides an alternative to the eating disorder, where individuals are assisted to establish supportive relationships that help build self-esteem and regulate affect.

CASE EXAMPLE

Eddie, an 18-year-old Indigenous man, presented for treatment following the funeral of a family member. Eddie reported nightly "visitations" by his deceased brother and 2 deceased friends. These experiences left him frightened and confused, and he had begun to resist sleep. Eddie described several significant losses over recent months and collaboratively decided that complex grief was the most accurate problem area. Eddie was able to see the connection between the recent losses and his depressed mood. He described his losses as: "like going surfing and being dumped by one wave, then another, then another. It all happens so fast that you can't get your breath back." Eddie acknowledged that having the space to talk about the people he had lost seemed to "take a bit of the sting out of it." However, the visitations continued to cause distress and discomfort talking about them. The therapist suggested talking to a local Aboriginal Elder (with whom the therapist had a previous connection) about these visitations, which he agreed. The following conversation took place after Eddie spoke to the Elder (referred to as Uncle).

THERAPIST: Eddie, were you able to see Uncle about your dreams?

EDDIE: Yeah. Saw him Monday. He said not to worry—they're from the Dreaming* – they were just checking on me. They were worried – I've been a bit of a mess lately and they were just trying to straighten things out.

THERAPIST: So is that OK with you?

EDDIE: Yeah. I talked to them a few times now. It's all right now. Uncle said they'll stay while I still need them.

THERAPIST: Are you going to talk to Uncle again?

EDDIE: No. He said it's OK. Just listen. And he said to tell you it's OK.

THERAPIST: Are they helping you straighten things out?

EDDIE: They will.

Once Eddy's anxious distress lessened following consultation with a culturally appropriate Elder from his community he was freed to focus on the losses within the problem area complex grief.

GROUP IPT FOR PERINATAL MENTAL HEALTH AND PTSD

A significant body of IPT research has focused on the treatment of perinatal depression, a natural fit for IPT. Rates of depression are highest from the reproductive years to preschool period.[16] Partner relationships become strained as well as friendships and social support. Depression can have profound effects on the infant, negatively influencing outcomes throughout their development.[17] IPT is ideally suited to address the issues that depressed parents experience, including losses, life changes, relationship issues, conflicts, and social isolation. My colleagues and I published the first randomized controlled trial of group IPT (IPT-G) for postnatal depression, establishing the feasibility and effectiveness of delivering a group intervention for mothers.[18] IPT-G mothers' depressive symptoms improved more rapidly in the short term and they were less likely to develop persistent symptoms, compared to the control group.[19] Later research by Forman and colleagues[20] in the United States revealed that treatment with individual IPT was not associated with improvements in child outcomes, recommending treatment should also target the mother-infant relationship. These findings posed significant challenges for those in the field. Grigoriadis and Ravitz[21] suggested that an IPT protocol could focus on the relationship between the parent and infant, supporting parental attunement and responsiveness to their child's needs and cues. In response, Australian

---

* Dreaming is First Nations people's understanding of the world and its creation, passed through storytelling. It represents the time when the Ancestral Spirits progressed over the land.

researchers began to experiment with modifying IPT-G for perinatal depression to include infants in the sessions and incorporate approaches from attachment theory and maternal sensitivity literature.[22] The changes closely overlapped with the IPT techniques of understanding and communicating needs and expectations, for example: (1) perceiving, interpreting, and responding to baby's signals of emotional state and needs; (2) responding to emotional requests and providing emotional plus instructional support; and (3) ensuring communication is developmentally appropriate, nonintrusive, and consistent. The manuals for group IPT treatment for PND (IPT-G) and mother-baby relationship (IPT-MB) are available from the respective authors. We have emphasized the importance of using both manuals flexibly, adapting it to each unique ethnic or cultural setting. Other creative ways that Australian researchers have adapted IPT include pioneering group treatment for post-traumatic stress disorder (PTSD).[23,24] Treatment consists of 10 sessions with groups of 4 to 8 patients who have experienced trauma in adult life. Given how pervasive trauma is among clients who access mental health services, IPT-G for PTSD provides a practical and flexible approach to addressing their difficulties.

ACCESS TO INTERPERSONAL PSYCHOTHERAPY IN AUSTRALIA

In 2006, the Australian government introduced the "Better Access" to mental health care scheme enabling patients with mental health disorders to receive up to 10 individual and 10 group Medicare-rebated treatment sessions per calendar year.[25] People experiencing mental health impacts from the pandemic can access an extra 10 sessions. The program aims to improve treatment and management for people experiencing mild-to-moderate mental health conditions with short-term, evidence-based interventions. The inclusion of psychological interventions under Medicare has been enormously successful in providing accessible, effective,[26] and relatively low-cost services to the public. The 5 approved treatments include cognitive behavioral therapy (CBT), IPT, psychoeducation, skills training, and relaxation training. Arguably, the inclusion of IPT and interpersonal counseling (IPC)[27] in this short list has accelerated demand for IPT training by psychiatrists, general practitioners, psychologists, and allied health professionals.

The framework of IPT, with its helpful problems areas, techniques, and strategies, has proven itself to be highly adaptable to a wide range of presenting problems. It is also easily compatible and effective when delivered via telehealth,[28] potentially extending its reach to underresourced, rural, and remote areas. New models of care in Australia propose less severe patients are directed to online, self-guided interventions as first-line treatments. Leading up to the pandemic, most of the digital psychological interventions on offer were based on CBT. Although there is a growing number of IPT self-help manuals available, Internet-delivered IPT has lagged behind CBT. Thus, one of the most creative areas of mental health research is likely to be the translation of IPT to online delivery, including guided or self-guided therapy. More research is needed on specific subgroups, such as those with low incomes, LGBTQIA, Indigenous, and ethnic minorities. Last, although IPT can still be improved and expanded, it has been remarkably successful at relieving aspects of human suffering and improving mental health.

ACKNOWLEDGMENT

I am very grateful to my colleagues for their contributions to this chapter, especially Rob McAlpine, Anthony Hillin, Michael Robertson, Carolyn Deans, Paul Rushton, Elizabeth Rieger, and Philip Keightley.

REFERENCES

1. Australian Bureau of Statistics (ABS). Population clock and pyramid. Commonwealth of Australia. Accessed April 23, 2022. https://www.abs.gov.au/ausstats/abs@.nsf/0/1647509ef7e25faaca2568a900154b63?OpenDocument

2. Australian Bureau of Statistics (ABS). Causes of death, Australia, 2020. 2021. Accessed April 23, 2022. https://www.abs.gov.au/statistics/health/causes-death/causes-death-australia/2020#intentional-self-harm-deaths-suicide-in-aboriginal-and-torres-strait-islander-people

3. ABS (Australian Bureau of Statistics). Australian Aboriginal and Torres Strait Islander Health Survey (AATSIHS): first results, Australia, 2012–13. Updated January 27, 2016. Accessed April 14, 2022. https://www.abs.gov.au/ausstats/abs@.nsf/Lookup/9F3C9BDE98B3C5F1CA257C2F00145721

4. Biddle N, Gray M. Tracking wellbeing outcomes during the COVID-19 pandemic (April 2021): continued social and economic recovery and resilience. ANU Center For Social Research & Methods. 2021. Accessed April 30, 2022. https://csrm.cass.anu.edu.au/research/publications/tracking-wellbeing-outcomes-during-covid-19-pandemic-april-2021-continued

5. Headspace. Insights. Loneliness over time. headspace National Youth Mental Health Survey 2020. 2020. Accessed March 24, 2022. https://headspace.org.au/assets/HSP10869-Loneliness-Report_FA01.pdf

6. Broadway B, Méndez S, Moschion J. Behind closed doors: the surge in mental distress of parents. Melbourne Institute. Updated August 2020. Accessed May 1, 2022. https://melbourneinstitute.unimelb.edu.au/__data/assets/pdf_file/0011/3456866/ri2020n21.pdf

7. Klerman GL, Weissman MM, Rounsaville BJ, Chevron ES. *Interpersonal therapy of depression*. Basic Books; 1984.

8. Elkin I, Shea MT, Watkins JT, et al. National Institute of Mental Health Treatment of Depression Collaborative Research Program. General effectiveness of treatments. *Arch Gen Psychiatry*. 1989;46:971–982.

9. Stuart S, Robertson M. *Interpersonal therapy: a clinician's guide*. Taylor and Francis; 2012.

10. Mufson L, Weissman M, Moreau D, Garfinkel R. Efficacy of interpersonal psychotherapy for depressed adolescents. *Arch Gen Psychiatry*. 1999;56:573–579.

11. Mufson LH, Dorta KP, Olfson M, Weissman MM, Hoagwood K. Effectiveness research: transporting interpersonal psychotherapy for depressed adolescents (IPT-A) from the lab to school-based health clinics. *Clin Child Fam Psychol Rev*. 2004;7:251–261.

12. Mufson L, Dorta KP, Moreau D, Weissman MM. *Interpersonal Psychotherapy for Depressed Adolescents*. 2nd ed. Guilford Press; 2011.

13. McAlpine R, Hillin A. *Interpersonal Psychotherapy for Adolescents: A Clinician's Guide*. Routledge; 2021.

14. Australian Institute of Health and Welfare & National Indigenous Australians Agency. Aboriginal and Torres Strait Islander Health Performance Framework. Tier 2 determinants of health. Updated December15, 2020. Accessed May 17, 2022. https://www.indigenoushpf.gov.au/measures/2-14-indigenous-people-access-trad itional-lands

15. Rieger E, Van Buren DJ, Bishop M, Tanofsky-Kraff M, Welch, R, Wilfley DE. An eating disorder-specific model of interpersonal psychotherapy (IPT-ED): causal pathways and treatment implications. *Clin Psychol Rev*. 2010;30:400–410.

16. Woolhouse H, Gartland D, Mensah F, Giallo R, Brown S. Maternal depression from pregnancy to 4 years postpartum and emotional/behavioural difficulties in children: results from a prospective pregnancy cohort study. *Arch Womens Ment Health*. 2016;19(1):141–151.

17. Center on the Developing Child at Harvard University. Maternal depression can undermine the development of young children. 2009. Working Paper No. 8. Accessed May 20, 2022. http://www.developingchild.harvard.edu

18. Mulcahy R, Reay RE, Wilkinson RB, Owen C. A randomised control trial for the effectiveness of group interpersonal psychotherapy for postnatal depression. *Arch Womens Ment Health*. 2010;13(2):125–139.

19. Reay RE, Owen C, Raphael B, Shadbolt B, Mulcahy R, Wilkinson RB. Trajectories of long-term outcomes for postnatally depressed mothers treated with group interpersonal psychotherapy. *Arch Womens Ment Health*. 2012;15(3):217–228.

20. Forman DR, O'Hara MW, Stuart S, Gorman LL, Larsen KE, Coy KC. Effective treatment for postpartum depression is not sufficient to improve the developing mother-child relationship. *Dev Psychopathol*. 2007;19(2):585–602.

21. Grigoriadis S, Ravitz P. An approach to interpersonal psychotherapy for postpartum depression. Focusing on interpersonal changes. *Can Fam Physician*. 2007;53:1469–1475.

22. Deans C, Reay RE, Buist A. Addressing the mother-baby relationship in interpersonal psychotherapy for depression: an overview and case study. *J Reprod Infant Psychol*. 2016;34(5):483–494.

23. Robertson M, Rushton PJ, Bartrum D, Ray R. Group-based interpersonal psychotherapy for posttraumatic stress disorder: theoretical and clinical aspects. *Int J Group Psychother*. 2004;54(2):145–175.

24. Robertson M, Rushton P, Batrim D, Moore E, Morris P. Open trial of interpersonal psychotherapy for chronic post traumatic stress disorder. *Australas Psychiatry*. 2007;15(5):375–379.

25. Department of Health, Australian Government. Better Access initiative. Updated May 20, 2022. Accessed May 25, 2022. https://www.health.gov.au/initiatives-and-programs/better-access-initiative

26. Pirkis J, Ftanou M, Williamson M. Australia's Better Access initiative: an evaluation. *Aust N Z J Psychiatry*. 2011;45:726–739.

27. Wilhelm K, May R. Interpersonal therapy in the general practice setting. *Medic Today*. 2017;18:41–49.

28. Reay RE, Looi JC, Keightley P. Telehealth mental health services during COVID-19: summary of evidence and clinical practice. *Australas Psychiatry*. 2020;28(5):514–516.

40

Interpersonal Psychotherapy in New Zealand

SUE LUTY AND DAWN NOLAN ■

In this chapter the evolution of IPT in New Zealand is described from research to training and dissemination, culminating in a description of a cultural adaptation of IPT for Māori, the indigenous culture of New Zealand.

INTRODUCTION

New Zealand, Aotearoa, is an island nation situated to the east of Australia with a land mass of 268,021 square kilometers, making it similar in size to Great Britain. There is a growing population, currently standing at 5,127,000, made up of 875,300 Māori and 707,600 Asian, with the remainder being mainly European.[1] The population is evenly split between males and females, with a mean age of 37 and 39 years, respectively. While the majority of the population are urban, those living rurally are thinly spread, with reduced access to services. New Zealand is considered to be a developed country with high rankings in civil liberties, education, and health, with an overall ranking of 14 from 189 countries.[2] It has a free trade economy with a focus on tourism, agriculture, and industry.

Originally a Polynesian nation, New Zealand developed a distinct Māori culture. Unique to New Zealand is the Treaty of Waitangi, signed by Māori chiefs in 1840 and representatives of the British government at the time of colonization. The treaty is based on the principles of protection, participation, and partnership in all matters of the people, with the aim of making New Zealand a truly bicultural society.

New Zealand has both private and publicly funded health services, with the majority of healthcare accessed through the public sector. The Health and Disability

Sue Luty and Dawn Nolan, *Interpersonal Psychotherapy in New Zealand* In: *Interpersonal Psychotherapy.* Edited by: Myrna M. Weissman and Jennifer J. Mootz, Oxford University Press. © Oxford University Press 2024. DOI: 10.1093/oso/9780197652084.003.0041

Commission NZ (HDCNZ) reported that 1 in 5 New Zealanders experience mental health issues, increasing to almost 1 in 3 for Māori, with the most prevalent disorders being mood disorders, anxiety, mental distress, eating disorders, addictions, post-traumatic stress disorder, and schizophrenia.[3] HDCNZ also noted access to mental health services has increased by 55% in the 10 years 2009–2019. However, the funding has increased by only 24%. This means an ever-increasing need to provide effective and efficient mental health services, including evidence-based talking therapies.

INTERPERSONAL PSYCHOTHERAPY RESEARCH IN NEW ZEALAND

Interpersonal psychotherapy (IPT) research and training initially developed at the Department of Psychological Medicine, University of Otago, Christchurch, in the South Island of New Zealand under the leadership of Professor Peter Joyce in the mid-1990s after Professor Chris Fairburn ran a training workshop. Since then, there have been a number of successful studies that have used IPT and adaptations of IPT and interpersonal and social rhythm therapy (IPSRT) to inform clinical practice. Beginning in the late 1990s with standard IPT in the psychotherapy for depression study (IPT vs. cognitive behavioral therapy [CBT])[4] and an adaptation for anorexia nervosa in the Anorexia Treatment Study,[5] these two studies not only gave further support to the effectiveness for depression but also outlined the challenges in adapting IPT for an eating disorder such as anorexia. Notable in this study was the increased length of therapy (20 sessions) and time taken to elicit the problem area with resultant improvement in functioning but less so the core features of the eating disorder. The suggestion was that further adaptations may be necessary.

After these, a number of projects have evaluated IPSRT with key investigators Dr. Marie Crowe, Maree Inder, and Katy Douglas, with several publications evolving from each. These include a randomized control trial of interpersonal psychotherapy in young people with bipolar disorder (2006); a randomized clinical effectiveness trial of a bipolar disorder clinic (2011); a pilot study of cognitively enhanced IPSRT for depression (2018); enhancing recovery for patients with recurrent mood disorders—IPSRT versus IPSRT plus cognitive remediation (2019); and the feasibility of delivering intensive rhythm stabilization therapy for patients with treatment-resistant bipolar disorder (2019); and teletherapy for recurrent mood disorders with IPSRT versus psychoeducation (2020).[6–14]

A key feature of these studies has been the understanding of a new problem area in IPSRT: "sense of self in relation to others." This replaces "grief for the loss of healthy self" in the context of treating both bipolar disorder and major depressive episode. Their experience suggested that there was less grief for loss of healthy self in depression and more problems associated with a sense of self in the context of here and now relationships with others (i.e., feelings of inadequacy, defectiveness, and incompetence in comparing oneself with others). Dr. Sue Luty has also led a small study evaluating the feasibility of delivering IPT by trained community support workers, proving its effectiveness and opening the possibility of further dissemination and training.[15]

Finally, a recent project under the leadership of Dr. Gary Cheung in Auckland is evaluating the effectiveness of group IPT for loneliness in the elderly. Unfortunately, COVID has both delayed this project and changed it to delivery via a Zoom platform, but it is already proving to be positively received by participants.

TRAINING AND DISSEMINATION

As Christchurch is situated in the South Island of New Zealand, most of the training, supervision, and dissemination has been based there. Training in IPT initially tended to occur within local research groups and via some workshops. However, Dr. Luty developed a postgraduate program in IPT at the University of Otago in the early 2000s, which allowed for distance-based training and supervision in IPT in addition to an academic component. The dissemination of IPT clinically has been slow, but many of the therapists trained for the above studies, and graduates of the postgraduate program continue to use IPT in their clinical practice. Dr. Luty continues to practice IPT in her private clinic and in a perinatal psychiatry service, where she has run successful group treatment of postpartum depression with IPT and IPT with reflective functioning enhancement. Dawn Nolan continues to practice IPT in her private practice, offering supervision and therapy for a number of adaptations for depression, bipolar disorder, personality disorder, anxiety, trauma, and couples across an age range from adolescence to older persons and for individuals and couples. Furthermore, a number of the research-trained therapists continue to practice IPT across the public and private sectors.

As discussed, funding has not kept pace with the significant increase in people wanting to access mental health services, resulting in limitations of resources. In the NZ rural settings where access to healthcare is further limited by thinly spread resources and the capacity for long-distance travel, the need for effective treatment that can be provided by clinicians from all disciplines has never been more relevant.

In 2007, clinical nurse specialist Dawn Nolan presented IPT to the Rural Specialist Mental Health Community Service in Canterbury as an evidence-based, time-limited treatment.

Supported by the Director of Nursing and senior management, IPT was slowly introduced, and a few clinicians in the service were funded to enroll for the University of Otago postgraduate IPT paper. IPT then became established in the service, with empirical and statistical data demonstrating that IPT-treated clients had a shorter length of stay and presented less frequently than clients offered a case management model alone.

Much of the success of the introduction of IPT in this Rural service may be attributed to the support of professional leads and the consultant psychiatrist of the team, but despite this team embracing the model, the practice of IPT did not appear to be growing at the same rate in other sectors of the mental health service. This led Dawn Nolan[16] to investigate "Factors That Influence the Uptake and Continuing Practice of Interpersonal Psychotherapy by Frontline Clinicians Following Formal Training" for her doctoral dissertation, in which she identified 3 areas of influence:

1. The therapist's experience of psychotherapeutic interventions in prior training
2. Team involvement and the role of senior clinicians in the implementation and dissemination of psychotherapeutic interventions in clinical practice
3. The perception and definition of roles across professional disciplines

Over the last 5 years, there has been a small increase in uptake of local training and practice across Canterbury, notably in the Child, Adolescent, and Family Service. In other areas of New Zealand, many of the students who have undertaken formal training continue to practice IPT and regularly attend a monthly peer supervision group set up as part of the training. Of the last 3 cohorts of IPT students, more than 80% have embedded IPT into their practice, with the majority choosing to leave the public sector to work in private practice, where they have more opportunity to offer IPT.

ADAPTATION OF IPT FOR MĀORI

In 2016, there was a devastating earthquake of 7.8 magnitude in Kaikoura, New Zealand, cutting off the town and limiting service access for more than a year. The Kaikoura district is served by the Rural Mental Health Community Team, who focused efforts to support the population, flying in a team and increasing the use of telehealth for IPT clients. Kaikoura has a higher-than-average population of Māori at 17.1%, as opposed to 14.6% throughout the rest of the country.[1] As previously outlined, mental health issues were already higher for the Indigenous population. Experience of the Christchurch earthquakes of 2010–2012 forewarned that access to mental health care would initially drop off but then spike rapidly 2 years later. It was essential to adapt IPT for Māori to uphold the Treaty of Waitangi principles of respect between Māori and non-Māori in partnership, participation, and protection.

Attending to cultural safety with Māori requires a respect and understanding of the connection between the people and land and acknowledgment of the importance of the unique concept of health and well-being. This was of particular significance to the community of rural Kaikoura, where many people live with their Iwi (tribe) and Hapu (kinship group of large families descended from common ancestors). Adapting IPT for Māori began with a consultation process, which followed the principles of the Treaty of Waitangi above. It was clear when talking with Māori cultural advisors, clinicians, and clients that colonization had left scars on the Indigenous population, which resulted in a lack of trust for Western medicine and stigma. This had become a barrier to accessing mental health care, particularly for talking therapies whose efficacy is dependent on a client's trust. Working in partnership with Pukenga Atawhai (Māori mental health workers) and Kaumatua (Elders) experienced in mental health, an adaptation of IPT for Māori was developed to incorporate the protocols of greeting, opening and closing the session.

Te Whare Tapa Wha (Māori model of well-being) was used as the foundation throughout all stages of IPT. This model incorporates 4 elements of health: spiritual connection with ancestors, the land, or spirits; physical well-being; *Whanau*, being family and community connection or reconnection; and mental, where health is only achieved when thoughts and feelings are integral components of body and soul. An example of how this was incorporated into the sessions was that the client brought in a number of rocks from the Kaikoura beach and discussed how their spirituality assisted her to deal with her family relationships.

Working with Māori also incorporated some practical differences. First, an aspect of Māori culture is establishing connection as part of developing a relationship, sharing details of ones Iwi and Hapu on first meeting, with an expectation that health workers will do the same. In Western health settings, this would be seen as a transgression of boundaries. Second, inviting Whanau (family) and Pukenga Atawhai into the session is highly desirable but raises issues of confidentiality, particularly in small communities when there has been a history of abuse. During the introduction and development of the model, clients were generous in their feedback and indicated areas that may be framed in a more cultural way. Permission was also sought to discuss aspects of therapy with the Kaumatua for cultural supervision.

In summary, the journey of IPT in New Zealand has been slow and steady with a strong localized focus on expert research in Christchurch. Pockets of training and clinical practice have been predominantly limited by access to accredited supervisors such as Sue and Dawn, but plans are underway to begin training more supervisors to extend the reach further across New Zealand. An adaptation for Māori with cultural consultation has been promising in its initial stages.

REFERENCES

1. StatsNZ Population. Home page. 2018. https://www.stats.govt.nz
2. United Nations Development Program. Human development report. 2020. https://hdr.undp.org/content/human-development-report-2020. Accessed September 6, 2022.
3. Ministry of Health. Annual update of key results 2018/19: New Zealand Health Survey. 2019. https://www.health.govt.nz/publication/annual-update-key-results-2018-19-new-zealand-health-survey. Accessed September 6, 2022.

4. Luty SE, Carter JD, McKenzie JM, et al. Randomised controlled trial of inter-personal psychotherapy and cognitive–behavioural therapy for depression. *Br J Psychiatry.* 2007;190(6):496–502.

5. McIntosh VV, Jordan J, Carter FA, et al. Three psychotherapies for anorexia nervosa: a randomized, controlled trial. *Am J Psychiatry.* 2005;162(4):741–747.

6. Crowe M, Inder M. Staying well with bipolar disorder: a qualitative analysis of five-year follow-up interviews with young people. *J Psychiatr Ment Health Nurs.* 2018;25(4):236–244.

7. Crowe M, Porter R, Inder M, et al. Clinical effectiveness trial of adjunctive in-terpersonal and social rhythm therapy for patients with bipolar disorder. *Am J Psychother.* 2020;73(3):107–114.

8. Crowe M, Inder M, Douglas K, et al. Interpersonal and social rhythm therapy for patients with major depressive disorder. *Am J Psychother.* 2020;73(1):29–34.

9. Crowe M, Inder M, Porter R, et al. Patients' perceptions of functional improvement in psychotherapy for mood disorders. *Am J Psychother.* 2021;74(1):22–29.

10. Crowe M, Porter R, Inder M, et al. Clinical effectiveness trial of adjunctive in-terpersonal and social rhythm therapy for patients with bipolar disorder. *Am J Psychother.* 2020;73(3):107–114.

11. Douglas KM, Groves S, Crowe MT, et al. A randomised controlled trial of psy-chotherapy and cognitive remediation to target cognition in mood disorders. *Acta Psychiatr Scand.* 2022;145(3):278–292.

12. Inder ML, Crowe MT, Luty SE, et al. Randomized, controlled trial of interper-sonal and social rhythm therapy for young people with bipolar disorder. *Bipolar Disorders.* 2015;17(2):128–138.

13. Inder ML, Crowe MT, Luty SE, et al. Prospective rates of suicide attempts and nonsuicidal self-injury by young people with bipolar disorder participating in a psychotherapy study. *Aust N Z J Psychiatry.* 2016;50(2):167–173.

14. Inder ML, Crowe MT, Moor S, et al. Three-year follow-up after psychotherapy for young people with bipolar disorder. *Bipolar Disord.* 2018;20(5):441–447.

15. Luty SE, Scalia S. Can interpersonal psychotherapy be delivered by a community agency? *Australas Psychiatry.* 2018;26(2):200–205.

16. Nolan D. *Factors That Influence the Uptake and Continuing Practice of Interpersonal Psychotherapy by Frontline Mental Health Clinicians Following Formal Training.* Doctoral dissertation. University of Otago; 2014.

PART IX

Interpersonal Counseling (IPC) in South America

41

Interpersonal Counseling in Brazil: A Task Shift Experience

MARCELO FEIJÓ MELLO, CAMILA MATSUZAKA, AND
ANNIKA C. SWEETLAND ■

Brazil is the fifth largest country in the world, with more than 214 million inhabitants (https://www.ibge.gov.br/apps/populacao/projecao/index.html). Despite being the thirteenth strongest economy in the world, inequality is significant. Brazil is the seventh most unequal country, where 10% of the wealthiest have 41.9% of the entire country's income, and 1% of the richest have 28.3% of the total income. An official survey from the Brazilian government reported in 2019 that more than 13 million Brazilians lived in extreme poverty (living with less than $1.9/day).[1] There is inequality between different regions. The North and Northeast regions are poorer than the wealthy Southeast. These disparities are a risk factor for psychiatric disorders in Brazil. Providing access to healthcare, specifically mental health services, is imperative.

The latest Global Health Estimates by the World Health Organization (WHO)[2] found that globally, depressive disorders ranked as the single largest contributor and anxiety disorders as the sixth most significant contributor to nonfatal health loss of all years living with a disability (YLD). In the WHO study, Brazil had the highest prevalence of depression and anxiety in the regions of the Americas. The current annual prevalence rate for depressive disorders was 5.8%, 9.3% for anxiety disorders, with a percentage YLD of 10.3% for depressive disorders and 8.3% for anxiety disorders.[3] Although there are effective treatments for both conditions, fewer than half of those affected receive such treatment.[4] The primary care services in Brazil have a scarcity of specialized mental health providers. The treatment coverage for depression is low.[5]

Marcelo Feijó Mello, Camila Matsuzaka, and Annika C. Sweetland, *Interpersonal Counseling in Brazil: A Task Shift Experience*
In: *Interpersonal Psychotherapy*. Edited by: Myrna M. Weissman and Jennifer J. Mootz, Oxford University Press.
© Oxford University Press 2024. DOI: 10.1093/oso/9780197652084.003.0042

INTERPERSONAL PSYCHOTHERAPY IN BRAZIL

The history of interpersonal psychotherapy (IPT) in Brazil began in the mid-1990s with Professor Dr. Feijó de Mello, an expert on chronic depression and post-traumatic stress disorder (PTSD), who applied IPT to both disorders. Having read the manuals and reviewed the literature, he took 2 IPT workshops with Dr. John Markowitz and 1 with Roy Mackenzie on group IPT at American Psychiatric Association meetings. He invited Prof. Markowitz to Sao Paulo for the first of several IPT workshops and began training IPT therapists himself. He subsequently received funding for a grant testing IPT as an adjunct to pharmacotherapy for chronic depression.[6]

Since 2005, Dr. Mello has organized IPT supervision and training with other mental health professionals. From 2007 to 2011, he coordinated a 63-hour IPT training course at the Federal University of Sao Paulo (UNIFESP), which included participation in seminars and 2 completed and supervised cases. Sixty-eight trainees completed the course during those years. To facilitate the access to IPT in Brazilian Portuguese, he published the IPT Brazilian manual in 2009 *Psicoterapia Interpessoal: Teoria e Prática* (by Aline Ferri Schoedl, Fernando Sargo Lacaz, Marcelo Feijó de Mello, Mariana Cadrobbi Pupo, and Rosaly F. Braga Campanini).

Since 2016, the UNIFESP IPT group (coordinated by Dr. Rosaly F. Braga Campanini and Dr. Euthymia Brandao de Almeida Prado) created a web-based IPT training for psychologists and organized a supervision group. Parallel to IPT training, another group of PTSD adaptation research[7] and IPT adaptation for patients with schizophrenia were developed.[8] Dr. Mello is carrying out a study examining IPT as a treatment for PTSD associated with sexual violence.[9]

BRAZILIAN IPT ADAPTATION FOR PRIMARY CARE: INTERPERSONAL COUNSELING

Brazil's Family Health Strategy (FHS) has made remarkable progress toward universal coverage of its population in primary care in the last decades, but only limited investments in mental health.[10] Specialized community-based psychosocial care centers were established to treat individuals with severe mental illness.[11] Community health workers (CHWs) are an essential human resource for health in Brazil. Still, no strategies were developed to integrate the treatment of common mental disorders within primary care. CHWs are employees of the public health system; each one is assigned to approximately 150 households within the catchment area of a given FHS outreach clinic. They visit each family monthly and gather information about health-promotion activities and primary clinical care.[10] They are also tasked with identifying potential warning signs of violence, neglect, truancy, or drug use. However, they receive no mental health training.[12]

There is strong evidence that the return on an investment after depression treatment is \$5.3 for each dollar invested.[13] Also, the investment must overcome human resources and infrastructure problems. The lack of specialized mental health professionals in primary care leads to a task-shifting or task-sharing solution that reassures specific mental health assessment and treatment procedures with abbreviated training and ongoing supervision to nonspecialists. There is evidence that trained and supervised nonspecialists can effectively deliver psychopharmacological and psychological treatments for mental disorders.[14,15] Globally, there is an increased focus on using lay CHWs to meet mental health needs.[16] Training these professionals to detect depressive disorders and offering an intervention can significantly decrease the mental health gap. Given the lack of mental health specialists in primary care and the unlikelihood of being able to engage individuals for an extended course of IPT, our team explored training CHWs in primary care to deliver the briefer and simpler version of IPT, interpersonal counseling (IPC).[17] IPC uses the same principles and techniques as IPT, but the language is simplified, and the format is considerably briefer (3–5 sessions), although the length can vary.

We carried out a randomized clinical trial (RCT) to test IPC administered by CHWs and compared it to enhanced treatment as usual (E-TAU). E-TAU involved referral to existing services and a follow-up call from a psychologist to further assist with the referral. We trained 42 CHWs to administer IPC using the IPC manual.[17,18] IPC comprised 3–4 weekly hourly sessions. Based on the individual's preference, sessions were provided at the clinic or during household visits. During the COVID pandemic, patients have been offered telephone sessions instead of a home visit. Delivering IPC in people's homes enhanced participation and retention care.

Interpersonal counseling training

The intensive 3-day training was delivered by two IPT therapists (Rosaly Campanini and Camila T. Matsuzaka). It included seminars on ethics and confidentiality, depressive disorders and symptoms, and IPC techniques described in the IPC manual.[17] The training process for the RCT is described in detail elsewhere.[19] CHWs were assigned to catchment areas that differed from their primary practice to avoid conflicts with usual work responsibilities and to enhance patient confidentiality. The trainers provided in-person clinical supervision for 2 hours twice a month and were available throughout the 23-month study period.

The RCT included 86 patients diagnosed with major depressive disorder confirmed by the Mini International Neuropsychiatric Interview MINI[20] and were randomized to receive either IPC or E-TAU. Assessment of depressive symptom severity using the Hamilton Depression Rating Scale (HDRS) occurred at baseline, end of the IPC, and 2 months after the end. Intention-to-treat analysis showed significant improvement in symptoms for both groups over 2 months, without significant treatment differences. However, there were significantly fewer symptoms on the HDRS-17 in the IPC group.

These preliminary results demonstrated feasibility and that IPC could be a low-cost and effective alternative to reduce the burden of depression in a setting that has inadequate specialist-led services. Our RCT was included in a recent global metanalysis[21] that showed a more robust finding for task sharing of psychological interventions across different groups of patients with depression.[22-24]

We also conducted a qualitative study using the research action qualitative method that collected data through focus groups and individual interviews with the CHWs. The data were collected 1 year after the end of the RCT. Discourse analysis was used based on the transcription of the focus group recording, organized into discourse and meaning analysis categories. The qualitative evaluation revealed that task shifting was acceptable to CHWs. They felt capable of detecting and managing mild-to-moderate depressive symptoms in primary care following a strict protocol under supervision. Regular supervision by a trained psychotherapist is essential following training.

In 2018–2019, we conducted another pilot study among primary care workers in Itaboraí, a midsize city located outside of Rio de Janeiro, to explore the acceptability and feasibility of implementing IPC in primary care for people with tuberculosis (TB) and depression. In this implementation pilot, we offered a 2-day workshop based on Mental Health Gap Action Program (mhGAP) (depression and suicide modules) and a 3-day training on IPC delivered by 2 IPT specialists (Camila Matsuzaka and Fatima de Silva), a psychiatrist and a psychiatric nurse, using the same methods described above. These trainings were open to all staff members (any level or role) in 2 FHS health outreach posts and the centralized TB program. Since this was an implementation science study seeking to explore the acceptability and feasibility of training existing primary care staff to deliver IPC, no incentives beyond transportation costs and refreshments were provided for either training or implementation throughout the 1-year pilot. Despite this, participation rates were high—including administrators, CHWs, nurses, and doctors—with 36 providers participating in both trainings. Over the course of 1 year, these primary care workers and TB providers were given weekly group supervision by 2 psychiatric nurses to implement IPC among their patients. Approximately one-third of the trainees (all levels) self-selected to deliver IPC with at least 1 patient (total ~ 40), often in pairs. Although clinical outcomes were not a focus of the study, it was notable that most patients (~80%) completed all 4 sessions, and of those, nearly all experienced depression remission.

Qualitative observations and interviews during and after the pilot revealed IPC as a highly acceptable and feasible intervention for patients and providers. Increased mental health sensitization at the clinic level and routine implementation of the Patient Health Questionnaire-9 (PHQ-9) as a screening tool had downstream implications as well; primary care providers were better able to more confidently identify patients that could be treated at the clinic level using IPC and more clearly refer patients with higher severity to specialists (using the PHQ-9 as a referral tool). Several providers even continued implementing IPC over a year after the pilot ended, providing peer supervision to one another. One physician was so excited about the work, she went on to pursue a master's degree in mental health.

The main limitations in implementing IPC were structural; Brazil's health system is significantly underresourced. Despite strong interest and perceived benefit, providers did not have time to conduct four 45-minute IPC sessions with patients. Frequent staff rotation at the nurse and doctor levels in the health outposts made it challenging to ensure continuity of care and retain IPC competencies. A more robust and stable workforce would be needed to bring the approach to scale. That said, if sufficiently resourced, the structure of the Brazilian Health System lends itself well to a task-shifting IPC approach at the primary care level, with clinical supervision potentially possible through nucleus of psychosocial support teams of specialists (including psychologists) that rotate among primary care facilities to provide consultation and supervision.[25]

In summary, some barriers to the IPC adaptation in this Brazilian study were identified:

1. Of the cases, 40.7% had severe depression at baseline (HDRS score $\geq$ 19), which was considered high for a primary care population. This points to the need for mental health treatment access in the primary care system.
2. Sustainability: In the Sao Paulo pilot study, the research grant provided weekly supervision and a small monetary compensation for the CHW to get involved valuing the time of work. CHW received 50 Brazilian reais (~US $15 by 2015) for each session completed as the provider. Political interests to develop a sustainable CHW specialization in mental health care is needed. In the Itoboraí pilot, while effective, weekly in-person supervision by 2 specialists was not replicable and scalable, and alternatives for clinical supervision using technology (e.g., WhatsApp, Zoom) would need to be explored.

Perceived facilitators were the following:

1. CHWs frequently reported feeling empowered during the research.
2. There was improved ability of CHWs to recognize depression, promoting assess to treatment and reducing stigma in the community.
3. The patients had an excellent adherence to IPC sessions: The mean number of IPC sessions completed was 2.26 ± 1.26.
4. Positive results received the attention of the stakeholders.

CASE EXAMPLES

Case 1

Maria is a 35-year-old woman, married, with incomplete primary school educa-tion, treated by clinician (general practitioner) for obesity and hypertension with a history of poor adherence to treatment. She complained of anxiety, unhappiness, loneliness, and a fear of dying. She could not identify when the depression symptoms had begun but suggested that it was since her son was born 10 years ago. As she grew into her new role as a mother, she found herself become increasingly overprotective of him. Maria attended 3 weeks of consecutive sessions. In the first session, the CHW observed that Maria had recently become more concerned about herself and her physical health. When exploring Maria's current relationships, the CHW learned about marital distance. In the second session, Maria elaborated further about her difficulties talking to her husband and blamed him for her depression symptoms. They had not spoken in a long time, except when he occasionally drank alcohol. Maria and the CHW jointly chose "role transition" as the relevant problem area since the birth of her son coincided with distance from her husband. Together, they thought of strategies to improve communication with the husband. In the third session, Maria still reported similar communication challenges, but during the session, Maria realized that she was not actually "in dispute" with her husband but wanted more closeness with him. She decided to change some attitudes toward her husband and her son.

Case 2

Lucia, a 45-year-old divorced woman with incomplete primary school education, was working for a company that went bankrupt. At the time of the first session, she had been unemployed for 7 months and had been experiencing mild symptoms of depression. She had a difficult life story, which included 2 failed marriages; however, her job and financial independence from her ex-spouses was extremely important to her. She lived with her 9-year-old son, who had recently been acting out at school. She still reported pain and limited movements from a car accident 4 years ago. She had recently tried some informal jobs as a house cleaner or babysitter but was unable to fulfill them because of her physical limitations. The CHW met her for 3 consecutive weekly sessions. Lucia was actively searching for a new job and meeting with a social worker from the Health Unit for assistance. She described feelings of sadness and crying but developed quick attachment to the CHW, which enabled her to share her feelings. Lucia and the CHW identified the primary problem area related to her transition after the unemployment. Lucia was also encouraged to get closer to her 21-year-old daughter and significant others. Lucia presented the therapist with a Christmas cake at the last session, expressing her gratitude for the assistance.

REFERENCES

1. IBGE. Extreme poverty reaches 13.5 million people and reaches highest level in 7 years (Extrema pobreza atinge 13,5 milhões de pessoas e chega ao maior nível em

7 anos). 2019. https://agenciadenoticias.ibge.gov.br/agencia-noticias/2012-agen cia-de-noticias/noticias/25882-extrema-pobreza-atinge-13-5-milhoes-de-pess oas-e-chega-ao-maior-nivel-em-7-anos. Accessed September 17, 2023.

2. World Health Organization. *Global Health Estimates 2019: Disease Burden by Cause, Age, Sex, by Country and by Region, 2000–2019.* World Health Organization; 2020.

3. World Health Organization. *Depression and Other Common Mental Disorders: Global Health Estimates.* World Health Organization; 2017.

4. Kohn R, Saxena S, Levav I, Saraceno B. The treatment gap in mental health care. *Bull World Health Org.* 2004;82(11):858–866.

5. Thornicroft G, Chatterji S, Evans-Lacko S, et al. Undertreatment of people with major depressive disorder in 21 countries. *Br J Psychiatry.* 2017;210(2):119–124.

6. de Mello MF, Myczcowisk LM, Menezes PR. A randomized controlled trial comparing moclobemide and moclobemide plus interpersonal psychotherapy in the treatment of dysthymic disorder. *J Psychother Pract Res.* 2001;10(2):117–123.

7. Campanini RF, Schoedl AF, Pupo MC, Costa AC, Krupnick JL, Mello MF. Efficacy of interpersonal therapy-group format adapted to post-traumatic stress disorder: an open-label add-on trial. *Depress Anxiety.* 2010;27(1):72–77.

8. Lacaz FS, Bressan RA, Mello MF. A psicoterapia interpessoal na depressão em pacientes com esquizofrenia: proposta de um modelo terapêutico a partir de três casos clínicos. *Trends Psychiatry Psychother.* 2005;27:252–261.

9. Proença CR, Markowitz JC, Prado EA, et al. Attrition in interpersonal psychotherapy among women with post-traumatic stress disorder following sexual assault. *Front Psychol.* 2019;10:2120.

10. Macinko J, Harris MJ, Phil D. Brazil's family health strategy—delivering community-based primary care in a universal health system. *N Engl J Med.* 2015;372(23):2177–2181.

11. Paim J, Travassos C, Almeida C, Bahia L, Macinko J. The Brazilian health system: history, advances, and challenges. *Lancet.* 2011;377(9779):1778–1797.

12. de Barros MM, Chagas MI, Dias MS. Knowledge and practices of the community health agent in the universe of mental disorder. *Cien Saude Colet.* 2009;14(1):227–232.

13. Chisholm D, Sweeny K, Sheehan P, et al. Scaling-up treatment of depression and anxiety: a global return on investment analysis. *Lancet Psychiatry.* 2016;3(5):415–424.

14. Rojas G, Fritsch R, Solis J, et al. Treatment of postnatal depression in low-income mothers in primary-care clinics in Santiago, Chile: a randomised controlled trial. *Lancet.* 2007;370(9599):1629–1637.

15. Patel V, Thornicroft G. Packages of care for mental, neurological, and substance use disorders in low-and middle-income countries: *PLoS Medicine* series. *PLoS Med.* 2009;6(10):e1000160.

16. Patel V, Chisholm D, Parikh R, et al. Addressing the burden of mental, neurological, and substance use disorders: key messages from disease control priorities. *Lancet.* 2016;387(10028):1672–1685.

17. Weissman MM, Hankerson SH, Scorza P, et al. Interpersonal counseling (IPC) for depression in primary care. *Am J Psychother.* 2014;68(4):359–383.

18. Klerman GL, Budman S, Berwick D, et al. Efficacy of a brief psychosocial intervention for symptoms of stress and distress among patients in primary care. *Med Care.* 1987;25(11):1078–1088.

19. Matsuzaka CT, Wainberg M, Norcini Pala A, et al. Task shifting interpersonal counseling for depression: a pragmatic randomized controlled trial in primary care. *BMC Psychiatry.* 2017;17:1–1.

20. Sheehan DV, Lecrubier Y, Sheehan KH, et al. The Mini-International Neuropsychiatric Interview (MINI): the development and validation of a structured diagnostic psychiatric interview for *DSM-IV* and *ICD-10. J Clin Psychiatry.* 1998;59(20):22–33.

21. Karyotaki E, Araya R, Kessler RC, et al. Association of task-shared psychological interventions with depression outcomes in low-and middle-income countries: a systematic review and individual patient data meta-analysis. *JAMA Psychiatry.* 2022;79(5):430–443.

22. Lund C, Schneider M, Garman EC, Davies T, et al. Task-sharing of psychological treatment for antenatal depression in Khayelitsha, South Africa: effects on antenatal and postnatal outcomes in an individual randomised controlled trial. *Behav Res Ther.* 2020;130:103466.

23. Spedding MF, Stein DJ, Naledi T, Myers B, Cuijpers P, Sorsdahl KR. A task-sharing intervention for prepartum common mental disorders: feasibility, acceptability and responses in a South African sample. *Afr J Prim Health Care Fam Med.* 2020;12(1):1–9.

24. Thirthalli J, Sivakumar PT, Gangadhar BN. Preventing late-life depression through task sharing: scope of translating evidence to practice in resource-scarce settings. *JAMA Psychiatry.* 2019;76(1):7–8.

25. Athié K, Delgado PG, Fortes S. Delgado mental health matrix support in primary care: a critical review (2000–2010). *Rev Bras Med Fam Comunidade Internet.* 2014;4:92.

42

Interpersonal Counseling for Internally Displaced Women in Bogotá, Colombia

ZELDE ESPINEL, JAMES M. SHULTZ, AND HELEN VERDELI ∎

OVERVIEW

In the Western Hemisphere, conflict-induced internal displacement has been focalized in Colombia, South America.[1,2] No other nation throughout the Americas has experienced internal displacement on a scale comparable to Colombia.[1-3] The Internal Displacement Monitoring Center estimated that, in 2021, there were 5.2 million internally displaced persons (IDPs) in Colombia, representing 84% of IDPs in the Americas and almost 9% of all IDPs worldwide.[4] About 2 in 3 Colombian IDPs are women and children.[1,5]

Colombian IDPs have a high prevalence of trauma exposure and correspondingly high rates of common mental disorders (CMDs),[2,5-9] especially among women.[10] We conducted a feasibility and acceptability pilot study to examine the potential efficacy of an evidence-based, stepped-care intervention adapted for depression, anxiety, and post-traumatic disorder (PTSD) in IDP women residing in Bogotá.[5] The study was named *OSITA* (meaning "little teddy bear" in Spanish), an acronym for Outreach, Screening, and Intervention for Trauma. OSITA implemented a brief version of interpersonal therapy (ITP)—interpersonal counseling (IPC)—as the mental health and psychosocial support intervention for the IDP women participants.[5]

Zelde Espinel, James M. Shultz, and Helen Verdeli, *Interpersonal Counseling for Internally Displaced Women in Bogotá, Colombia* In: *Interpersonal Psychotherapy.* Edited by: Myrna M. Weissman and Jennifer J. Mootz, Oxford University Press.
© Oxford University Press 2024. DOI: 10.1093/oso/9780197652084.003.0043

CONFLICT-INDUCED INTERNAL DISPLACEMENT IN COLOMBIA

The driver behind Colombia's burgeoning numbers of IDPs is the prolonged insurgency, dating from the 1960s, involving multiple armed actors, including left-wing guerrilla factions and right-wing paramilitary battling each other and the Colombian National Police and armed forces.[1-3] From the 1970s through the early 2000s, Colombia became a veritable geographic checkerboard of shifting control. Power and leadership of towns and municipalities changed hands frequently. People were displaced, at the level of the household or the community, as new armed groups took charge or new codes of conduct were issued by armed groups coming into power.[11] Most IDPs have not been able to return to their homes. As internal displacement has been ongoing for multiple decades at a variable pace, the total numbers of IDPs have continuously accrued.

To date, the armed conflict is estimated to have claimed 260,000 lives and to have displaced almost 7 million individuals. The government of Colombia has officially designated IDPs as "victims of the armed conflict"—protected citizens who are eligible for medical, mental health, social, and legal services, as well as support for reclaiming their properties ("restitution of the lands").[12] The reality is that the vast majority of IDPs, most of whom originally resided in rural communities, have resettled in large urban centers and adapted to a new lifestyle. Among the 7 million IDPs ever displaced over multiple decades, some have died and a small proportion have returned to their homes, but most live displaced and adapted to their new environs, as the 2021 estimate of 5.2 million IDPs makes clear.[4]

Following years of negotiations, the government of Colombia and the largest guerrilla group, the Revolutionary Armed Forces of Colombia signed "the Peace" in 2016. The Nobel Prize was awarded to Colombian President Juan Manuel Santos for this achievement. With peace declared, Colombia officially ushered in the "postconflict" era. Indeed, the level of internecine violence has diminished. Nevertheless, internal displacement has continued even after the peace accords because other nonstate armed groups, including the National Liberation Army—nonsignatories to "the Peace"—have remained intact and active, particularly along Colombia's Pacific coast.[8,9,13]

TESTING INTERPERSONAL COUNSELING TO WOMEN IDPS IN COLOMBIA

Methods

With funding from Grand Challenges Canada, OSITA aimed to *recruit and enroll* women IDPs residing in Bogota and assess their displacement-related trauma/loss exposures across all phases of displacement, *screen* for CMDs (major depressive disorder, generalized anxiety disorder, and PTSD), and using validated Spanish language measures, *intervene* using a locally adapted version of IPC, *follow up* participants, ideally to the point of symptom resolution, and *refer* women with severe symptoms or suicidality to specialized services.

Team

Expert researchers from multiple international universities (Columbia University, London School of Hygiene and Tropical Medicine, University of Miami Miller School of Medicine) identified a Colombian university partner to be the local research partner and recipient of the grant funding.

Over the course of the study, 3 types of counselors were hired. The university partner originally stipulated the hiring of *public health graduate students* to act as OSITA counselors. To increase sustainability, community-connected IDP women were added as counselors. These IDP women had no health background. Following review of counselor performance 6 months into the implementation phase, OSITA's original contingent of student counselors was replaced with *experienced outreach workers* and medical students (to fulfill university expectations); all of them met competency criteria. The IDP women continued for the full duration of the intervention and were found to be effective counselors.

Participants

The OSITA team worked intensively, ultimately using 18 recruitment sources, to identify and enroll 279 eligible IDP women. Some of the more productive recruitment sources included vocational education centers, community health centers, public sector hospitals, and governmental "victims of the armed conflict" processing centers. OSITA participants were women IDPs with a mean age of 37 years. About half (53%) had completed secondary education, and an additional 18% had vocational or higher education beyond the secondary level. Approximately half of the participants (50%) were single (never married, separated, divorced); 31% lived with a partner in civil union; and 10% were married. Eleven percent were indigenous, and 18% were Afro-Colombian.

Goals

OSITA goals were to assess ease of participant recruitment and retention, ability to deliver IPC with fidelity, efficacy of IPC in reducing symptom levels of CMDs, and sustainability of the intervention.

Language

All OSITA components, and delivery of IPC sessions, were conducted in Spanish.

Intervention

Multiple forms of IPT, including IPC, are interventions with proven effectiveness for populations of adults and youth experiencing CMD symptom elevations related to potentially traumatizing exposures (PTEs) in humanitarian emergency situations worldwide.[14,15] IPC's focus on loss, conflict, and disruption of social networks fit well for the Colombian context and the forced migration experiences of IDP women participants in the OSITA study.

OSITA COUNSELORS: SELECTION, TRAINING, AND SUPERVISION

The OSITA counselors, along with Bogotá government psychosocial professionals working with victim populations, were trained for a week on site in Bogotá by an IPC master trainer and supervisor from Columbia University (H. V.). Subsequently, counselors were supervised weekly, in person or online, by 2 IPC-certified professionals, 1 based in the United States (H. V.), and the other a Spanish-fluent supervisor, who provided periodic on-site supervision in Bogotá.

TRAUMA/LOSS EXPOSURES AND CMD SYMPTOM ELEVATIONS

Data from the OSITA baseline assessment and initial intervention visit revealed a very high prevalence of CMD symptom elevations. Symptom elevations were related to the extraordinary magnitude of trauma/loss exposures experienced by the IDP women participants.

CMD symptom elevations

In our targeted recruitment sample, 177 participants (63.4%) had symptoms in the moderate/severe range for at least 1 CMD at baseline assessment. Half of the participants (50.9%) had moderate or severe symptom levels for depression at baseline, as measured by the Patient Health Questionnaire-9 (PHQ-9), which has been locally validated. Forty percent had moderate or severe levels of anxiety symptoms (measured by the Generalized Anxiety Disorder-7), and 39.4% had post-traumatic stress symptoms (measured by PTSD Checklist—Civilian Version). Among these 177 participants with CMD symptom elevations, moderate/severe scores were found on a single CMD measure for 61 participants, on 2 CMD measures for 44, and on all 3 CMD measures for 72. These 177 participants with symptom elevations were referred for IPC.

Trauma/loss exposures

Colombian IDPs have experienced extreme adversities throughout each phase in the trajectory of forced migration, most simply conceived as predisplacement, characterized by PTEs to extreme violence and brutality; peridisplacement is defined by cascades of losses (of their homes, land, livestock, community, status); and postdisplacement, during which they had to navigate a place both foreign and frigid, living in poverty, and trying to adapt to the urban life, unable to rely on job skills acquired and refined over their rural lifetimes.

In sequence, the principal types of stressors encountered during each of the 3 phases of displacement can be summarized as exposures to predisplacement *trauma*, peridisplacement *loss*, and postdisplacement *life change*. On average, these women had experienced throughout these phases 2 dozen exposures of such impact that a single such event could have enduring, life-changing impact.

ADAPTATION OF IPC

Feedback from IPC trainees and participants confirmed that the 4 therapeutic foci of IPC were highly relevant to the target population. The participants had frequently experienced multiple violent deaths of loved ones, which were at times not accompanied by community rituals given the circumstances of the displacement; cascades of role transitions (life changes) from their former identity and place in the community of origin to the current impoverished and marginalized urban life; disputes with family members that included instances of domestic violence by and toward the participants, as well as covert disputes with the host community around incidents of exploitation or humiliation that were not expressed openly due to the power differential; and loneliness and social isolation that was fueled by suspicion related to the political backdrop. IPC was implemented as designed.[14,15] Mobilization of resources, which is an integral part of assigning the sick role in the initial sessions, played a prominent role: In addition to persons in the participants' environment, the counselor made them aware of networks of designated victim support centers for registered IDPs, offering economic, health, vocational, and educational support. Stress inoculation and grounding techniques were added for those participants with significant anxiety. Another type of adaptation was related to the delivery of IPC: The protocol specified that the participants would be followed until they had 2 consecutive sessions at or below subsyndromal threshold cutoff (treatment to target).[5]

OUTCOMES

Analyses of symptom changes in the sample of completers with baseline, last session, and follow-up data points revealed significant decreases over time in depression, anxiety, and PTSD symptom levels from baseline to last IPC session and further significant decreases in depression from last IPC session to follow-up. IDP women who were referred for second and subsequent IPC sessions were those with moderate/severe symptom levels on 1 or more measures at baseline. By the last IPC session and the follow-up session, the great majority of these women scored in the subsyndromal range, below the moderate symptom cutoff point.

MAJOR BARRIERS TO AND FACILITATORS OF IMPLEMENTATION

As a feasibility pilot study, OSITA encountered several challenges that precluded the possibility of scaling the intervention for broader dissemination in its original form. First, participant recruitment proved to be much more problematic than foreseen by our local collaborators. Their government contacts who were charged with working with conflict victims were reluctant to provide access to women IDPs as had been anticipated. Seeking alternative recruitment sources was unsystematic and inefficient. OSITA fell short of the recruitment goal of 300 participants. Recruitment was hampered by the understandable lack of trust on the part of IDPs, who were reticent to enroll, layers of governance barriers, and lack of protocols for accessing IDPs.

Second, the insistence on the part of the university partner to hire graduate students as counselors in the first year limited the geographic scope of recruitment to near-campus areas, and safety concerns further restricted outreach.

Third, referrals for psychiatric consultation services for women participants with severe CMD symptoms and high suicidal risk was very problematic. Six separate referral sources and pathways were sought and employed, ranging from government programs to hospitals with mental health services, to individual practitioners, yet only one-quarter of OSITA's high suicide risk participants received a professional consultation. Therefore, developing a safety plan for participant follow-up was essential.

Fourth, participant attrition and loss to follow-up were a major issue. Although some of the dropouts may have been related to participants feeling better after several IPC sessions and not returning, practical impediments were prominent. Many women participants were unable to return for follow-up IPC sessions due to lack of time, bus fare, or childcare. Other barriers included family interference or failure to receive employer permission as well as stigma and discrimination for seeking mental health support.

CONCLUSIONS AND RECOMMENDATIONS

One of the most powerful findings from the OSITA study was confirmation that IDP women participants had extremely high levels of trauma exposure that were likely causally related to the burden of psychological symptoms consistent with CMDs. Almost two-thirds presented at baseline with moderate or severe symptoms.

The OSITA intervention appeared to be feasible as a stepped-care intervention for this high-risk population, but any future version would need to be adapted in terms of partner selection, counselor selection, recruitment mechanisms, active outreach to participants, and safety precautions for those who have severe or suicidal symptoms. Using validated screening instruments for CMDs was effective for being able to detect baseline levels of CMD symptoms for IPC eligibility and to track progress on symptom reduction and resolution over time, in part for determining when to terminate the IPC intervention. The overall trend of marked declines in CMD symptoms among those receiving the intervention was extremely encouraging but needs to be confirmed with a more definitive application of IPC that achieves a high level of participant retention.

Based on the OSITA experience, key recommendations for future work in Colombia are as follows:

1. IDPs should be reached directly instead of going through government intermediaries.
2. Since IDP women have firsthand knowledge of forced migration and have the potential to build rapport and trust among participants, they can be trained to effectively assume the counselor role. With adequate training and supervision, IDP women do not need a mental health/health background to deliver IPC effectively.
3. To minimize attrition, online or telephone or telehealth consultations can be provided to IDP participants.
4. Interventions should be linked to sustainability and scalability from the beginning.

REFERENCES

1. Shultz JM, Ceballos ÁM, Espinel Z, Oliveros SR, Fonseca MF, Florez IJ. Internal displacement in Colombia: fifteen distinguishing features. *Disaster Health*. 2014;2(1):13–24.
2. Shultz JM, Garfin DR, Espinel Z, et al. Internally displaced "victims of armed conflict" in Colombia: the trajectory and trauma signature of forced migration. *Curr Psychiatry Rep*. 2014;16(10):475.
3. Chaskel R, Gaviria SL, Espinel Z, Taborda E, Vanegas R, Shultz JM. Mental health in Colombia. *BJPsych Int*. 2015;12(4):95–97.
4. Internal Displacement Monitoring Center. 2022 Global Report on Internal Displacement (GRID). Accessed December 27, 2022. https://www.internal-displacement.org/publications/2022-global-report-on-internal-displacement
5. Shultz JM, Verdeli H, Gómez Ceballos Á, et al. A pilot study of a stepped-care brief intervention to help psychologically-distressed women displaced by conflict in Bogotá, Colombia. *Glob Ment Health (Camb)*. 2019;6:e28.

6. Lagos-Gallego M, Gutierrez-Segura JC, Lagos-Grisales GJ, Rodriguez-Morales AJ. Post-traumatic stress disorder in internally displaced people of Colombia: an ecological study. *Travel Med Infect Dis.* 2017;16:41–45.

7. Lagos-Gallego M, Gutiérrez-Segura JC, Lagos-Grisales GJ, Rodríguez-Morales AJ. Alcoholism in internally displaced people of Colombia: an ecological study. *Travel Med Infect Dis.* 2019;31:101315.

8. Santaella-Tenorio J, Bonilla-Escobar FJ, Nieto-Gil L, et al. Mental health and psychosocial problems and needs of violence survivors in the Colombian Pacific Coast: a qualitative study in Buenaventura and Quibdó. *Prehosp Disaster Med.* 2018;33(6):567–574.

9. Bonilla-Escobar FJ, Osorio-Cuéllar GV, Pacichana-Quinayaz SG, et al. Impacts of violence on the mental health of Afro-descendant survivors in Colombia. *Med Confl Surviv.* 2021;37(2):124–145.

10. Wirtz AL, Pham K, Glass N, et al. Gender-based violence in conflict and displacement: qualitative findings from displaced women in Colombia. *Confl Health.* 2014;8:10.

11. Ramirez E, Gomez AP, Gesteira C, Chaskel R, Espinel Z, Shultz JM. Ghosts in the big city: surviving and adapting to internal displacement in Colombia, South America. *Intervention: Journal of Mental Health and Psychosocial Support in Conflict Affected Areas.* 2016;14(3):320–329.

12. Republica de Colombia, Ministerio del Interior. *Law of the Victims (Law 1448): Ley de Víctimas y Restitución de Tierras y Sus Decretos Reglamentarios: LEY 1448 de 2011.* Republica de Colombia, Ministerio del Interior; 2011. Accessed December 27, 2022. http://www.centrodememoriahistorica.gov.co/micrositios/caminosParaLa Memoria/descargables/ley1448.pdf

13. Reardon S. Colombia: after the violence. *Nature.* 2018;557:19–24.

14. Gomez Ceballos AM, Andrade AC, Markowitz T, Verdeli H. "You pulled me out of a dark well": a case study of a Colombian displaced woman empowered through interpersonal counseling (IPC). *J Clin Psychol.* 2016;72(8):839–846.

15. Weissman MM, Hankerson SH, Scorza P, et al. Interpersonal counseling (IPC) for depression in primary care. *Am J Psychother.* 2014;68(4):359–383.

Interpersonal Psychotherapy in Different Populations in the United States

43

Family-Based Interpersonal Psychotherapy (FB-IPT) for Depressed Preadolescents

LAURA DIETZ ■

Sixty years ago, the psychiatric community widely accepted the understanding that depression in prepubertal children (e.g., ages 12 and under) was developmentally inconsistent with the deep-rooted psychodynamic theory that children lacked the meta-cognitive and self-reflective skills to experience many of the depressive symptoms seen in adults. Pioneering work by clinical scientists[1-3] documented the phenomenology of depressive symptoms in children and the developmental sequelae of these symptoms that contributed to validating the relevance of depressive disorders in children. This research spurred further exploration of the ways that preadolescent depression may present and the constellation of risk factors that may contribute to its onset. Developmental psychopathologists hypothesized that early onset depressive disorders in children often went "undiagnosed and undertreated" and argued for future treatment models that addressed family risk factors and interpersonal impairment with peers as targets for reducing symptoms and teaching skills that could reduce the likelihood or delay the onset of a more severe depression in adolescence.[4,5]

As the validity and acceptance of depression in children increased, so did the lack of effective treatments and best practices for addressing preadolescent depression. The first studies of psychological treatments for preadolescents with depression focused on downward extension models of cognitive behavior therapy (CBT) in community samples of youth with elevated depressive symptoms. While CBT demonstrated effective symptom reduction compared to wait list or no treatment, it surprisingly did not outperform less sophisticated interventions, such as relaxation exercises and attention control support from school nurses or other

Laura Dietz, *Family-Based Interpersonal Psychotherapy (FB-IPT) for Depressed Preadolescents* In: *Interpersonal Psychotherapy*. Edited by: Myrna M. Weissman and Jennifer J. Mootz, Oxford University Press. © Oxford University Press 2024. DOI: 10.1093/oso/9780197652084.003.0044 professionals not trained in mental health.[6-8] These findings halted the progress of evidence-based treatments for prepubertal depression and left mostly unstructured supportive and individual models of psychotherapy to fill the void as the standard of treatment for depression in children under 12 years.

Psychological interventions for depression in preadolescent children continued to lag behind the growing need for evidence-based treatments at the approach of the millennium. Although psychotherapy for depressive disorders in preadolescent children was regarded as the first line of treatment, some children with depression were treated with medications, most notably the selective serotonin reuptake inhibitors (SSRIs), which were effective in treating depression in adults and were beginning to be studied in depressed adolescents. The "black box" warning on SSRIs in 2004 in the United States was related to concerns of increasing suicidality in children under 18 and resulted in a dramatic decrease in physicians' willingness to prescribe SSRIs to children. At the same time, outpatient mental health services began seeing an increase in children under 12 presenting for psychological treatment with depressive symptoms and/or suicidality and again highlighted the lack of evidence-based interventions for this population.[9-11]

In 2008, Drs. Laura Dietz and Laura Mufson published an open-trial pilot study of family-based interpersonal psychotherapy (FB-IPT),[12] a 14-session psychological intervention for depressed children ages 12 and under that used the conceptual framework and structure of interpersonal psychotherapy for adolescents (IPT-A)[13] while incorporating developmentally appropriate techniques and approaches germane to addressing the risk factors associated with preadolescent depression. The rationale behind FB-IPT is to reduce preadolescents depressive symptoms by increasing social support, to reflect on affective changes associated with interpersonal events, and to improve communication and problem-solving skills in interpersonal relationships.

Both adult and adolescent models of IPT provided a conceptual foundation for understanding preadolescents' developmental transitions and for addressing their interpersonal contexts, namely their family relationships, that may contribute to emotional distress and difficulties. Inherent to IPT is the understanding that role transitions are often related to depressive symptoms, and treatment focuses on helping clients recognize how changes in routines, circumstances, and social/developmental roles necessitate changes in behavior to meet new challenges and responsibilities that come with the new role. This treatment focus is particularly germane to preadolescents, who are in the process of developmental transitions as they move from childhood to adolescence. Important role transitions seen in preadolescents include balancing changes in their relationships with parents, as they are becoming more independent and need to take on more responsibilities, the experience of moving from primary to secondary schools, the beginning of physical changes associated with puberty, and the associated social and emotional experiences of becoming an adolescent, including changes in peer relationships. Preadolescents' peer relationships become increasingly important during this period of development, and there are increased expectations for more skilled behavior in friendships. Bullying peaks during this period, and the consequences of peer rejection and exclusion are particularly difficult for preadolescents. Acceptance by friends becomes increasingly important for preadolescents' emotional well-being, and often preadolescents need to learn more mature interpersonal skills for communicating their feelings and managing conflict.

In this chapter, we review the clinical adaptations present in the FB-IPT psychotherapy model used with depressed preadolescents as related to both the original adult model of IPT and modifications to IPT-A. Next, we provide an overview of the model and a brief review of the *empirical evidence that supports FB-IPT*, which includes an open study and 2 randomized controlled trials.

AN OVERVIEW OF FB-IPT ADAPTATIONS AND MODIFICATIONS TO ADULT AND ADOLESCENT MODELS OF IPT

Family-based IPT is conceptually rooted in an interpersonal model of depression[14] and in developmental research on the antecedents of depression in youth. FB-IPT focuses on improving 2 domains of interpersonal impairment in depressed preadolescents, parent-child conflict and peer impairment, as a means to decrease preadolescents' depressive symptoms. We focus on improving communication and problem-solving skills in the parent-child relationship, the primary context for children's social and emotional development, to model effective interpersonal behavior with peers and to improve the quality of the parent-child relationship to buffer depressed preadolescents from the effects of peer stress.

Family0-based IPT is a developmental adaptation of the adult model of IPT and a modification of IPT-A.[15] As in the adult model, FB-IPT divides treatment into 3 phases and structures treatment around 1 of 4 "problem areas" temporally associated with the onset of depressive symptoms (loss, role disputes, role transitions, and interpersonal deficits). Many of the core clinical activities in the adult model of IPT are retained and incorporated into FB-IPT, including the interpersonal inventory, sharing the problem area formulation with the client, and utilizing strategies such as communication analysis and decision analysis in the middle phase of treatment to improve interpersonal interactions and find ways to increase social support networks. FB-IPT also includes a termination phase.

Although the content across the 3 phases of treatment is retained with modifications, FB-IPT differs from the adult and adolescent models in structure of the sessions across phases. Most notably, sessions are structured to involve individual meeting time with the preadolescent, as well as individual meeting time with the parent or dyadic meeting time with the preadolescent and parent. Below we outline the structure of sessions in FB-IPT that provide a foundation for other developmental modifications to facilitate treatment with preadolescent children.

Initial phase of FB-IPT

In the initial phase of FB-IPT (sessions 1–5), the therapist "checks in" with the preadolescent and parent for 10 minutes, before dividing the remainder of the session into individual meetings with the preadolescent (approximately 20 minutes) and then the parent (20 minutes). In meetings with preadolescents, FB-IPT therapists explore the relationship between depressive symptoms and negative experiences in family and peer relationships and complete the Closeness Circle and Interpersonal Inventory, an interactive mapping of preadolescents' relationships. Parent meetings focus on psychoeducation about depression, helping preadolescents maintain routines with reasonable expectations for their performance, and parenting strategies for responding to increased irritability, interpersonal avoidance, and/or anergia in preadolescents ("Parenting Tips"). Session 5, when the interpersonal problem area is identified and case formulation shared with the preadolescent and parent, begins with the dyad together for 25 minutes and then the therapist meeting individually with the preadolescent for 25 minutes to ensure understanding of the identified problem area and goals for the middle phase of treatment.

Middle phase (sessions 6–10)

Therapists meet individually with the preadolescent (25 minutes) and then with the parent-child dyad (25 minutes). The primary interventions of FB-IPT include teaching communication and problem-solving skills to preadolescents and parents. During dyadic sessions, preadolescents and parents role-play communication skills that are relevant to the identified problem area. Parent-child problem-solving is facilitated by the therapist to help parent-child dyads negotiate solutions to difficulties. Dyadic sessions also focus on increasing preadolescents' positive experiences with peers. Preadolescents are coached to initiate social experiences with peers and rehearse new communication skills for interpersonal approach with both therapists and parents. Parents engage in problem-solving with the preadolescent to increase opportunities for peer interaction; with preadolescents' approval, parents are sometimes enlisted to initiate peer initiation for their children.

Termination phase (sessions 10–12)

Therapists meet individually with preadolescents (35 minutes) and then with the dyad (25 minutes). Preadolescents and parents reflect on the progress in treatment and, in collaboration with the FB-IPT therapist, discuss next steps in treatment planning, as well as consolidate skills, discuss prevention strategies, and identify a plan for depression recurrence. Both the preadolescent and parent reflect on their feelings in ending the treatment relationship with the FB-IPT therapist, who models a "good" good-bye for both while maintaining the ability for the family to reach out again should the need arise.

Family-based IPT incorporates several developmental modifications for 7- to 12-year-olds as compared to IPT-A, which include (1) increased parental involvement and structured dyadic sessions, (2) visual representations of the mood ratings and communication analysis, and (3) an increased focus on comorbid anxiety in the problem area of interpersonal deficits. We elaborate on these modifications below:

Increased parental involvement and structured dyadic sessions

Family-based IPT actively involves parents in both conjoint and dyadic sessions with preadolescents during different phases of treatment. Individual meetings with parents address psychoeducation about preadolescent depression and the challenges experienced in parenting their depressed preadolescent. As in IPT-A, the limited sick role is a primary theme for conjoint sessions with parents during the initial phase of treatment (sessions 1–5), with the goal of placing the blame for the preadolescent's problems in functioning and behavior on the depression. The therapist enlists the parent to support the preadolescent to try to engage in as many of their normal activities as possible with revised expectations. The expanded limited sick role focuses on the challenges in parenting a depressed preadolescent and is personalized to the specific struggles within a parent-child dyad. In FB-IPT, we have developed a complementary set of Parent Tips to guide parents to interact with their depressed preadolescents in ways that reduce negative emotionality and parent-child escalation. The FB-IPT uses the Parent Tips to personalize strategies for reducing parenting challenges during the initial phase of treatment to stabilize conflict in the family and promote increased support for the preadolescent.

During the middle phase of FB-IPT (sessions 6–11), therapists introduce and role-play new communication skills and problem-solving strategies in individual meetings with the preadolescent and then in dyadic meeting with the preadolescent and parent. FB-IPT utilizes the skills presented in IPT-A but has streamlined and simplified them for use with preadolescents who often present with less sophisticated abstract reasoning and perspective taking skills ("Tween Tips"). The Tween Tips often are presented as directives for behavior in interactions with parents and peers ("use good timing" or make "I feel" statements) in order remind preadolescents of the skills and how they are employed in interpersonal interactions. Similarly, aspects of problem-solving have been expanded into more specific guidelines for how preadolescents can use compromise ("meet in the middle") or negotiation ("let's make a deal"). In individual meetings with preadolescents, the FB-IPT therapist introduces these communication skills and provides an example of how the preadolescent could use them in interactions with family members or peers. The communication is often scripted and role-played during individual meetings with preadolescents. In dyadic meetings, parents learn the same skills as their preadolescents and engage in practice utilizing different Tween Tips in role plays with both the FB-IPT therapist and their preadolescents. These dyadic sessions are used to increase the parents' communication skills and give the parent-preadolescent dyad a common language for using different ways of communicating or solving problems. It also allows the FB-IPT therapist to directly address any concerns between the dyad that may be contributing to conflict in the family.

Mood rating scale, communication analysis, and communication skills

Family-based IPT relies heavily on visual materials to help preadolescents at different cognitive levels synthesize and integrate both concrete and abstract information from interpersonal interactions (e.g., event information, affective responses, perspective taking about the other's experience of the event) for later problem-solving. Preadolescents learn to track changes in their mood using a mood thermometer, a 1–10 rating scale anchored at 3 points with emotional faces (see Figure 43.1).

Communication analysis is mapped out on paper helping depressed preadolescents identify events in recent interactions and their affective consequences. Communication skills are presented sequentially in the middle phase of treatment, accompanied by visual reminders of these communication strategies for rehearsal outside of therapy sessions.

Focus on comorbid anxiety

Family-based IPT is also rooted in an understanding of the phenomenology of preadolescent depression; specifically, that comorbid anxiety disorders, particularly those related to separation or social anxiety, are associated with early-onset depression. Some preadolescents have anxious temperaments that predispose them to anxiety disorders that involve social or interpersonal contexts, such as social phobia and separation anxiety, and usually involve avoidance of anxiety-producing interpersonal situations. Other preadolescents experience anxiety that is secondary to the social withdrawal and anhedonia that often accompanies depression. Interpersonal avoidance is a common feature among depressed preadolescents with comorbid anxiety. When preadolescents stop socializing, their friendships suffer, which may make approaching friends more difficult in the future. Interpersonal avoidance also can stem from co-occurring anxiety associated with the identified problem area. Losses, transitions, and conflict also produce anxiety in preadolescents, who are more affected by changes and/or distress in family environments. In addition, preadolescents with interpersonal deficits also frequently experience anxiety in social contexts.

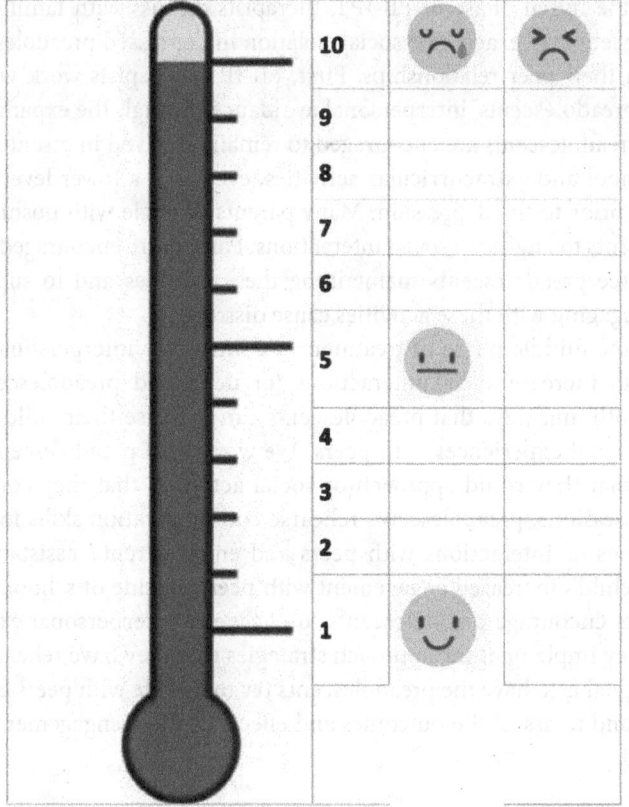

Figure 43.1 Mood thermometer.
CREDIT: Laura Dietz, PhD, asked Oxford University Press permission to reproduce for this chapter.

Family-based IPT seeks to increase preadolescents' social interaction with peers by teaching them new communication and problem-solving skills for initiating social interactions and handling conflict, as well as encouraging them to practice these strategies with peers outside of sessions in "interpersonal experiments." Like in an experiment, preadolescents initiate a previously rehearsed social interaction with a peer to determine whether the strategy is helpful in producing a positive social outcome. While engaging in interpersonal experiments and practicing interpersonal approach strategies aim to reduce preadolescents' depressive symptoms and social isolation, it also decreases preadolescents' anxiety about initiating interactions with peers. With increased practice, preadolescents develop increased confidence and less discomfort in approaching friends. With improved communication skills, depressed preadolescents may experience positive social interactions and subsequently may demonstrate increased interpersonal approach behaviors. With increased confidence and renewed motivation for social engagement, depressed preadolescents may be more likely to increase their social contacts and successes, which results in improved mood and the preadolescents may be less apt to avoid interpersonal situations in the future.

During the initial phase of FB-IPT, therapists discuss with families how co-morbid anxiety may exacerbate social isolation in depressed preadolescents, par-ticularly in their peer relationships. First, FB-IPT therapists work with parents to reduce preadolescents' interpersonal avoidance through the expanded limited sick role. Preadolescents are encouraged to remain involved in essential routines, such as school and extracurricular activities, even if at a lower level of engage-ment than prior to the depression. Many parents struggle with pushing anxious preadolescents to engage in social interactions. Parents are encouraged to support and reinforce preadolescents maintaining these routines and to support them when re-engaging with these activities cause distress.

During the middle phase of treatment, we introduce interpersonal approach strategies to increase social interactions for depressed preadolescents. These focus on outlining ways that preadolescents can increase their child's initiation of interpersonal experiences with peers. We work with preadolescents to iden-tify peers that they could approach or social activities that they could partici-pate in. In sessions, preadolescents rehearse communication skills for initiating conversations or interactions with peers and enlist parents' assistance to sup-port their child's increased engagement with peers outside of school. Therapists and parents encourage preadolescents to engage in interpersonal experiments, wherein they implement the approach strategies that they have rehearsed in ses-sions. The goal is to have the preadolescents try to initiate with peers as practiced in session and to assess the outcomes and effects of these engagement efforts on their mood.

EMPIRICAL EVIDENCE FOR FB-IPT

Support for FB-IPT as an efficacious treatment for preadolescents diagnosed as having depression includes an open treatment trial,[12] a randomized controlled trial,[16] and a small randomized controlled trial among overweight and obese preadolescents with loss-of-control (LOC) eating.[17] The results from the open treatment trial of FB-IPT ($N = 20$) demonstrated the feasibility and acceptability of FB-IPT as a psychosocial intervention for preadolescents with depression and their parents, as evidenced by high treatment compliance, low attrition rates, and favorable clinical outcomes for preadolescents completing treatment. The trial also demonstrated that preadolescents who received FB-IPT by itself were as likely as those receiving combination treatment (SSRI and FB-IPT) to have significant reductions in depressive and anxiety symptoms and to experience sig-nificant improvement in global functioning.[12]

In a follow-up study,[16] 42 treatment-seeking preadolescents who met *Diagnostic and Statistical Manual of Mental Disorders, Fourth Edition (DSM-IV)*[17] criteria for a depressive disorder were randomly selected to FB-IPT or child-centered therapy (CCT), a supportive and nondirective treatment that closely approximates the standard of care for pediatric depression in community mental health. Preadolescents receiving FB-IPT were more likely to have achieved re-mission posttreatment than those receiving CCT (66% vs. 31%) and evidenced greater reductions in anxiety symptoms and interpersonal impairment across treatment. A significant indirect effect for decreased social impairment mediated the association between the FB-IPT and the preadolescents' depressive symptoms posttreatment. This result suggests that reducing social impairment is one mechanism by which FB-IPT may decrease preadolescents' depressive symptoms.[16]

Most recently, FB-IPT was tested as an effective intervention for reducing depressive and anxiety symptoms in overweight and/or obese preadolescents with monthly episodes of LOC eating.[18] Compared with those treated with family-based health education, those randomized to receive FB-IPT demonstrated greater decreases in depressive and anxiety symptoms after a 12-week course of treatment, and the reductions in depressive symptoms were maintained at the 1-year follow-up. Although no differences in weight-related outcomes were found, preadolescents receiving FB-IPT were less likely to endorse LOC eating posttreatment and evidenced greater reductions in disordered-eating attitudes at the 6-month follow-up.[18] Although these preadolescents' depressive and anxiety symptoms did not reach diagnostic levels, the reduction of these comorbid symptoms may be significant in improving their LOC eating as they enter adolescence. Taken together, these findings support FB-IPT as a promising and effective treatment for anxiety and depression in preadolescents.

SUMMARY

Family-based FB-IPT is an adaptation of IPT that has been developmentally modified for use with preadolescent children between the ages of 7 and 12 who are seeking treatment for clinically significant depressive symptoms. The model of treatment aligns conceptually with adult IPT and includes three phases of treatment, treatment formulation around 1 of 4 problem areas, and techniques such as communication analysis. Differences between FB-IPT and the adult model of psychological treatment include the way sessions are structured and the dyadic nature of parental involvement in sessions. Developmental modifications to IPT-A allow for increased parental involvement in sessions with structured tasks for working with parents, visual representations of mood rating and communication analysis, and an increased focus on developmental transitions and comorbid anxiety in depressed preadolescents. Empirical studies in depressed preadolescents and those with LOC eating support the efficacy of FB-IPT to reduce depressive and anxiety symptoms in this age group.

REFERENCES

1. Kovacs M, Feinberg TL, Crouse-Novak M, Paulauskas SL, Pollock M, Finkelstein R. Depressive disorders in childhood: II. A longitudinal study of the risk for a subsequent major depression. *Arch Gen Psychiatry.* 1984;41(7):643–649.
2. Puig-Antich J, Lukens E, Davies M, Goetz D, Brennan-Quattrock J, Todak G. Psychosocial functioning in prepubertal major depressive disorders: I.

Interpersonal relationships during the depressive episode. *Arch Gen Psychiatry.* 1985;42(5):500–507.

3. Puig-Antich J, Lukens E, Davies M, Goetz D, Brennan-Quattrock J, Todak G. Psychosocial functioning in prepubertal major depressive disorders: II. Interpersonal relationships after sustained recovery from affective episode. *Arch Gen Psychiatry.* 1985;42(5):511–517.

4. Angold A, Costello EJ, Farmer EM, Burns BJ, Erkanli A. Impaired but undiagnosed. *J Am Acad Child Adolesc Psychiatry.* 1999;38(2):129–137.

5. Hammen C, Rudolph K, Weisz J, Rao U, Burge D. The context of depression in clinic-referred youth: neglected areas in treatment. *J Am Acad Child Adolesc Psychiatry.* 1999;38(1):64–71.

6. Kahn JS, Kehle TJ, Jenson WR, Clark E. Comparison of cognitive-behavioral, relaxation, and self-modeling interventions for depression among middle-school students. *School Psychol Rev.* 1990;19(2):196–211.

7. Vostanis P, Feehan C, Grattan E. Two-year outcome of children treated for depression. *Eur Child Adolesc Psychiatry.* 1998;7:12–18.

8. Vostanis P, Feehan C, Grattan E, Bickerton WL. A randomised controlled outpatient trial of cognitive-behavioural treatment for children and adolescents with depression: 9-month follow-up. *J Affect Disord.* 1996;40(1-2):105–116.

9. Bridge JA, Greenhouse JB, Weldon AH, Campo JV, Kelleher KJ. Suicide trends among youths aged 10 to 19 years in the United States, 1996–2005. *JAMA.* 2008;300(9):1025–1026.

10. Bridge JA, Horowitz LM, Fontanella CA, et al. Age-related racial disparity in suicide rates among US youths from 2001 through 2015. *JAMA Pediatr.* 2018;172(7):697–699.

11. Whalen DJ, Dixon-Gordon K, Belden AC, Barch D, Luby JL. Correlates and consequences of suicidal cognitions and behaviors in children ages 3 to 7 years. *J Am Acad Child Adolesc Psychiatry.* 2015;54(11):926–937.

12. Dietz LJ, Mufson L, Irvine H, Brent DA. Family-based interpersonal psychotherapy for depressed preadolescents: an open-treatment trial. *Early Interv Psychiatry.* 2008;2(3):154–161.

13. Mufson L, Dorta KM, Moreau D, Weissman MM. *Interpersonal Psychotherapy for Depressed Adolescents.* 2nd ed. Guilford Publications; 2004.

14. Klerman GL, Weissman MM, Rounsaville BJ, Chevron ES. *Interpersonal Psychotherapy of Depression.* Basic Books; 1984.

15. Dietz LJ, Weinberg RB, Mufson L. *Family Based Interpersonal Psychotherapy (FB-IPT) for Depressed Preadolescents.* Oxford University Press; 2018.

16. Dietz LJ, Weinberg RJ, Brent DA, Mufson L. Family-based interpersonal psychotherapy for depressed preadolescents: examining efficacy and potential treatment mechanisms. *J Am Acad Child Adolesc Psychiatry.* 2015;54(3):191–199.

17. American Psychiatric Association. *Diagnostic and statistical manual of mental disorders (4th ed.).* 1994.

18. Shomaker LB, Tanofsky-Kraff M, Matherne CE, et al. A randomized, comparative pilot trial of family-based interpersonal psychotherapy for reducing psychosocial symptoms, disordered-eating, and excess weight gain in at-risk preadolescents with loss-of-control-eating. *Int J Eating Disord.* 2017;50(9):1084–1094.

Interpersonal Psychotherapy
for Adolescents (IPT-A)

**LAURA MUFSON, ANAT BRUNSTEIN KLOMEK,
GLENDA GARCIA, AND VALASÍA MAKRIDIS ■**

Depression in adolescence is common and if untreated can result in impairment in functioning across multiple domains.[1,2] Rates of depression in adolescents are increasing, so it is more important than ever to disseminate effective treatments for adolescent depression.

INTERPERSONAL PSYCHOTHERAPY FOR ADOLESCENTS

Interpersonal psychotherapy for adolescents (IPT-A) maintains the same premise and problem areas and adapts them developmentally to treat adolescents ages 12 through 18 years of age with unipolar depression.[3] Developmental adaptations were undertaken to address the parental role in treatment, adolescent tasks of individuation and establishing autonomy from parents, and describe transitions such as parental divorce, changing schools or childhood home, as well as initial experiences with grief. Specific adaptations include (1) family involvement in all 3 phases of treatment, (2) delineation of a limited sick role, (3) inclusion of the closeness circle, (4) more focus on skills training in the middle phase, and (5) the codification of the Teen Tips, a set of communication strategies taught to the adolescent and sometimes parents/caretakers as well.

Laura Mufson, Anat Brunstein Klomek, Glenda Garcia, and Valasía Makridis, *Interpersonal Psychotherapy for Adolescents (IPT-A)* In: *Interpersonal Psychotherapy.* Edited by: Myrna M. Weissman and Jennifer J. Mootz, Oxford University Press.
© Oxford University Press 2024. DOI: 10.1093/oso/9780197652084.003.0045

IPT-A ADAPTATIONS

Family involvement

In IPT-A, parent/caretaker involvement is recommended in the initial and termination phase, with middle phase involvement dependent on the identified problem area. In the initial phase, parents/caretakers are educated about depression and its impact on adolescent functioning and the parameters of IPT-A treatment. At the end of treatment, parents/caretakers learn about the adolescent's progress in treatment, impact of treatment on their relationships, warning signs of depression and strategies for managing potential recurrence. In the middle phase, their participation provides adolescents with opportunities to practice skills with their parents/caretakers or for the clinician to update them on how they can continue to support their adolescent.

Limited sick role

IPT-A psychoeducation includes acknowledging the impact that depression has on functioning and how the context of the illness may also contribute to symptoms, thereby removing blame from the adolescent. The adolescent is encouraged to *do* as many of their normal activities as possible (e.g., attending school) with the recognition that they may not perform them as well while depressed, and that their performance and motivation will improve as they begin to feel better. It is very important to share this concept with parents/caretakers to enlist their support for their teen.[3]

Closeness circle

In IPT-A, the closeness circle provides a visual diagram of the adolescent's significant relationships as the starting point for the interpersonal inventory.[3] The adolescent is asked to identify the most important people in their life, both positive and negative, specifically those people who feature in their current story that includes their depression. The adolescent identifies 4 or 5 people who would be most important to discuss to understand the role they may play in the adolescent's depression, including both supportive and stressful relationships, to set the stage for the Interpersonal Inventory.[3]

Teen Tips

In the middle phase of treatment, the therapist uses the problem area as the context for teaching new interpersonal skills. One focus is on how communicating differently might have resulted in more positive interactions and conversations, which could have led to less negative emotions. The clinician identifies specific interactions to teach new communication skills that have been codified as Teen Tips in IPT-A.[3] The Teen Tips are practiced during session role plays so the adolescent will be successful in implementing them during their interpersonal experiments conducted outside of sessions to create new more positive interpersonal interactions.

IPT-A EMPIRICAL SUPPORT

Interpersonal psychotherapy for adolescents has been demonstrated to be effective in reducing depression and improving social and global functioning in studies of depressed adolescents in the United States, Puerto Rico, and Australia.[4,5-8] Recently, a meta-analysis and systematic review of the effectiveness of psychotherapies for treating depression in youth found that IPT-A was significantly more effective than control conditions.[9,10] Additionally, a significantly larger effect size for IPT-A in comparison to cognitive behavioral therapy (CBT)was reported.[9] IPT-A also has been found to be particularly effective for older adolescents and those who report high levels of parent-adolescent conflict.[4,11] When using IPT-A with ethnically diverse low-income adolescent girls with a history of depression and child maltreatment, IPT-A was more effective at reducing depressive symptoms when compared to other methods of treatment.[12] Additionally, IPT has been adapted to target different cultural factors that play a role in the treatment of depressed adolescents.[6,7]

IPT-A FOR GROUPS

Interpersonal psychotherapy for adolescents was adapted to be delivered in a group format in a hospital-based outpatient clinic setting.[13] Group IPT-A (IPT-AG) consists of a combination of individual and group therapy sessions delivered over the course of 14 weeks, including 12 group sessions and 2 to 3 individual pregroup sessions with each adolescent and parent/caretaker participating in part of these sessions.[13] The group provides a place for adolescents to practice their communication and problem-solving skills with their peers. In addition to the initial IPT-AG model,[13] a World Health Organization (WHO) version of group IPT[14] has been used to treat depressed adolescents in several countries, including Nepal and Uganda.[15-17]

Empirical support

Group IPT-A has been more frequently adapted and disseminated internationally. In Australia, adolescents treated with IPT-AG reported significant reductions in depression severity, internalizing problems, anxiety symptoms, number of comorbid diagnoses, and number of depressed adolescents no longer meeting full criteria for depression at posttreatment.[8] IPT-AG has been adapted for adolescent populations in Africa.[18,19] In a qualitative study in Nepal, participants related depression to interpersonal problem areas of grief, dispute, role transition, and social isolation. Sharing one's experiences and relationships were more culturally consistent as the first step in alleviating distress.[17]

INTERPERSONAL PSYCHOTHERAPY—ADOLESCENT SKILLS TRAINING

Adolescent skills training for IPT (IPT-AST) was adapted from the group model and designed as an indicated preventive intervention for adolescents with elevated symptoms of depression.[20] It is typically delivered in the school setting and includes the 3 phases of treatment: 1 or 2 individual pregroup sessions, 8 group sessions, and an individual midgroup session. The adolescent is not assigned a particular problem area and instead may set a goal for improving a specific set of skills that can be applied to different relationships.[20] Parents/caretakers are invited to participate in a pregroup session as well as the midgroup session to practice the interpersonal strategies with their adolescent. IPT-AST also has been delivered as a universal prevention program,[21] as well as for adolescents who are at risk for depression based on high parent-child conflict or low peer support.[22]

Empirical support

School-based trials that compare IPT-AST to group counseling have also demonstrated its efficacy as a school-based depression prevention program.[23,24] IPT-AST also showed significant reduction in adolescent reported conflict with mothers at postintervention and 12-month follow-up.[25] Research on IPT-AST in an urban primary care setting found patients to have high fidelity, high attendance rates, high rates of satisfaction, and modest improvements in depression and anxiety symptoms.[26] Similarly, an adaptation of IPT-AST that incorporates strategies for dealing with social anxiety and peer victimization demonstrated significant declines in adolescent and evaluator-rated social anxiety, depression, and reports of peer victimization.[27] IPT-AST has been implemented primarily in the United States but is currently being used in the United Kingdom and in schools in India.

ADAPTATIONS AND IMPLEMENTATION FOR DIFFERENT SETTINGS

Interpersonal psychotherapy for adolescents also has been adapted for other healthcare delivery settings, cultural populations, and diagnostic profiles.

School context

IPT-A has been adapted and delivered in school-based health clinics[4] modified to be delivered as 12 sessions in 16 weeks to accommodate the school schedule. There is decreased parental involvement along with flexibility to include parents by telephone rather than in person. IPT-AST also was designed for delivery in the school context.[20] Students at risk are identified from classroom screenings for elevated depression symptoms. IPT-AST has been delivered by expert clinicians as well as by existing school personnel and been shown to be effective in preventing the development of depression diagnoses[28-30] and had preliminary effectiveness in a pediatric primary care setting.[26]

Primary care setting

IPT-A has been adapted for delivery in the pediatric primary care setting as a stepped-care model. The sessions focus on the same content but in stepped fashion: 8 sessions in the initial phase (step 1) and another 8 sessions in step 2 if not significantly improved after step 1. Step 1 sessions focus on the initial and middle phase of IPT-A, including psychoeducation about depression, an abbreviated Interpersonal Inventory, and teaching interpersonal skills. If significantly improved after step 1, step 2 would be 3 maintenance sessions over the next 8 weeks to provide support and consolidation of skills. If not significantly improved after step 1, step 2 sessions continue the work of the middle phase, providing the opportunity for ongoing practice of communication and problem-solving skills as well as relapse prevention. Parent involvement remains flexible. IPT-A appears feasible, acceptable, and potentially beneficial to this sample of urban, mostly Latino adolescents who typically experience significant barriers to receiving care.[31]

IPT-AG for lay providers

Group IPT has been adapted for use in low- and middle-income countries to be delivered by lay providers due to a shortage of trained mental health care professionals in these countries. One of the initial studies of group IPT with adolescents was conducted in Uganda.[15] A second study examined the adaptation of the group model of IPT for use with depressed adolescents in Nepal.[16,17] This experience suggested a number of modifications, such as involvement of parents/caregivers, extension of group duration from 8 to 12 sessions, single-gender groups, and reframing the intervention as a life skills training program to destigmatize the treatment.[16] Studies are needed to fully assess feasibility and effectiveness of the adapted intervention. Most recently, Mufson and colleagues have undertaken an adaptation of the WHO Group IPT manual for adults (used in Uganda and Nepal) for the treatment of adolescents with depression in Mozambique. Working with people familiar with the culture and healthcare systems in Mozambique, experts in IPT-A revised the manual to structure it for delivery by lay community providers, with implementation details included in the manual. The manual was then reviewed by mental health providers in Mozambique to identify aspects that needed additional cultural adaptations. Last, a cohort of mental health providers and lay providers will be trained in the intervention and several initial groups will be conducted, followed by a manual review for additional adaptations that may be needed to make the treatment most culturally relevant and beneficial for the community.

ADAPTATIONS FOR DIFFERENT POPULATIONS

IPT-A for PTSD (post-traumatic stress disorder)

There are new efforts to examine the efficacy of IPT-A for adolescents with PTSD or subsyndromal symptoms of PTSD in both the United States[32] and the United Kingdom.[33] The general adaptation of IPT-A for PTSD follows the same tenets as the adult model.[34] In the United States, treatment modifications also include (1) extended duration of treatment to 14–16 individual sessions with an option for up to 4 additional collateral parent or family sessions within 16 weeks; (2) psychoeducation focused on trauma and trauma reactions and the concept of affective attunement; and (3) weekly ratings for depression and for anxiety, irritability, or anger as it pertains to the particular adolescent's trauma profile. Parents/caregivers are provided with psychoeducation about the intergenerational transmission of trauma and involved in safety planning as needed.

Interpersonal psychotherapy for adolescents with trauma in the United Kingdom includes a greater focus on the elucidation of the brain, emotion, and interpersonal behavior connection. The focus is on strengthening attachments and formation of trusting relationships, identifying the physiological underpinnings of their emotions, and improving physiological reactivity to increase the feeling of safety, which ultimately leads to increased social engagement and regulation of emotions.[33]

Across both implementation settings, considerations are being made to address safety concerns, potential need for longer duration of care, as well as the impact of the adolescent's familial context to support the use of new skills. More studies and specifically randomized control studies of IPT-A for PTSD are needed.

IPT-A adapted for suicide

The first adaptation of IPT-A for suicide prevention was in Taiwan.[35] Mufson and colleagues later adapted the IPT-A manual for adolescents recruited from the emergency room after suicidal behavior or significant ideation that required treatment in an intensive day program; treatment was delivered as a twice-a-week intervention for 8 weeks and then weekly for next 12 weeks for a total of 20 weeks.[36] The depression clinic at Schneider's Children Medical Center in Israel initiated work with both a 12-week IPT-A adaptation for suicide as well as Ultra-Brief Crisis IPT-A Based Intervention for Suicidal Children and Adolescents (IPT-A-SCI)[37] with the same 3 goals: reducing suicide risk; building a treatment plan based on understanding the emotional and interpersonal aspects underlying suicidal behavior; and increasing hope among patients and their parents.

Intended for children and adolescents ages 6–18 years old, IPT-A-SCI comprises an intensive phase of 5 weekly sessions and a follow-up phase consisting of 4 emails across a 3-month period. We require parental attendance at the first and final sessions and invite parents to attend additional sessions as needed. For children under 10 years of age, parents are present during all 5 sessions. The emails are sent to both the adolescent and their parents. The intensive phase is based on IPT-A with the addition of some elements adapted from CBT for suicide prevention[38] and dialectical behavioral therapy,[39] including an interpersonal safety plan,[40] additional work with parents, and a greater focus on affective work.

IMPLEMENTATION

Interpersonal psychotherapy for adolescents is designed to be delivered once a week for 12 weeks in an outpatient setting, although the treatment schedule can be more flexible if necessary. IPT-A has been delivered in schools in a 16-week model, which allows for changes in frequency to accommodate school vacations and events as well as clinician choice to meet less frequently after week 8 if indicated. Similarly, duration can be extended or sessions can be temporarily scheduled more frequently than once a week if necessary. However, it is important to keep the time-limited nature of the intervention by explicitly resetting the treatment contract with the modified timetable of sessions.

TRAINING AND SUPERVISION

Training and supervision vary depending on setting and providers. The training workshop can vary from 1 to 2 full days of training or 4our half-days of training; in settings such as primary care or school-based clinics, it was done in 1 day or 2 half-days. In all settings, it generally is best to have a weekly supervision in which to discuss clinicians' cases with 3–4 people per group to have time to review each person's session. However, depending on the setting, the group can be larger if necessary due to the cost constraints of an organization supporting the work. Ideally, ongoing supervision and consultation of treatment cases includes monitoring audio recordings of sessions. When recording is not possible, it is more important to do role playing in sessions to have clinicians demonstrate their skills as well as have them write out their problem area formulation to ensure appropriate case conceptualization. There is less experience in training and supervising lay providers in IPT-A. This is important future work as lay providers are a potential solution to address the shortage of mental health providers in the United States and other countries.

It also is crucial to consider the cultural context in which the intervention is being implemented, especially when providing psychoeducation about depression and discussing styles and strategies for communication and problem-solving. Using a stance of cultural humility is recommended—ask the adolescent how they feel their parent/caretaker would respond to certain strategies. Similarly, when meeting with parents, clinicians should ask about their beliefs regarding family roles, communication styles, and expectations, as well as assess their openness to new forms of communication and problem-solving. Role playing during training and supervision can help to clarify the cultural differences that may impact implementation of the strategies.

CASE EXAMPLE

In treating a 14-year-old adolescent girl from a religiously observant family, the therapist formulated the problem area as a role transition since the adolescent wanted gradually to become secular. The work with the adolescent and her parents included working on accepting the adolescents' new role and level of observance within the family and validating the significance of this transition within their culture and community. In addition, the therapist focused on allowing both the adolescent and the parents to express the various feelings, which were both negative (anger, shame, frustration) and positive (pride that she knows what she wants) toward one another. The therapist also worked with the parents on directly and openly communicating to the adolescent what they wanted her to do (respect the house rules) and avoid doing (try to convince her younger sister to be like her). Since many daily situations became very challenging, the work included practicing the process of decision analysis so that they could engage in constructive problem-solving and find solutions to their differences.

SUMMARY

The efficacy and effectiveness studies demonstrate IPT-A and its adaptations' acceptability, efficacy and effectiveness for diverse populations of adolescents from the United States to Japan, Australia, and Africa. Work in progress focuses on adapting the intervention for new populations, including adolescents with trauma and those at risk for suicide. To address the worldwide shortage of mental health providers, new initiatives emphasize training lay providers to deliver existing and new models of interpersonal psychotherapy for adolescents.

REFERENCES

1. Daly M. Prevalence of depression among adolescents in the US from 2009 to 2019: analysis of trends by sex, race/ethnicity, and income. *J Adolesc Health.* 2022;70:496–499.
2. Thapar A, Collishaw S, Pine DS, Thapar AK. Depression in adolescence. *Lancet.* 2012;379(9820):1056–1067.
3. Mufson L, Dorta KP, Moreau D, Weissman MM. *Interpersonal Psychotherapy for Depressed Adolescents.* Guilford Press; 2004.
4. Mufson L, Dorta KP, Wickramaratne P, Nomura Y, Olfson M, Weissman MM. A randomized effectiveness trial of interpersonal psychotherapy for depressed adolescents. *Arch Gen Psychol.* 2004;61(6):577–584.
5. Mufson L, Weissman MM, Moreau D, Garfinkel R. Efficacy of interpersonal psychotherapy for depressed adolescents. *Arch Gen Psychiatry.* 1999;56(6):573–579.
6. Rossello J, Bernal G. The efficacy of cognitive-behavioral and interpersonal treatments for depression in Puerto Rican adolescents. *J Consult Clin Psychology.* 1999;67(5):734–745.
7. Rossello J, Bernal G, Rivera-Medina C. Individual and group CBT and IPT for Puerto Rican adolescents with depressive symptoms. *Cultur Divers Ethnic Minor Psychol.* 2008;14(3):234–254.
8. O'Shea, G, Spence SH, Donovan CL. Group versus individual psychotherapy for depressed adolescents. *Behav Cogn Psychother.* 2015;43:1–19.
9. Eckshtain D, Kuppens S, Ugueto A, et al. Meta-analysis: 13-year follow-up of psychotherapy effects of youth depression. *J Am Acad Child Adolesc Psychiatry.* 2020;59(1):45–63.
10. Weersing VR, Jeffreys M, Do MT, Schwartz KT, Bolano C. Evidence base update of psychosocial treatments for child and adolescent depression. *J Clin Child Adolesc Psychol.* 2017;46(1):11–43.
11. Gunlicks-Stoessel M, Mufson L, Jekal A, Blake Turner J. The impact of perceived interpersonal functioning on treatment for adolescent depression: IPT-A versus treatment as usual in school-based health clinics. *J Consult Clin Psychology.* 2010;78(2):260–267.
12. Toth SL, Handley SD, Manly JT, et al. The moderating role of child maltreatment in treatment efficacy for adolescent depression. *J Abnorm Child Psychol.* 2020;48:1351–1365.
13. Mufson L, Gallagher T, Dorta KP, et al. A group adaptation of interpersonal psychotherapy for depressed adolescents. *Am J Psychother.* 2004;58(2):220–237.
14. World Health Organization and Columbia University. *Group Interpersonal Therapy (IPT) for Depression.* WHO; 2016. (WHO generic field-trial version 1.0).
15. Bolton P, Bass J, Betancourt T, et al. Interventions for depression symptoms among adolescent survivors of war and displacement in northern Uganda: a randomized controlled trial. *JAMA.* 2007;298(5):519–527.
16. Rose-Clarke K, Pradhan I, Shrestha P, et al. Culturally and developmentally adapting group interpersonal therapy for adolescents with depression in rural Nepal. *BMC Psychol.* 2020;8(83):1–15.
17. Rose-Clarke K, Hassan E, Bk P, et al. A cross-cultural interpersonal model of adolescent depression: a qualitative study in rural Nepal. *Soc Sci Med.* 2021;270:113623.

18. Yator O, Khasakhala LI, John-Steward G, Kumar M. Acceptability and feasibility of group interpersonal therapy (IPT-G) for depressed HIV+ postpartum adolescents delivered by community health workers: a protocol paper. *Clin Med Insights: Psychiatry.* 2020;11:1–11.

19. Thurman TR, Nice J, Taylor TM, Luckett B. Mitigating depression among orphaned and vulnerable adolescents: a randomized controlled trial of interpersonal psychotherapy for groups in South Africa. *Child Adolesc Ment Health.* 2017;22(4):224–231.

20. Young JF, Mufson L, Schueler CM. *Preventing Adolescent Depression Interpersonal Psychotherapy Adolescent Skills Training.* Oxford University Press; 2016.

21. Horowitz JL, Garber J, Ciesla JA, Young JF, Mufson L. Prevention of depressive symptoms in adolescents: a randomized trial of cognitive-behavioral and interpersonal prevention programs. *J Consult Clin Psychol.* 2007;75(5):693.

22. Young JF, Jones JD, Gallop R, et al. Personalized depression prevention: a randomized controlled trial to optimize effects through risk-informed personalization. *J Am Acad Child Adolesc Psychiatry.* 2021;60(9):1116–1126.

23. Young JF, Makover HB, Cohen JR, Mufson L, Gallop RJ, Benas JS. Interpersonal psychotherapy-adolescent skills training: anxiety outcomes and impact of comorbidity. *J Clin Child Adolesc Psychol.* 2012;41(5):640–653.

24. Young JF, Jones JD, Sbrilli MD, et al. Long-term effects from a school-based trial comparing interpersonal psychotherapy-adolescent skills training to group counseling. *J Clin Child Adolesc Psychol.* 2019;48(1):362–370.

25. Young JF, Gallop R, Mufson L. Mother-child conflict and its moderating effects on depression outcomes in a preventative intervention for adolescent depression. *J Clin Child Adolesc Psychol.* 2009;38(5):696–704.

26. Kanine RM, Bush ML, Davis M, Jones JD, Sbrilli MD, Young JF. Depression prevention in pediatric primary care: implementation and outcomes of interpersonal psychotherapy—adolescent skills training. *Child Psychiatry Hum Dev.* 2023;54(1):96–108.

27. La Greca AM, Ehrenreich-May J, Mufson L, Chan S. Preventing adolescent social anxiety and depression and reducing peer victimization: intervention development and open trial. *Child Youth Care Forum.* 2016;45(6):905–926.

28. Young JF, Mufson L, Davies M. Efficacy of interpersonal psychotherapy–adolescent skills training: an indicated preventive intervention for depression. *J Child Psychol Psychiatry.* 2006;47(12):1254–1262.

29. Young JF, Mufson L, Gallop R. Preventing depression: a randomized trial of interpersonal psychotherapy-adolescent skills training. *Depress Anxiety.* 2010;27(5):426–433.

30. Young JF, Benas JS, Schueler CM, Gallop B, Gilham J, Mufson L. A randomized depression prevention trial comparing interpersonal psychotherapy adolescent skills training to group counseling in schools. *Prev Sci.* 2016;17(3):314–324.

31. Mufson L, Rynn M, Yanes-Lukin P, et al. Stepped care interpersonal psychotherapy treatment for depressed adolescents: a pilot study in pediatric clinics. *Adm Policy Ment Health.* 2018;45:417–431.

32. Ragbeer S, Mufson L. Interpersonal psychotherapy for depressed adolescents (IPT-A): initial adaptations for PTSD. Oral presentation at: 8th Conference of the International Society of Interpersonal Psychotherapy; November 2019; Budapest, Hungary.

33. Cestaro V. Implementation of interpersonal psychotherapy for PTSD adaptations for adolescents—successes and challenges. Online workshop at: 9th Conference of the International Society of Interpersonal Psychotherapy; November 2021; Zoom.

34. Markowitz, JC. *Interpersonal Psychotherapy for Posttraumatic Stress Disorder*. Oxford University Press; 2016.

35. Tang TC, Jou SH, Ko CH, Huang SY, Yen CF. Randomized study of school-based intensive interpersonal psychotherapy for depressed adolescents with suicidal risk and parasuicide behaviors. *Psychiatry Clin Neurosci*. 2009;63(4):463–470.

36. Mufson L, Brunstein-Klomek A, Ortin A, Rapp A, DiCola L, Goldberg Rynn M. IPT-A adapted for depressed youth engaging in suicidal behavior: preliminary outcomes and experiences. Oral presentation at: ISIPT Conference; June 2013; Iowa City, Iowa.

37. Catalan LH, Frenk ML, Spigelman EA, et al. Ultra-brief crisis IPT-A based intervention for suicidal children and adolescents (IPT-A-SCI) pilot study results. *Front Psychiatry*. 2020;11:553422.

38. Stanley B, Brown G, Brent DA, et al. Cognitive-behavioral therapy for suicide prevention (CBT-SP): treatment model, feasibility, and acceptability. *J Am Acad Child Adolesc Psychiatry*. 2009;48(10):1005–1013.

39. Miller LA, Rathus HJ, Linehan MM, Wetzler S, Leigh E. Dialectical behavior therapy adapted for suicidal adolescents. *J Psychiatr Pract*. 1997;3(2):78.

40. Stanley B, Brown GK. Safety planning intervention: a brief intervention to mitigate suicide risk. *Cogn Behav Pract*. 2012;19:256–264.

45

Interpersonal Psychotherapy for the Prevention of Excess Weight Gain in Black/African American Adolescent Girls

NATASHA L. BURKE, TRACY SBROCCO, LAUREN B. SHOMAKER, AND MARIAN TANOFSKY-KRAFF ■

Interpersonal psychotherapy (IPT) may be especially salient for Black/African American adolescent girls with high weight and disordered eating. This chapter reviews the rationale for preventing adult obesity in Black/African American teenagers and the preliminary research supporting IPT for this underrepresented group. Then, we provide an overview of a culturally adapted IPT program for the prevention of excess weight gain in Black/African American teenagers. We present the adaptations proposed as well as their foundation on empirically derived data. Finally, we present a brief case example.

HEALTH DISPARITIES FOR BLACK/AFRICAN AMERICAN ADOLESCENTS

There are major health disparities in obesity and cardiometabolic health among Black/African American individuals. Prior to the COVID-19 pandemic, population-wide stabilization of obesity rates were not observed among Black/African American females.[1] Though overweight/obesity rates are high for adolescents and adults across the United States, the prevalence for Black/African American individuals is disproportionately high due to myriad reasons, including

Natasha L. Burke, Tracy Sbrocco, Lauren B. Shomaker, and Marian Tanofsky-Kraff, *Interpersonal Psychotherapy for the Prevention of Excess Weight Gain in Black/African American Adolescent Girls* In: *Interpersonal Psychotherapy*. Edited by: Myrna M. Weissman and Jennifer J. Mootz, Oxford University Press. © Oxford University Press 2024. DOI: 10.1093/oso/9780197652084.003.0046 enduring structural factors (e.g., structural racism), chronic stress, and related biospsychosocial factors.[2] Indeed, 43% of Black/African American adolescent girls are estimated to have overweight/obesity (body mass index, BMI, kg/m^2, ≥85th percentile for age and gender), in contrast to 31% of non-Hispanic White adolescent girls.[3,4] Prevalence of high weight concerns rises dramatically by adulthood, with 82% of Black/African American women having overweight or obesity, compared to the US adult average of 67%.[4] Having about 10%–20% higher rates of overweight/obesity puts Black/African American females at disproportionate risk for serious adverse health outcomes, including cardiovascular disease, type 2 diabetes, and multiple cancers.[2,5] However, most weight-based interventions have not been successful for this population, with attrition particularly problematic.[2] As obesity in adolescence predicts obesity in adulthood,[6] and the risk of continued excess weight gain into adulthood increases with age and degree of excess weight,[7,8] adolescence offers a crucial window for the prevention of excess weight gain and its associated adverse health concerns for Black/African American girls.[9]

OBESITY MANAGEMENT IN ADOLESCENTS

The standard approach to prevent excess weight gain is lifestyle-based intervention to decrease total caloric intake and increase energy expenditures.[10] Yet, lifestyle interventions unfortunately have been insufficiently effective in adolescents, and they particularly have fallen short with youth identifying as underrepresented racial/ethnic groups.[11-15] To date, Black/African American girls/families are largely missing from the efficacy studies that make up the evidence base for treatments. Because of this omission, questions arise about whether it is appropriate to advocate for using an evidence base for this population when they were not part of efficacy trials and whether resulting treatments generalize to this population. For instance, lifestyle approaches are plagued by much higher attrition for Black/African American youth as compared with their White peers.[16,17] It is likely that such programs are not ideal or may not be acceptable to many Black/African American adolescents and their families.[18] Reasons for this lack of acceptance vary and can include minimal cultural tailoring of program rationale and materials as well as convenience of treatment approaches, as commonly cited barriers to engagement include time constraints, transportation, and lack of child care. Consequently, to date, there is no gold standard weight loss/stabilization approach for Black/African American adolescents.

IPT FOR EATING AND WEIGHT ISSUES IN UNDERREPRESENTED RACIAL/ETHNIC MINORITY GROUPS

Interpersonal psychotherapy may be an alternative that addresses culturally salient enablers and barriers to effective weight stabilization in Black/African

American adolescent girls at risk for adult obesity. While no research has specifically tested IPT for weight loss in samples of Black/African American teenagers, a small body of preliminary data in adults with eating disorders supports this general notion. The majority of IPT treatments for disordered eating have been conducted with samples of White adults. In a multisite study testing a variety of treatments for recurrent binge eating among adults with heterogeneous ethnic/racial identities, attrition for racial/ethnic minority adults in treatments *other than* IPT was higher than for White adults.[19] There was a pattern for substantially better retention among those identifying as an underrepresented ethnic/racial group in IPT in contrast to the other treatment modalities of cognitive behavioral guided self-help or behavioral weight loss treatment. Findings from another study suggest that IPT may be especially effective for Black/African American adults with bulimia nervosa.[20] Chui and colleagues[20] reported that adults with bulimia nervosa in a large multicenter trial responded, overall, with higher abstinence rates when randomized to cognitive behavioral therapy as opposed to IPT. However, Black/African American participants specifically showed greater reductions in binge-eating episode frequency when treated with IPT compared to cognitive behavioral therapy. These initial findings in adults with binge-type eating disorders suggest that it is possible that IPT might be a preferred treatment of choice for underrepresented ethnic/racial groups.

IPT FOR THE PREVENTION OF EXCESS WEIGHT GAIN

For over a decade, we have been studying an adapted IPT program for the prevention of excess IPT for adolescents (IPT-A) weight gain in a group format for adolescents at risk for adult obesity. This adaptation was based on IPT Adolescent Skills Training for the prevention of depression[21] and IPT for binge-eating disorder.[22] Aspects taken from Adolescent Skills Training[21] included the prevention (of full-syndrome) aspect of treatment with removal of the "sick role"; the developmental tailoring of treatment to adolescents (e.g., including interpersonal aspects such as peer pressure, developing autonomy, etc.); and the general structure of the program. Similar to IPT for binge-eating disorder,[22] however, the focus of the adapted IPT program was eating disorder behaviors, with rationale for therapy focusing on the interpersonal mechanisms leading to eating disorder behaviors and structuring the group therapy sessions as an "interpersonal laboratory." However, the focus of the adapted program was not binge eating itself, but loss-of-control (LOC) eating, a behavior commonly reported by adolescents with high weight. LOC eating, the hallmark feature of binge eating, refers to episodes characterized by a subjective lack of control over eating regardless of the amount of food consumed.[23] While full-syndrome binge-eating disorder affects only approximately 1% of adolescents, subthreshold LOC, referring to LOC eating that does not meet full-syndrome frequency and/or duration criteria, is far more common.[23] Further, a greater proportion of Black/African American youth and a greater proportion of adolescent girls report LOC eating in comparison to those identifying as White and males, respectively.[24-26] In community samples of varying weight, LOC is endorsed by approximately 25% of Black/African American girls,[27] with higher estimates (40%–50%) among those with overweight or obesity.[23] Our group and others have demonstrated that subthreshold LOC eating is a prospective risk factor for gaining excess body weight and excess body fat or adiposity over time as youth grow.[23,28-32] Mechanistically, reported LOC eating episodes likely represent a propensity for recurring excess caloric intake in an effort to cope with a variety of life stressors.[27,33-35] As IPT for binge-eating disorder has resulted in weight stabilization or modest weight loss in those who are effectively treated,[19,36] reducing LOC eating via IPT has been proposed to prevent excess weight gain.[37]

In a single-site randomized controlled trial, we compared our adaptation of IPT to a standard-of-care health education group, matched for time/attention (twelve 90-minute adolescent group sessions) and facilitator expertise (psychologists), in adolescent girls of all ethnic/racial backgrounds who were generally healthy, but had above-average BMI (≥75th percentile for age) and endorsed LOC eating. LOC eating and BMI outcomes were equivocal.[38,39] However, in post hoc analyses, ethnic/racial minority adolescents, the majority (60%) of whom identified as Black/African American, evidenced lower odds of LOC eating 3 years later after IPT, as compared to health education.[40] Moreover, we observed a signal that Black/African American participants in IPT also stabilized BMI gain 3 years later, as compared to those assigned to health education. One possible interpretation is that promoting positive social relationships and healthy social functioning through delivery of IPT positively impacts eating behavior and weight over time as adolescents develop because interpersonal connection affects many dimensions of health, including eating, obesity, and associated health comorbidities.[41] Based on these data, we have proposed further culturally adapting IPT to decrease LOC eating through strengthening social ties to stabilize BMI and body fat gain in Black/African American adolescent girls. To date, our preliminary quantitative data and clinical experience have supported this approach.

CULTURALLY ADAPTED IPT FOR BLACK/AFRICAN AMERICAN ADOLESCENT GIRLS

We have used a team science approach and partnerships to address the obesity inequities faced by Black/African American youth. This has included transdisciplinary partnerships (e.g., experts from public health, psychology, medicine, policy, nutrition) in addition to academic-community partnerships.[42] Of note, in contrast to the prevailing, White cultural framework that views LOC eating as occurring in response to individualized failed dieting attempts to achieve thinness,[43,44] Black/African American adolescents and parents perceived LOC eating as precipitated by, in part, sociocultural barriers to healthy eating. Specifically, these barriers included psychological distress that can arise in response to racism, discrimination, changes in family structure, social isolation, and interpersonal conflict,[45,46] which are recognized social determinants of health that disproportionately affect Black/African American communities.[47-53]

Recognizing important structural, environmental, and cultural differences among Black/African American families, we sought to further adapt IPT, an approach already suggesting promising outcomes with this population. Following the literature suggesting the importance of family involvement in working to improve the health of Black/African American youth with high weight,[54,55] we used focus groups to identify parameters of IPT to be culturally adapted (Table 45.1). In doing so, we expect to be better positioned to encourage this demographic group to enter and engage in care to produce outcomes similar to our findings from our larger, mixed race/ethnicity trial.

Key themes across 14 focus groups[45,46] with Black/African American girls, parents, and community leaders demonstrated 4 messages pertinent to delivery of IPT with Black/African American adolescent girls. First, though

Table 45.1 CULTURALLY INFORMED MODIFICATIONS TO
CULTURALLY ADAPTED IPT PROGRAM[a]

Key qualitative themes	Culturally informed IPT program adaptations for adolescents identifying as Black or African American
- Focus on social stress (*not* dieting) as precipitant of LOC eating (i.e., "being greedy," "pigging out," "throwin' down") - Aversion to stigma of weight *loss* program	- Advertise program as a way to improve relationships and eating habits for healthy growth - Incorporate Black/African American cultural vernacular terms for LOC eating in recruitment, assessment, manual, and clinical vignettes
- Parental desire to improve parent/caregiver-daughter relationships - Adolescents uncertain about how parents will receive more direct communication about conflict/disagreement	- Addition of a parallel parent group at the first IPT session to provide information on nutrition, behavioral weight management, and relationship skills that adolescents will learn to promote more positive parent-adolescent communication
- Most compelling program offers foundational nutrition-activity knowledge and relationship skills	- Inclusion of standard behavioral recommendations for nutrition and physical activity at start of intervention
- Call for ideal program facilitator with expertise in Black/African American culture, but not from immediate community	- Psychologist facilitator identifying as Black/African American with personal and professional knowledge of obesity and the culture

[a] Data from References 45 and 46.

dietary restriction in response to interpersonal conflict is common for some racial/ethnic groups,[56] Black/African American individuals in our focus groups noted that *LOC eating in response to interpersonal conflict is common*. The concept of LOC eating highly resonated with Black/African American girls. Girls emphasized eating in response to conflicts with relatives and others in their social milieu. Factors such as sociocultural isolation and a lack of self-efficacy also were raised as risk factors for LOC eating. Second, *it is not about thinness/dieting*. Responses centered on relationships and reducing LOC eating as it relates to the sociocultural/physical isolation that can be eliciting of psychological distress, with little commentary on body size. Of import, focus group participants did not articulate a desire for thinness, an explicit and implicit element of many programs for obesity or LOC eating. Reducing stress or distress is a component of some existing programs, yet a primary focus on sociocultural/interpersonal stressors as triggers of LOC eating is a departure from the norm and central to adapted IPT. Approaches (e.g., cognitive behavioral therapy) predicated on the notion that body dissatisfaction and dietary restraint trigger LOC eating have been less effective in racial/ethnic minorities.[57] Third, *parental involvement is important*. Black/African American adolescents desired an informational session preparing parents to understand communication skills (e.g., "I feel" statements) so that new dialogue would not be interpreted as disrespectful. Also, Black/African American parents expressed a desire for a parent session providing core nutrition and behavioral guidance. Fourth, *group leaders' identities matter*. Girls expressed that group leaders should be female, identify as Black/African American, young, and ideally someone who had lost weight successfully herself. Leaders should be someone from outside of the immediate community to allow girls to speak more freely.

Responding to focus group themes and concerns, we culturally tailored the existing adapted IPT program for delivery to Black/African American families as it is well suited to address the LOC eating, a behavioral phenotype for obesity, that occurs in response to interpersonal conflict and communication difficulties.[45,46]

CASE EXAMPLE

Katia was a 14-year-old African American girl who reported LOC eating. During the pregroup interpersonal inventory, Katia noted that her first LOC eating episodes occurred in response to her soccer coach's ongoing comments about her body shape and size relative to her smaller framed White and Asian teammates. Though Katia was an excellent soccer player, she felt ashamed, sad, and angry for being singled out for her bigger, curvier shape and used food as a coping mechanism by "pigging out" after each soccer practice. Recent news events focused on police violence against Black/African American people in the United States already had Katia and her family on edge and exacerbated her LOC eating of late. She felt isolated as well, feeling that she could not talk with her teammates about the issues she was facing as they would "not understand." During the pregroup meeting (and again in the initial phase of group), Katia was educated about the mechanisms through which LOC eating occurs in an interpersonal framework (i.e., in response to interpersonal conflicts to deal with negative emotions), and goals were set focusing on interpersonal role disputes and interpersonal deficits. Through IPT with a Black, female therapist and group members similarly affected by recent sociopolitically publicized events against Black individuals, Katia found a safe space to articulate her concerns and learned to use communication skills—specifically focusing on the communication skills[21] of "What you don't say speaks volumes," "I" statements, and "Strike while the iron is cold"—to address her goals. She also learned through the group that comparisons of Black female bodies to other racial/ethnic groups is not uncommon, helping her to feel less isolated. Through in-group role plays and using the group as an interpersonal laboratory during the middle phase of group, she successfully utilized communication strategies for speaking with her mother for emotional support and with her coach to respectfully address the issue that led to her initial LOC eating episodes, leading to a significant reduction in LOC eating over time.

In this case, the interpersonal role conflict was situated within race-based body comparisons and exacerbated by race-based current events, highlighting culturally specific stressors (vs. thinness/dieting concerns) precipitating LOC eating.[45,46] Though sociocultural matching does not account fully account for therapeutic outcomes,[58,59] having a Black/African American therapist[45,46] was particularly salient given the stressors and conflicts Katia and other girls in her group faced. Involving Katia's mother as an emotional support, such as versus her friends, was in line with focus groups that highlighted the importance of family in intervention.[45,46] Indeed, this support helped both Katia and her mother to speak openly about current sociopolitical events and address issues with Katia's coach.

CONCLUSION

Though one specific type of individual-level intervention will not stem the tide of obesity and mental/physical health inequities, culturally adapted IPT may be especially effective for preventing excess weight gain among Black/African American youth. It is feasible, acceptable, and flexible enough to address culturally specific interpersonal issues that lead to LOC eating and excess weight gain. Future research will include randomized clinical trials to examine the efficacy of culturally adapted IPT for Black/African American families.

DISCLAIMER

The opinions and assertions expressed herein are those of the authors and are not to be construed as reflecting the views of the United States Department of Defense.

REFERENCES

1. Carnethon MR, Pu J, Howard G, et al. Cardiovascular health in African Americans: a scientific statement from the American Heart Association. *Circulation*. 2017;136(21):e393–e423.
2. Pickett S, Burchenal CA, Haber L, Batten K, Phillips E. Understanding and effectively addressing disparities in obesity: a systematic review of the psychological determinants of emotional eating behaviours among Black women. *Obes Rev*. 2020;21(6):e13010.
3. Ogden CL, Carroll MD, Lawman HG, et al. Trends in obesity prevalence among children and adolescents in the United States, 1988–1994 through 2013–2014. *JAMA*. 2016;315(21):2292–2299.
4. Ogden CL, Carroll MD, Kit BK, Flegal KM. Prevalence of childhood and adult obesity in the United States, 2011–2012. *JAMA*. 2014;311(8):806–814.
5. Pi-Sunyer FX. Medical complications of obesity in adults. In: Fairburn CG, Brownell KD, eds. *Eating disorders and obesity*. 2nd ed. Guilford Press; 2002:467–472.
6. Styne DM. A plea for prevention. *Am J Clin Nutr*. 2003;78(2):199–200.
7. Field AE, Cook NR, Gillman MW. Weight status in childhood as a predictor of becoming overweight or hypertensive in early adulthood. *Obes Res*. 2005;13(1):163–169.
8. Whitaker RC, Wright JA, Pepe MS, Seidel KD, Dietz WH. Predicting obesity in young adulthood from childhood and parental obesity. *N Engl J Med*. 1997;337(13):869–873.
9. Alberga AS, Sigal RJ, Goldfield G, Prud'homme D, Kenny GP. Overweight and obese teenagers: why is adolescence a critical period? *Pediatr Obes*. 2012;7(4):261–273.
10. O'Connor EA, Evans CV, Burda BU, Walsh ES, Eder M, Lozano P. Screening for obesity and intervention for weight management in children and adolescents: evidence report and systematic review for the US Preventive Services Task Force. *JAMA*. 2017;317(23):2427–2444.
11. Kamath CC, Vickers KS, Ehrlich A, et al. Behavioral interventions to prevent childhood obesity: a systematic review and meta-analyses of randomized trials. *J Clin Endocrinol Metab*. 2008;93(12):4606–4615.
12. Klesges RC, Obarzanek E, Kumanyika S, et al. The Memphis Girls' Health Enrichment Multi-site Studies (GEMS): an evaluation of the efficacy of a 2-year obesity prevention program in African American girls. *Arch Pediatr Adolesc Med*. 2010;164(11):1007–1014.
13. Resnicow K, Yaroch AL, Davis A, et al. GO GIRLS! results from a nutrition and physical activity program for low-income, overweight African American adolescent females. *Health Educ Behav*. 2000;27(5):616–631.
14. Stevens CJ. Obesity prevention interventions for middle school-age children of ethnic minority: a review of the literature. *J Spec Pediatr Nurs*. 2010;15(3):233–243.
15. Resnicow K, Taylor R, Baskin M, McCarty F. Results of Go Girls: a weight control program for overweight African-American adolescent females. *Obes Res*. 2005;13(10):1739–1748.
16. Dolinsky DH, Armstrong SC, Østbye T. Predictors of attrition from a clinical pediatric obesity treatment program. *Clin Pediatr (Phila)*. 2012;51(12):1168–1174.

17. Ligthart KA, Buitendijk L, Koes BW, van Middelkoop M. The association between ethnicity, socioeconomic status and compliance to pediatric weight-management interventions: a systematic review. *Obes Res Clin Pract.* 2017;11(5 Suppl 1):1–51.

18. Cassidy O, Sbrocco T, Tanofsky-Kraff M. Utilizing non-traditional research designs to explore culture-specific risk factors for eating disorders in African American adolescents. *Adv Eat Disord.* 2015;3(1):91–102.

19. Wilson GT, Wilfley DE, Agras WS, Bryson SW. Psychological treatments of binge eating disorder. *Arch Gen Psychiatry.* 2010;67(1):94–101.

20. Chui W, Safer DL, Bryson SW, Agras WS, Wilson GT. A comparison of ethnic groups in the treatment of bulimia nervosa. *Eat Behav.* 2007;8(4):485–491.

21. Young JF, Mufson L, Schueler CM. *Preventing Adolescent Depression: Interpersonal Psychotherapy—Adolescent Skills Training.* Oxford University Press; 2016.

22. Wilfley DE, MacKenzie KR, Welch RR, Ayres VE, Weissman MM. *Interpersonal Psychotherapy for Group.* Basic Books; 2000.

23. Byrne ME, LeMay-Russell S, Tanofsky-Kraff M. Loss-of-control eating and obesity among children and adolescents. *Curr Obes Rep.* 2019;8(1):33–42.

24. Swanson SA, Crow SJ, Le Grange D, Swendsen J, Merikangas KR. Prevalence and correlates of eating disorders in adolescents: results from the national co-morbidity survey replication adolescent supplement. *Arch Gen Psychiatry.* 2011;68(7):714–723.

25. Goldschmidt AB, Loth KA, MacLehose RF, Pisetsky EM, Berge JM, Neumark-Sztainer D. Overeating with and without loss of control: associations with weight status, weight-related characteristics, and psychosocial health. *Int J Eat Disord.* 2015;48(8):1150–1157.

26. Lee-Winn AE, Reinblatt SP, Mojtabai R, Mendelson T. Gender and racial/ethnic differences in binge eating symptoms in a nationally representative sample of adolescents in the United States. *Eat Behav.* 2016;22:27–33.

27. Cassidy OL, Matheson B, Osborn R, et al. Loss of control eating in African-American and Caucasian youth. *Eat Behav.* 2012;13(2):174–178.

28. Tanofsky-Kraff M, Yanovski SZ, Schvey NA, Olsen CH, Gustafson J, Yanovski JA. A prospective study of loss of control eating for body weight gain in children at high risk for adult obesity. *Int J Eat Disord.* 2009;42(1):26–30.

29. Field AE, Austin SB, Taylor CB, et al. Relation between dieting and weight change among preadolescents and adolescents. *Pediatrics.* 2003;112(4):900–906.

30. Stice E, Cameron RP, Killen JD, Hayward C, Taylor CB. Naturalistic weight-reduction efforts prospectively predict growth in relative weight and onset of obesity among female adolescents. *J Consult Clin Psychol.* 1999;67(6):967–974.

31. French SA, Story M, Neumark-Sztainer D, Downes B, Resnick M, Blum R. Ethnic differences in psychosocial and health behavior correlates of dieting, purging, and binge eating in a population-based sample of adolescent females. *Int J Eat Disord.* 1997;22(3):315–322.

32. Tanofsky-Kraff M, Cohen ML, Yanovski SZ, et al. A prospective study of psychological predictors of body fat gain among children at high risk for adult obesity. *Pediatrics.* 2006;117(4):1203–1209.

33. Ranzenhofer LM, Engel SG, Crosby RD, et al. Using ecological momentary assessment to examine interpersonal and affective predictors of loss of control eating in adolescent girls. *Int J Eat Disord.* 2014;47(7):748–457.

34. Ranzenhofer LM, Hannallah L, Field SE, et al. Pre-meal affective state and laboratory test meal intake in adolescent girls with loss of control eating. *Appetite*. 2013;68:30–37.

35. Vannucci A, Tanofsky-Kraff M, Shomaker LB, et al. Construct validity of the Emotional Eating Scale Adapted for Children and Adolescents. *Int J Obes*. 2012;36(7):938–943.

36. Wilfley DE, Welch RR, Stein RI, et al. A randomized comparison of group cognitive-behavioral therapy and group interpersonal psychotherapy for the treatment of overweight individuals with binge-eating disorder. *Arch Gen Psychiatry*. 2002;59(8):713–721.

37. Tanofsky-Kraff M, Wilfley DE, Young JF, et al. Preventing excessive weight gain in adolescents: interpersonal psychotherapy for binge eating. *Obesity (Silver Spring)*. 2007;15(6):1345–1355.

38. Tanofsky-Kraff M, Shomaker LB, Wilfley DE, et al. Excess weight gain prevention in adolescents: three-year outcome following a randomized controlled trial. *J Consult Clin Psychol*. 2017;85(3):218–227.

39. Tanofsky-Kraff M, Shomaker LB, Wilfley DE, et al. Targeted prevention of excess weight gain and eating disorders in high-risk adolescent girls: a randomized controlled trial. *Am J Clin Nutr*. 2014;100(4):1010–1018.

40. Burke NL, Shomaker LB, Brady S, et al. Impact of age and race on outcomes of a program to prevent excess weight gain and disordered eating in adolescent girls. *Nutrients*. 2017;9(9):947.

41. Holt-Lunstad J, Robles TF, Sbarra DA. Advancing social connection as a public health priority in the United States. *Am Psychol*. 2017;72(6):517–530.

42. Stokols D, Hall KL, Taylor BK, Moser RP. The science of team science: overview of the field and introduction to the supplement. *Am J Prev Med*. 2008;35(2 suppl):S77–S89.

43. Herman CP, Mack D. Restrained and unrestrained eating. *J Pers*. 1975;43(4):647–660.

44. Nathan PE, Gorman JM. *A Guide to Treatments That Work*. 4th ed. Oxford University Press; 2015.

45. Cassidy O, Eichen DM, Burke NL, et al. Engaging African American adolescents and stakeholders to adapt interpersonal psychotherapy for weight gain prevention. *J Black Psychol*. 2018;44(2):128–161.

46. Cassidy O, Sbrocco T, Vannucci A, et al. Adapting interpersonal psychotherapy for the prevention of excessive weight gain in rural African American girls. *J Pediatr Psychol*. 2013;38(9):965–977.

47. Brody GH, Chen YF, Murry VM, et al. Perceived discrimination and the adjustment of African American youths: a five-year longitudinal analysis with contextual moderation effects. *Child Dev*. 2006;77(5):1170–1189.

48. Lambert SF, Herman KC, Bynum MS, Ialongo NS. Perceptions of racism and depressive symptoms in African American adolescents: the role of perceived academic and social control. *J Youth Adolesc*. 2009;38(4):519–531.

49. Sue DW, Capodilupo CM, Torino GC, et al. Racial microaggressions in everyday life: Implications for clinical practice. *Am Psychol*. 2007;62(4):271–286.

50. Ahye BA, Devine CM, Odoms-Young AM. Values expressed through intergenerational family food and nutrition management systems among African American women. *Fam Community Health*. 2006;29(1):5–16.

51. Liburd LC. Food, identity, and African-American women with type 2 diabetes: an anthropological perspective. *Diabetes Spectr.* 2003;16(3):6.

52. Wilfley DE, Pike KM, Striegel-Moore RH. Toward an integrated model of risk for binge eating disorder. *J Gender Cult Health.* 1997;2:1–3.

53. Kumanyika SK, Whitt-Glover MC, Gary TL, et al. Expanding the obesity research paradigm to reach African American communities. *Prev Chronic Dis.* 2007;4(4):A112.

54. Barr-Anderson DJ, Adams-Wynn AW, DiSantis KI, Kumanyika S. Family-focused physical activity, diet and obesity interventions in African-American girls: a systematic review. *Obes Rev.* 2013;14(1):29–51.

55. Kumanyika SK, Whitt-Glover MC, Haire-Joshu D. What works for obesity prevention and treatment in black Americans? Research directions. *Obes Rev.* 2014;15(suppl 4):204–212.

56. Cain AS, Bardone-Cone AM, Abramson LY, Vohs KD, Joiner TE. Refining the relationships of perfectionism, self-efficacy, and stress to dieting and binge eating: examining the appearance, interpersonal, and academic domains. *Int J Eat Disord.* 2008;41(8):713–721.

57. Huey SJ Jr, Polo AJ. Evidence-based psychosocial treatments for ethnic minority youth. *J Clin Child Adolesc Psychol.* 2008;37(1):262–301.

58. Sue DW, Sue D, Neville HA, Smith L. *Counseling the Culturally Diverse: Theory and Practice.* John Wiley & Sons; 2019.

59. Smith TB, Trimble JE. Matching clients with therapists on the basis of race or ethnicity: a meta-analysis of clients' level of participation in treatment. In: *Foundations of Multicultural Psychology: Research to Inform Effective Practice.* American Psychological Association; 2016:115–128.

46

Interpersonal Psychotherapy in Older Adults With Major Depression

CHARLES F. REYNOLDS III ■

SPECIAL POPULATIONS AND MAJOR FINDINGS

Over the past 3 decades, starting in 1989, my research group at the University of Pittsburgh Department of Psychiatry has conducted randomized clinical trials sponsored by the National Institute of Mental Health using interpersonal psychotherapy (IPT) for the treatment of older adults living with major depression. We have addressed acute and maintenance treatment with IPT,[1,2] treatment of depression in primary care settings,[3] and treatment of bereavement-related depression.[4] We have also addressed the impact of IPT on social role performance in older adults with major depression.[5] We have found that monthly maintenance IPT in "young older" adults (mean age 68) with recurrent major depressive episodes is effective in preventing recurrence over a 3-year period, as compared with supportive care and pill placebo.[1] Combined pharmacotherapy and IPT was also superior to monotherapy in maintaining social adjustment and health-related quality of life over 1 year.[5] In a second maintenance trial involving an older sample (mean age 78), we did not see evidence of IPT efficacy against recurrence—possibly because of cognitive impairment involving executive functions.[2] In primary care settings, we have seen that IPT combined with antidepressant pharmacotherapy is superior to care as usual in bringing about response of major depression and in more quickly reducing suicidal ideation.[3] Older patients in primary care receiving combination treatment with IPT and antidepressant medication also experienced a 24% reduction in mortality risk over an 8- to 9-year period, as compared with patients in usual care, reflecting reduced cancer-related mortality.[6]

Charles F. Reynolds III, *Interpersonal Psychotherapy in Older Adults With Major Depression* In: *Interpersonal Psychotherapy.* Edited by: Myrna M. Weissman and Jennifer J. Mootz, Oxford University Press. © Oxford University Press 2024. DOI: 10.1093/oso/9780197652084.003.0047

Finally, patients with bereavement-related major depression responded well to combined IPT and antidepressant pharmacotherapy, but continued to show some unresolved grief symptoms. This observation led to the construct of prolonged grief disorder, as distinct from major depression[7] and to randomized clinical trials investigating treatment with a grief-specific psychotherapy (prolonged grief disorder therapy, PGDT) which incorporated some IPT elements.[8]

By way of further context, the hallmarks of major depression in older adults are its co-occurrence with medical disorders and increasing frailty; mild cognitive impairment (particularly of executive functioning); social determinants of illness (e.g., bereavement, transitions in major social roles, loneliness, and social isolation); exposure to polypharmacy; and increased risk for suicide. Late-life depression is also a risk factor for dementia and may in some cases be an early or prodromal expression of dementia, particularly after the age of 75 or 80. Major depression in older adults also occasions considerable caregiver burden in family members.

We have found that older adults with major depression readily engage with IPT, which addresses the interpersonal and social contexts of depression, related variously to bereavement and grief, transitions in social roles such as retirement and the concurrent need to establish new purpose in life, interpersonal conflict, and loneliness and social isolation. A major strength of IPT in late-life depression is that it fosters personalization of treatment and does so at a deep, existential level, allowing patient and therapist to engage in problem-solving where patients are suffering the most. In addition, our studies with IPT have also involved the use of antidepressant pharmacotherapy. Because IPT encourages the acceptance of the patient role and therewith adherence to the use of antidepressant medication, research participants in our randomized controlled trials have typically received combination treatment—both to get well during acute treatment and then to stay well during maintenance treatment for up to 3 years.

ADAPTATIONS OF IPT AND OF TRAINING AND SUPERVISION IN THE CONTEXT OF LATE-LIFE MAJOR DEPRESSION

Our IPT therapists have come from diverse clinical backgrounds, including clinical psychology with expertise in psychodynamic psychotherapy, psychiatric nursing, and social work. Although we have encountered no insurmountable challenges in the use of IPT for older depressed patients, IPT therapists have occasionally found it necessary to slow the pace of IPT work to accommodate patients with slowing of information-processing speed and mild executive impairments (common in late-life depression and a hallmark of more treatment-resistant forms of depression). It may be that executive function deficits in older adults after the age of 75 pose obstacles to IPT efficacy because of impairments in working memory and cognitive flexibility. We have also found that repetition of key messages and specific behavioral strategies across therapy sessions are useful in reinforcing learning how to cope with depression and with bereavement. Review and repetition of key messages in consecutive IPT sessions helps to reinforce learning, together with encouragement to practice new coping and communication strategies between sessions. Engaging family caregivers to encourage new communication strategies is also helpful in strengthening the therapeutic alliance. Our IPT therapists have typically engaged family members early during treatment by means of a conjoint or dyadic interview, with follow-up dyadic sessions if felt to be needed or requested. This strategy has proved helpful where the major problem focus of IPT dealt with interpersonal conflict or changes in social roles. Brief telephone calls between sessions can be a useful way of offering encouragement and is welcomed by patients. Our therapists have encouraged patients to call, if needed, or call patients to check in and encourage continued focus on issues raised during in-person therapy sessions. We have found that the use of such strategies—dyadic interviews and telephone calls—have supported engagement with IPT and helped to build a supportive therapeutic alliance. Patients have frequently told us that they value their IPT sessions and the relationship with IPT therapists. And IPT therapists themselves enjoy administering the treatment with older adults.

We have used weekly group-based supervision of IPT therapists to ensure adherence to manualized IPT protocols. These groups have matured into collaborative sessions in which therapists learn from each other, while working under the supervision of faculty investigators in case-based discussion to address strategies for deepening engagement in therapy. IPT naturally encourages such learning processes grounded in interactions among therapists.

CHALLENGES OF IMPLEMENTATION AND HOW CHALLENGES WERE ADDRESSED

We audio-record IPT sessions, and approximately 10%–20% of the sessions are rated by blinded research assistants for the presence of IPT strategies and for focus on specific IPT problem areas, such as bereavement, social role transitions, interpersonal conflict, or social isolation. These ratings inform supervision of IPT therapists, allowing supervisors to correct drift and to strengthen focus on specific IPT problem areas. Specific problem focus is key to IPT's efficacy in both acute and maintenance treatment.[1] Ratings are also used to document differentiation of IPT sessions from supportive medication-clinic visits.

CASE EXAMPLE

The patient is a 75-year-old Black woman who serves as a caregiver for her husband, now living with moderately severe dementia, motor disturbances, and psychotic symptoms diagnosed as Parkinson disease (PD). Our patient presented with a Structured Clinical Interview for DSM Disorders diagnosis of recurrent major depression and a Hamilton Depression Rating Scale score of 21 on the

17-item scale, indicating moderate severity. She endorsed suicidal ideation (with no history of attempt), feelings of caregiver burnout, and complaints of conflicts with her husband, who required but resisted her help with many activities of daily living (ADL). (He had been a fiercely independent man before coming down with PD.) The IPT therapist had a background in geropsychiatric social work and carried out several interventions: (1) neurologic consultation (which resulted in a medication change for the spouse with PD, including the use of pimavanserin for psychotic symptoms); (2) a house call to observe the patient's communication with her spouse and supervision of his ADL; and (3) arrangements for respite care to provide a breather for the patient several times a week. As a result of the IPT therapist's house call and psychoeducational intervention, addressing a simpler, more focused, and slower communication style, the patient was better able to regulate her own emotional responses to her husband's difficult behaviors and, also importantly, to acknowledge and cope with feelings of grief over the gradual loss of her partner. The patient accepted a course of antidepressant pharmacotherapy with sertraline. Over the course of 16 weeks of IPT and medication, she reported feeling better, with a decrease in her Hamilton Depression Rating to 6. She described far fewer conflicts with her dementing husband, attributing benefit to her increased understanding of and patience with his disabilities.

FUTURE PLANS

Our use of IPT in the context to bereavement-related major depression led to additional research into complicated or chronic grieving. In collaboration with Holly Prigerson, we developed diagnostic criteria for prolonged grief disorder (now recognized in the *Diagnostic and Statistical Manual of Mental Disorders, Fifth Edition Text Revision, DSM-5-TR*), which is distinct from but often accompanied by major depressive disorder (MDD).[7] IPT is part of the foundation of PGDT, developed by Katherine Shear and colleagues. PGDT is highly effective in treating prolonged grief disorder.[8,9] PGDT combines elements of IPT, cognitive behavioral therapy, and other strategies from exposure-based treatment and motivational interviewing. Like IPT, PGDT helps grieving depressed patients to both accept the finality of loss and engage in restoration-focused coping. An important component of PGDT is the focus on reestablishing interpersonal relationships as bereaved older adults come to terms with their loss and work to rebuild a life of purpose and meaning. PGDT is superior to IPT in relieving the symptoms and suffering of prolonged grief disorder in older adults, which is distinct from bereavement-related major depression.[8] IPT is an appropriate treatment for the latter.[4] Differential treatment response of PGD to PGDT and to IPT has helped to validate the construct of prolonged grief disorder as a stress disorder in *DSM-5-TR*, distinct from MDD.

Going forward, we plan to use IPT and PGDT as probes of underlying brain changes seen in chronic grieving among older adults, to identify via functional magnetic imaging biomarkers of risk for chronic grieving and mediators and moderators of successful treatment outcomes. This work will address theories of attachment in grief, issues of emotion dysregulation, the role of the brain's reward circuitry (nucleus accumbens) in chronic grieving symptoms such as yearning, and the interplay with such neuromodulators as the endocannabinoid system and hormones such as vasopressin and oxytocin.[10-12]

In conclusion, both IPT and PGDT are essentially learning-based treatments that help patients cope adaptively and actively with loss-focused and restoration-focused challenges.[12] Because MDD is increasingly recognized as a risk factor for prolonged grief disorder, treating bereavement-related MDD with IPT soon after the loss may serve to prevent the subsequent development of prolonged grief disorder and its complications.

REFERENCES

1. Reynolds CF III, Frank E, Perel JM, et al. Nortriptyline and interpersonal psychotherapy as maintenance therapies for recurrent major depression: a randomized controlled trial in patients older than 59 years. *JAMA*. 1999;281(1):39–45.
2. Reynolds CF III, Dew MA, Pollock BG, et al. Maintenance treatment of major depression in old age. *N Engl J Med*. 2006;354(11):1130–1138.
3. Bruce ML, Ten Have TR, Reynolds CF, et al. Reducing suicidal ideation and depressive symptoms in depressed older primary care patients: a randomized controlled trial. *JAMA*. 2004;291(9):1081–1090.
4. Reynolds CF, Miller MD, Pasternak RE, et al. Treatment of bereavement-related major depressive episodes in later life: a controlled study of acute and continuation treatment with nortriptyline and interpersonal psychotherapy. *Am J Psychiatry*. 1999b;156(2):202–208.
5. Lenze EJ, Dew MA, Mazumdar S, et al. Combined pharmacotherapy and psychotherapy as maintenance treatment for late life depression: effects on social adjustment. *Am J Psychiatry*. 2002;159(3):466–468.
6. Gallo JJ, Morales KH, Bogner HR, et al. Long term effect of depression care management on mortality in older adults: follow-up of cluster randomized clinical trial in primary care. *BMJ*. 2013;346:f2570.
7. Prigerson HG, Boelen PA, Xu J, Smith KV, Maciejewski PK. Validation of the new *DSM-5-TR* criteria for prolonged grief disorder and the PG-13-revised (PG-13-R) scale. *World Psychiatry*. 2021;20(1):96–106.
8. Shear MK, Wang Y, Skritskaya N, Duan N, Mauro C, Ghesquiere A. Treatment of complicated grief in elderly persons: a randomized clinical trial. *JAMA Psychiatry*. 2014;71(11):1287–1295.
9. Shear MK, Reynolds CF, Simon NM, et al. Optimizing treatment of complicated grief: a randomized clinical trial. *JAMA Psychiatry*. 2016;73(7): 685–694.
10. Reiland H, Banerjee A, Claesges SA, et al. The influence of depression on the relationship between loneliness and grief trajectories in bereaved older adults. *Psychiatry Res Commun*. 2021;1:100006.
11. Kang M, Bohorquez-Montoya L, McAuliffe T, et al. Loneliness, circulating endocannabinoid concentrations and grief trajectories in bereaved older adults: a longitudinal study. *Front Psychiatry*. 2021;12:783187.
12. O'Connor M-F. *The Grieving Brain*. Harper Collins Publishers; 2022.

47

A Culturally Grounded Interpersonal Psychotherapy With American Indians/Alaska Natives

MARIA YELLOW HORSE BRAVE HEART, JOSEPHINE CHASE, JENNIFER ELKINS, AND JENNIFER MARTIN ■

BACKGROUND

American Indians and Alaska Natives (AIANs) face pervasive trauma exposure, collective histories of communal suffering, and elevated risk for depression and post-traumatic stress disorder (PTSD). Few evidence-based treatments exist,[1-3] and access to culturally grounded treatment is limited. AIANs also face disproportionate socioeconomic barriers (e.g., unemployment, limited income, lack of health insurance, lower educational attainment, limited Indian Health Service funding) and sociocultural barriers (e.g., few AIAN therapists, distrust of Western interventions, cultural differences in symptoms) that complicate treatment engagement.

The health, well-being, and service utilization of AIANs should be understood within the context of *historical trauma* (HT), the cumulative emotional and psychological wounding across generations. HT provides context for current trauma, grief, and loss across the life span by rooting it in the collective psychosocial suffering across generations. This empowers AIAN survivors by reducing stigma and isolation. The *historical trauma response* (HTR) refers to the constellation of features that have been observed among massively traumatized populations, including depression, psychic numbing, self-destructive behavior, and identification with the dead. Individual trauma responses are viewed as emerging from genocide, oppression, and racism. Historical unresolved grief is a component of HTR that includes the generational collective experience of unresolved grief.

Maria Yellow Horse Brave Heart, Josephine Chase, Jennifer Elkins, and Jennifer Martin, *A Culturally Grounded Interpersonal Psychotherapy With American Indians/Alaska Natives* In: *Interpersonal Psychotherapy*. Edited by: Myrna M. Weissman and Jennifer J. Mootz, Oxford University Press. © Oxford University Press 2024. DOI: 10.1093/oso/9780197652084.003.0048

Selected as a tribal best practice,[4] the *historical trauma and unresolved grief intervention* (HTUG) is a short-term, culturally grounded intervention for grief resolution and trauma mastery. HTUG was developed as a group intervention incorporating traditional culture, language, ceremonies, and clinical intervention strategies in a 4-day psychoeducational experience in the Black Hills of South Dakota.[5]

The Iwankapiya (healing) study combined HTUG with group interpersonal psychotherapy (IPT) and compared it to IPT. IPT focuses on the interpersonal context for depression, and the relationship of current life events to mood[6] is effective for treating depression and PTSD in diverse non-AIAN groups.[6–10]

ADAPTATIONS

The *IPT Uganda model*[10] was selected for modification due to its congruence with AIAN cultures (e.g., collectivist societies, rural populations, valuing interdependency, and strong kinship bonds). Most AIAN healing practices take place in a group setting, with family and other tribal members providing support. IPT's focus on interpersonal triggers for depression aligns with AIAN cultural values and the emphasis on interdependence. Additional modifications were made to tailor this for AIAN communities.

The *HTUG model* comprises 4 components: (a) addressing collective trauma history, along with the historical underpinning grounded in current reality, (b) offering psychoeducation regarding grief and trauma, (c) focusing on trauma and grief resolution in the group format, and (d) experiential practices incorporating traditional healing and therapeutic modalities, including smudging with sage and sweetgrass, traditional song, prayer, and talking circles.[11] HTUG incorporates the HTR, which does not pathologize the features. This leads to more support, reduction in depression and anxiety, opportunities to reach out to others, and decreased isolation and stigma. The "sick role" in IPT was modified to derive from HTR because it is experienced by tribal communities as pathologizing. By contrast, HTR was not stigmatizing. Because of this, some participants eagerly stated: "I have that," "Me too," and they spoke freely and openly about their trauma response features.

Because AIANs are pathologized, it is important that HTR are normalized as a reaction to the history of genocide. For example, in the response to the original implementation of HTUG, one elder (a leader of the Sitting Bull and Big Foot Memorial Ride) expressed that he had sacrificed for the 4 previous years to prepare for the final ride in 1990 to heal from the assassination of Sitting Bull, Big Foot, and the Wounded Knee Massacre. The ride was a traditional way to mourn and heal from the massacre—until that day no one had ever wiped his tears. Acceptance of HT in AIAN communities is widespread and plays a critical role in facilitating engagement with evidence-based interventions such as IPT. As exhibited in Table 47.1, the required additional cultural-related content from HTUG enhanced IPT, but the time frame was the same.

Table 47.1 SESSION TOPICS

Session	IPT	HTUG + IPT
1–5	• *Sick Role* orientation re: depression and not the person's fault • Diagnose primary interpersonal problem area • Focus on interpersonal issues and their influence on mood • Help participants externalize depression • Establish group safety and cohesion • Sharing about symptoms and relationship issues • Listening and sharing about symptoms and relationship issues	• *HTR* orientation • Confronting the history • Group processing • Psychoeducation about trauma, grief, and depression, use of AIAN videos • Foster group identity/cohesion, safety • Traditional cultural review of protective factors and Indigenous ways of dealing with trauma, grief, and depression • Diagnose primary HTR and interpersonal problem area • Interpersonal issues and historical trauma and influence on mood • Help member see mental health symptoms as part of HTR and not the individual's "fault" • Cultural emphasis on listening and sharing about symptoms and relationship issues
6–10	• Group problem-solving and practice about interpersonal conflicts • Work through grief and loss • Increasing capacity to address role transitions • Members help one another • Members focus on changing what they can in their lives	• Releasing the pain: trauma graph exercise • Group problem-solving and practice about interpersonal conflicts • Work through grief and loss • Facilitating increased capacity to address role transitions • Traditional cultural releasing • Members help one another • Members focus on changing what they can in their lives
11, 12	• Group ending, summarize changes in symptoms and problems • Review relationship losses • Discuss possible new issues that could trigger depression and how to cope with these • Review group process and experiences • Discuss feelings about ending and continued group member support	• Group ending, summarize changes in symptoms and problems • Reviewing relationship losses • Discuss possible new issues that could trigger depression and how to cope with these • Review group process and experiences • Discuss feelings about ending and continued group member support • Transcending the trauma: *Wiping the Tears* traditional practice and formation of extended family kinship bond

Abbreviation: HTUG, Historical Trauma and Unresolved Grief Intervention.

·CHALLENGES

HTUG + IPT facilitators received additional training and education. This aspect presented challenges in terms of additional time and a unique set of dynamics to the concept of the wounded healer. This approach required group cofacilitators to address their own traumatic tribal, family, and individual history to support other traumatized individuals in their healing process. Coming from the same background of wounding offers both challenges and strengths: Traditionally, healers approached other healers for help, acknowledging that healers need help as well as validating the value of healing. Another issue during the study was the ongoing trauma that occurred in the community that affected both the participants and the facilitators. In addition to seeking approval from multiple internal review boards, challenges included remoteness, long distances, lack of structural facilities, scarcity of reliable services such as no child care, unreliable cell phone coverage, lack of transportation, and the endemic effects of intergenerational trauma experienced in the daily lives of participants and sometimes the researchers themselves.

The lack of basic infrastructure made finding suitable spaces to meet scarce. In addition, limited cell phone coverage made communication difficult. Nonexistent child care resources made it impossible for some women to attend. Due to not having reliable public or personal transportation, it was common for participants to drive long distances, have frequent vehicle breakdowns, and encounter bad road conditions. Project staff faced challenges of trauma exposure and grief and loss. Group members and staff experienced trauma within their communities, such as having to withdraw from the project to reflect on personal trauma. Unfortunately, domestic violence is not uncommon and can be traced back to the boarding school era, with the legacy of violence, abuse, and neglect.[12]

Some recommended strategies to help support and engage successfully with AIAN communities are to practice cultural humility, become aware of one's bias and privilege, and employ decolonizing research strategies. Use the practice of your own cultural experience and theoretical and cultural wisdom practices, such as ceremonies and culture, to guide healing work. Respect and recognize the intelligence and wisdom of AIAN people. Prepare for contingency plans, be able to leverage resources in poverty settings in creative ways, adapt, and be prepared to play multiple roles. Be flexible and patient, as remote rural settings with high rates of traumatic exposure often need rescheduling, crisis intervention outreach, and compassionate sensitivity. Community loss and trauma will impact research. Add trauma-informed care into the research framework. Try to create some form of sustainability. Once the research work has been implemented, there is a need for continuation of care and support for participants who live in communities with limited resources. Starting a peer group for ongoing support or encouraging traditional cultural resources is also helpful.[13]

NEXT STEPS

As stated above, the HTUG model is a stand-alone model that has been developed over 30 years.[13,14] The recommendations for continuing work with HTUG, and HTUG + IPT are as follows:

- **Continue training and education** regarding HT with diverse tribal populations.
- **Conduct further research** to determine the efficacy of HTUG compared to the efficacy of HTUG + IPT. This is especially important because qualitative feedback from group facilitators indicated a particular relevance and preference for HTUG. Future research will focus on comparing HTUG + IPT, HTUG, and IPT to tease out the unique effects of each intervention. Further research should also examine the contributing role of group facilitator demographics (i.e., gender, race, age, prior trauma history).
- **Possible replication of the Iwankapiya study** to build the evidence base for the applicability of HTUG + IPT with tribal populations.
- **Publish the *HTUG Model Training Manual*** to ensure fidelity to the model.
- **Train-the-Trainers.** Given the unique nature and impact of the HTUG model, and the importance in fidelity to the model when using it, we are establishing a formal certification for HTUG.
- **Further development of HTUG and HTUG + IPT.** Next steps include tailoring these interventions to address parenting given the unique impact of HT and complex boarding school legacy on parenting.
- **Advocacy on continuing awareness and healing efforts.** This is especially important given the increased awareness and attention to boarding school trauma and violence in the news.

CASE EXAMPLE

John (pseudonym) is an AIAN male military veteran and a boarding school survivor who is in his 80s. He has been in recovery from substance abuse and in counseling for many years. John disclosed experiencing grief for his family when he was placed in boarding school at a young age, where he also suffered neglect and physical abuse. John shared that the HTUG + IPT intervention was his first opportunity to share his traumatic history and begin to process how it was a significant contributor to his traumatic history, depression, and subsequent self-medicating with substances.

John shared that he feels HTUG is the missing link in therapy for AIANs. John felt that in addition to the assessments in HTUG that ask about boarding school experiences and other HTR features, and the education that HTUG provides about HT effects that allowed him the opportunity and support to discuss his traumatic past. Additionally, John felt the support and understanding of the group members gave him the encouragement to address these issues. The integration of HTUG with IPT enhanced the efficacy and relevancy of both models for addressing depression, trauma, and anxiety. However, HTUG added a distinct and important component related to the intergenerational trauma and HT in AIANs that was not present in IPT.

Implementing evidence-based interventions in AIAN communities can be challenging for myriad reasons. This study validated that centering a culturally tailored approach of HTUG—developed by and for AIANs—is the most effective strategy. Our work demonstrates the potential for lasting healing when traditional practices are respected and acknowledged at the same level as evidence-based Western practices. AIAN practitioners and researchers have been historically mandated to approach evidence-based practice through a Western lens, and our work reveals that traditional tribal healing practices are just as effective.

ACKNOWLEDGMENTS

We acknowledge Oglala Sioux Tribe Research Review Board, Oglala Lakota College Institutional Review Board, Great Plains Area Indian Health Service Institutional Review Board, First Nations Community Health Source Behavioral Health, and the University of New Mexico Human Research Protection Office.

REFERENCES

1. Beitel M, Myhra LL, Gone JP, et al. Psychotherapy with American Indians: an exploration of therapist-rated techniques in three urban clinics. *Psychotherapy.* 2018;55(1):45.
2. Pearson CR, Parker M, Zhou C, Donald C, Fisher CB. A culturally tailored research ethics training curriculum for American Indian and Alaska Native communities: a randomized comparison trial. *Crit Public Health.* 2019;29(1):27–39.
3. Pomerville A, Burrage RL, Gone JP. Empirical findings from psychotherapy research with indigenous populations: a systematic review. *J Consult Clin Psychol.* 2016;84(12):1023.
4. Echo-Hawk H, Erickson J, Naquin V, et al. *Compendium of Behavioral Health Best Practices for Indigenous American India/Alaska Native and Pacific Island Populations: A Description of Selected Best Practices and Cultural Analysis of Local Evidence Building.* First Nations Behavioral Health Association; 2011.
5. Heart MY. Oyate Ptayela. Rebuilding the Lakota Nation through addressing historical trauma among Lakota parents. *J Hum Behav Soc Environ.* 1999;2(1–2):109–126.
6. Weissman MM, Markowitz JC, Klerman G. *Comprehensive Guide to Interpersonal Psychotherapy.* New York: Basic Books; 2008.
7. Krupnick JL, Green BL, Stockton P, Miranda J, Krause E, Mete M. Group interpersonal psychotherapy for low-income women with posttraumatic stress disorder. *Psychotherapy Res.* 2008;18(5):497–507.

8. Markowitz JC, Patel SR, Balan IC, et al. Toward an adaptation of interpersonal psychotherapy for Hispanic patients with *DSM-IV* major depressive disorder. *J Clin Psychiatry*. 2009;70(2):214.

9. Markowitz JC, Petkova E, Neria Y, et al. Is exposure necessary? A randomized clinical trial of interpersonal psychotherapy for PTSD. *Am J Psychiatry*. 2015;172(5):430–440.

10. Verdeli H, Clougherty K, Bolton P, et al. Adapting group interpersonal psychotherapy for a developing country: experience in rural Uganda. *World Psychiatry*. 2003;2(2):114–120.

11. Brave Heart MY, Chase J, Myers O, et al. Iwankapiya American Indian pilot clinical trial: historical trauma and group interpersonal psychotherapy. *Psychotherapy*. 2020;57(2):184–196.

12. Brave Heart MYH. The return to the sacred path: healing the historical trauma and historical unresolved grief response among the Lakota through a psychoeducational group intervention. *Smith College Stud Soc Work*. 1998;68(3):287–305.

13. Heart MY, Chase J, Elkins J, Martin MJ, Nanez MJ, Mootz JJ. Women finding the way: American Indian women leading intervention research in Native communities. *Am Indian Alask Native Men Health Res*. 2016;23(3):24.

14. Chase JA. *Native American Elders' Perceptions of the Boarding School Experience on Native American Parenting: an Exploratory Study*. 2012. Unpublished doctoral dissertation; Smith College, Northampton, MA. https://scholarworks.smith.edu/theses/390. Accessed September 17, 2023.

48

Interpersonal Psychotherapy With Hispanic/Latinx Individuals

SAPANA R. PATEL, LAURA MUFSON, AND
ROBERTO LEWIS-FERNÁNDEZ ■

HISPANIC/LATINX INDIVIDUALS

Individuals of Hispanic/Latinx descent comprise 8.9% of the world population[1] and 18.7% of the national population, representing the largest US minoritized ethnoracial group.[2] Relative to non-Hispanic Whites, and considering their own mental health needs, Hispanics/Latinxs experience disparities in care, including underutilization of mental health services[3-5] involving both entry and retention in care.[6] Strategies to mitigate these disparities include enhancing the cultural fit between clients and treatments, as attending to treatment preferences and cultural alignment between the therapy and the client's views and practices influence engagement and retention.[7-10] Responding to minimal involvement of Hispanics/Latinxs in psychotherapy studies,[11-14] evidence-based interventions (EBIs) such as interpersonal psychotherapy (IPT) have been adapted to this population to determine fit and effectiveness for Hispanic/Latinx adolescents and adults.[14,15]

HISPANIC/LATINX INDIVIDUALS AND INTERPERSONAL PSYCHOTHERAPY

The term *Hispanic/Latinx* refers to multiple cultural groups originating from the Spanish-speaking countries of Central and South America, as well as Mexico, the Caribbean, and Spain. In the United States, the term refers to an ethnicity that has common attributes but encompasses diverse cultural backgrounds varying in sociopolitical histories, practices, and values.[16] Given this diversity, clinicians

Sapana R. Patel, Laura Mufson, and Roberto Lewis-Fernández, *Interpersonal Psychotherapy With Hispanic/Latinx Individuals*
In: *Interpersonal Psychotherapy*. Edited by: Myrna M. Weissman and Jennifer J. Mootz, Oxford University Press.
© Oxford University Press 2024. DOI: 10.1093/oso/9780197652084.003.0049

are expected to develop knowledge about, and skill interacting with, their clients' health-related views and practices (cultural competence) and evidence curiosity and genuine interest when exploring clients' identities while remaining aware of their own possible biases (cultural humility).

Based on experience implementing IPT with Hispanic/Latinx adults and adolescents in New York City,[17-22] we discuss evidence on cultural fit and clinical effectiveness of IPT for this population. Several initial points are warranted. First, research suggests that Hispanic/Latinx individuals tend to value their ability to function, contribute to society, and engage in interpersonal relationships beyond symptom remission.[23-25] These goals are highly congruent with the IPT focus on interpersonal relations and psychosocial functioning and on linking improvements in those domains to symptom reduction. Second, the typical Hispanic/Latinx emphasis on interpersonal relatedness in social interactions makes IPT a well-suited treatment modality. Interpersonal conflicts in marriage and the family are common issues in psychotherapy for this population.[26-28] For instance, parent-child generational gaps regarding acculturating to US society may result in acculturative stress that contributes to role disputes.[17-19,22] Third, the IPT emphasis on maintaining a personal and emotionally expressive clinical relationship is congruent with typical Hispanic/Latinx value of *personalismo*,[28] a value for interacting with persons with whom one has a warm, caring, and trusting personal relationship.

ADAPTATIONS TO IPT FOR HISPANIC/LATINX INDIVIDUALS

Cultural adaptation of EBIs involves the modification of intervention protocols to consider language, cultural background, and social context to better align with the client's cultural views and practices.[29] Several meta-analyses have found cultural adaptations more efficacious and effective than the parent, unadapted interventions.[30] In our work treating Hispanic/Latinx adults with major depression in New York City, we conducted a preliminary adaptation of IPT to address the stressors, views, and coping strategies of this population based on focus groups with IPT clinicians and their Hispanic/Latinx clients.[22]

We made several adaptations to IPT based on these qualitative data. First, we integrated an abbreviated cultural assessment based on the *Diagnostic and Statistical Manual of Mental Disorders (DSM-V)*[31] Cultural Formulation (CF) approach[32,33] into the initial evaluation and treatment-planning sessions of IPT. The CF informed the Interpersonal Inventory and IPT formulation, allowing the clinician to present the formulation using the client's language and notions of illness.[27] Second, we focused on interpersonal relationships and de-emphasized depression as a treatable medical illness. This follows general IPT practice of tailoring the treatment focus to the client's perspective, such as by de-emphasizing the medical model for a client who believes that depression is a test from God. Third, given that Hispanic/Latinx clients usually rely strongly on their families for psychological, social, and security needs, usually termed *familismo*,[34] we highlighted the family as a source of motivation for solving problems in interpersonal functioning; we also noted that the family can serve as a treatment barrier, such as when relatives oppose a client's behaviors that seem to run counter to family needs. Last, since therapy was viewed as a relationship that was not expected to end in the short term and some clients perceived the time limit as a form of abandonment, we provided education about time-limited psychotherapy and acknowledged that this approach differed from usual handling of problems in their social network.

Interpersonal psychotherapy for adolescents (IPT-A) was also developed and evaluated in the context of community-based outpatient mental health services while working with a Hispanic/Latinx immigrant population in New York City.[17-19] The adaptation took a culturally humble and iterative approach by working directly with adolescents and families to explore how IPT problem-solving strategies and techniques might be adapted to align with Hispanic/Latinx cultural views and practices. After treating 14 adolescents with the first manual draft, additional refinements were made in response to clinical experiences.

The focus of IPT-A on role transitions and role disputes provides a natural framework for addressing acculturative stresses.[17] Clinicians can use the framework to help adolescents communicate with family members about culturally based differences in expectations for behavior. It can also guide negotiation of conflicts stemming from differences between parents' more traditional viewpoints and adolescents' desire for greater assimilation into the usually more permissive and individualistic New York City society.[17-19] These conflicts often present over issues such as curfews, dating, sexuality, gender roles, and difficulties explaining family behavior to peers if it is considered by them to be antiquated or oppressive. IPT-A clinicians work with adolescents to develop communication and problem-solving strategies to help navigate this interpersonal terrain while remaining respectful of Hispanic/Latinx values and customs.[17-19]

IPT RESEARCH WITH HISPANIC/LATINX INDIVIDUALS

Research shows that IPT reduces depressive symptoms among Hispanic/Latinx adults.[35,36] Five randomized controlled trials on the effectiveness of IPT have been conducted among Hispanic/Latinx youth in outpatient clinics in the United States and Puerto Rico and in US school-based health and primary care clinics.[17-21] IPT-A was found to be effective largely in Hispanic/Latinx samples of depressed adolescents.[17-19] In the school-based effectiveness study treatment, IPT-A resulted in better outcomes in depression symptom reduction (Cohen's $d = 0.50$), improved social functioning ($d = 0.55$), and global functioning ($d = 0.54$) compared to treat-. ment as usual (supportive psychotherapy).[18] Clinical trials in Puerto Rico[20,21] used a different IPT manual than the US studies but similarly showed support for IPT as an effective treatment for Hispanic/Latinx youth. One of the 2 studies showed mixed findings for IPT, possibly due to low IPT fidelity and client adherence.[21]

In the school-based study, US-born Hispanic/Latinx adolescents had significantly greater depression symptoms and worse social and overall functioning posttreatment than foreign-born adolescents,[18] suggesting poorer outcomes for these youth, who likely have experienced greater acculturative stress and been aware of discrimination than more recent immigrants, a consistent research finding.[37-39] We also found that family interpersonal functioning accounted for a larger proportion of the indirect effect of IPT-A on depression than peer functioning, suggesting that family and peer functioning are key targets of psychotherapy for depressed Hispanic/Latinx youth.[40] IPT-A's fit with the cultural priorities of familismo and personalismo[28,34] provides a positive therapeutic context in which to address the roles of acculturation and family cohesion in adolescent depression and interpersonal adjustment.[18,40]

IMPLEMENTATION OF IPT FOR HISPANIC/ LATINX ADOLESCENTS

Hispanic/Latinx adolescents have the lowest utilization of clinical services for depression among US ethnoracial groups, based on data from the National Comorbidity Survey Adolescent Supplement (NCS-A).[41] Reasons for this include logistical access barriers (e.g., limited transportation, child care, and English proficiency), stigma of mental health services (usually leading to lack of support from family and peers), and mistrust of formal services due to previous negative experiences with therapy.[42]

Logistical and stigma-related barriers may be reduced by implementing treatments in youth-serving settings, such as schools or primary care clinics, which are more accessible and less stigmatizing.[43-45] However, despite increased availability of school-based mental health care,[46] Hispanic/Latinx youth, especially those with Spanish-monolingual parents,[47] are less likely than non-Hispanic/Latinx White and Black students to attend schools that provide these services or to obtain treatment even when the schools do provide services.[48-51] In this context, it is particularly meaningful that IPT-A demonstrated good session attendance by students and was effective in decreasing depression and improving social and global functioning when delivered in school-based health clinics in urban Hispanic/Latinx communities.[18]

Implemented in pediatric primary care clinics, the stepped-care model of IPT-A (SCIPT-A) consists of beginning with 8 weekly sessions of IPT-A followed by either 3 maintenance sessions of IPT-A if significantly improved at 8 weeks or, if not improved, followed by 8 more weekly IPT-A sessions combined with the initiation of medication treatment. When implemented, Hispanic/Latinx adolescents demonstrated high session attendance (82%), including their parents (>50%), who participated in at least 1 phone or individual session; all participants reported that treatment duration was adequate and that they derived benefit from treatment.[19] Depressive symptom reduction and overall illness severity improvement showed medium-to-large effect sizes relative to treatment as usual (Cohen's $d = 0.35$ and $d = 0.85$, respectively), suggesting that SCIPT-A can be feasibly and acceptably implemented in a pediatric primary care setting serving Hispanic/Latinx youth and families.[19]

CASE EXAMPLE

The conflicting expectations in Hispanic/Latinx families between adolescent girls and their parents are a frequent precipitant of role disputes associated with depressive symptoms in teens. This "problem area" is illustrated by the case of Ana, a 15-year-old US-born young woman of Dominican descent who lives with her parents and her 14-year-old brother. During the Interpersonal Inventory, Ana expressed being upset about the markedly different family expectations regarding chores between her and her brother. She felt that her mother, Altagracia, did not understand how the fact that Ana has many more chores than her brother makes her feel, so she withdrew from interacting, feeling unsupported and misunderstood. In the middle phase of treatment, the goal became to help clarify Ana's and Altagracia's expectations for Ana's role in the home and for their relationship. Using the Teen Tips, a set of communication strategies (e.g., using "I statements," aim for the right timing),[52] the clinician helped Ana to clarify that she wanted her mother to treat her and her brother more equally. The therapist also helped Ana to explore with her family whether her mother's parenting approach is typical of traditional Hispanic/Latinx gender roles whereby Dominican daughters are expected to do more around the house than sons. During collateral sessions with Altagracia, the clinician helped her clarify the acculturation differences between her and her daughter, given the fact that younger members of immigrant families, especially when they are US born, typically acculturate to US society more quickly and fully than older members.[53] This led to clarification of Altagracia's expectations for Ana, including perceived differences in gender roles between Ana and her son, and to consider how Altagracia could be responsive to Ana's emotions without completely abandoning her expectations of filial behavior. Once expectations were clarified, the clinician brought Ana and Altagracia together in two dyadic sessions to coach them on communicating their expectations and associated feelings to negotiate their different perspectives. Coaching on how to verbalize the other person's perspective ("Give to Get") and on one's own feelings (I statement) allowed them to feel more validated and empowered. This led them to identify potential solutions, such as Altagracia sharing information equally with the siblings and expecting Ana's brother to clean his own room instead of Ana. Over time, Ana reported improvements in mood and in her relationship with her mother. The dyadic sessions allowed Ana and Altagracia to communicate more clearly and openly, an approach they continued to practice until the end of treatment.

RECOMMENDATIONS

Given workforce limitations, linguistic, ethnoracial, and/or cultural matching between clinician and client is often unavailable. For groups seeking to train and supervise clinicians in using IPT with Hispanic/Latinx clients, we propose several recommendations. First, provide training in methods for cultural assessment using brief interviews like the CF Interview (e.g., see https://nyculturalcompete

nce.org/cfionlinemodule/). This taps clients' expectations of care, clarifying their illness models and cultural practices. Second, help clinicians access culturally adapted forms of IPT, preferably manualized interventions that enable fidelity assessment. Third, encourage clinicians to reflect on their own biases, especially when encountering cultural differences regarding gender roles, filial expectations, and other aspects of interpersonal relationships. Fourth, include attention to structural and systemic elements in identifying causes and precipitants of mental health problems and barriers to improvement. Attention to all these factors allows clinicians to respond sensitively and flexibly—and to iteratively adapt and personalize treatment—to the cultural views and circumstances of each client.

REFERENCES

1. United Nations Department of Economics and Social Affairs, Population Division. World population prospects 2022. Updated 2019. Accessed June 1, 2022. https://population.un.org/wpp/
2. United States Census Bureau. Quick facts United States. Updated 2021. Accessed June 1, 2022. https://www.census.gov/quickfacts/fact/table/US/RHI725220
3. Alexandre PK, Martins SS, Richard P. Disparities in adequate mental health care for past-year major depressive episodes among Caucasian and Hispanic youths. *Psychiatr Serv*. 2009;60(10):1365–1371.
4. Blanco C, Patel SR, Liu L, et al. National trends in ethnic disparities in mental health care. *Med Care*. 2007;45(11):1012–1019.
5. Sorkin DH, Pham E, Ngo-Metzger Q. Racial and ethnic differences in the mental health needs and access to care of older adults in California. *J Am Geriatr Soc*. 2009;57(12):2311–2317.
6. Miranda J, Azocar F, Organista KC, Muñoz RF, Lieberman A. Recruiting and retaining low-income Latinos in psychotherapy research. *J Consult Clin Psychol*. 1996;64(5):868–874.
7. Dwight-Johnson M, Unutzer J, Sherbourne C, Tang L, Wells KB. Can quality improvement programs for depression in primary care address patient preferences for treatment? *Med Care*. 2001;39(9):934–944.
8. Cooper LA, Gonzales JJ, Gallo JJ, et al. The acceptability of treatment for depression among African-American, Hispanic, and White primary care patients. *Med Care*. 2003;41(4):479–489.
9. Fairhurst K, Dowrick C. Problems with recruitment in a randomized controlled trial of counseling in general practice: causes and implications. *J Health Serv Res Policy*. 1996;1:77–80.
10. Jaycox LH, Asarnow JR, Sherbourne CD, Rea MM, LaBorde AP, Wells KB. Adolescent primary care patients' preferences for depression treatment. *Admin Policy Ment Health Serv Res*. 2006;33:198–207.
11. Elkin I, Shea MT, Watkins JT, et al. National Institute of Mental Health Treatment of Depression Collaborative Research Program: general effectiveness of treatments. *Arch Gen Psychiatry*. 1989;46:971–982.

12. Navarro AM. Efectividad de las psicoterapias con Latinos en los Estados Unidos: Una revision meta-analitica. *Interam J Psychol.* 1993;27:131–146.

13. Bernal G, Scharrón-del-Río MR. Are empirically supported treatments valid for ethnic minorities? Toward an alternative approach for treatment research. *Cultur Divers Ethnic Minor Psychol.* 2001;7(4):328–342.

14. Miranda J, Nakamura R, Bernal G. Including ethnic minorities in mental health intervention research: a practical approach to a long-standing problem. *Cult Med Psychiatry.* 2003;27(4):467–486.

15. Bernal G, Bonilla J, Padilla-Cotto L, Pérez-Prado EM. Factors associated to outcome in psychotherapy: an effectiveness study in Puerto Rico. *J Clin Psychol.* 1998;54(3):329–342.

16. Laria AJ, Lewis-Fernández R. Issues in the assessment and treatment of Latino patients. In Lim RF, ed. *Clinical Manual of Cultural Psychiatry.* American Psychiatric Publishing; 2015:183–249.

17. Mufson L, Weissman MM, Moreau D, Garfinkel R. Efficacy of interpersonal psychotherapy for depressed adolescents. *Arch Gen Psychiatry.* 1999;56:573–579.

18. Mufson L, Dorta KP, Wickramaratne P, Nomura Y, Olfson M, Weissman MM. A randomized effectiveness trial of interpersonal psychotherapy for depressed adolescents. *Arch Gen Psychiatry.* 2004;61:577–584.

19. Mufson L, Rynn M, Yanes-Lukin P, et al. Stepped care interpersonal psychotherapy treatment for depressed adolescents: a pilot study in pediatric clinics. *Admin Policy Ment Health Ment Health Serv Res.* 2018;45(3):417–431.

20. Rosselló J, Bernal G. Efficacy of cognitive-behavioral and interpersonal treatments for depression in Puerto Rican adolescents. *J Couns Clin Psychol.* 1999;67(5):734–745.

21. Rosselló J, Bernal G, Rivera-Medina C. Individual and group CBT and IPT for Puerto Rican adolescents with depressive symptoms. *Cultur Divers Ethnic Minor Psychol.* 2008;14(3):234–245.

22. Markowitz JC, Patel SA, Balan I, et al. Towards an adaptation of interpersonal psychotherapy for depressed Hispanic Patients. *J Clin Psychiatry.* 2009;70(2):214–222.

23. Bernal G, Bonilla J, Bellido C. Ecological validity and cultural sensitivity for outcome research: issues for the cultural adaptation and development of psychosocial treatments with Hispanics. *J Abnorm Child Psychol.* 1995;23(1):67–82.

24. Martínez Pincay IE, Guarnaccia PJ. "It's like going through an earthquake": anthropological perspectives on depression among Latino immigrants. *J Immigr Minor Health.* 2007;9(1):17–28.

25. Szapocznik J, Williams RA. Brief strategic family therapy: twenty-five years of interplay among theory, research and practice in adolescent behavior problems and drug abuse. *Clin Child Fam Psychol Rev.* 2000;3(2):117–134.

26. Comas-Diaz L, Duncan JW. The cultural context: a factor in assertiveness training with mainland Puerto Rican women. *Psychol Women Q.* 1985;9(4):463–476.

27. Patel SR, Lewis-Fernández R. *Interpersonal Therapy and Cultural Issues. Casebook of Interpersonal Psychotherapy.* Oxford University Press; 2012.

28. Delgado M. Hispanics and psychotherapeutic groups. *Int J Group Psychother.* 1983;33(4):507–520.

29. Bernal G, Domenech Rodríguez MM. Advances in Latino family research: cultural adaptations of evidence-based interventions. *Fam Process.* 2009;48(2):169–178.

30. Hall GC, Ibaraki AY, Huang ER, Marti CN, Stice E. A meta-analysis of cultural adaptations of psychological interventions. *Behav Ther.* 2016;47(6):993–1014.

31. American Psychiatric Association. *Diagnostic and statistical manual of mental disorders (5th ed.).* 2013. Accessed June 1, 2022. https://doi.org/10.1176/appi.books.9780890425596

32. Lewis-Fernández R, Díaz N. The cultural formulation: a method for assessing cultural factors affecting the clinical encounter. *Psychiatr Q.* 2002;73(4):271–295.

33. Aggarwal NK, Lewis-Fernández R. An introduction to the cultural formulation interview. *Focus.* 2015;13(4):426–431.

34. Sabogal F, Marín G, Otero-Sabogal R, Marín BV, Perez-Stable EJ. Hispanic familism and acculturation: what changes and what doesn't? *Hisp J Behav Sci.* 1987;9(4):397–412.

35. Markowitz JC, Spielman LA, Sullivan M, Fishman B. An exploratory study of ethnicity and psychotherapy outcome among HIV-positive patients with depressive symptoms. *J Psychother Prac Res.* 2000;9:226–231.

36. Toth SL, Rogosch FA, Oshri A, et al. The efficacy of interpersonal psychotherapy for depression among economically disadvantaged mothers. *Dev Psychopathol.* 2013;25(4 pt 1):1065–1078.

37. Alegría M, Canino G, Shrout PE, et al. Prevalence of mental illness in immigrant and non-immigrant US Latino groups. *Am J Psychiatry.* 2008;165(3):359–369.

38. Peña JB, Wyman PA, Brown CH, et al. Immigration generation status and its association with suicide attempts, substance use, and depressive symptoms among Latino adolescents in the USA. *Prev Sci.* 2008;9(4):299–310.

39. Smokowski PR, Bacallao ML. Acculturation, internalizing mental health symptoms and self-esteem: cultural experiences of Latino adolescents in North Carolina. *Child Psychiatry Hum Dev.* 2007;37:273–292.

40. Reyes-Portillo JA, McGlinchey EL, Yanes-Lukin PK, Turner JB, Mufson L. Mediators of interpersonal psychotherapy for depressed adolescents on outcomes in Latinos: the role of peer and family interpersonal functioning. *J Latina/o Psychol.* 2017;5(4):248–260.

41. Merikangas KR, He J, Burstein M, et al. Lifetime prevalence of mental disorders in US adolescents: results from the National Comorbidity Study—Adolescent Supplement (NCS-A). *J Am Acad Child Adolesc Psychiatry.* 2010;49:980–989.

42. Barrera I, Longoria D. Examining cultural mental health care barriers among Latinos. *Journal for Leadership, Equity, and Research.* 2018;4(1):1–12.

43. Asarnow JR, Rozenman M, Wiblin J, Zeltzer L. Integrated medical-behavioral care compared with usual primary care for child and adolescent behavioral health: a meta-analysis. *JAMA Pediatr.* 2015;169(10):929–937.

44. Brown JD, Wissow LS, Zachary C, Cook BL. Receiving advice about child mental health from a primary care provider: African American and Hispanic parent attitudes. *Med Care.* 2007;45(11):1076–1082.

45. Ishikawa RZ, Cardemil EV, Alegría M, Schuman CC, Joseph RC, Bauer AM. Uptake of depression treatment recommendations among Latino primary care patients. *Psychol Serv.* 2014;11(4):421–432.

46. Ali MM, West K, Teich JL, Lynch S, Mutter R, Dubenitz J. Utilization of mental health services in educational setting by adolescents in the United States. *J Sch Health.* 2019;89:393–401.

47. Kim G, Loi CXA, Chiriboga DA, Jang Y, Parmelee P, Allen RS. Limited English proficiency as a barrier to mental health service use: a study of Latino and Asian immigrants with psychiatric disorders. *J Psychiatr Res.* 2011;45(1):104–110.

48. Bear L, Finer R, Guo S, Lau AS. Building the gateway to success: an appraisal of progress in reaching underserved families and reducing racial disparities in school-based mental health. *Psychol Serv.* 2014;11(4):388–397.

49. Guo S, Kataoka SH, Bear L, Lau AS. Differences in school-based referrals for mental health care: understanding racial/ethnic disparities between Asian American and Latino youth. *Sch Ment Health.* 2014;6(1):27–39.

50. Kim RE, Becker KD, Stephan SH, et al. Connecting students to mental health care: pilot findings from an engagement program for school nurses. *Adv Sch Ment Health Promot.* 2015;8(2):87–103.

51. Bains RM, Cusson R, White-Frese J, Walsh S. Utilization of mental health services in school-based health centers. *J Sch Health.* 2017;87(8):584–592.

52. Mufson L, Dorta KP, Moreau D, Weissman MM. *Interpersonal Psychotherapy for Depressed Adolescents.* Guilford Press; 2004.

53. Portes A, Rumbaut RG. Introduction: the Second Generation and the Children of Immigrants Longitudinal Study. *Ethn Racial Stud.* 2005;28(6):983–999.

Brief Interpersonal Psychotherapy (IPT-B) for Perinatal Depression

HOLLY A. SWARTZ, MARY CURRAN, AND
NANCY K. GROTE (DECEASED) ∎

INTRODUCTION

Depression is a prevalent illness affecting 20% of individuals over their lifetime[1]; however, few receive adequate treatment.[2-4] This problem is magnified for women, who are twice as likely as men to experience a depressive episode[5] and are unlikely to engage in care.[6] Depression during pregnancy is common[7] and the most potent predictor of postpartum depression.[8] It is linked to low birth weight and prematurity, especially for socioeconomically disadvantaged women in the United States.[9] Maternal postpartum depression, in turn, has potential lasting adverse effects on maternal, infant, and child well-being.[10-13] Thus, detecting and treating depression during pregnancy is essential to the health of both mothers and children.[12,14]

Fortunately, treating maternal depression has downstream benefits for families.[15-17] Interpersonal psychotherapy (IPT), an excellent treatment for depression,[18] has demonstrated efficacy for postpartum depression.[19,20] Depressed women of childbearing age, however, are often overwhelmed by the demands of caring for their families and therefore may have difficulty engaging in treatment.[21-23] Putting their own needs behind those of everyone else for whom they feel responsible, many mothers do not prioritize their own mental health and are less likely to commit to a full course of psychotherapy.[24,25] These challenges are compounded when mothers are living on low incomes.[1,26] Thus, adapting IPT to meet the needs of depressed women of childbearing age, especially those on low incomes, requires systematic attention to practical and psychological barriers to care.

Holly A. Swartz, Mary Curran, and Nancy K. Grote (deceased), *Brief Interpersonal Psychotherapy (IPT-B) for Perinatal Depression* In: *Interpersonal Psychotherapy*. Edited by: Myrna M. Weissman and Jennifer J. Mootz, Oxford University Press. © Oxford University Press 2024. DOI: 10.1093/oso/9780197652084.003.0050

ADAPTING IPT FOR DEPRESSED MOTHERS ON LOW INCOMES

To address practical barriers to care, our team developed a shorter version of IPT,[27] Brief IPT (IPT-B),[28,29] which is designed to deliver a full course of IPT in 8 sessions, roughly half the length of "full-dose" 16-session IPT.[28] IPT-B offers the dual advantages of rapid relief from suffering and reduced practical barriers (time commitment) for overwhelmed populations. In IPT-B, time limits enhance intrinsic motivation for change by activating both therapist and patient to move quickly toward a resolution of interpersonal difficulties. Although encouragement to make rapid changes is part of standard IPT, in IPT-B the process is intensified and emphasized because of the foreshortened time course. The initial phase of IPT is limited to 2 (rather than 3) sessions, and the middle phase of treatment focuses on 1 of 3 (rather than 4) possible IPT problem areas. More so than in standard IPT, the IPT-B therapist moves quickly to explore potential avenues to help patients re-engage in positive interpersonally focused activities, often working on these tasks before addressing the complexities of the interpersonal problem area. Achieving a small amount of relief from depression (presumably by re-engaging in pleasurable activities) makes it easier for patients to then undertake the more challenging tasks required to resolve their interpersonal problems in 8 sessions.

THE ENGAGEMENT SESSION

We typically pair IPT-B with an engagement session based on principles of motivational interviewing (MI)[30] and ethnographic interviewing.[31] It precedes the first session of IPT-B and focuses on both the patient's perceptions of her problem(s) and specific impediments (psychological and practical) to participation in psychotherapy.[21,32] In the engagement session, therapists explore practical, psychological, and cultural barriers to depression treatment. Engagement session goals are to address and resolve ambivalence about treatment seeking and to increase motivation for change. It assumes patients will be more receptive to treatment when therapists communicate understanding of their individual and culturally embedded needs, perspectives, and experiences.

During the engagement session and IPT-B that follows, therapists use open-ended questions to build an alliance and create a person-centered therapeutic experience. Clinicians suspend their cultural biases and assumptions, adopt a stance of cultural humility,[33] and respect patients' autonomy and right of self-determination, even if some patient choices conflict with clinicians' core personal beliefs. This stance allows clinicians to develop an accurate understanding of the patient's experience from her own perspective.

The engagement session is organized into 5 sections that can be administered in a sequence that makes sense for each patient-clinician dyad: (1) *The Story*: The clinician explores the central dilemma as conceptualized by the patient, with special attention paid to the patient's mood symptoms (and how they impact her life) and the social context in which the story is unfolding (i.e., the impact of poverty, racism, etc. on her experiences); (2) *Treatment History and Hopes for Treatment:* Because so many patients have had prior experiences with treatment—both good and bad—it is imperative to explore these prior experiences and help patients voice their hopes for current treatment, either as a contrast to prior negative experiences or as follow-up to prior favorable experiences. It includes an exploration of formal mental health treatment as well as help-seeking activities such as pastoral support, traditional healers, or self-directed remedies; (3) *Feedback and Psychoeducation:* Using the MI strategy of elicit-provide-elicit (i.e., asking patients' permission before offering information and eliciting their reaction to the material once the information is given), the clinician summarizes information derived from the story, treatment hopes, and a standardized depression inventory such as the Patient Health Questionnaire-9 (PHQ-9)[34]; (4) *Barriers to Treatment Seeking:* Includes a systematic exploration of potential barriers to treatment seeking, with a focus on psychological and cultural factors; and (5) *Elicit Commitment:* The session ends with an outline of the next steps in seeking treatment.

Paired with an engagement session, IPT-B has been tested for depressed mothers of children with psychiatric disorders.[17] It was subsequently adapted by Nancy Grote and colleagues as an intervention for depressed pregnant women.[27] Further adaptations include delivering care in obstetrics and gynecology offices, flexible scheduling of treatment sessions at the clinic or on the phone, facilitation of access to social services, and use of maintenance IPT during the postpartum period to reduce risk for recurrence of depression.[35] This comprehensive approach to caring for depressed, low-income, women during the perinatal period is described below.

MOMCARE INTERVENTION

MOMCare, developed and tested by Nancy K. Grote, is a collaborative care intervention for perinatal depression delivered in public health clinics where women received social and maternity support services.[36] The MOMCare model focuses on the social context of current interpersonal functioning, chronic stressors associated with living in poverty, and biologic and psychological factors that contribute to perinatal depression. Women enter MOMCare while pregnant and are followed longitudinally for a year postdelivery. MOMCare includes the engagement session described above to help resolve practical, psychological, and cultural barriers to care; patient choice of IPT-B and/or pharmacotherapy from her obstetrics or primary care provider for acute treatment; telephone sessions in addition to in-person visits; outreach for women missing sessions, including texting, telephone calls; and utilizing depression care specialists (DCSs), who are part of the routine care team. The DCS follows participants every 1–2 weeks (in person or by telephone) during the acute phase of treatment (about 3–6 months postbaseline) and monthly during the maintenance phase of treatment (about 1 year postpartum) once a clinical response has been achieved.

Participants in the MOMCare study were depressed, pregnant women living on low incomes. Compared to usual care, MOMCare showed significant improvement in quality of care, depression severity, and remission rates from before birth to 18 months postbaseline for socioeconomically disadvantaged women.[36] MOMCare also mitigated the risk of postpartum depressive symptoms and impaired functioning among those with an adverse birth event.[37] Investigators further showed that MOMCare had an even greater impact on perinatal depressive outcomes for socioeconomically disadvantaged women with comorbid posttraumatic stress disorder (PTSD) than for those without PTSD.[38]

CASE EXAMPLE

Amika (name and identifying features changed to protect patient privacy) was a 20-year-old, first-time parent, 18 weeks pregnant, who identified as mixed race (African American/Hispanic). Amika worked full time at a pharmacy chain and lived with the father of the baby (FOB). A maternity support services (MSS) social worker referred her to MOMCare after she screened positive for depression on the PHQ-9, with a score of 15 (moderate severity).

During the engagement session, Amika endorsed feeling stressed with low energy, low mood, poor sleep, and worries about how her feelings might impact her baby. Stressors included an unplanned pregnancy, precarious finances, FOB unemployed, car breaking down, and conflict with FOB and her father around religious differences. Amika described a prior history of depression, which she managed through drawing, being in school, and prayer. She outlined barriers to treatment, such as time, unreliable transportation, and FOB not wanting her "talking about their business to other people." She had an unhelpful experience with counseling following a sexual assault, where the "counselor didn't understand [her]" and "just wanted to diagnose and medicate [her]." Amika and the therapist collaboratively addressed barriers to care, identifying need for flexibility in scheduling due to work and unreliable transportation as well as a preference for treatment by phone or at the clinic where she was receiving MSS. The therapist affirmed her wish to feel better before the baby was born and honored her self-efficacy in choosing whether to participate in treatment.

Initial IPT-B sessions focused on gathering a biopsychosocial-cultural history, understanding Amika's depression timeline, conducting the interpersonal inventory, and determining the IPT problem area. Amika's mood worsened after learning she was pregnant, compounded by financial worries and increased fighting with the FOB. The therapist and Amika explored supportive and stressful people in her life. Amika indicated that the FOB was supportive at times and hoped to be part of the baby's life. Amika's relationship with her parents, who divorced in her early teens, was tenuous. They also had financial challenges. Her dad, who was a devout Christian, provided practical support but wished Amika to return to the church, which was a source of conflict. Amika was unable to rely consistently on her mom, who also suffered from depression. Amika was close with her maternal grandmother, who helped raise her but was now deceased. The FOB's family was supportive. Amika identified coworkers and old high school friends as potential sources of support.

"Complicated pregnancy" is an additional IPT problem area relevant to some pregnant women and considered a subtype of role transition.[39] It was originally described by Spinelli and colleagues and refers to "unplanned, untimely, or overvalued pregnancy."[40] For Amika, the identified IPT problem area was a complicated pregnancy involving an unplanned pregnancy and limited social/financial resources. Treatment focused on helping Amika explore her feelings around the role transition, realistically assess what was lost, build social supports, connect with her baby, and learn ways to ask for what she wanted and needed to better manage the new social role. To build social support, Amika was encouraged to call old friends as a between-session homework assignment. Problem-solving around chronic stressors was integrated into each session by asking: "Who in your life might be helpful and in what ways?" Amika decided to ask her dad to help her fix her car and apply for a free cell phone and minutes. Amika identified her grandma as a source of strength, and she was sad that her grandma would not meet this baby. Amika identified supportive strategies her grandma might have recommended, such as "slow down, take one thing at a time, save money, and think before you act." Amika found her grandma's imagined words comforting, and they allowed her to feel less alone. As treatment progressed, she focused on the goals of feeling better, reducing stress, building support, and joining with the FOB around preparing for the baby. To promote treatment engagement and retention, we communicated with Amika regularly by text messages and offered flexible scheduling in the public health setting, which she found less stigmatizing than a mental health center.

Amika completed a full course of IPT-B (8 sessions), and her PHQ-9 score dropped to a 4 (not depressed range) before giving birth to a healthy, full-term baby boy, with the FOB and her mom in attendance. She engaged well with her baby and continued monthly maintenance sessions during the first postpartum year. Through IPT-B, she realized her feelings gave her important information about what she needed and helped her feel more able to ask for help from appropriate people. Though the FOB was not supportive of her decision, she decided to go back to school for a technical degree with the encouragement of the FOB's mother and grandmother. During the first postpartum year, she navigated numerous stressors without a recurrence of depression. This included an incident where the FOB physically assaulted her, leading to their breakup and eviction from their apartment. Despite these challenges, she completed her schooling, safely negotiated visitations with the FOB, managed expectations from her parents, and reconnected with supportive friends.

SUMMARY

The MOMCare pragmatic adaption of IPT-B strives to meet the needs of underserved communities, specifically socioeconomically disadvantaged, depressed individuals during the perinatal period. Significant adjustments to IPT include decreased duration of treatment, flexible delivery of care, the addition of maintenance IPT sessions in the postpartum period, and systematic attention to barriers to care and chronic stressors. Therapists employ engagement strategies throughout treatment, adopting a stance of cultural humility[33] to prioritize patients' lay expertise, culturally informed practices, and patient-centered strengths and resources. The MOMCare adaptation of IPT advances the health and well-being of those least likely to receive treatment.

ACKNOWLEDGMENTS

We would like to acknowledge the contributions of Nancy K. Grote, PhD. Dr. Grote was a seminal contributor to the work described in this chapter. She was the principal investigator for several projects funded by the National Institute of Mental Health to develop, test, and disseminate brief IPT for perinatal depression, especially for women on low incomes. Her wisdom and compassion continue to inspire many.

REFERENCES

1. Hasin DS, Sarvet AL, Meyers JL, et al. Epidemiology of adult *DSM-5* major depressive disorder and its specifiers in the United States. *JAMA Psychiatry.* 2018;75(4):336–346.
2. Kessler RC, Chiu WT, Demler O, Merikangas KR, Walters EE. Prevalence, severity, and comorbidity of 12-month *DSM-IV* disorders in the National Comorbidity Survey Replication. *Arch Gen Psychiatry.* 2005;62(6):617–627.
3. Moitra M, Santomauro D, Collins PY, et al. The global gap in treatment coverage for major depressive disorder in 84 countries from 2000–2019: a systematic review and Bayesian meta-regression analysis. *PLoS Med.* 2022;19(2):e1003901
4. Wang PS, Lane M, Olfson M, Pincus HA, Wells KB, Kessler RC. Twelve-month use of mental health services in the United States: results from the National Comorbidity Survey Replication. *Arch Gen Psychiatry.* 2005;62(6):629–640.
5. Kessler RC. Epidemiology of women and depression. *J Affect Disord.* 2003;74(1):5–13.
6. Swartz H, Shear M, Wren F, et al. Depression and anxiety among mothers who bring their children to a pediatric mental health clinic. *Psychiatric Serv.* 2005;56(9):1077–1083.
7. Norhayati MN, Hazlina NH, Asrenee AR, Emilin WM. Magnitude and risk factors for postpartum symptoms: a literature review. *J Affect Disord.* 2015;175:34–52.
8. O'Hara MW, McCabe JE. Postpartum depression: current status and future directions. *Annu Rev Clin Psychol.* 2013;9:379–407.
9. Grote NK, Bridge JA, Gavin AR, Melville JL, Iyengar S, Katon WJ. A meta-analysis of depression during pregnancy and the risk of preterm birth, low birth weight, and intrauterine growth restriction. *Arch Gen Psychiatry.* 2010;67(10):1012–1024.

10. Slomian J, Honvo G, Emonts P, Reginster JY, Bruyere O. Consequences of maternal postpartum depression: a systematic review of maternal and infant outcomes. *Womens Health (Lond)*. 2019;15:1745506519844044.

11. Weissman MM, Gammon GD, John K, et al. Children of depressed parents: increased psychopathology and early onset of major depression. *Arch Gen Psychiatry*. 1987;44(10):847–853.

12. Weissman MM, Olfson M. Translating intergenerational research on depression into clinical practice. *JAMA*. 2009;302(24):2695–2696.

13. Field TM. Infants of depressed mothers. In Johnson SL, Hayes AM, eds. *Stress, coping, and depression*. Lawrence Erlbaum Associates Publishers; 2000:3–22.

14. O'Hara MW, Engeldinger J. Treatment of postpartum depression: recommendations for the clinician. *Clin Obstet Gynecol*. 2018;61(3):604–614.

15. Weissman MM, Pilowsky DJ, Wickramaratne PJ, et al. Remissions in maternal depression and child psychopathology: a STAR*D-child report. *JAMA*. 2006;295(12):1389–1398.

16. Swartz HA, Frank E, Zuckoff A, et al. Brief interpersonal psychotherapy for depressed mothers whose children are receiving psychiatric treatment. *Am J Psychiatry*. 2008;165(9):1155–1162.

17. Swartz HA, Cyranowski JM, Cheng Y, et al. Brief psychotherapy for maternal depression: impact on mothers and children. *J Am Acad Child Adolesc Psychiatry*. 2016;55(6):495–503.

18. Weissman MM, Markowitz JC, Klerman GL. *The Guide to Interpersonal Psychotherapy*. Oxford University Press; 2018.

19. O'Hara MW, Pearlstein T, Stuart S, Long JD, Mills JA, Zlotnick C. A placebo controlled treatment trial of sertraline and interpersonal psychotherapy for postpartum depression. *J Affect Disord*. 2019;245:524–532.

20. O'Hara MW, Stuart S, Gorman LL, Wenzel A. Efficacy of interpersonal psychotherapy for postpartum depression. *Arch Gen Psychiatry*. 2000;57(11):1039–1045.

21. Swartz HA, Zuckoff A, Grote NK, et al. Engaging depressed patients in psychotherapy: integrating techniques from motivational interviewing and ethnographic interviewing to improve treatment participation. *Prof Psychol Res Pract*. 2007;38(4):430–439.

22. Ferro T, Verdeli H, Pierre F, Weissman MM. Screening for depression in mothers bringing their offspring for evaluation or treatment of depression. *Am J Psychiatry*. 2000;157(3):375–379.

23. Swartz HA, Shear MK, Greeno C, et al. Depression and anxiety among mothers bringing their children to a pediatric mental health clinic. *Psychiatric Serv*. 2005;56:1077–1083.

24. Swartz HA, Shear MK, Frank E, Cherry CR, Scholle SH, Kupfer DJ. A pilot study of community mental health care for depression in a supermarket setting. *Psychiatr Serv*. 2002;53(9):1132–1137.

25. Swartz HA, Shear MK, Wren FJ, et al. Depression and anxiety among mothers who bring their children to a pediatric mental health clinic. *Psychiatr Serv*. 2005;56(9):1077–1083.

26. Marmot M, Bell R. Fair society, healthy lives. *Public Health*. 2012;126(suppl 1): S4–S10.

27. Grote NK, Bledsoe SE, Swartz HA, Frank E. Feasibility of providing culturally relevant, brief interpersonal psychotherapy for antenatal depression in an obstetrics clinic: a pilot study. *Res Soc Work Pract*. 2016;14(6):397–407.

28. Swartz HA, Grote NK, Graham P. Brief interpersonal psychotherapy (IPT-B): overview and review of the evidence. *Am J Psychother*. 2014;68(4):443–462.

29. Swartz HA, Frank E, Shear MK, Thase ME, Fleming MAD, Scott J. A pilot study of brief interpersonal psychotherapy for depression in women. *Psychiatr Serv*. 2004;55:448–450.

30. Miller WR, Rollnick S. *Motivational Interviewing: Helping People Change*. 3rd ed. Guilford Press; 2013.

31. Schensul SL, Schensul JJ, LeCompte MD. *Essential Ethnographic Methods: observations, Interviews, and Questionnaires. Ethnographer's Toolkit 2*. Alta Mira Press; 1999.

32. Grote NK, Zuckoff A, Swartz HA, Bledsoe SE, Geibel SL. Engaging women who are depressed and economically disadvantaged in mental health treatment. *Social Work*. 2007;52(4):295–308.

33. Lekas HM, Pahl K, Fuller Lewis C. Rethinking cultural competence: shifting to cultural humility. *Health Serv Insights*. 2020;13:1178632920970580.

34. Kroenke K, Spitzer RL, Williams JB. The PHQ-9: validity of a brief depression severity measure. *J Gen Intern Med*. 2001;16(9):606–613.

35. Grote NK, Bledsoe SE, Swartz HA, Frank E. Culturally relevant psychotherapy for perinatal depression in low-income Ob/Gyn patients. *Clin Soc Work J*. 2004;32(3):327–347.

36. Grote NK, Katon WJ, Russo JE, et al. Collaborative care for perinatal depression in socioeconomically disadvantaged women: a randomized trial. *Depress Anxiety*. 2015;32(11):821–834.

37. Bhat A, Grote NK, Russo J, et al. Collaborative care for perinatal depression among socioeconomically disadvantaged women: adverse neonatal birth events and treatment response. *Psychiatr Serv*. 2017;68(1):17–24.

38. Grote NK, Katon WJ, Russo JE, et al. A randomized trial of collaborative care for perinatal depression in socioeconomically disadvantaged women: the impact of comorbid posttraumatic stress disorder. *J Clin Psychiatry*. 2016;77(11):1527–1537.

39. Spinelli MG, Endicott J. Controlled clinical trial of interpersonal psychotherapy versus parenting education program for depressed pregnant women. *Am J Psychiatry*. 2003;160(3):555–562.

40. Spinelli MG. *Interpersonal Psychotherapy for Perinatal Depression*. CreateSpace Independent Publishing Platform; 2017.

50

Telephone Interpersonal Psychotherapy Delivered by Nurses for Postpartum Depression

SOPHIE GRIGORIADIS, CINDY-LEE DENNIS, AND PAULA RAVITZ ■

THE CONTEXT OF THE WORK, INCLUDING GEOGRAPHIC AREA AND POPULATION

Our team conducted a randomized controlled trial (RCT) to evaluate interpersonal psychotherapy (IPT) delivered over the telephone by nurses for postpartum depression (PPD). PPD is a long-standing, global public health concern that affects the whole family unit.[1-3] Women prefer psychotherapy over pharmacological treatments.[4] Despite this, many do not seek psychotherapy as only 20% of those referred uptake psychotherapy treatment, and many drop out.[5] Numerous barriers limit access to psychotherapies for PPD, including the availability of mental health specialists and geographic barriers, especially in underserved rural areas.[6] Telephone delivery is an underutilized format that has demonstrated depression treatment efficacy.[7] It has flexibly in its delivery, is private and nonstigmatizing, and has the potential to reduce costs and the barriers to care access. Although advances in technology, such as the Internet, have enhanced the range of options available for communication, the telephone remains the most accessible to the majority of individuals.[8] IPT is recommend as a first-line treatment for PPD[9] given its demonstrated effectiveness.[10] Several telephone-IPT studies have showed promising results.[11-13] To address a gap in psychotherapy uptake, we adapted IPT

Sophie Grigoriadis, Cindy-Lee Dennis, and Paula Ravitz, *Telephone Interpersonal Psychotherapy Delivered by Nurses for Postpartum Depression* In: *Interpersonal Psychotherapy*. Edited by: Myrna M. Weissman and Jennifer J. Mootz, Oxford University Press. © Oxford University Press 2024. DOI: 10.1093/oso/9780197652084.003.0051 to be delivered by nonspecialist health workers over the telephone. To improve clinical utility, scalability, and accessibility of IPT for PPD, we changed both the specialized *provider* to trained nurses and the *medium* to telephone delivery and conducted an RCT to determine the effect of telephone-delivered IPT by trained public health nurses on PPD following 12 weeks of treatment. Our hypothesis was that fewer women who received nurse-delivered telephone-IPT would remain clinically depressed at 12 weeks than those who received standard PPD care in their community, with follow-up at 24 and 36 weeks.

The participants in the RCT were mothers who were between 2 and 24 weeks' postpartum and clinically depressed. They were recruited from across Canada, a multicultural country with vast rural areas where specialized healthcare is often difficult to access. Almost all Canadians, however, have access to a telephone.[14] Although Canada is a bilingual country, the trial was only offered in English as we did not have the funds for a bilingual trial, and it was conducted out of the University of Toronto.

We received 961 referrals between January 2009 and May 2012, with 241 women eligible and randomized. Public health departments from 36 health regions in 6 provinces across Canada screened and referred postpartum women, and women were also accepted following self-referral from advertisements. The majority (93.8%) of the participants were referrals from public health nurses and other health professionals (e.g., social workers, lactation consultants). We recruited our sample from across Canada, so we demonstrated the feasibility of providing the intervention nationally. Participants identified themselves as diverse in ethnicity. A third had low- or poverty-level annual household income, and a quarter had an educational level of high school or less. Thus, the generalizability of this study was excellent. Women were recruited on average at 12 weeks' postpartum (SD = 6.74). At 12 weeks' postrandomization, 204 (84.7%) participants completed the follow-up telephone interview, with 202 (83.8%) at 24 weeks and 197 (81.7%) at 36 weeks.

We found nurse-delivered telephone-IPT to be an effective treatment for diverse urban and rural postpartum women with clinical depression that can improve treatment access disparities. Compared to standard local care, nurse-delivered telephone-IPT significantly improved PPD, anxiety, and partner relationship quality at 12 weeks' postrandomization, with between group-differences in symptoms sustained to 36 weeks.

THE IPT TECHNOLOGY AND DELIVERY METHODS

Women allocated to the intervention group received 12 weekly 1-hour IPT sessions delivered by a trained nurse, with the first contact to initiate treatment occurring within 72 hours after trial enrollment. The 3 phases of IPT were administered according to the manual by Weissman et al.[15,16] In early sessions, the IPT nurses established a therapeutic alliance, provided psychoeducation about depression and IPT, placed the depression in an interpersonal context, reviewed the mother's current and past interpersonal relationships, identified the interpersonal problem area(s) most related to the current depressive episode, and set treatment goals. During the middle phase, treatment focused on resolving interpersonal difficulties, such as conflicts with a partner or extended family (interpersonal disputes) and changes in social roles associated with the challenges of new parenthood and needed support (role transitions). The concluding phase reinforced the mother's efforts, gains, and competence in working through the interpersonal problems and overcoming depression, with contingency planning in the event of depression recurrence. This trial defined intervention compliance as completing an IPT course of at least ten 30- to 60-minute sessions within 16 weeks.

The intervention was delivered over the telephone and digitally audio recorded to enable supervision and adherence. Women had no travel time to the session and could be anywhere to receive treatment, although we asked them to be in a private area away from distractions. Thus, they could receive the therapy in the comfort of their own home. The sessions were scheduled at a mutually convenient time for the mother and research nurse-therapist. Mothers came to describe the nurses as the "safe voice."

ADAPTATIONS MADE FOR DELIVERY THROUGH THE TECHNOLOGY AND FOR TRAINING AND SUPERVISION

IPT adaptation for nurse-delivered telephone delivery

As the telephone provides only an auditory medium, the lack of visual cues was a challenge. The therapists could not "see" the mother's emotions and whether she was close to tears or her behavior (i.e., sudden increased agitation or restlessness). Psychotherapy involves the pursuit of affect, and we needed to teach the nurses how to actively listen and ask for any cues. For example, the nurses asked the mothers what they were feeling when they heard a change in the mother's tone of voice and/or when discussing a potentially emotionally charged experience, such as struggles with breastfeeding, sleep, or marital conflict. In addition, nurses are skilled at problem-solving, and it was important not to automatically give advice. Alternatively, the nurses guided the mothers to reflect on the challenges of role transitions and/or role disputes and support them in generating their own ideas and options for coping. Although being in one's home provides an advantage to the mother of not having to hire child care, this often worked as a disadvantage for us as she may have had to interrupt therapy to attend to a child, which may have delayed the session. Once again, listening carefully during these times was used as a source of further psychosocial information. Confidentiality could not be guaranteed by us, and this could have affected the mother's willingness or ability to safely participate. At the outset, the nurses were instructed to inform the mothers to ensure no other adult was in the room, and the therapist had to learn to recognize signs that others, including family members with whom they may have been in conflict, with were present (e.g., pauses, one-word answers).

Silences, which are often useful in therapy, were more difficult to be patient with, and we trained the nurses to resist asking: "Are you still there?"

Safety was a potential issue, as is the case in all clinical care. We ensured the nurses had access to one of the supervisors 24 hours per day, and we needed to lower our threshold to make use of the public emergency response system if necessary. The trial being national made it challenging to keep the nurses abreast of community resources to inform the mothers in the termination phases for follow-up support if needed. Thus, our research assistant engaged in frequent searches to ensure we were up to date. One of the benefits of mental health experts providing in-person care from an office is that our credentials are displayed for our participants to be reminded, and thus the therapist has instant face validity of "expert." The telephone delivery, combined with the use of trained nurses, lacked this inherent positive attribute, which can work as a positive placebo. However, the nurses may have been alternatively experienced by the mothers as trustworthy and caring with less of a power differential, enabling them to feel safe to openly speak of their emotional experiences. Overall, we believe that the adaptations made to overcome the barriers strengthened the nurses' delivery of IPT.

IPT training and supervision

Seven registered female nurses based in Toronto were trained to provide the IPT intervention. The nurses were selected based on references and clinical experience initially. Only the public health nurses had clinical experience working with women with PPD; however, they did not use structured psychotherapies in their practice. The 3 mental health nurses had some experience of using psychotherapy in practice, but not for PPD. None of the nurses had clinical expertise in IPT. What was pivotal in the selection process was the nurse completing a telephone mock engagement session with an actor who portrayed a depressed mother. In this session, it was important that they conveyed empathy and understanding as this capacity is vital for an effective therapist. The nurses were then trained and clinically supervised by us, of which 2 were subsequently trained to become peer supervisors. Each nurse attended 8 hours of didactics followed by conducting two 12-session, clinically supervised telephone-IPT training cases with women experiencing PPD who were not involved in the trial. The nurses were required to achieve satisfactory competence and adherence prior to treating any trial participants, with adherence ratings on use of required IPT techniques.[17,18] During the trial, to enhance treatment fidelity, the nurses were continuously monitored for IPT adherence and used treatment-tracking forms with IPT phase- and focus-specific practice checklists. Examples of phase-specific checklist practice reminders included the following:

- conducting an interpersonal inventory with attention to the inclusion of the relationship with the baby (beginning phase)

- exploring the role transition changes, challenges, and what the mothers missed; conducting communication analyses in role disputes; recruiting or connecting with social supports (middle phase)
- reviewing progress, takeaways, and contingency plans in the event of relapse (termination phase).

Over the course of the trial, the nurse-therapists noted specific wording of questions and expressions of empathy for "just-in-time" practice reminders to aid them in their own "role transitions" from being nurses to being IPT therapists (see Figure 50.1).

Telephone-IPT sessions were digitally audio recorded to guide supervision and for adherence ratings. In-person or teleconferenced group supervision occurred weekly to uphold competence and the quality of the IPT being delivered. In addition, 25% of IPT session recordings were randomly selected from each of the 3

Interpersonal Inventory

- *Reflecting on relationships in the Interpersonal Inventory helps us to understand how having a baby has impacted your life and your relationships.*
- *Who: are the important people in your life? do you turn to or turns to you for comfort, help, or support? How has the relationship changed with the baby's birth, or been affected by your depression?*
- *What about with your relationship with you baby? and their states of feeling settled, happy, or not; how do you respond, and how does this affect your mood?*

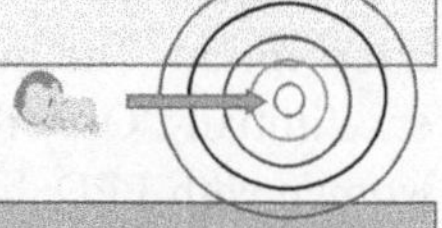

Role Transitions

- *You're experiencing a different side of yourself as a new mother along with a different sense of your partner as a co-parent.*
- *Ask/explore: how have things changed or affected you (ask for examples to tell you more about the changes they noticed).*
- *Ask/explore: how were things before the baby was born? what do you miss?*

To enhance therapeutic process, elicit affect and express empathy

- *It seems like you are really struggling to figure out how to adjust to being a parent of your son/daughter.*
- *I encourage you to be patient with yourself; people rarely snap out of depression; they gradually feel better with increasing connection to supportive others. Our goal is to actively work to ward helping you remit this depression. Tell me more about your struggles...*
- *If client is tearing-up, ask: What are in you in touch with right now? What's behind the tears?*

Figure 50.1 Practice examples of just-in-time reminders.
CREDIT: Adapted from training manual co-created with public health nurses, and baby image adapted from https://stock.adobe.com/sk/search/images?k=baby+diaper+cart oon&asset_id=295396603

treatment phases, and nurses were reviewed by an independent IPT-trained rater for treatment fidelity using an IPT adherence checklist. The rater was trained to achieve over 90% agreement with an IPT expert trainer on the adherence scale used for this trial. IPT nurses documented all intervention activities (telephone discussions, left messages, missed sessions) in an activity log. Strict safety protocols were developed, and adverse events were assessed through weekly IPT nurse discussions and a review of completed questionnaires by the trial coordinator. All these steps were taken to ensure the nurses delivered high-fidelity IPT.

BARRIERS TO AND FACILITATORS OF IMPLEMENTATION

Barriers

Out of the 120 women randomized to telephone-IPT, 104 (86.7%) complied by receiving 10 or more sessions lasting more than 30 minutes. There were 16 noncompliers, of which 7 received no sessions, 4 had 1–3 sessions, and 5 completed 4–6 sessions. Stated reasons for disinterest or inability to continue from participant interviews conducted by the trial coordinator included starting in-person therapy ($n = 1$), being too busy ($n = 1$), feeling better ($n = 2$), inability to connect with participants after repeated attempts ($n = 6$), repeated missed appointments ($n = 3$), and maternal choice to discontinue after an IPT nurse contacted a provincial child welfare agency as required by law due to safety concerns for the infant ($n = 3$). Of the 1216 IPT sessions provided in the trial, 909 (74.8%) were initiated as scheduled. Once initiated, 1189 (97.8%) sessions were completed.

Our most crucial challenge was to ensure the nurse became a proficient therapist. We recognized the core therapeutic foundational skills required empathy and understanding of the mother's life stage and devised our mock interview for the selection of the study therapists for this ability. Regardless, the nurse selection and training processes were initially labor intensive, and the supervisors' needed to be available constantly; developing 2 of the nurses into peer supervisors eased some of the workload and increased feasibility and scalability.

Facilitators

There was high treatment fidelity, as demonstrated through the intervention adherence ratings (86%). Of the 98 (81.7%) women who evaluated their IPT experience with a satisfaction questionnaire, the majority reported liking the telephone treatment (97.9%) and finding it to be convenient (94.9%). They also perceived the IPT nurses to be competent and well trained (99%) and the quality of the IPT sessions to be excellent (99%). They endorsed that IPT helped with their problems (96.9%), and that they would like to receive it again if they became depressed in the future (96%). Interestingly, 57 (58.2%) women indicated that they would have liked more than the planned 12 IPT sessions. The telephone-based intervention was thus highly acceptable to women, with a low dropout rate of less than 14%. In addition, we were able to access women from across the country through our use of the public health system.

FUTURE PLANS AND RECOMMENDATIONS

Future research should address questions regarding infant and interparental outcomes and potential moderators and mediators of acute and long-term treatment outcomes. We know that treatment is essential to prevent untoward infant outcomes, and demonstrating this for telephone delivered IPT will further increase its dissemination.

PUBLICATIONS RESULTING FROM THE WORK

The work based on the trial can be found in 3 sources. The first is the paper where our trial protocol was published. The second is the results of our trial, which were published in the *British Journal of Psychiatry*.[19,20] Our work was presented in many workshops in local venues to international scientific meetings. Currently, there are no translations, but our unpublished treatment manual, co-authored with some of the study nurses, was adopted by the Toronto Public Health organization, where nurses were subsequently trained to deliver IPT.[21] In summary, telephone-based IPT delivered by trained nurses for the treatment of clinically depressed mothers recruited across Canada was found to overcome many barriers to treatment access and to be highly effective with exemplary levels of patient satisfaction.

DECLARATION OF INTERESTS

None of us report any disclosures. All of us declare no support from any organization for the submitted work; no financial relationships with any organizations that might have an interest in the submitted work in the previous 3 years; no other relationships or activities that could appear to have influenced the submitted work.

REFERENCES

1. Howard LM, Molyneaux E, Dennis CL, Rochat T, Stein A, Milgrom J. Perinatal mental health 1 non-psychotic mental disorders in the perinatal period. *Lancet*. 2014;384(9956):1775–1788.
2. Netsi E, Pearson RM, Murray L, Cooper P, Craske MG, Stein A. Association of persistent and severe postnatal depression with child outcomes. *JAMA Psychiatry*. 2018;75(3):247–253.

3. Stein A, Pearson RM, Goodman SH, et al. Effects of perinatal mental disorders on the fetus and child. *Lancet*. 2014;384(9956):1800–1819.

4. McHugh RK, Whitton SW, Peckman AD, Welge JA, Otto MW. Patient preference for psychological vs pharmacologic treatment of psychiatric disorders: a meta-analytic review. *J Clin Psychiatry*. 2013;74(6):595–602.

5. Weddington WW Jr. Adherence by medical-surgical inpatients to recommendations for outpatient psychiatric treatment. *Psychother Psychosom*. 1983;39(4):225–235.

6. Ko JY, Farr SL, Dietz PM, Robbins CL. Depression and treatment among US pregnant and nonpregnant women of reproductive age, 2005–2009. *J Womens Health*. 2012;21(8):830–836.

7. Mohr DC, Vella L, Hart S, Heckman T, Simon G. The effect of telephone-administered psychotherapy on symptoms of depression and attrition: a meta-analysis. *Clin Psychol.* 2008;15(3):243–253.

8. Horton R, Peterson MG, Powell S, Engelhard E, Paget SA. Users evaluate LupusLine, a telephone peer counseling service. *Arthritis Care Res*. 1997;10(4):257–263.

9. Parikh SV, Quilty LC, Ravitz P, et al. Canadian Network for Mood and Anxiety Treatments (CANMAT) 2016 clinical guidelines for the management of adults with major depressive disorder: section 2. Psychological treatments. *Can J Psychiatry*. 2016;61(9):524–539.

10. O'Hara MW, Stuart S, Gorman LL, Wenzel A. Efficacy of interpersonal psychotherapy for postpartum depression. *Arch Gen Psychiatry*. 2000;57(11):1039–1045.

11. Heckman TG, Markowitz JC, Heckman BD, et al. A randomized clinical trial showing persisting reductions in depressive symptoms in HIV-infected rural adults following brief telephone-administered interpersonal psychotherapy. *Ann Behav Med*. 2018 Mar 15;52(4):299–308.

12. Neugebauer R, Kline J, Bleiberg K, et al. Preliminary open trial of interpersonal counseling for subsyndromal depression following miscarriage. *Depress Anxiety*. 2007;24(3):219–222.

13. Posmontier B, Neugebauer R, Stuart S, Chittams J, Shaughnessy R. Telephone-administered interpersonal psychotherapy by nurse-midwives for postpartum depression. *J Midwifery Womens Health*. 2016;61(4):456–466.

14. Canadian Radio-television and Telecommunications Commission. *Communications Monitoring Report 2018*. Canadian Radio-television and Telecommunications Commission; 2019.

15. Weissman M, Markowitz J, Klerman GL. *The Guide to Interpersonal Psychotherapy*. Oxford University Press; 2018.

16. Stuart S, Robertson M. *Interpersonal Psychotherapy: A Clinician's Guide*. Arnold; 2003.

17. Ravitz P, Grigoriadis S. *IPT for PPD: Phase-Specific Adherence Checklist* (adapted from Laura Mufson). University of Toronto; 2008.

18. Mufson L, Clougherty KF, Young JF, Verdeli H. *IPT-A Consultation Checklist*. State Psychiatric Institute, Columbia University College of Physicians and Surgeons; 2004.

19. Dennis CL, Ravitz P, Grigoriadis S, et al. The effect of telephone-based interpersonal psychotherapy for the treatment of postpartum depression: study protocol for a randomized controlled trial. *Trials*. 2012;13:38.

20. Dennis CL, Grigoriadis S, Zupancic J, Kiss A, Ravitz P. Telephone-based nurse-delivered interpersonal psychotherapy for postpartum depression: nationwide randomised controlled trial. *Br J Psychiatry.* 2020;216(4):189–196.

21. Ravitz P, Grigoriadis S, Biglieri S, Antunes M, Dennis CL. *Integrating IPT into Toronto Public Health Nursing: Toronto Public Health; 2015.* Unpublished manuscript.

51

Interpersonal Psychotherapy Delivered by Nurses

DANIEL WESEMANN AND TERESA JUDGE-ELLIS ∎

INTRODUCTION

Interpersonal psychotherapy (IPT) has been closely linked to nursing since its inception. Hildegard Peplau has been referred to as the mother of psychiatric-mental health nursing by developing one of the first advanced practice nursing programs in the 1950s.[1,2] Peplau tailored her educational program around her theory of nursing (theory of interpersonal relations).[3] For Peplau, one of the principles of nursing is that interpersonal relationships are foundational to the overall health of the individual.[1,3] Along with the emphasis away from the intrapersonal to the interpersonal, the phases of treatment are similar between the theories.

Other nurse theorists (i.e., Martha Rogers and Jean Watson) can also be connected to IPT as sharing theoretical foundations (i.e., Harry Sullivan) and focusing on the importance of the nurse-patient relationship as being transformational in the process of providing therapy and overcoming the challenges of clients.[1] Over time, nursing's use of IPT within practice and research has continued.

POSTPARTUM DEPRESSION TREATMENT

Postpartum depression can affect between 7% and 13% of all childbearing women and can have negative effects for the mother, child, and entire family system.[4,5] Caring for postpartum depression can be complicated as pharmacological interventions can be problematic for women wishing to breastfeed their infants since most psychopharmacological agents are expressed in the breast milk.[6] IPT

Daniel Wesemann and Teresa Judge-Ellis, *Interpersonal Psychotherapy Delivered by Nurses* In: *Interpersonal Psychotherapy*. Edited by: Myrna M. Weissman and Jennifer J. Mootz, Oxford University Press. © Oxford University Press 2024. DOI: 10.1093/oso/9780197652084.003.0052 has a long-standing history of addressing the needs of women with postpartum depression due to multiple issues with IPT's core focus of treatment (interpersonal disputes, role transitions, grief, and interpersonal deficits) in this population.[1,7] IPT has continued to have a high level of evidence in treating postpartum depression. A meta-analysis of depressed mothers with infants in neonatal intensive care units found that multiple nursing interventions were beneficial in providing support. One of the interventions that was most effective was IPT.[8] Nurses have begun using IPT remotely to provide telehealth treatment to effectively care for women with postpartum depression. With the COVID-19 pandemic forcing many to provide treatment remotely, nurse and nurse midwives used remote training methods effectively to employ psychological interventions such as IPT.[9] Dennis et al.[4] used registered nurses to provide IPT to new mothers with postpartum depression and found that the group receiving IPT was 4.5 times less likely to have depression. This study has significant impact due to the nurses coming from various clinical backgrounds (e.g., public health, emergency room, and pediatric) and none were from mental health. This underscores the ability of IPT to be trained to nurses without graduate education as a cost-effective intervention. Posmontier et al.[5] also provided IPT remotely using telephones and facilitated by nurse-midwives. This study found that the nurse midwives adhered to the IPT protocol and overcame the apprehension of the women engaging in IPT to use psychotherapy and not medication for their postpartum depression. The study found statistically significant improvement with depression levels but did not find improvement with their global assessment of functioning and mother-infant bonding scores. While postpartum depression can affect women across the socioeconomic spectrum, low-income women can have more restrictions to access to care and worse outcomes even into the child's early developmental years. A randomized controlled study led by a nurse researcher demonstrated using IPT as effective in increasing bonding between low-income mothers and their infant and toddler children.[10]

INTERPERSONAL COUNSELING

Interpersonal counseling (IPC) was developed in 2000 for medical providers who do not have mental health expertise.[11] IPC has been effective as depressed patients have reported a preference for IPC over taking psychotropic medications for their depression.[12] A recent study has also shown that IPC compared to IPT can be effectively implemented by psychiatric nurses at a primary care clinic, who then refer patients to psychologists providing IPT after using IPC as an initial phase treatment alternative.[13] The implications for nurses using IPC are significant as nurses are already working within medical clinics, and an estimated 60% of mental health care delivery is within the primary care provider office.[14] There is also a growing number of primary care nurse practitioners (family nurse practitioners, adult-gerontology nurse practitioners, and pediatric nurse practitioners) who are seeking dual certification within primary care and psychiatric-mental health.[15] These dually certified nurse practitioners provide integrated medical and mental health services within their practice. IPC could have a significant impact for these dually certified nurse practitioners. The case example in this chapter provides greater context for this clinical application.

EDUCATION OF NURSES PERFORMING IPT

In 1979, the American Nurses Association developed certification for the psychiatric-mental health certified nurse specialist (PMHCNS).[16] The PMHCNS was to use psychotherapy as the primary intervention in graduate nursing programs and the advance practiced registered nurses (APRNs) to receive primary training as psychotherapists. In 2014, the PMHCNS certification was discontinued, and the psychiatric-mental health nurse practitioner (PMHNP) certification became the only path for APRNs wanting psychiatric-mental health certification.[2] This left PMHNP programs with the difficult task of teaching their students how to prescribe medications and provide psychotherapy to their clients without significantly increasing their plans of study and clinical requirements.[17]

The PMHNPs have been moving away from the role of psychotherapist engaging in more prescriber roles enticed by allure of higher salaries related to higher billing for medication management appointments.[2,17] According to the Centers for Medicare Services (CMS) reimbursement rates, in 2019 the difference between doing just medication management and psychotherapy for 1 hour is around $170 in favor of prescribing medications (99213 = $61.93 per 15 minutes and 90834 = $78.69 per 45–0 minutes, respectively).

The 2019 CMS reimbursement rates for PMHNPs[18-20] caused concern that PMHNP programs were emphasizing the psychopharmacology content over the psychotherapy content due to graduates going into prescribing-only roles. In 2022, a national survey found that PMHNP programs were still providing psychotherapy content within their program but with significant variance. PMHNP program directors who responded ($N = 39$; 26%) to the survey reported that they were most often teaching cognitive behavioral therapy and motivational interviewing as their top two psychotherapy theories. IPT was found to be in third place with 59% of the PMHNP programs teaching their students IPT to a level of competency[21] (Figure 51.1).

The PMHNP programs continue to struggle with either providing in-depth education and experience to 2 psychotherapy theories or providing a broad approach to psychotherapy education and teaching several theories to a basic level of competency.[21] One strategy that PMHNP programs could use to ensure their students would have a strong background in performing IPT would be to offer an intensive weekend course of IPT training. The course would be for 16 hours over 2 days and provided by an IPT-certified supervisor or certified trainer (level D or E). The PMHNP student would then be at level A certification and could move into advanced supervision and work toward level B certification and higher once the PMHNP student graduates from their respective PMHNP program. The difficulty with this is finding an IPT supervisor or trainer to do this for the students. The financial difficulties are several as well with either having the trainer volunteer

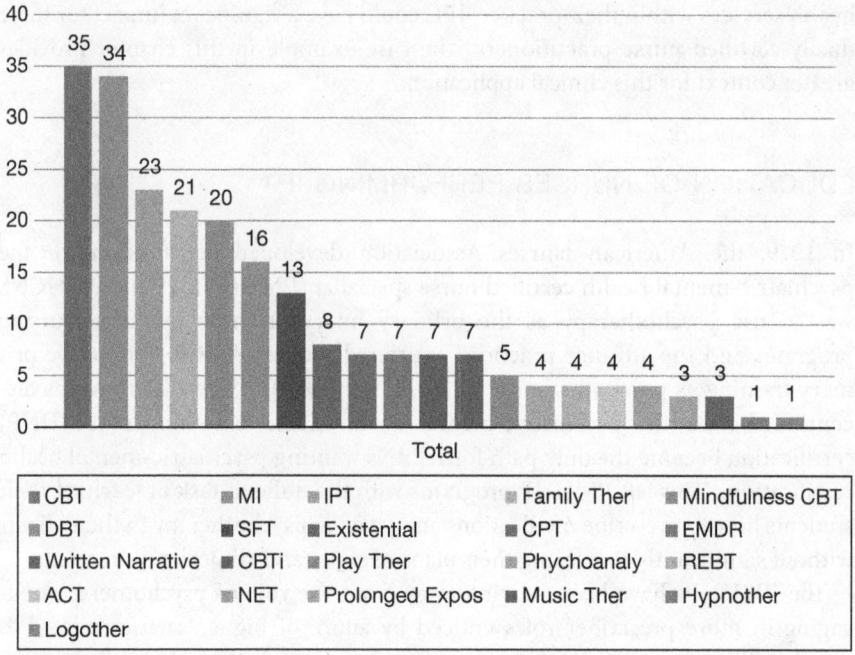

Figure 51.1 Psychotherapy theories reported to be taught by PMHNP program directors.[21] CBT, cognitive behavioral therapy; DBT, dialectical behavioral therapy; MI, motivational interviewing.
CREDIT: Wesemann D (the first author of this chapter), Convoy S, Goldstein D, Melino K. How PMHNP program directors facilitate psychotherapeutic skill acquisition. *Journal of the American Psychiatric Nurses Association.* 2022:10783903221091980.

their time or adding an expense to PMHNP students to attend this training. If PMHNP programs can navigate this complication, then their program can graduate PMHNPs into the workforce with an appreciation and understanding for the evidence-based approach of IPT.

CASE EXAMPLE

The following case study illustrates the use of IPT in a nurse-led integrated primary care/psychiatry practice in a rural Midwestern town. The nurse therapist in this case study is a dually certified family nurse practitioner and PMHNP.

Assessment phase

B. N., a 78-year-old woman, presented to the clinic with the chief complaint of urinary incontinence. This was her first visit to the dually certified nurse practitioner (hereafter referred to as NP).

B. N. stated that her friends from church had told her that the NP was easy to talk to and a good listener. Even though B. N. had a "regular doctor" in town 25 miles away, NP listened to and processed B. N.'s symptoms about her urinary issues. Throughout the interview, NP noted B. N.'s affect to be blunted, her speech slow and of normal volume, and her thoughts linear, however not quick to initiate or clearly define their character, needing mild direction to narrow the urinary incontinence symptoms and give a clear history of symptom progression. Through gentle clarification, it appeared that the urinary incontinence symptoms were chronic in nature. NP noted that B. N. had chosen not to fill out any of the previsit paperwork, which included a Patient Health Questionnaire-2 screen for depression.

NP assessed that other health issues might have been driving B. N.'s visit. First, she had been referred to NP because she was a "good listener." Second, B. N.'s symptoms were not pointing to an acute exacerbation or dramatic change of a chronic condition. Third, although this was the first visit with B. N., her mental status exam along with an unfinished depression screening tool pointed toward the need for further evaluation of B. N.'s mental health.

NP: B. N., it sounds as though you have a chronic issue with urinary incontinence and that these symptoms have remained constant, meaning there has not been a pattern change in the past several months.

B. N.: Yes, I suppose that is accurate.

NP: OK, well we can revisit these symptoms and do a further exam or work up in the future at any time.

B. N.: [*nods in agreement*]

NP: I am interested in how else you are doing. What have you been up to these days?

Long silence

B. N.: Not much. Usually I am more excited about Christmas.

NP: [*silence*]

B. N.: I can't think about it, but my son died last November. Things won't be the same and I just can't think about it.

[*B. N. disclosed that her son, previously healthy, had died suddenly of a pulmonary embolus the day before Thanksgiving just over 1 year ago.*]

[*NP noted that there were no thoughts of suicide or passive death wish and confirmed this with B. N. NP also included B. N. in the process of naming her symptoms as those of depression and grief.*]

B. N.: I came in for urinary incontinence and now I have depression and grief?

NP: You feel confused because you hadn't considered that we would end up talking about mental health.

B. N.: Yes, now what do I do?

NP: We could work on this together, address this as another health issue.

B. N.: What would that look like? Could you do that? I don't have a lot of time to travel out of town for more visits.

NP asked B. N. to return to the clinic within the next week for another visit focused on her depression and grief. B. N. was adamantly opposed to psychiatric medications and chose to begin therapy sessions with the NP.

Middle phase

The following two sessions focused on B. N.'s memories at the time of her son's death. IPT techniques and goals of facilitating the grief process and increasing socialization became an agreed on focus. B. N. had been out shopping when her son had died. She was told of his death by her son's wife, Lisa. B. N. recalled this as a loving experience with Lisa, however, was frustrated with herself that she then became "numb" throughout the rest of the immediate grieving time. She felt guilty that she hadn't thanked Lisa. NP engaged B. N. in the process of gaining courage to meet with Lisa and visualizing the encounter as one to help B. N. with her goal of "thanking" Lisa for her support. Together NP and B. N. worked on the "script" for the phone call and did small role play conversations.

B. N. returned for the fifth session after a successful visit with Lisa.

B. N.: I feel like a veil is lifted and I can have a good relationship with her again. That was a good decision. Lisa said she was glad that I called her! She had been sad too and so we talked a lot about that.

NP: While at times uncomfortable, sharing an intimate, painful experience can be worth the risk as it increases intimacy and enhances relationships.

[*B. N. agreed that she felt improved mood. The positive encounter and sharing with Lisa provided an opportunity to learn more about B. N.'s other relationships.*]

[*B. N.'s main social outlet was her church's women's group, which met monthly. Through that, B. N. knew 3 other women, all widows, who were her closest friends. They met weekly to sew and have lunch.*]

[*B. N. said that she had cut back and had missed the last monthly group meeting. B. N. acknowledged that it might be helpful to speak with her friends about her grief.*]

B. N.: We just don't talk about this. We all know that it's hard. We support one another; we just don't talk like this.

Termination phase

Three weeks passed before B. N. was able to get in for her sixth session. Each session started with: "What have you been up to since the last time you were here?" In earlier sessions, B. N. had a difficult time retrieving activities to report, often saying: "I am watching TV" or "I'm not sure, I went to church and the grocery store."

B. N. (sixth session): Well, you won't believe it, but I did it. It was very scary. You know we don't talk about this sort of thing. We were in our sewing time, and I said that I was still very sad about my son's death. We all kept sewing. I asked them what they remembered about the funeral. They each told me something different. I know I started to cry, but I just focused on my sewing. We didn't talk about this for a long time; we talked about other things, too. But as we were leaving, 2 of my friends stayed back and each gave me a hug and told me that it was good to talk like that and that they missed me in the group and were glad I was back.

B. N.: Grief is hard. It does help me to get back to my activities, and I'm so glad that I can talk to my daughter-in-law again. That has been helpful. [*NP offered a return appointment for follow up, and B. N. declined. NP asked B. N. whether she had any overall concerns about her health to review. B. N. said no and that the urinary incontinence was no longer a major concern, but that she would follow up with NP about this.*]

NP: B. N., I'm glad that you came in.

B. N.: Thank you. It's good that people like you exist to help people like me.

NP: You worked hard. Grief work is hard.

B. N.: I'm glad I talked to the people I did. Thank you for your help.

REFERENCES

1. Wheeler K. *Psychotherapy for the Advanced Practice Psychiatric Nurse: A How-to Guide for Evidence-Based Practice.* Springer Publishing Company; 2013:419–440.

2. Jones JS, Tusaie K, eds. *Fast Facts for the Nurse Psychotherapist: The Process of Becoming.* Springer Publishing Company; 2019.

3. Fawcett J. Peplau's theory of interpersonal relations. In *Contemporary Nursing Knowledge: Analysis and Evaluation of Nursing Models and Theories.* 2nd ed. F. A. Davis Company; 2005.

4. Dennis CL, Grigoriadis S, Zupancic J, Kiss A, Ravitz P. Telephone-based nurse-delivered interpersonal psychotherapy for postpartum depression: nationwide randomised controlled trial. *Br J Psychiatry.* 2020;216(4):189–196.

5. Posmontier B, Neugebauer R, Stuart S, Chittams J, Shaughnessy R. Telephone-administered interpersonal psychotherapy by nurse-midwives for postpartum depression. *J Midwifery Womens Health.* 2016;61(4):456–166.

6. Stahl S. *Prescriber Guide: Stahl's Essential Psychopharmacology.* 7th ed. Cambridge University Press; 2020.

7. Stuart S, Robertson M. *Interpersonal Psychotherapy: A Clinician's Guide.* 2nd ed. Hodder Education; 2012.

8. Maleki M, Mardani A, Harding C, Basirinezhad MH, Vaismoradi M. Nurses' strategies to provide emotional and practical support to the mothers of preterm infants in the neonatal intensive care unit: a systematic review and meta-analysis. *Womens Health.* 2022;18:17455057221104674.

9. Wang TH, Tzeng YL, Teng YK, Pai LW, Yeh TP. Evaluation of psychological training for nurses and midwives to optimise care for women with perinatal depression: a systematic review and meta-analysis. *Midwifery*. 2022;104:103160.

10. Beeber LS, Schwartz TA, Holditch-Davis D, Canuso R, Lewis V, Hall HW. Parenting enhancement, interpersonal psychotherapy to reduce depression in low-income mothers of infants and toddlers: a randomized trial. *Nurs Res*. 2013;62(2):82–90.

11. Weissman MM, Markowitz JC, Klerman G. *Comprehensive Guide to Interpersonal Psychotherapy*. Basic Books; 2008.

12. Magnani M, Sasdelli A, Bellino S, et al. Treating depression: what patients want; findings from a randomized controlled trial in primary care. *Psychosomatics*. 2016;57(6):616–623.

13. Kontunen J, Timonen M, Muotka J, Liukkonen T. Is interpersonal counselling (IPC) sufficient treatment for depression in primary care patients? A pilot study comparing IPC and interpersonal psychotherapy (IPT). *J Affect Disord*. 2016;189:89–93.

14. Park LT, Zarate CA Jr. Depression in the primary care setting. *N Engl J Medic*. 2019;380(6):559–568.

15. Wesemann DE, Dirks MS, Van Cleve SN. Dual-track education for nurse practitioners: current and future directions. *J Nurse Pract*. 2021;17(6):732–736.

16. Wheeler K. *The Nurse Psychotherapist and a Framework for Practice*. Springer Publishing; 2022:419–440.

17. Wesemann DE, Handrup C. Where is the psychotherapy content in PMHNP programs? *Perspect Psychiatr Care*. 2022;58(3):1077–1081.

18. Wesemann D. Maximizing the use of psychotherapy with PMHNP: a call to action for nurse leaders. *Nurse Leader*. 2019;17(6):537–541.

19. American Medical Association. Fee schedule for community/private mental health centers effective July 1, 2019. 2017. https://medicaid.ms.gov/wp-content/uploads/2014/03/CommunityMentalHealthCenter.pdf. Accessed September 17, 2023.

20. American Medical Association. Fee schedule for psychiatrist and psychiatric mental health nurse practitioners for mental health/psychiatric services. 2019. https://medicaid.ms.gov/wp-content/uploads/2014/03/MentalHealthPsychiatry.pdf

21. Wesemann D, Convoy S, Goldstein D, Melino K. How PMHNP program directors facilitate psychotherapeutic skill acquisition. *J Am Psychiatr Nurses Assn*. 2022:10783903221091980.

Interpersonal Psychotherapy for Post-traumatic Stress Disorder (PTSD)

JOHN C. MARKOWITZ ■

We live in a violent world beset by all too many natural and human traumas. A significant percentage of these traumas result in post-traumatic stress disorder (PTSD), a debilitating syndrome of rising prevalence.[1,2] Patients with PTSD suffer from anxiety, mistrust, depressive symptoms, emotional detachment, and reexperiencing of painful memories.[3] They often try to ignore or suppress these traumatic memories, feelings, and symptoms, leading to delay in seeking treatment.[4]

Post-traumatic stress disorder is treatable. Evidence-based treatments include pharmacotherapy with serotonin reuptake inhibitors and other medications and principally with exposure-based treatments. Exposure, based on simple behavioral principles, requires patients to face their fears of traumas that they have desperately tried to avoid, so much so that almost everything has come to remind them of it. Facing one's fears leads to habituation, with decreased anxiety and recognition that one has experienced something horrible, but that the memory and its associated cues are not themselves dangerous. Exposure-based therapy is the best studied approach to PTSD, benefits many people, and gets primary recommendations in PTSD guidelines. On the other hand, this grueling, painful treatment has high rates of patient refusal and high dropout. Moreover, no treatment approach benefits all patients.

Two decades ago, we began to explore the expansion of interpersonal psychotherapy (IPT) to anxiety disorders, a *Diagnostic and Statistical Manual of Mental Disorders* (*DSM*)[3] category that then included PTSD. In fact, PTSD appeared the ideal target for a therapy that focuses on the connection between mood symptoms

John C. Markowitz, *Interpersonal Psychotherapy for Post-traumatic Stress Disorder (PTSD)* In: *Interpersonal Psychotherapy.*
Edited by: Myrna M. Weissman and Jennifer J. Mootz, Oxford University Press. © Oxford University Press 2024.
DOI: 10.1093/oso/9780197652084.003.0053

and life events. PTSD was the only *DSM* disorder specifically defined by a traumatic life event (Criterion A), and patients with PTSD clearly have affect-related difficulties. They characteristically show little or no affect, reporting that they feel numb, as they actively detach themselves from their emotions. Further, research had shown that social support is both a risk factor for and at risk from PTSD: Patients, feeling frightened and unsafe, mistrust other people and isolate themselves, whereas social support is an important protective factor against developing PTSD and an aid in recovery. Because IPT addresses affect in the context of a distressing life event and has been shown to mobilize social support, it appeared a good fit for PTSD.[5]

It was clear from the outset that IPT, as an affect-focused therapy, would approach PTSD differently from exposure-based treatments. There would be no homework or exposure exercises. The goal would not be to relive the details of the trauma, but rather to explore how the trauma had affected the patient's feelings and social life. To do this, it was necessary to first elicit how patients felt, to reclaim feelings patients were pushing out of their awareness. We suggested that "feelings are powerful, but not dangerous," and that a key to determining whom one could trust was knowing how you felt about another person.[5]

Early sessions were spent in large part on "affective attunement," helping benumbed patients to let upsetting feelings (negative affects) register in social situations, and then to parse that "upset" into specific emotions, such as anxiety, sadness, and anger. Having elicited these emotions, the therapist let the patient sit with them and helped to normalize them. This led to exploring why a patient might be annoyed by another person and what options he or she had to detail with it. A key sequence often arose wherein a patient would initially reluctantly acknowledge anger toward someone, then agree that the anger made sense, role play expressing it, and later confront the offending person. This confrontation often led to an apology and knowledge that the other person might be trustworthy; or a brushoff and evidence of untrustworthiness. So IPT for PTSD focused on the present, not the traumatic past, and on how the traumatized patient could optimally interact to test and build trust with other people. We incorporated this adaptation of IPT, a radical departure from exposure-based therapies, into a treatment manual.[5] Aside from the need for affective attunement of patients, the therapist needs background knowledge of PTSD and a tolerance of strong negative affect. Otherwise, this is standard IPT.

Even in the immediate aftermath of September 11, 2001, when the National Institute of Mental Health (NIMH) was issuing emergency trauma grants to deal with PTSD, grant reviewers were skeptical. The dogma in the field was that exposure was necessary to treat PTSD. "How will IPT handle flashbacks?" one grant reviewer wanted to know. Despite our argument that most disorders responded to more than one treatment approach, and that relieving symptoms in one (here, interpersonal) domain led to generalized syndromal improvement, NIMH declined to fund an IPT study.

In collaboration with Kathryn Bleiberg, PhD, in New York, I conducted a small open trial of IPT for PTSD, which yielded highly positive results (including improvement in flashbacks).[6] This led to NIMH funding our 14-week randomized controlled trial comparing IPT to prolonged exposure (PE), the best tested exposure therapy; and to relaxation therapy (RT), an active control condition, for 110 unmedicated patients with chronic PTSD. We found IPT improved PTSD symptoms more than did RT and no less well than PE.[7] Moreover, patients preferred[8] and were (nonsignificantly) less likely to drop out of IPT.[7] IPT also had advantages for the 50% of patients who had comorbid major depression[7] and for patients whose trauma involved sexual abuse.[9] Patients who responded (≥30% improvement) or remitted after 14 weeks of IPT were likely to remain better at 3-month follow-up.[10]

One controlled trial is encouraging, but demonstrating efficacy requires multiple trials from multiple research groups. Thankfully, this has been forthcoming. Janice Krupnick, PhD, and colleagues published the first randomized controlled trial of IPT, in group format, and found it more efficacious than a waiting list control for multiply traumatized, non-treatment-seeking women in medical and gynecological clinics.[11] Marcelo Feijo de Mello, MD, PhD, and his group have now published 2 related studies: In the first, IPT showed benefit for patients who received it in addition to antidepressant medication, compared to medication alone.[12] They have just published a randomized controlled trial finding IPT and sertraline equally effective for patients with PTSD following a recent sexual assault.[13] Our group published an open trial of IPT for combat veterans with PTSD, a high-risk group for PTSD with historically poor response to exposure therapy, and we again found encouraging results.[14] We await the first controlled trial for veterans, a comparison of IPT with PE,[15] which Drs. M. Tracie Shea, Krupnick, and colleagues are on the verge of publishing. It also purportedly shows IPT to be no less effective than exposure therapy, with possible advantages.

It has taken 2 decades, but IPT has now been mentioned in the latest US Department of Defense/Veterans Administration treatment guidelines as a treatment for PTSD.[16] How does IPT help patients? It may work by repairing disrupted attachment and affect dysregulation[17] and possibly through effects in the anterior hippocampus.[18] IPT provides a more comfortable, patient-preferred alternative to exposure-based treatments and to medication, and it is likely to be accepted in cultures that might find exposure therapy inimical or off-putting, as Dr. Susan Meffert and colleagues have found.[19,20] IPT may also help address the new or reawakened PTSD symptoms many patients have suffered under the stresses of the COVID-19 pandemic.[21]

We hope that further research will test IPT for PTSD in different settings, formats, and different treatment populations, and that this now evidence-based treatment can be disseminated around the world for populations in need.

REFERENCES

1. Mental Health America. 2021 The state of mental health in America. 2020. Accessed May 4, 2023. https://mhanational.org/sites/default/files/2021%20State%20of%20Mental%20Health%20in%20America_0.pdf

2. Markowitz JC. *In the Aftermath of the Pandemic: Interpersonal Psychotherapy for Anxiety, Depression, and PTSD.* Oxford University Press; 2021.

3. American Psychiatric Association. *Diagnostic and Statistical Manual of Mental Disorders (DSM-5)* 5th ed. American Psychiatric Association; 2013.

4. Wang PS, Berglund P, Olfson M, Pincus HA, Wells KB, Kessler RC. Failure and delay in initial treatment contact after first onset of mental disorders in the National Comorbidity Survey Replication. *Arch Gen Psychiatry.* 2005;62(6):603–613.

5. Markowitz JC. *IPT for PTSD: Interpersonal Psychotherapy for Posttraumatic Stress Disorder.* Oxford University Press; 2016.

6. Bleiberg KL, Markowitz JC. Interpersonal psychotherapy for posttraumatic stress disorder. *Am J Psychiatry.* 2005;162(1):181–183.

7. Markowitz JC, Petkova E, Neria Y, et al. Is exposure necessary? A randomized clinical trial of interpersonal psychotherapy for PTSD. *Am J Psychiatry.* 2015;172(5):430–440.

8. Markowitz JC, Meehan KB, Petkova E, et al. Treatment preferences of psychotherapy patients with chronic PTSD. *J Clin Psychiatry.* 2016;77(3):363–370.

9. Markowitz JC, Neria Y, Lovell K, Van Meter PE, Petkova E. History of sexual trauma moderates psychotherapy outcome for posttraumatic stress disorder. *Depress Anxiety.* 2017;34(8):692–700.

10. Markowitz JC, Choo T, Neria Y. Stability of improvement after psychotherapy of posttraumatic stress disorder. *Can J Psychiatry/La Revue Canadienne de Psychiatrie* 2018;63:37–43.

11. Krupnick JL, Green BL, Stockton P, Miranda J, Krause E, Mete M. Group interpersonal psychotherapy for low-income women with posttraumatic stress disorder. *Psychother Res.* 2008;18(5):497–507.

12. Campanini RF, Schoedl AF, Pupo MC, Costa AC, Krupnick JL, Mello MF. Efficacy of interpersonal therapy-group format adapted to post-traumatic stress disorder: an open-label add-on trial. *Depress Anxiety.* 2010;27(1):72–77.

13. Proença CR, Markowitz JC, Coimbra BM, et al. Interpersonal psychotherapy versus sertraline for women with posttraumatic stress disorder following recent sexual assault: a randomized clinical trial. *Eur J Psychotraumatol.* 2022;13(2):2127474.

14. Pickover A, Lowell A, Lazarov A, et al. Interpersonal psychotherapy of posttraumatic stress disorder for veterans and family members: an open trial. *Psychiatr Serv.* 2021;72(8):866–873.

15. Shea MT, Krupnick JL, Sautter FJ, et al. Rationale, design, and methods of a two-site randomized controlled trial: effectiveness of two treatments for posttraumatic stress disorder in veterans. *Contemp Clin Trials.* 2021;105:106408.

16. Department of Veterans Affairs. *VA/DoD Clinical Practice Guideline for the Management of Posttraumatic Stress Disorder and Acute Stress Disorder.* US Department of Veterans Affairs; 2017. Accessed May 4, 2023.https://www.health quality.va.gov/guidelines/MH/ptsd/VADoDPTSDCPGClinicianSummaryFi nal.pdf.

17. Milrod B, Keefe JR, Choo T-H, et al. Separation anxiety in PTSD: a pilot prevalence and treatment study. *Depress Anxiety.* 2020;37(4):386–395.

18. Suarez-Jimenez B, Zhu X, Lazarov A, et al. Anterior hippocampal volume predicts affect-focused psychotherapy outcome. *Psychol Med.* 2020;50(3):396–402.

19. Jiang RF, Tong HQ, Delucchi KL, Neylan TC, Shi Q, Meffert SM. Interpersonal psychotherapy versus treatment as usual for PTSD and depression among Sichuan earthquake survivors: a randomized clinical trial. *Confl Health*. 2014;8:14.

20. Meffert SM, Neylan TC, McCulloch CE, et al. The Mental Health, HIV, and Domestic Violence (MIND) study: a randomized, controlled trial of scalable, non-specialist mental health care for HIV-positive women affected by gender based violence. *PloS Med*. 2021;18(1):e1003468.

21. Markowitz JC. *In the Aftermath of the Pandemic: Interpersonal Psychotherapy for Anxiety, Depression, and PTSD*. Oxford University Press; 2021.

53

Interpersonal Psychotherapy With Sexual and Gender Minority Individuals

JEREMY D. KIDD, ROMA KACZMARKIEWICZ, S. J. LANGER, CLAIRE KOLJACK, AND TONDA L. HUGHES ■

OVERVIEW AND DEFINITION OF TERMS

Sexual minority (SM) includes lesbian, gay, bisexual, queer, or any otherwise nonheterosexual people. *Gender minority* (GM) refers to transgender, nonbinary, and gender diverse people whose gender identity (i.e., internal sense of being a man, woman, another gender, or no gender) differs from the sex they were assigned at birth. *Cisgender, cisman,* and *ciswoman* describe people whose gender identity aligns with sex assigned at birth. Importantly, SM and GM are not always mutually exclusive because sexual and gender identity are distinct concepts (e.g., GM individuals might also identify as sexual minority).

We begin with a brief overview of the epidemiology of mental illness among SGM (sexual and gender minority) populations. Next, we discuss minority stress, a major contributor to SGM health disparities that is often interpersonally mediated. We then propose strategies for delivering interpersonal psychotherapy (IPT) to SGM clients.

MENTAL HEALTH DISPARITIES AMONG SGM POPULATIONS

The National Institutes of Health has identified SGM people as a health disparities population.[1] SM adults are more likely than heterosexual adults to

Jeremy D. Kidd, Roma Kaczmarkiewicz, S. J. Langer, Claire Koljack, and Tonda L. Hughes, *Interpersonal Psychotherapy With Sexual and Gender Minority Individuals* In: *Interpersonal Psychotherapy.* Edited by: Myrna M. Weissman and Jennifer J. Mootz, Oxford University Press. © Oxford University Press 2024. DOI: 10.1093/oso/9780197652084.003.0054 meet Diagnostic and Statistical Manual of Mental Disorders: DSM-5[2] criteria for major depressive disorder, bipolar disorder, anxiety disorders, post-traumatic stress disorder, eating disorders,[3-7] and substance use disorders.[8,9] Compared to other SM subgroups, bisexual people are even more heavily impacted by mental health problems. For example, bisexual individuals have higher risk of depressive and anxiety symptoms and heavy drinking than lesbian or gay people.[5,6,10,11] While most population-based, representative sample studies do not ask about gender identity, multiple studies have reported higher levels of depression, anxiety disorders, and disordered eating among GM people, compared to cisgender people.[3,4,12-14] For example, one study of over 120,000 adolescents found that GM youth were more likely to have attempted suicide than cisgender youth: 51% transgender boys, 30% transgender girls, and 42% nonbinary adolescents versus 10%–18% cisgender adolescents.[15] Despite these alarming statistics, the majority of SGM individuals are mentally healthy, highlighting individual and community-level resilience factors such as social support[14,16,17] that can serve as a focus in IPT.

MINORITY STRESS AS THE MAJOR CONTRIBUTOR TO SGM HEALTH DISPARITIES

Researchers and public health experts often use minority stress theory to explain SGM health disparities.[18-20] In this framework, people with marginalized identities experience unique stressors derived from identity-based stigma and discrimination, which are often interpersonal (e.g., medical discrimination, verbal or physical harassment). This can lead to internalized stigma, identity concealment, and anticipatory fear of mistreatment. These further increase minority stress and worsen health outcomes. SGM people with multiple marginalized identities (e.g., SGM people of color) often experience even greater levels of minority stress, which may relate to the confluence and interaction of minority stressors.[21,22] Minority stress also occurs via systems that privilege heterosexuality and being cisgender over SGM identities (e.g., implicitly assuming clients are heterosexual and cisgender unless they say otherwise, health systems' lack of attention to SGM people and their health needs).

Chronic exposure to minority stress increases vulnerability to poorer health. For example, among GM individuals, minority stress is associated with increased risk for depression and suicidality[23,24]and physical health problems.[25] In critiquing minority stress theory, Diamond and colleagues[26] noted that SGM people who experience everyday discrimination report less social safety and connectedness, factors that are associated with poorer health and well-being. This suggests that interventions are needed to alleviate minority stress *and* increase social safety— aims that IPT is well suited to accomplish.

EXISTING IPT RESEARCH WITH SGM AND RELATED POPULATIONS

To our knowledge, there is no published research on IPT with SGM people, apart from a few studies that evaluated IPT in the treatment of depression among cisgender men living with HIV, many of whom identified as gay or bisexual. These studies provided insight into how IPT might be applied more broadly with SM individuals. For example, between 1993 and 1998, Markowitz and colleagues conducted two pilot trials[27,28] and a randomized controlled trial (RCT)[29] in which they modified standard IPT for men living with HIV. First, they expanded the "sick role" to include depression and HIV (e.g., "The difficulties you're experiencing are due to having depression and a chronic medical condition."). Second, they utilized the "here-and-now" focus of IPT to help clients shift from counterfactual, ruminative thinking about past events that may have led to HIV infection. Third, they distinguished between normative distress after HIV diagnosis and depressive symptoms that arose due to interpersonal problems related to the diagnosis (e.g., sexual stigma). Finally, they allowed case formulations to include multiple interpersonal problem areas. For example, for participants with depression who tested positive for HIV after a partner died of AIDS, IPT would focus on both grief and role transition (i.e., the HIV diagnosis). In a 4-arm RCT,[29] participants who received tailored IPT or supportive therapy with imipramine experienced greater reductions in depressive symptoms than participants who received cognitive behavioral therapy r supportive therapy alone. Although these trials[30-32] focused on a subgroup of SM individuals, they can inform adaptations of IPT for SGM individuals more broadly.

THEORY-DRIVEN CONSIDERATIONS WHEN CONDUCTING IPT WITH SGM CLIENTS

The previous section and more general SGM health research support several modifications that could improve IPT's acceptability with SGM clients. First, we discuss adaptations to the Interpersonal Inventory, sick role, and interpersonal case formulation. We then review universal principles of SGM-affirming psychotherapy. We then propose strategies to help clients identify sources of identity affirmation, which can mitigate the negative impact of minority stress.

Expanding the Interpersonal Inventory

At the beginning of treatment, IPT therapists complete the Interpersonal Inventory to understand the client's current relationships and how they relate to the presenting concern. This inventory includes questions about the same types of relationships (e.g., friends, family, coworkers) for SGM and cisgender heterosexual people, with several additional considerations. For SGM clients, important "family" relationships may extend beyond their childhood family (i.e., family of origin), particularly because it is still common for parents to be unsupportive or even hostile toward their SGM child. Consequently, nonfamilial relationships are often important supports for SGM people (i.e., chosen family).[33-35] SGM individuals might even refer to specific friends as "mother," "sister," or "brother." While romantic and sexual partners are often important sources of support, SGM clients' relationships may be subjected to social stigma or lack legal recognition. Research suggests that nonmonogamous relationships may be more common among SGM people than cisgender heterosexual people.[36,37]

When completing the Interpersonal Inventory, therapists should strive to understand how relationships have been impacted by the client's sexual/gender identity and minority stress. For example, if a transgender woman states that her parents do not know she is transgender, the therapist could ask how not being able to live authentically affects how she feels when spending time with her parents.

Reconceptualizing the sick role

Interpersonal psychotherapy therapists use the sick role to emphasize that a client's current emotional state and functional impairment are attributable to a "disease" (e.g., major depressive disorder) rather than personal failings or immutable personality traits. While externalizing blame is a helpful approach for SGM clients, modifications to this paradigm may improve acceptability. For example, our preliminary research indicated that many SGM people disapprove of language that places them in a passive position vis-à-vis their health. Such framing overlooks the ways that SGM people overcome obstacles daily to live authentically in a society that systematically marginalizes them. It also runs counter to research that suggests that, for some SGM individuals, taking an active role in promoting the health and well-being of the SGM community (e.g., advocacy) is protective against negative mental health outcomes.[38] Furthermore, given psychiatry's role in pathologizing SGM individuals,[39-41] clients may bristle at the sick role conceptualization.

Minority stress theory[18-20] offers a dialectical approach to the sick role that combines externalizing the source of impairment and promoting agency to address it. For example, an IPT therapist might formulate a client's depressed mood as resulting from conflict with a family member after "coming out" as bisexual (role dispute). In our adapted sick role, the therapist would attribute the client's symptoms to their family's stigmatizing attitudes (externalizing) and ask the client to consider times in the past when they experienced stigma and how they responded (promoting agency). This preserves the original intent of the sick role while avoiding pathologizing SGM status and recognizing the everyday resilience of SGM people.

"Coming out" and gender transition: Culturally tailored case formulations

A key element of IPT is the interpersonal case formulation, in which a therapist assigns the client's symptoms to a problem area: grief, role transition, role dispute, or interpersonal deficits. Therapists typically choose a single problem area on which to focus. However, this approach may not encapsulate the life experiences of SGM clients. In this section, we consider sexual and gender identity/expression disclosure as examples of the dynamic interplay between role transitions and role disputes.

In Western society, it is generally assumed from birth that an individual will be heterosexual and cisgender.[42,43] This assumption is so pervasive that we internalize it as children, expecting that these characterizations will describe our identities. Being SGM means actively challenging these assumptions on intrapersonal and interpersonal levels. Even before SGM people share their identities with others, they often spend a substantial amount of time considering how their sexuality- or gender-related feelings differ from what is expected of them. Understanding and accepting a SGM identity for oneself is a *role transition* and can be stressful. Longitudinal research with SM youth showed that earlier identity awareness is associated with better mental health outcomes,[44] but only when others react with support and validation.[45,46] *Role disputes* may arise when a client's SGM identity conflicts with what was expected by others. For example, when a bisexual woman's coworkers learn that she has a girlfriend, their reactions could range from surprise to rejection to hostility. Navigating these situations increases interpersonal stress. There is a dynamic relationship between role transitions and role disputes. For example, a transgender man who has resolved the role transition-related stress of accepting his own identity may experience another role transition if he begins to view himself as inferior (i.e., internalized stigma) after a series of role disputes with transphobic family members. For the IPT therapist to accurately conceptualize this, the case formulation needs to reflect the relationships among multiple IPT focus areas. Because coming out is an iterative process for SGM individuals as they meet new people and adopt new social roles (e.g., parent, spouse, coworker), this approach can have enduring benefits. Conversely, some GM individuals may not need or want their transgender history to be known and choose to live "stealth," so there may be variability in what information is shared and with whom. However, that does not minimize the need to adapt to new social roles.

Beyond coming out there are multiple transition-related stressors that GM individuals face that are different from those faced by cisgender SM clients. These include asking others to use one's gender pronouns and correcting them if they do not, negotiating gender-segregated spaces, adjusting to physical changes resulting from hormonal/surgical interventions, or adapting to the interpersonal and societal expectations of one's affirmed gender.[25] For instance, a Black trans man might struggle with a role dispute due to racist stereotypes his neighbor holds about Black men, whereby the neighbor conflates assertiveness with aggressiveness.

Therapy may involve survival-focused coping[47] by practicing new assertiveness skills that allow him to live more safely in a society that can be dangerous for men of color. Several articles are available that discuss other considerations for the IPT therapist working with GM clients.[48,49]

Universal affirmation

At the start of treatment, IPT therapists can reduce stigma by asking all clients their sexual and gender identity. This signals to clients an interest and openness to discussing identity-related topics. Therapists can ask on intake forms or verbally alongside other demographic questions. Similarly, therapists can establish rapport and communicate respect by offering their own gender pronouns (e.g., he, she, they) and then asking clients about theirs. Once a therapist knows a client's name and pronouns, it is important to use them consistently when speaking to or about that person. This includes clinical documentation. Using a client's correct name can itself be an intervention to reduce depressive symptoms and suicidality.[50] Therapists may slip and forget to use correct pronouns. When that happens, we should correct ourselves and continue the conversation. The goal is to do better next time and be prepared that it may create a rupture in the therapeutic alliance.

It is also important to avoid assuming the gender of other people in a client's life (e.g., spouse, partner, friends). Use either the person's name or the pronoun "they" until the client states their gender. Similarly, remember that the words someone uses to describe their sexual identity may not correlate with current or past behavior. For example, a gay man may have sexual partners who are nonbinary. When discussing children and pregnancy, remember that some nonbinary individuals and transgender men can become pregnant, and that there are multiple pathways to building a family (e.g., adoption, surrogacy). By maintaining a nonassuming and nonjudgmental stance, therapists will better understand clients' lives and experiences, a key ingredient in successful psychotherapy.

Facilitating identity affirmation

One key strategy for helping SGM clients manage minority stress-related role transitions and disputes is increasing access to affirming social support. Developing relationships with other SGM people can decrease isolation and provide a counternarrative to the societal privileging of heterosexual and cisgender identities.[14,16,17] IPT is well suited for this because it encourages therapists to actively assist clients to identify practical solutions to interpersonal problems (e.g., applying for jobs, creating a date app profile). For SGM people, this might include joining community support groups or other SGM-focused activities (e.g., sports teams, book clubs). Online SGM communities can also be useful, particularly for clients who are not "out" or who live in areas without an established SGM community (e.g., rural areas). Some clients (e.g., SGM older adults, SGM people of color) may desire support that reflects their intersectional identities.

Gender-affirming medical and social interventions can be an important part of gender transition for some GM individuals. For those who need them, they are associated with improved mental health and quality of life, including reduced risk of suicide.[51-54] Similar to the active role that IPT therapists take with clients who are applying for jobs (e.g., reviewing resumes, role-playing interviews), therapists can help GM clients navigate interactions with medical providers and health systems as well as with partners and families. Clients may need to advocate for themselves, assert their needs, or educate medical providers (many providers lack education regarding trans health), or develop questions about procedures for surgical consultations. Additionally, a client may need to negotiate the timing of medical or social interventions with a partner who is adjusting to the physical and social changes. Providers need to remember not to reinforce gender stereotypes about appearance and behavior related to gender roles and expression, taking a nuanced and client-centered approach to clients' individualized goals and how they express their gender.[55]

CONCLUSION

Interpersonal psychotherapy therapists are well positioned to address SGM mental health disparities, which are substantially attributable to interpersonal stigma and discrimination. The adaptations proposed in this chapter are intended to generate hypotheses for future studies and to assist IPT therapists in increasing social safety and mitigating the impact of minority stress on SGM clients.

REFERENCES

1. National Institute on Minority Health and Health Disparities. Sexual and gender minorities formally designated as a health disparity population for research purposes. 2016. Accessed August 20, 2022. https://www.nimhd.nih.gov/about/directors-corner/messages/message_10-06-16.html
2. American Psychiatric Association. *Diagnostic and Statistical Manual of Mental Disorders (DSM-5)*. 5th ed. American Psychiatric Association; 2013.
3. Parker LL, Harriger JA. Eating disorders and disordered eating behaviors in the LGBT population: a review of the literature. *J Eat Disord*. 2020;8:51.
4. Nagata JM, Ganson KT, Austin SB. Emerging trends in eating disorders among sexual and gender minorities. *Curr Opin Psychiatry*. 2020;33(6):562–567.
5. Kerridge BT, Pickering RP, Saha TD, et al. Prevalence, sociodemographic correlates and *DSM-5* substance use disorders and other psychiatric disorders among sexual minorities in the United States. *Drug Alcohol Depend*. 2017;170:82–92.
6. Ploderl M, Tremblay P. Mental health of sexual minorities. A systematic review. *Int Rev Psychiatry*. 2015;27(5):367–385.

7. Gonzales G, Henning-Smith C. Health disparities by sexual orientation: results and implications from the Behavioral Risk Factor Surveillance System. *J Community Health*. 2017;42(6):1163–1172.

8. Medley G, Lipari RN, Bose J, et al. Sexual orientation and estimates of adult substance use and mental health: results from the 2015 National Survey of Drug Use and Health. 2016. Accessed October 13, 2018. https://www.samhsa.gov/data/sites/default/files/NSDUH-SexualOrientation-2015/NSDUH-SexualOrientation-2015/NSDUH-SexualOrientation-2015.htm

9. Kidd JD. Substance use and related disorders in sexual and gender minority populations. In Galanter M, Kleber HD, Brady KT, Levin FR, eds. *The American Psychiatric Publishing Textbook on Substance Abuse Treatment*. American Psychiatric Association; 2021:591–608.

10. Chan RCH, Operario D, Mak WWS. Bisexual individuals are at greater risk of poor mental health than lesbians and gay men: the mediating role of sexual identity stress at multiple levels. *J Affect Disord*. 2020;260:292–301.

11. Pakula B, Shoveller J, Ratner PA, Carpiano R. Prevalence and co-occurrence of heavy drinking and anxiety and mood disorders among gay, lesbian, bisexual, and heterosexual Canadians. *Am J Public Health*. 2016;106(6):1042–1048.

12. Witcomb GL, Bouman WP, Claes L, Brewin N, Crawford JR, Arcelus J. Levels of depression in transgender people and its predictors: results of a large matched control study with transgender people accessing clinical services. *J Affect Disord*. 2018;235:308–315.

13. Millet N, Longworth J, Arcelus J. Prevalence of anxiety symptoms and disorders in the transgender population: a systematic review of the literature *Int J Transgend*. 2017;18(1):27–38.

14. Budge SL, Adelson JL, Howard KA. Anxiety and depression in transgender individuals: the roles of transition status, loss, social support, and coping. *J Consult Clin Psychol*. 2013;81(3):545–557.

15. Toomey RB, Syvertsen AK, Shramko M. Transgender adolescent suicide behavior. *Pediatrics*. 2018;142(4):e20174218.

16. Kidd JD, Jackman KB, Wolff M, Veldhuis CV, Hughes TL. Risk and protective factors for substance use among sexual and gender minority youth. *Curr Addict Rep*. 2018;5(2):158–173.

17. Pflum SR, Testa RJ, Balsam KF, Goldblum PB, Bongar B. Social support, trans community connectedness, and mental health symptoms among transgender and gender nonconforming adults. *Psychol Sex Orientat Gend Divers*. 2015;2(3):281–286.

18. Meyer IH. Prejudice, social stress, and mental health in lesbian, gay, and bisexual populations: conceptual issues and research evidence. *Psychol Bull*. 2003;129(5):674–697.

19. Hendricks ML, Testa RJ. A conceptual framework for clinical work with transgender and gender nonconforming clients: an adaptation of the minority stress model. *Prof Psychol-Res Pr*. 2012;43(5):460–467.

20. Rich AJ, Salway T, Scheim A, Poteat T. Sexual minority stress theory: remembering and honoring the work of Virginia Brooks. *LGBT Health*. 2020;7(3):124–127.

21. Lett E, Asabor EN, Beltran S, Dowshen N. Characterizing health inequities for the US transgender Hispanic population using the Behavioral Risk Factor Surveillance System. *Transgend Health*. 2021;6(5):275–283.

22. Everett BG, Steele SM, Matthews AK, Hughes TL. Gender, race, and minority stress among sexual minority women: an intersectional approach. *Arch Sex Behav.* 2019;48(5):1505–1517.

23. Bockting WO, Miner MH, Swinburne Romine RE, Hamilton A, Coleman E. Stigma, mental health, and resilience in an online sample of the US transgender population. *Am J Public Health.* 2013;103(5):943–951.

24. Tebbe EA, Moradi B. Suicide risk in trans populations: an application of minority stress theory. *J Couns Psychol.* 2016;63(5):520–533.

25. DuBois LZ, Juster RP. Lived experience and allostatic load among transmasculine people living in the United States. *Psychoneuroendocrinology.* 2022;143:105849.

26. Diamond LM, Alley J. Rethinking minority stress: a social safety perspective on the health effects of stigma in sexually-diverse and gender-diverse populations. *Neurosci Biobehav Rev.* 2022;138:104720.

27. Markowitz JC, Klerman GL, Perry SW. Interpersonal psychotherapy of depressed HIV-positive outpatients. *Hosp Community Psychiatry.* 1992;43(9):885–890.

28. Markowitz JC, Klerman GL, Clougherty KF, et al. Individual psychotherapies for depressed HIV-positive patients. *Am J Psychiatry.* 1995;152(10):1504–1509.

29. Markowitz JC, Kocsis JH, Fishman B, et al. Treatment of depressive symptoms in human immunodeficiency virus-positive patients. *Arch Gen Psychiatry.* 1998;55(5):452–457.

30. Heckman TG, Heckman BD, Anderson T, et al. Tele-interpersonal psychotherapy acutely reduces depressive symptoms in depressed HIV-infected rural persons: a randomized clinical trial. *Behav Med.* 2017;43(4):285–295.

31. Heckman TG, Markowitz JC, Heckman BD, et al. A randomized clinical trial showing persisting reductions in depressive symptoms in HIV-infected rural adults following brief telephone-administered interpersonal psychotherapy. *Ann Behav Med.* 2018;52(4):299–308.

32. Moosa MYH, Jennah FY. Antidepressants versus interpersonal psychotherapy in treating depression in HIV-positive patients. *S Afr J Psychiatry.* 2012;18(2):47–52.

33. Levin NJ, Kattari SK, Piellusch EK, Watson E. "We just take care of each other": Navigating "chosen family" in the context of health, illness, and the mutual provision of care amongst queer and transgender young adults. *Int J Environ Res Public Health.* 2020;17(19):7346.

34. Breder K, Bockting W. Social networks of LGBT older adults: an integrative review. *Psychol Sex Orient Gend Divers.* 2023;10(3):473–489.

35. Hull KE, Ortyl TA. Conventional and cutting-edge: definitions of family in LGBT communities. *Sex Res Social Policy.* 2018;16:31–43.

36. Moors AC, Gesselman AN, Garcia JR. Desire, familiarity, and engagement in polyamory: results from a national sample of single adults in the United States. *Front Psychol.* 2021;12:619640.

37. Levine EC, Herbenick D, Martinez O, Fu TC, Dodge B. Open relationships, nonconsensual nonmonogamy, and monogamy among US adults: findings from the 2012 National Survey of Sexual Health and Behavior. *Arch Sex Behav.* 2018;47(5):1439–1450.

38. Matsuno E, Israel T. Psychological interventions promoting resilience among transgender individuals: transgender resilience intervention model (TRIM). *Couns Psychol.* 2018;46(5):632–655.

39. Drescher J. Out of *DSM*: depathologizing homosexuality. *Behav Sci (Basel)*. 2015;5(4):565–575.

40. Drescher J. Queer diagnoses revisited: the past and future of homosexuality and gender diagnoses in *DSM* and *ICD*. *Int Rev Psychiatry*. 2015;27(5):386–395.

41. Ashley F. The misuse of gender dysphoria: toward greater conceptual clarity in transgender health. *Perspect Psychol Sci*. 2021;16(6):1159–1164.

42. Collins KM, Levitt HM. Heterosexism and the self: a systematic review informing LGBQ-affirmative research and psychotherapy. *J Gay Lesbian Soc Serv*. 2021;33(3):376–405.

43. Barnett M, Fotheringham F, Hutton V, O'Loughlin K. Heterosexism and cisgenderism. In Hutton V, Sisko S, eds. *Multicultural Responsiveness in Counseling and Psychology*. Palgrave MacMillan; 2021:153–178.

44. Fish JN, Pasley K. Sexual (minority) trajectories, mental health, and alcohol use: a longitudinal study of youth as they transition to adulthood. *J Youth Adolesc*. 2015;44(8):1508–1527.

45. Pearson J, Wilkinson L. Family relationships and adolescent well-being: are families equally protective for same-sex attracted youth? *J Youth Adolesc*. 2013;42(3):376–393.

46. Austin A, Craig SL. Support, discrimination, and alcohol use among racially/ethnically diverse sexual minority youths. *J Gay Lesbian Soc Serv*. 2013;25(4):420–442.

47. Goodman LA, Fels Smyth K, Borges AM, Singer R. When crises collide: how intimate partner violence and poverty intersect to shape women's mental health and coping? *Trauma Violence Abuse*. 2009;10(4):306–329.

48. Budge SL. Interpersonal psychotherapy with transgender clients. *Psychotherapy*. 2013;50(3):356–359.

49. Barbisan GK, Moura DH, Lobato MIR, da Rocha NS. Interpersonal psychotherapy for gender dysphoria in a transgender woman. *Arch Sex Behav*. 2020;49(2):787–791.

50. Russell ST, Pollitt AM, Li G, Grossman AH. Chosen name use is linked to reduced depressive symptoms, suicidal ideation, and suicidal behavior among transgender youth. *J Adolesc Health*. 2018;63(4):503–505.

51. Tordoff DM, Wanta JW, Collin A, Stepney C, Inwards-Breland DJ, Ahrens K. Mental Health outcomes in transgender and nonbinary youths receiving gender-affirming care. *JAMA Netw Open*. 2022;5(2):e220978.

52. Baker KE, Wilson LM, Sharma R, Dukhanin V, McArthur K, Robinson KA. Hormone therapy, mental health, and quality of life among transgender people: a systematic review. *J Endocr Soc*. 2021;5(4):bvab011.

53. Nguyen HB, Chavez AM, Lipner E, et al. Gender-affirming hormone use in transgender individuals: impact on behavioral health and cognition. *Curr Psychiatry Rep*. 2018;20(12):110.

54. Turban JL, King D, Kobe J, Reisner SL, Keuroghlian AS. Access to gender-affirming hormones during adolescence and mental health outcomes among transgender adults. *PLoS One*. 2022;17(1):e0261039.

55. Langer SJ. *Theorizing Transgender Identity for Clinical Practice: A New Model for Understanding Gender*. Hachette UK/Jennifer Kingsley Publishers; 2019.

54

Telephone Interpersonal Psychotherapy (Tele-IPT) for Rural Persons With HIV and Comorbid Depression

TIMOTHY G. HECKMAN, TIMOTHY ANDERSON, AND
BERNADETTE D. HECKMAN ■

THE NEED FOR TELE-IPT FOR RURAL PERSONS LIVING WITH HIV AND COMORBID DEPRESSION

In December 2020, there were 58,898 persons living with HIV (PLWH) infection in nonmetropolitan areas of the United States, for a rate of 129.4 infections per 100,000 persons.[1] Rural areas of the southern United States have been particularly hard hit by HIV, largely because the opioid epidemic has gone unchecked in this region.[2]

HIV-related stigma, HIV criminalization laws, the lack of transportation, and a shortage of mental health practitioners in rural areas exacerbate psychiatric disorders and prevent many rural PLWH from obtaining mental health care and adhering to medical treatments.[3] Unfortunately, compared to their urban counterparts, rural PLWH are less likely to have seen a mental health provider in the past year[4] and make fewer annual visits to mental health professionals in general.[5] Because of these barriers and the lack of social supports, it is not surprising that rural PLWH are 1.3 times more likely to be diagnosed with depression than their metropolitan counterparts,[6] and mortality is significantly higher in rural (10.4%) than urban PLWH (6.0%).[7]

Timothy G. Heckman, Timothy Anderson, and Bernadette D. Heckman, *Telephone Interpersonal Psychotherapy (Tele-IPT) for Rural Persons With HIV and Comorbid Depression* In: *Interpersonal Psychotherapy*. Edited by: Myrna M. Weissman and Jennifer J. Mootz, Oxford University Press. © Oxford University Press 2024. DOI: 10.1093/oso/9780197652084.003.0055

TECHNOLOGY AND METHODS USED TO DELIVER TELE-IPT TO RURAL PLWH

In response to high rates of depressive disorders and geographic and psychological barriers to mental health care, and in light of the depression treatment efficacy of interpersonal psychotherapy (IPT) in a variety of clinical populations,[8] a randomized clinical trial was conducted to determine if brief telephone-administered IPT (tele-IPT) provided depressive symptom relief in rural PLWH and comorbid depressive disorders compared to usual care (UC). The clinical trial's inclusion criteria were (1) 18 years of age or older; (2) a self-reported diagnosis of HIV infection or AIDS; (3) residence in a county with US Department of Agriculture Rural-Urban Continuum Code of 4 through 9; (4) diagnosis of major depressive disorder (MDD), MDD in partial remission, or dysthymic disorder based on the Mood Module of the PRIME-MD (per the *Diagnostic and Statistical Manual of Mental Disorders, Fourth Edition*); and (5) written informed consent.

The first patient was enrolled into the clinical trial in August 2010, and intervention outcome data were collected through December 2015. A total of 147 patients completed the trial. The average patient was 52.0 years of age, Caucasian (74%), and self-identified as gay/bisexual (50.3%). Slightly more than one-third lived in a county with a population of 2500 to 19,999 that was adjacent to a metropolitan area. Approximately 15% of patients were attending self-help groups, and 30% were receiving services from healthcare professionals in their community during their participation in the clinical trial.

Tele-IPT patients received 9 weekly 1-hour tele-IPT sessions. Sessions 1 and 2 consisted of patient-therapist introductions and an overview of the therapy protocol. Teletherapists and patients also explored patients' depressive symptoms and discussed the nature of depression and the IPT sick role. Therapists also collaborated with patients, via the Interpersonal Inventory, to link their depressive distress with their current interpersonal relationships, leading to identifying the most central problematic relationship(s) or circumstance that served as the interpersonal focus for the remainder of treatment.

Applying core IPT treatment principles,[9] therapists framed each patient's primary interpersonal concern using 1 of 4 focal areas: interpersonal role dispute (e.g., conflict with partner); role transition (e.g., loss of employment, moving from an urban to a rural environment); grief (death of loved one); or interpersonal sensitivities (chronic difficulties forming or maintaining close relationships). Sessions 3 through 9 addressed the problematic relationship/issue identified in sessions 1 and 2. Sessions 8 and 9 addressed issues of therapy termination and maintenance of treatment gains. On average, tele-IPT patients participated in 7.8 of the 9 teletherapy sessions; 82% attended all 9 sessions. The primary interpersonal focal problems identified in patients were role transition (54%), interpersonal sensitivity (16%), interpersonal role disputes (15%), and unresolved grief/bereavement (15%). Role transitions commonly voiced by patients included a sudden shift from full-time employment to being unemployed (either through retirement or involuntary separation), becoming single or divorced after being in a serious long-term committed relationship, and vacillating between periods of good and poor health.

Initial intervention-outcome analyses that focused on short-term changes on the Beck Depression Inventory (BDI) found that tele-IPT patients reported significant reductions in depressive symptoms from preintervention (M = 26.0) through postintervention (M = 20.2), whereas UC controls reported no significant reductions in BDI values from pre- (M = 27.0) through postintervention (M = 25.6), t = 2.84, P < .005, d = 0.53 (Heckman et al., 2017). Analyses of longer term changes found that between-group difference on the BDI at 4-month follow-up were marginally significant (tele-IPT = 21.71, UC controls = 25.08, Cohen d = 0.41, P = .058), and that, at 8-month follow-up, tele-IPT patients reported significantly fewer depressive symptoms than UC controls (tele-IPT = 20.55, UC controls = 24.43, Cohen d = 0.47, P = .029; Heckman et al., 2018).[10] Taken together, the clinical trial found that 9 sessions of tele-IPT produced significant and sustained reductions in depressive symptoms in rural PLWH compared to UC, with "medium" treatment effect sizes.

ADAPTING IPT FOR TELEPHONE ADMINISTRATION WITH HIV-INFECTED PERSONS WITH DEPRESSION

Our choice of tele-IPT for use with rural PLWH was based on several reasons, including (1) IPT is time limited, not long-term; (2) IPT is focused, not open ended; (3) IPT addresses current interpersonal relationships, not past ones; (4) IPT takes an interpersonal rather than intrapsychic approach; (5) IPT takes an interpersonal rather than cognitive behavioral approach; and (6) while personality is recognized, it is not the focus of IPT.[11] Given the lack of social supports in rural areas, IPT was considered an appropriate treatment that was intended to enable patients to maintain or repair ruptured relationships. It was also surmised that providing IPT to rural PLWH via standard or cellular telephones would make the treatment accessible to a greater number of persons and negate any requirements for patients to have high-speed broadband, Internet connectivity, or other necessities associated with videoconferencing (e.g., Zoom or Skype).[12,13]

Initial sessions focused on working with tele-IPT patients to create an environment during therapy that optimized privacy/confidentiality and reduced the likelihood of technical complications. These measures included (1) identifying a location where privacy was heightened and distractions were unlikely (e.g., a setting in which there was no television or other computer devices); (2) weekly therapy sessions were scheduled at times when distractions were unlikely; (3) having a plan to manage call waiting during therapy sessions; (4) identifying and eliminating potential multitasking activities (e.g., driving during therapy sessions) that would be distracting or hazardous for the patient; (5) when possible, using traditional landline telephones to reduce the likelihood of "dropped" calls; (6) avoiding use of the speakerphone feature; and (7) if using a cell phone, ensuring a fully charged battery.

ADAPTATIONS TO THE REMOTE IPT INTERVENTION

Our decades-long work with rural PLWH[10] advised that tele-IPT would have greater depression treatment efficacy if contextualized for the unique life circumstances of this group. Many rural PLWH report that HIV infection is not their primary life stressor; it is just one of many challenges they routinely confront. Family crises (e.g., unresolved family conflict, domestic violence, etc.), personal financial difficulties, and living with other comorbid health conditions, such as hypertension, migraine headaches, active alcohol/substance use disorders are common struggles for many rural PLWH. As such, teletherapists focused on the patient's focal point of treatment (most often role transitions) within the larger context of unpredictable life events, financial challenges, and other health concerns.

Regarding technology, all sessions were delivered via audio-only telephone for teletherapy. Because all patients lived in geographically remote regions, there were significant obstacles to transportation, and many patients had not previously received mental health services. Furthermore, patients often lacked high-speed Internet, which made video-based teletherapy impossible. Our group had pilot tested video-based IPT[14] but discovered that videoconferenced IPT was impractical for rural areas. Specifically, "dropped" videoconference calls were common, and a significant lag time between what the therapist appeared to be saying and what the patient was hearing was too disruptive to the therapeutic alliance. Additionally, significant delays in video-feed interfered with clients' processing their emotional reactions to interpersonal events during IPT-based communication analysis. We discovered that maintaining continuity of experiential processes was better maintained during a clear audio form of teletherapy connection for remotely located patients.

In our randomized clinical trial of tele-IPT,[15] all tele-IPT therapists were PhD-level clinical psychologists, licensed in one or more states, and experienced in administering treatments via telephone. Specifically, therapists had administered IPT, motivational interviewing, supportive-expressive therapy, and coping effectiveness training to individuals and/or groups living with HIV as part of previous clinical trials. All tele-IPT sessions were audio recorded and reviewed to verify fidelity to tele-IPT protocol. On a regular basis, teletherapists convened through standard conference calls to discuss current patients, challenges to conducting therapy over the telephone, and other issues relevant to the tele-IPT treatment.

BARRIERS TO AND FACILITATORS OF IMPLEMENTATION

There were minor challenges to conducting tele-IPT with rural PLWH, but these challenges were not insurmountable. Some patients had limited data plans and were reluctant to allocate a significant proportion of their cellular data plan to the tele-IPT treatment. For these few patients, additional funds were added to their incentive payments to defray additional costs to their data plans. Understanding patient data plan barriers prior to initiating teletherapy is crucial so that support can be provided to mitigate or eliminate this barrier. One goal of IPT is to increase social support resources. In many rural areas, however, there are very few (and sometimes no) in-person social support resources. Given the lack of social supports in rural areas, patients and teletherapists often discussed the use of remote support systems, such as social media platforms (e.g., Facebook). Remote support is likely preferable to no support for persons living with a chronic health condition and depression. Finally, while working remotely with any vulnerable group, articulated threats of harm to self or others were monitored carefully by teletherapists. In this clinical trial, teletherapists always had in their possession contact information for patients' family members, friends, and local emergency departments in the event that immediate intervention was necessary. While no adverse events were reported during the project clinical trial, for the teletherapist conducting therapy in rural areas, it is critical to have a thorough understanding of available local crises resources in the rural community in which their patient resides.

Issues of privacy and confidentiality were somewhat common. Some patients were participating in tele-IPT with significant others or family members in close proximity, while others received tele-IPT while in public settings. These instances, however, tended to be exceptions and even provided in vivo situations to work through patients' privacy concerns. Other relational treatments (e.g., psychodynamic) might have considered these relational situations as transference, but we worked with these barriers to privacy as part of needed privacy and boundaries for effective interpersonal communication. Similar to in-person IPT, some patients were not responsive to tele-IPT because their problems with interpersonal sensitivity were more severe and left them isolated and without meaningful relationships. However, the tele-IPT format seemed to work well for other persons with few relationships and otherwise interpersonally avoidant tendencies. We found that accompanying changes in unique interpersonal problems occurred during tele-IPT; specifically, changes in socially avoidant interpersonal problems were significantly and uniquely co-occurring with decreases in depressive symptoms.[16]

While rural PLWH have significant confidentiality concerns, the anonymity of the tele-IPT treatment gave most patients an increased and immediate sense of safety. As such, teletherapists reported that many clients actively engaged in treatment from the very first session. The flexibility of tele-IPT enabled clients to engage in therapy from most any location, resulting in high session attendance rates. In addition to geographic remoteness, some patients displayed long-standing agoraphobic symptoms, and tele-IPT provided needed therapeutic services and hope to find new ways to re-engage and initiate social relationships within their more limited social environment.

Tele-IPT was also effective for PLWH in remote communities because of the significant experience of stigma surrounding one's HIV status. Relatedly, some patients were even concerned about receiving other medical services for fear that their medical information was not truly private in their small community (regardless of Health Insurance Portablity and Accountability Act assurances). Some patients felt judged and stigmatized by community and family members for their HIV infection. This stigma could be multiplied for some clients with lesbian, gay, bisexual, transgender, queer/questioning, and other sexuality identity (LGBTQ+ sexual identity), as well as other ways in which they experienced rejection and shame for their personhood. Tele-IPT worked well during these unfortunate, even dire, social circumstances because the treatment focused on discovering hopeful avenues for positive interpersonal support and addressing their fears and concerns with trusted others.

The treatment also benefited patients who were more socially gregarious but had felt repeatedly damaged in past interpersonal relationships. The seclusion of remote telecommunicating provided a safe space to explore these interpersonal disputes. Because these clients were so highly emotionally activated by these relational conflicts, tele-IPT provided a safe space to consider their relational experiences. Some patients also reported they were able to immediately apply role plays from tele-IPT because the context of the sessions had greater proximity to the persons involved with conflicts.

FUTURE PLANS FOR TELE-IPT

Interpersonal psychotherapy administered via telephone is an efficacious treatment for depression[8] and appears to be a particularly apt treatment for rural PLWH.[15] As the evidence base for IPT (and tele-IPT) continues to grow, future implementation science research should investigate how tele-IPT can be scaled up and offered to large numbers of individuals in need of brief and easily accessible depressive symptom relief. Future efforts should also formally train students in mental health professions (e.g., psychiatry, psychology, and social work) to provide remotely administered treatments early in their careers. This is important because mental health practitioners who receive training or have real-world experiences in teletherapy feel more self-efficacious and prepared to administer remote therapies than those without formal or experiential training.[17]

Formal training in teletherapy can naturally intersect with tele-IPT training because therapists worry that their interpersonal skills are less effective during teletherapy than during in-person therapy.[12] Furthermore, a significant problem for therapists who conduct teletherapy involves processing emotional communication.[18] Because teletherapy patient outcomes are no different from in-person therapy during RCT studies,[17] training therapists to accept and translate their existing skills within a tele-IPT context is recommended. Training therapists in both interpersonal skills and emotional communication processes could help boost effective communication analysis techniques within tele-IPT. As the number of rural PLWH continues to increase, and as additional research highlights tele-IPT's depression treatment efficacy, it is critically important to transition this promising treatment from the research arena into community settings.

REFERENCES

1. Centers for Disease Control and Prevention. HIV Surveillance Report. May 2022. Accessed May 25, 2022. http://www.cdc.gov/hiv/library/reports/hiv-surveillance.html

2. WebMD. 2022. HIV in rural areas. Accessed May 25, 2022. https://www.webmd.com/hiv-aids/hiv-rural-areas

3. Kalichman SC, Katner H, Banas E, Hill M, Kalichman MO. HIV-related stigma and non-adherence to antiretroviral medications among people living with HIV in a rural setting. *Soc Sci Med.* 2020;258:113092.

4. Reif S, Whetten K, Ostermann J, Raper JL. Characteristics of HIV-infected adults in the Deep South and their utilization of mental health services: a rural vs. urban comparison. *AIDS Care.* 2006;18(suppl):10–17.

5. van Luenen S, Garnefski N, Spinhoven P, Spaan P, Dusseldorp E, Kraaij V. The benefits of psychosocial interventions for mental health in people living with HIV: a systematic review and meta-analysis. *AIDS Behav.* 2018;22(1):9–42.

6. Sheth SH, Jensen PT, Lahey T. Living in rural New England amplifies the risk of depression in patients with HIV. *BMC Infect Dis.* 2009;9:1–8.

7. Lahey T, Lin M, Marsh B, et al. Increased mortality in rural patients with HIV in New England. *AIDS Res Hum Retroviruses.* 2007;23(5):693–698.

8. Cuijpers P, Geraedts AS, van Oppen P, Andersson G, Markowitz JC, van Straten A. Interpersonal psychotherapy for depression: a meta-analysis. *Am J Psychiatry.* 2011;168(6):581–592.

9. Weissman MM, Markowitz JC, Klerman G. *Comprehensive Guide to Interpersonal Psychotherapy.* Basic Books; 2008.

10. Heckman TG, Somlai AM, Peters J, et al. Barriers to care among persons living with HIV/AIDS in urban and rural areas. *AIDS Care.* 1998;10(3):365–375.

11. Wilfley DE, MacKenzie KR, Welch RR, Ayres VE, Weissman MM. *Interpersonal Psychotherapy for Group.* Basic Books; 2000.

12. Lin T, Stone S, Heckman T, Anderson T. Zoom-in to zone-out: therapists report less therapeutic skill in telepsychology versus face-to-face therapy during the COVID-19 pandemic. *Psychotherapy.* 2021;58(4):449–459.

13. Markowitz JC, Milrod B, Heckman TG, et al. Psychotherapy at a distance. *Am J Psychiatry.* 2021;178(3):240–246.

14. Ransom D, Heckman TG, Anderson T, Garske J, Holroyd K, Basta T. Telephone-delivered, interpersonal psychotherapy for HIV-infected rural persons with depression: a pilot trial. *Psychiatr Serv.* 2008;59(8):871–877.

15. Heckman TG, Markowitz JC, Heckman BD, et al. A randomized clinical trial showing persisting reductions in depressive symptoms in HIV-infected rural adults following brief telephone-administered interpersonal psychotherapy. *Ann Behav Med.* 2018;52(4):299–308.

16. Anderson T, McClintock AS, McCarrick SS, et al. Working alliance, interpersonal problems, and depressive symptoms in tele-interpersonal psychotherapy for HIV-infected rural persons: evidence for indirect effects. *J Clin Psychol.* 2018;74(3):286–303.

17. Lin T, Heckman TG, Anderson T. The efficacy of synchronous teletherapy versus in-person therapy: a meta-analysis of randomized clinical trials. *Clin Psychol Sci Pract.* 2022;29(2):167.

18. Békés V, Aafjes-van Doorn K, Luo X, Prout TA, Hoffman L. Psychotherapists' challenges with online therapy during COVID-19: concerns about connectedness predict therapists' negative view of online therapy and its perceived efficacy over time. *Front Psychol*. 2021;12:705699.

RELEVANT PUBLICATIONS FOR TELE-IPT WITH RURAL PEOPLE LIVING WITH HIV

Anderson T, McClintock AS, McCarrick SS, et al. Working alliance, interpersonal problems, and depressive symptoms in tele-interpersonal psychotherapy for HIV-infected rural persons: evidence for indirect effects. *J Clin Psychol*. 2018;74(3):286–303.

Heckman TG, Markowitz JC, Heckman BD, et al. A randomized clinical trial showing persisting reductions in depressive symptoms in HIV-infected rural adults following brief telephone-administered interpersonal psychotherapy. *Ann Behav Med*. 2018;52(4):299–308.

Interpersonal Psychotherapy in Prisons and Jails for Major Depression

JENNIFER E. JOHNSON ■

HIGH MENTAL HEALTH NEEDS AND LOW MENTAL HEALTH RESOURCES IN CORRECTIONAL SETTINGS

The United States has the highest incarceration rate in the world, with almost 2 million adults incarcerated on any given day.[1] Individuals who are incarcerated report high rates of past year substance use disorders (66%)[2] and mental health problems, including major depressive episode (24%–30%)[2]; post-traumatic stress disorder (28%–29%)[3]; antisocial personality disorder (35%)[4]; borderline personality disorder (17%–32%)[5]; psychosis (15%–24%)[2]; mania or hypomania (7%–14%+)[2,6–8]; chronic health conditions[9,10]; stressful life events (e.g., death of loved ones, divorce, job loss, loss of rights to children)[11–15]; prolonged stress (abuse,[16,17] assault, racism,[18] violent neighborhoods)[19]; low social belongingness[20,21]; and suicidal ideation or behavior (40%–50%).[22–27] In addition to causing distress, major depressive disorder (MDD) increases risk of victimization,[28] prison recidivism,[29] and substance use relapse.[30,31]

Individuals with MDD who are incarcerated often have severe, treatment-resistant depression and multiple comorbidities.[20,32] The largest randomized trial of any MDD treatment in an incarcerated population ($n = 181$) tested interpersonal psychotherapy (IPT) versus prison treatment as usual.[20] The average intake Hamilton Depression Rating Scale score of participants was in the "severe" range, despite more than 70% already receiving prison mental health treatment (including medications). The median number of past depressive episodes was "too many to count"; 6% were experiencing a psychotic depressive episode.[20] A majority

Jennifer E. Johnson, *Interpersonal Psychotherapy in Prisons and Jails for Major Depression* In: *Interpersonal Psychotherapy.* Edited by: Myrna M. Weissman and Jennifer J. Mootz, Oxford University Press. © Oxford University Press 2024. DOI: 10.1093/oso/9780197652084.003.0056

(72%) of participants met criteria for antisocial personality disorder, and 38% met criteria for borderline personality disorder.[20] Many (42%) participants had attempted suicide in their lifetime.[20] Most (87%) had experience lifetime physical assault, and more than half (58%) had experienced sexual assault.[20] Nationally, individuals who are male, are low income, did not complete high school, and come from racial and ethnic minority groups are overrepresented in the justice system.[33]

Because correctional systems have a primary goal of public safety (i.e., to keep the public safe from harm) rather than public health, resources for health and behavioral health services in correctional settings tend to be sparse. Less than 10% of justice-involved individuals are able to access mental health or substance use services (including medication) on any given day.[34] Few incarcerated individuals receive individual psychotherapy (or psychotherapy at all), and the few licensed mental health providers at the facilities are typically busy addressing acute psychiatric crises. Prison treatment as usual typically consists of antidepressant medications, if anything.[35] One of our goals in adapting, testing, and implementing IPT in prisons was to find an inexpensive way to provide a community standard dose of psychosocial MDD treatment (i.e., group IPT delivered by available prison providers) that was effective and low cost enough to promote its widespread adoption in prisons.[20]

IPT PROBLEM AREAS ARE A GOOD FIT BUT LOGISTICAL ADAPTATIONS FOR LOW-RESOURCE SETTINGS ARE NEEDED

Interpersonal psychotherapy problem areas are a good fit for individuals who are incarcerated because life stressors, relationship challenges, and social isolation are common and salient in this population.[20,32,36] *Role disputes* (or conflicts) include aggressive confrontations by others in prison; conflictual, abusive, or exploitative relationships outside prison; and negotiation with caretakers to ensure their children's well-being.[37] Individuals who are incarcerated are also attempting to make several *role transitions*: from the community to the prison and back again, to being away from loved ones, from a criminally involved or drug-abusing to a crime-free lifestyle, and sometimes to or from jobs or providing primary care for their children.[14,38] The *average* "life change unit" score of individuals newly sentenced to prison was more than twice the clinical cutoff.[11] Individuals who are incarcerated are also disproportionately likely to have lost a friend or family member through suicide or homicide (*grief*).[11,13,14] Bereavement-related distress may be exacerbated by other loss-related life transitions, such as family dissolution and loss of parental rights to children.[15] In our studies, acceptability of IPT to prison patients and providers was high.[20,39] IPT's relational focus was seen as a good fit.[40,41] Individuals in prison often receive highly structured, psychoeducational interventions (i.e., "classes"), if anything. However, it is our experience that it is the relational and life change issues that keep them up at night.

Unlike a class, group IPT (a semistructured group therapy) gave them a place to have their feelings and address these issues.

The primary adaptations made to IPT and to our IPT manual over a series of studies[20,32,36,39,42,43] related to limited prison mental health resources. We used group IPT. We used both master's level mental health counselors and non-mental health-trained prison health services staff, such as re-entry planners, as IPT counselors. At the request of prison counselors who were not mental health treatment specialists, we created a more detailed, structured, plain-language IPT manual from principles in published IPT manuals.[44,45] We added sections describing reflective listening in detail. We changed the names of the IPT problem areas to "grief, life changes, conflicts, and problem patterns" rather than "grief, role transitions, role conflicts, and interpersonal deficits." We scripted group sessions in each of these areas (4 grief sessions, 4 life changes sessions, 6 conflicts sessions, 4 problem patterns sessions, plus opening and closing group sessions) to be delivered in a flexible order to help counselors cover relevant IPT steps for each group member's IPT problem area (see Table 55.1).

Group IPT consisted of twenty 90-minute sessions over 10 weeks, with 4 individual (pregroup, midgroup, postgroup, and 1 month booster) sessions.[20] The individual sessions were used to orient patients to IPT, collaboratively set treatment goals, prepare patients to use group effectively, and keep group members focused on their interpersonal goals. All participants set treatment goals in 1 or 2 IPT problem areas in the first pregroup session. Counselors summarized the goals in writing, gave them to participants at the first group session, and referenced them periodically during group treatment. Instructions for creating the written goals summaries and examples are provided in Table 55.2. Some refinement of group members' treatment goals took place during the first 5 group sessions. Group members practiced supporting others during sessions unrelated to their own problem area/s.

In creating the more detailed manual, we also fleshed out how to apply IPT problem areas to individuals experiencing incarceration.[42] We added examples relevant to individuals in prison (e.g., loss of children, loss of partner) to grief and life changes sessions. We included sections on managing anger during conflicts, how to handle getting bad news from others, and avoiding physical confrontations in conflict sessions. Similar to others,[46,47] we adapted the interpersonal deficits to address current problematic relationship patterns (including isolation) that often result from trauma, including isolation and attachment to abusive relationships. Efforts to improve social support were aimed at supports outside and inside the prison. Treatment heavily utilized IPT techniques of empathy and encouragement/acceptance of affect given high rates of interpersonal trauma, negative life events, and Axis II disorders. Non-mental health counselors (i.e., reentry workers and bachelor's-level prison substance use counselors) and master's-level mental health professionals were able to conduct IPT adherently, competently, and effectively using this manual.[20,39,42] The manual is available at no cost by contacting the chapter author.[48]

Table 55.1 ORGANIZATION OF SESSIONS FOR GROUP IPT FOR MDD
AMONG INDIVIDUALS IN PRISON

Week 0	*Individual pregroup interviews* *(write up goals sheets for first group session)*
Week 1	Group introduction session Grief session 1 (Tell the story and feel the feelings)
Week 2	Conflicts session 1 (Learning about the disagreement) Life Changes session 1 (Tell the story and feel the feelings)
Week 3	Problem Patterns session 1 (Isolation) Grief session 2 (Revisit the relationship and feel the feelings)
Week 4	Conflicts session 2 (Exploring and practicing communication) Life Changes session 2 (What was lost)
Week 5	Problem Patterns session 2 (Healthy and unhealthy ways to fight isolation part 1) Grief session 3 (Revisit the relationship) *Midgroup individual sessions*
Week 6	Conflicts session 3 (Exploring and practicing communication) Conflicts session 4 (Exploring relationship options)
Week 7	Problem Patterns session 3 (Healthy and unhealthy ways to fight isolation part 2) Life Changes session 3 (What was gained, lessons learned, new opportunities)
Week 8	Grief session 4 (Going forward) Life Changes session 4 (Succeeding in the new situation)
Week 9	Conflicts session 5 (Practicing changes) Problem Patterns session 4 (Identifying positive sources of social support)
Week 10	Conflicts session 6 (Handling difficult situations) Closing group session
Postgroup	*Individual postgroup interviews* *Individual booster session 1 month later*

EFFECTIVENESS

The 2 largest randomized trials of any treatment (including medications) for MDD in an incarcerated population evaluated IPT. The first (smaller) trial of 38 incarcerated women with MDD who were attending prison substance use treatment found that IPT significantly reduced in-prison depressive symptoms relative to an attention-matched control condition.[32] The subsequent (larger) study[20] found that IPT reduced depressive symptoms, hopelessness, and post-traumatic stress disorder symptoms, and increased rates of MDD remission relative to

Table 55.2 STEPS FOR CREATING AND CASE EXAMPLES OF WRITTEN
IPT TREATMENT GOALS SUMMARIES

Steps for creating the summary	It is important to have a mutually agreed-on written case conceptualization/treatment contract ("goals summary") before the beginning of group. The goals summary is written for the patient in lay terms. It provides a brief description of the problem leading to the current depressive episode and ways of using the IPT group to address it. In the pregroup individual session: (1) Determine when the person's most recent (not first) depressive episode started. (2) Ask open-ended questions about what was going on in the person's life around that time. Ask about their relationships, any losses, any changes in their circumstances. (3) Listen carefully for interpersonal conflicts, life changes, grief, and isolation. With individuals in prison, there are usually many potential triggers. (4) Reflect potential triggers for the depressive episode back to the patient: "So, it seems like there were a lot of stressful things going on in your life at the time"; list them, then ask: "Which of them bothered you or is currently bothering you the most?" (5) Discuss the most salient triggers for the current depressive episode, and then once 1 (or 2) are identified, ask: "Would you like to work on that issue in group?" (6) Once a troublesome issue that the person would like to work on is identified, describe the IPT steps for working with that issue, how s/he could use the group, and ask him/her if that makes sense. (7) Negotiate and renegotiate as necessary. After the individual session, write up a user-friendly paragraph describing the issue and another short paragraph describing how to address it. Bring the statement to the first group, run it by the patient for accuracy and fit, and revise as necessary.
Example treatment goal in life change problem area	Steve, You told me that your depression gets bad when major things change in your life. From what you told me, it sounds like a lot has changed for you in the past year and a half. First, your wife split up with you and filed a restraining order. Second, you told me that this year you lost your apartment, your job, and your life because you started using more after your wife left and because she seems to be trying to make your life hard. Being back in prison is tough for you because you worked very hard over the last 10 years to put your life back together. It is discouraging to think about starting over again. *Goal*: As you said, major life changes can trigger depression. Your goal will be to come to terms with what has happened to you over the last year, including letting yourself express guilt, anger, and loss. You understandably have a lot of mixed feelings about what has happened. After you have let yourself have these feelings, we can start thinking about what you can get from this experience that is positive and what might be good about your new life going forward. We can also talk about the steps you will need to take and help you get the positive support you will need to succeed in rebuilding a productive, positive life.

Table 55.2 CONTINUED

Example treatment goal in conflicts problem area	Jennifer,
	You describe your current depression as being directly connected to your relationship with your boyfriend, about which you have mixed feelings. On the one hand, even after all you've been through with him, you do still love him, and you are afraid of being able to support yourself and your children if you leave. On the other hand, you are angry with him for selling your car, cheating on you, and not communicating with you. You also admit to doing things that hurt him, too. You wonder whether there is too much water under the bridge for the 2 of you to ever be happy together. You feel stuck and afraid, unsure what to do when you leave prison, and this uncertainty affects your feelings about yourself and your future.
	Goal: No one can make this decision for you, but it may be helpful to work through what you hope to do when you leave here. This may involve steps you will try to take to improve the relationship, or it may include steps you can take to leave the relationship. It is important to get out of the stuck position in which you have felt yourself trapped for the last several years. The group will provide an opportunity to explore the basis of this relationship, the emotions it creates within you, and different ways to either try to improve the relationship or leave it. Talking about the implications of the 2 alternatives and getting ideas from others in the group may help you in your decision. Having a clear plan will help reduce your worry and depression.

prison treatment alone. Effects on hopelessness were particularly strong.[20] The trial concluded that IPT is effective and cost-effective and recommended to treat MDD among prisoners.[20] It is currently the only treatment of any kind (including psychosocial or pharmacological) for MDD evaluated among incarcerated individuals.[20]

IPT IMPLEMENTATION

Facilitators and barriers were identified through a planned quantitative and qualitative analysis.[39] Analyses were guided by the Consolidated Framework for Implementation Research,[49] a common implementation science conceptual framework. Intervention-related implementation facilitators included IPT's acceptability to prisoner participants and to prison study counselors. Both groups were enthusiastic about IPT. They described IPT as a good fit for the needs of individuals in prison because it allowed for affectively laden discussion of personal issues in safety, and it was time limited, practical, and solution focused. Potential inner setting implementation facilitators included unmet mental health needs among prisoners and the priority that prisoners, providers, and administrators put on improving prisoner mental health. Individual-level facilitators of IPT implementation included prison administrators and providers who were interested in evidence-based practices for MDD, open to feedback and to learning new treatments, committed to helping their clients, viewed rehabilitation (vs. punishment) as the prison's primary goal, and were competent in many of the skills needed to deliver IPT (e.g., helping clients set goals and respecting client preferences). Prison providers and administrators also described large mental health needs in their facilities and limited resources to address them; some were motivated to the point of being almost desperate to improve services. There was high tension for change and high relative priority.

Barriers to IPT implementation in prisons may include mental health stigma (i.e., prisoners not wanting to be labeled as having MDD).[39] Another may be the need to help counselors, who are used to highly structured interventions, learn reflective listening and balance listening and addressing goals in a semistructured intervention. Counselors were able to learn these strategies and reported liking them once they learned them, but mastery and comfort took time.[39] Potential inner setting barriers include a shortage of treatment staff (which is why we developed a group intervention that could be used by non-mental health specialist counselors), challenges obtaining additional resources, stressful collegial relationships, space shortages, and varied organizational readiness.[39] Potential outer setting barriers included rules that led some prisoners to deny mental health symptoms for fear they would not be paroled. Finally, although there was no differential effectiveness of IPT by sex,[20] men's groups often took longer than did women's groups to become comfortable discussing emotionally sensitive issues (which some were concerned would be seen as "admitting weakness") in front of the other group members.[39] Addressing mental health stigma (especially in men's facilities and with parole boards), scalable provider training models, strategies to improve organizational and implementation climate, and financial strategies (to provide resources to hire additional providers, provide additional supervision, and reduce stress on existing providers) may help address these barriers.[39]

Cost-effectiveness

Cost-effectiveness analyses in the largest trial of IPT for MDD in prison[20] provided insights into the costs and benefits of newer versus more established IPT programs. Effects of IPT, though significant in the overall sample, were driven by differences observed in IPT participants who were assigned to (mental health specialist and nonspecialist) counselors on their second or subsequent set of IPT groups.[20] Counselors (regardless of their level of prior mental health training) understood IPT and how it works much better on their second and subsequent sets of groups, rather than their first. However, most (72%) of the costs of IPT were training and supervision costs.[20] Cost per patient for the entire IPT treatment was $2,054, including costs for IPT training and supervision or $575 without these costs.[20] For providers running their second or subsequent IPT group, cost per additional patient week in remission from MDD (relative to treatment as usual alone) was $524 ($148 excluding training and supervision costs, which would not be needed for established programs).[20]

Training needs and recommendations

The most challenging skills for prison counselors (with or without previous therapy training) to learn were getting an initial IPT case conceptualization and treatment contract in the first pregroup session and holding on to the IPT frame in terms of managing structure and flexibility of discussion topics over group sessions. The group setting required counselors to track work on multiple group members' goals simultaneously, which could be challenging. Managing group processes (e.g., group conflicts with Axis II comorbidity in more than half of participants) could also be challenging. Despite these challenges, group IPT was effective,[20] and group work may be the only option in some settings.

Based on our experiences training prison counselors,[20,32,36,39,42,43] we recommend an initial training and a refresher training 6 months later that focus on (1) the steps of IPT case conceptualization (e.g., how to involve patients in treatment planning while still guiding treatment; understanding which components should be counselor contributions and which should be patient contributions to the plan, making a written IPT goals summary with each patient); (2) how the steps of addressing each problem area (e.g., tell the story, feel the feelings, explore what is gained and what is lost, hold the memory, and find new supports in the present) guide when to change gears or stay on course in a planned session; and (3) psychotherapy basics (reflective listening, open-ended questions, getting specifics of experiences, and communication). Given the centrality of the written case conceptualization for group IPT, we have provided 2 de-identified examples of these written case conceptualizations in Table 55.2. We recommend providing supervision for the first 2 rounds of groups, including review of written case conceptualizations and at least some audio recordings. However, given this initial investment in supervision, our results suggest that cost-effectiveness of IPT programs will improve with more established IPT programs versus newer programs because (a) counselors would have led at least 1 set of IPT groups, and (b) training and supervision costs, which accounted for 72% of the costs of IPT,[20] would diminish or end with time as therapists became more experienced in IPT.

FUTURE PLANS AND RECOMMENDATIONS

Given the motivation and enthusiasm expressed by administrators, providers, and clients for IPT for MDD in prison, a primary IPT implementation task for the future is finding scalable training and supervision models for resource-poor prison systems.[39] Ongoing supervision by the study team cost more than study counselor time to provide IPT.[20] Prisons can sometimes afford a 1- or 2-day training, but ongoing consultation and supervision are harder.[39] Unfortunately, studies of implementation of other psychosocial interventions found that single workshops typically have little effect on provider competence.[50] Therefore, efforts to implement IPT in prisons may benefit from examining scalable on-going training models.[39] Low-cost, scalable methods of training professional and paraprofessional counselors are needed to help get mental health treatment to individuals who need it most in many settings. This is a mental health ac-cess and equity issue. From a systemic perspective, incarcerating fewer people and better funding criminal justice and affiliated community treatment settings (e.g., community mental health centers) would also help to reduce unnecessary mental health-related morbidity, mortality, and continuing mental health-related incarceration.

Explanation of session structure

Group sessions are organized around themes: building social support and then doing work on each of the interpersonal problem areas (grief, conflicts, transitions, and problem patterns). The suggested schedule of sessions was chosen because it rotates work on problem areas, giving each group member a turn to work on the issues most salient to them and time to do interpersonal homework between ses-sions related to that problem area. This is a suggested order for the group sessions. Leaders may want to adjust this order, including to more directly address crises as they arise.

If you have a group with no members with goals in 1 of the topic areas, we rec-ommend not using those sessions and spending more time on the issues/sessions relevant to group members' goals. If you plan to stretch out some sessions, make a tentative schedule ahead of time about how that will happen, knowing that it can change based on what is salient in group members' lives at the time.

REFERENCES

1. Sawyer W, Wagner P. Mass incarceration: the whole pie 2022. 2022. Accessed June 13, 2022. https://www.prisonpolicy.org/reports/pie2022.html
2. James D, Glaze LE. Mental health problems of prison and jail inmates. US Department of Justice, Office of Justice Programs, Bureau of Justice Statistics; 2006. Bureau of Justice Statistics Special Report.
3. Trestman RL, Ford J, Zhang W, Wiesbrock V. Current and lifetime psychiatric ill-ness among inmates not identified as acutely mentally ill at intake in Connecticut's jails. *J Am Acad Psychiatry Law Online*. 2007;35(4):490–500.
4. Black DW, Gunter T, Loveless P, Allen J, Sieleni B. Antisocial personality disorder in incarcerated offenders: psychiatric comorbidity and quality of life. *Ann Clin Psychiatry*. 2010;22(2):113–120.
5. Conn C, Warden R, Stuewig J, et al. Borderline personality disorder among jail inmates: how common and how distinct? *Correct Compend*. 2010;35(4):6.

6. Quanbeck CD, Stone DC, Scott CL, McDermott BE, Altshuler LL, Frye MA. Clinical and legal correlates of inmates with bipolar disorder at time of criminal arrest. *J Clin Psychiatry*. 2004;65(2):198–203.

7. Kemp DE, Hirschfeld RM, Ganocy SJ, et al. Screening for bipolar disorder in a county jail at the time of criminal arrest. *J Psychiatr Res*. 2008;42(9):778–786.

8. Schnittker J, Massoglia M, Uggen C. Out and down: incarceration and psychiatric disorders. *J Health Soc Behav*. 2012;53(4):448–464.

9. Fazel S, Baillargeon J. The health of prisoners. *Lancet*. 2011;377(9769):956–965.

10. Maruschak LM, Berzofsky M, Unangst J. *Medical Problems of State and Federal Prisoners and Jail Inmates, 2011–12*. US Department of Justice, Office of Justice Programs, Bureau of Justice Statistics; 2015.

11. Keaveny M, Zauszniewski, JA. Life events and psychological well-being in women sentenced to prison. *Issues Ment Health Nurs*. 1999;20(1):73–89.

12. Klein DN, Santiago NJ. Dysthymia and chronic depression: introduction, classification, risk factors, and course. *J Clin Psychol*. 2003;59(8):807–816.

13. Weissman MM, Markowitz JC, Klerman GL. *Comprehensive Guide to Interpersonal Psychotherapy*. Basic Books; 2000.

14. Hurley W, Dunne MP. Psychological distress and psychiatric morbidity in women prisoners. *Aust N Z J Psychiatry*. 1991;25:461–470.

15. Genty PM. Permanency planning in the context of parental incarceration: legal issues and recommendations. In Seymour C, ed. *Children With Parents in Prison: Child Welfare Policy, Program, & Practice Issues*. Transaction Publishers; 2001:75–92.

16. US Department of Justice, Bureau of Justice Statistics. *Women Offenders*. BJS Clearinghouse; 1999.

17. Browne A, Miller, B, Maguin E. Prevalence and severity of lifetime physical and sexual victimization among incarcerated women. *Int J Law Psychiatry*. 1999;22:301–322.

18. Turney K, Lee H, Comfort M. Discrimination and psychological distress among recently released male prisoners. *Am J Men's Health*. 2013;7(6):482–493.

19. Freudenberg N. Jails, prisons, and the health of urban populations: a review of the impact of the correctional system on community health. *J Urban Health*. 2001;78(2):214–235.

20. Johnson JE, Stout RL, Miller TR, et al. Randomized cost-effectiveness trial of group interpersonal psychotherapy (IPT) for prisoners with major depression. *J Consult Clinical Psychol*. 2019;87(4):392–406.

21. Richie FJ, Bonner J, Wittenborn A, Weinstock LM, Zlotnick C, Johnson JE. Social support and suicidal ideation among prisoners with major depressive disorder. *Arch Suicide Res*. 2021;25(1):107–114.

22. Hayes LM, Rowan JR. *National Study of Jail Suicides: Seven Years Later*. National Center for Institutions and Alternatives; 1988.

23. Charles DR, Abram KM, McClelland GM, Teplin LA. Suicidal ideation and behavior among women in jail. *J Contemp Crim Justice*. 2003;19:65–81.

24. Sarchiapone M, Jovanovic N, Roy A, et al. Relations of psychological characteristics to suicide behavior: results from a large sample of male prisoners. *Pers Individ Dif*. 2009;47(4):250–255.

25. DuRand CJ, Burtka GJ, Federman EJ, Haycox JA, Smith JW. A quarter century of suicide in a major urban jail: implications for community psychiatry. *Am J Psychiatry*. 1995;152(7):1077–1080.

26. Fazel S, Benning R. Suicides in female prisoners in England and Wales, 1978–2004. *Br J Psychiatry*. 2009;194:183–184.

27. Daniel A, Fleming J. Serious suicide attempts in a state correctional system and strategies to prevent suicide. *J Psychiatry Law*. 2005;33:227–247.

28. Blitz C, Wolff N, Shi J. Physical victimization in prison: the role of mental illness. *Int J Law Psychiatry*. 2008;31:385–393.

29. Baillargeon J, Binswanger IA, Penn JV, Murray OW, Williams BA. Psychiatric disorders and repeat incarcerations: the revolving prison door. *Am J Psychiatry*. 2009;166(1):103–109.

30. Samet S, Fenton MC, Nunes E, Greenstein E, Aharonovich E, Hasin D. Effects of independent and substance-induced major depressive disorder on remission and relapse of alcohol, cocaine and heroin dependence. *Addiction*. 2013;108(1):115–123.

31. McKay JR, Pettinati HM, Morrison R, Feeley M, Mulvaney FD, Gallop R. Relation of depression diagnoses to 2-year outcomes in cocaine-dependent patients in a randomized continuing care study. *Psychol Addict Behav*. 2002;16:225–235.

32. Johnson JE, Zlotnick C. Pilot study of treatment for major depression among women prisoners with substance use disorder. *J Psychiatr Res*. 2012;46(9):1174–1183.

33. Wang L, Sawyer W, Herring T, Widra E. Beyond the count: a deep dive into state prison populations. *Prison Policy Initiative*; 2022. Accessed June 13, 2022. https://www.prisonpolicy.org/reports/beyondthecount.html#childhood

34. Taxman FS, Perdoni M, Caudy M. The plight of providing appropriate substance abuse treatment services to offenders: modeling the gaps in service delivery. *Victims Offenders*. 2013;8(1):70–93.

35. Baillargeon J, Contreras S, Grady JJ, Black SA, Murray O. Compliance with antidepressant medication among prison inmates with depressive disorders. *Psychiatr Serv*. 2000;51(11):1444–1446.

36. Johnson JE, Zlotnick C. A pilot study of group interpersonal psychotherapy for depression in substance abusing women prisoners. *J Subst Abuse Treat*. 2008;34:371–377.

37. Enos S. *Mothering From the Inside: Parenting in a Women's Prison*. SUNY Press; 2001.

38. Garcia Coll C, Surrey JL, Buccio-Notaro P, Molla B. Incarcerated mothers: crimes and punishments. In Surry JL, Coll CG, et al., ed. *Mothering Against the Odds: Diverse Voices of Contemporary Mothers*. Guilford Press; 1998:255–274.

39. Johnson JE, Hailemariam M, Zlotnick C, et al. Mixed methods analysis of implementation of interpersonal psychotherapy (IPT) for major depressive disorder in prisons in a hybrid type I randomized trial. *Adm Policy Ment Health*. 2020;47(3):410–426.

40. Johnson JE, Schonbrun YC, Nargiso JE, et al. "I know if I drink I won't feel anything": substance use relapse among depressed women leaving prison. *Int J Prisoner Health*. 2013;9(4):1–18.

41. Johnson JE, Schonbrun YC, Peabody ME, et al. Provider experiences with prison care and aftercare for women with co-occurring mental health and substance use disorder: treatment, resource, and systems integration challenges. *J Behav Health Serv Res*. 2015;42(4):417–436.

42. Johnson JE, Williams C, Zlotnick C. Development and feasibility of a cell phone-based transitional intervention for women prisoners with comorbid substance use and depression. *Prison J*. 2015;95(3):330–352.

43. Johnson JE, Miller T, Stout RL, et al. Study protocol: hybrid type I cost-effectiveness and implementation study of interpersonal psychotherapy (IPT) for men and women prisoners with major depression. *Contemp Clin Trials*. 2016;47:266–274.

44. Wilfley D, MacKenzie KR, Welch RR, Ayres VE, Weissman MM. *Interpersonal Psychotherapy for Group*. Basic Books; 2000.

45. Weissman M, Markowitz J, Klerman G. *Comprehensive Guide to Interpersonal Psychotherapy*. Basic Books; 2000.

46. Krupnick JL, Green BL, Stockton P, Miranda J, Krause E, Mete M. Group interpersonal psychotherapy for low-income women with posttraumatic stress disorder. *Psychother Res*. 2008;18(5):497–507.

47. Duberstein PR, Ward EA, Chaudron LH, et al. Effectiveness of interpersonal psychotherapy-trauma for depressed women with childhood abuse histories. *J Consult Clin Psychol*. 2018;86(10):868–878.

48. Johnson JE, Zlotnick C, Nargiso C, Gamble S. Manual for IPT for major depressive disorder in prisons. 2015. Unpublished manuscript.

49. Damschroder L, Aron DC, Keith RE, Kirsh SR, Alexander JA, Lowery JC. Fostering implementation of health services research findings into practice: a consolidated framework for advancing implementation science. *Implement Sci*. 2009;4:50–64.

50. Herschell A, Kolko DJ, Baumann BL, Davis AC. The role of therapist training in the implementation of psychosocial treatments: a review and critique with recommendations. *Clin Psychol Rev*. 2010;30(4):448–466.

CHRONOLOGICAL LIST OF PUBLICATIONS RELATED TO IPT FOR MDD IN PRISONS AND JAILS

1. Johnson JE, Zlotnick C. A pilot study of group interpersonal psychotherapy for depression in substance abusing women prisoners. *J Subst Abuse Treat*. 2008;34:371–377.

2. Johnson JE, Zlotnick C. Pilot study of treatment for major depression among women prisoners with substance use disorder. *J Psychiatr Res*. 2012;46(9):1174–1183.

3. Johnson JE, Schonbrun YC, Nargiso JE, et al. "I know if I drink I won't feel anything": substance use relapse among depressed women leaving prison. *Int J Prisoner Health*. 2013;9(4):1–18.

4. Johnson JE, Schonbrun YC, Peabody ME, et al. Provider experiences with prison care and aftercare for women with co-occurring mental health and substance use disorder: treatment, resource, and systems integration challenges. *J Behav Health Serv Res*. 2015;42(4):417–436.

5. Nargiso JE, Kuo C, Zlotnick C, Johnson JE. Social support network characteristics of incarcerated women with co-occurring major depressive and substance use disorders. *J Psychoactive Drugs*. 2014;46(2):93–105.

6. Kao JC, Chuong A, Reddy MK, Gobin RL, Zlotnick C, Johnson JE. Associations between past trauma, current social support, and loneliness in incarcerated populations. *Health Justice*. 2014;2:7.

7. Johnson JE, Williams C, Zlotnick C. Development and feasibility of a cell phone-based transitional intervention for women prisoners with comorbid substance use and depression. *Prison J*. 2015;95(3):330–352.

8. Johnson JE, Miller T, Stout RL, et al. Study protocol: hybrid type I cost-effectiveness and implementation study of interpersonal psychotherapy (IPT) for men and women prisoners with major depression. *Contemp Clin Trials*. 2016;47:266–274.

9. Johnson JE, Stout RL, Miller TR, et al. Randomized cost-effectiveness trial of group interpersonal psychotherapy (IPT) for prisoners with major depression. *J Consult Clin Psychol*. 2019;87(4):392–406.

10. Wittenborn AK, Natamba BK, Rainey M, Zlotnick C, Johnson JE. Suitability of the Multidimensional Scale of Perceived Social Support as a measure of functional social support among prisoners with major depressive disorder. *J Community Psychol*. 2020;48(3):960–976.

11. Felton JW, Hailemariam M, Richie F, et al. Preliminary efficacy and mediators of interpersonal psychotherapy for reducing posttraumatic stress symptoms in an incarcerated population. *Psychother Res*. 2020;30(2):239–250.

12. Johnson JE, Hailemariam M, Zlotnick C, et al. Mixed methods analysis of implementation of interpersonal psychotherapy (IPT) for major depressive disorder in prisons in a hybrid type I randomized trial. *Adm Policy Ment Health*. 2020;47(3):410–426.

13. Moore K, Siebert S, Brown G, Felton J, Johnson JE. Stressful life events among incarcerated women and men: association with depression, loneliness, hopelessness, and suicidality. *Health Justice*. 2021;9(1):22.

ENGAGE NYC

Interpersonal Counseling in New York City Community Settings

SARAH CHIAO, MIRIAM TEPPER, ANNIKA C. SWEETLAND,
JENNIFER J. MOOTZ, KATHLEEN F. CLOUGHERTY,
JENNIFER L. STEELE, WILLIAM TARRANT, MICHELLE GARCIA,
JORGE PETIT, SASHA-MARIE ROBINSON, SANTIAGO W.
BUENO-LÓPEZ, AND MILTON L. WAINBERG ■

INTRODUCTION

Mental illnesses constitute a major health burden in the United States.[1] While around half of the people living in the United States will be diagnosed with a mental illness in their lifetime, only half of those diagnosed will have access to treatment, and a fraction will receive high-quality evidence-based care.[1–3] Underserved communities, including racial and ethnic minorities, have long faced significant disparities in treatment access, service utilization, and mental health outcomes compared to the general population.[4] These disparities, exacerbated during the COVID-19 pandemic, have shed light on the many challenges of the current mental health treatment system nationwide.[5]

The US mental health treatment system has struggled to address these critical disparities in access and quality of care. Preexisting challenges, including workforce shortages, limited access to services, and variable availability and quality of community-based services, have worsened since the pandemic's onset.[5] These challenges are amplified by additional barriers to service access among underserved groups, such as inadequate insurance coverage and mistrust of the healthcare system.[6–8] Collaborative care for depression involves primary care physician referral to on-site mental health care managers who recommend antidepressant medications, track adherence, or offer evidence-based psychotherapy

Sarah Chiao, Miriam Tepper, Annika C. Sweetland, Jennifer J. Mootz, Kathleen F. Clougherty, Jennifer L. Steele, William Tarrant, Michelle Garcia, Jorge Petit, Sasha-Marie Robinson, Santiago W. Bueno-López, and Milton L. Wainberg, *ENGAGE NYC*
In: *Interpersonal Psychotherapy*. Edited by: Myrna M. Weissman and Jennifer J. Mootz, Oxford University Press.

(e.g., problem-solving). Even though collaborative care for depression studies have shown important improvements in treatment access for depressed patients from racial and ethnic minority groups,[9–12] in real-world settings collaborative care has exhibited low enrollment of minority populations, perhaps due to stigma, low awareness, and a lack of client and community engagement.[13] There is, therefore, a dire need to innovate the existing mental health treatment system to achieve more equitable access and outcomes for underserved communities in the United States.

Task sharing (i.e., moving responsibility for certain elements of care delivery to individuals who do not have specialized training in mental health care delivery) with lay providers is a successful approach that is commonly employed in low- and middle-income countries (LMICs) to address workforce shortages for mental health specialists.[14] Historically, uptake of a task-sharing approach in the United States had been limited due to licensure regulatory requirements and scope of practice. Yet, the increased disparities and clinical needs resulting from the pandemic highlight the potential value of utilizing such an approach.[15]

The Columbia University/New York State Psychiatric Institute educational, training, clinical, and research Mental Wellness Equity Center established by Dr. Milton Wainberg in 2020 aims to end the mental and substance use disorders disparity gap among populations designated by the National Institutes of Health that experience these disparities in the United States. To do so, the Mental Wellness Equity Center introduces innovative solutions to ensure that clinically and culturally effective care is available, addresses social determinants of health (SDoH; i.e., nonmedical factors, such as unemployment, that can contribute to mental distress and impact mental health outcomes[16]), and promotes policies that create and sustain a scalable blueprint for the nation.

In January 2022, the Mental Wellness Equity Center launched ENGAGE (Engaging CommuNities to Gain MentAl WellbeinG and Equity), an initiative funded by and developed with the New York State Office of Mental Health (NYS-OMH). ENGAGE seeks to train a new cadre of lay workers ("Community Wellness Workforce") to deliver accessible and high-quality mental health assessments and interventions, as well as address SDoH among New York State residents. The model of ENGAGE builds on a successful community health initiative developed in Mozambique (led by Dr. Milton Wainberg; see Chapter 19 on Mozambique) that utilized task sharing and a digitized measurement-based application to optimize resource allocation, enhance rigor, and match interventions with needs.[17,18] Taking the lessons learned from this work, ENGAGE aims to leverage digital tools to reduce mental health disparities, thereby facilitating the transformation of the public mental health system locally and nationally.

Currently in its pilot implementation phase, ENGAGE has partnered with 2 community-based organizations, each with 2 clinic sites, to serve residents in 4 underserved urban areas in New York City: Harlem, Brooklyn, Bronx, and Washington Heights (northern Manhattan). In the ENGAGE model, lay providers will reduce wait lists for care by engaging and screening clients with the Electronic Mental Wellness Tool, a validated brief tool used to guide stratified care.[19] Lay providers will also offer brief evidence-based interventions to address common mental health concerns, hazardous alcohol and substance use, suicide risk, and SDoH. In this chapter, we discuss the training and credentialing process of teaching lay providers (community wellness workers; CwWs), as well as their supervisors with mental health licensure, within the 2 partner agencies to deliver interpersonal counseling (IPC) for the treatment of common mental health conditions.

THREE-DAY IPC TRAINING WORKSHOP

The first cohort of CwWs began their IPC training in September 2022. Two IPC expert trainers, Kathleen Clougherty, MSW, and Jennifer Mootz, PhD, facilitated a 3-day in-person workshop with 14 CwWs from ENGAGE's 2 partner organizations. The CwWs had diverse professional backgrounds, having worked previously as peer specialists, crisis counselors, case managers, and employment specialists. Three clinical supervisors who are licensed mental health clinicians with master's degrees were also trained. Most of the CwWs represented the communities their agencies serve (i.e., Latinx, Black/African American, LGBTQ+ [lesbian, gay, bisexual, transgender, queer/questioning], etc.), a feature that has been critical in enhancing workforce diversity and cultural relevance of care delivery.[15]

ENGAGE's IPC training follows the apprenticeship model for teaching lay providers to offer mental health treatments in LMICs.[20] This includes a 3-day intensive workshop (9 hours of didactic learning and 6 hours of experiential practice in small groups), followed by weekly group supervision, during which time trainees discuss their cases, practice their skills, and get feedback from certified IPC supervisors. The CwWs are credentialed in IPC when they have completed and received supervision on a minimum of 3 training cases.

During the in-person workshop, CwWs discussed the cultural beliefs and norms of mental health and interpersonal struggles faced by Latinx and Black/African American communities. In addition, they considered COVID-19's impact on mental well-being and interpersonal relationships among communities in Brooklyn, Harlem, Bronx, and Washington Heights. For instance, CwWs shared that many immigrants, including those from the Dominican Republic, could not return to their home countries to perform funeral rituals for deceased loved ones because of travel restrictions.

Several features of the IPC workshop contributed to its success. To promote active learning, facilitators included the use of case examples that reflected the communities that CwWs serve, and experiential practice was woven into IPC didactic content. To explore the nuances of offering IPC by bilingual staff in Spanish-speaking communities, 5 Spanish-speaking CwWs formed a single breakout group and role-played IPC in both English and Spanish. Additionally, since this IPC cohort included both supervisors and supervisees, a designated breakout group for supervisors was created to prevent supervisees from feeling self-conscious role-playing in front of their supervisors. CwWs exhibited strong enthusiasm about ENGAGE's vision to achieve mental health care equity, reflected through their active engagement during training.

After CwWs completed the 3-day workshop, they moved into the apprenticeship phase to become credentialed in IPC. Five weekly clinical supervision groups, facilitated by IPC expert trainers Kathleen Clougherty, MSW, and Jennifer Steele, LCSW, were formed. Each group included 2 to 4 CwWs, and each supervision spanned 60 to 90 minutes.

TAILORING IPC TO THE ENGAGE CONTEXT

Through the ENGAGE initiative, IPC is delivered by CwWs to address common mental health conditions such as depression, anxiety, and post-traumatic stress. In 4 weekly sessions and a follow-up fifth session 1 month later, CwWs work with clients to address interpersonal events linked with distress. The goal is to reduce symptoms and manage the identified problem area. In the context of the current initiative, there are several advantages to having a lay workforce offer IPC. First, it helps overcome structural barriers to receiving care in traditional settings and enables clients to get immediate help for transient reactions to life stressors (e.g., COVID-19) linked with common mental health problems. IPC also meets many individuals' preference for talk therapy over medication while circumventing high dropout rates with long-term talk therapy.[21] Additionally, having community members deliver IPC enhances the quality and cultural relevance of service delivery.[15] Finally, a lay workforce can help expand and diversify the current mental health field by encouraging more individuals to pursue mental health care as a career path. Several CwWs in our first IPC cohort have already expressed an interest in being guided to pursue additional mental health and social work training.

Given the increased demand and acceptability of telehealth, ENGAGE has tailored IPC by piloting hybrid services (i.e., a mixture of in-person and remote care) to broaden the reach and accessibility of this intervention.[22] To ensure the smooth administration of IPC via telehealth, IPC supervisors have emphasized the importance for CwWs to establish ground rules (e.g., engaging in sessions in a private space and keeping distractions to a minimum) for remote services with clients. In addition, we created and distributed electronically fillable PDFs of IPC assessment tools (e.g., the mood rating scale) to CwWs, such that they can share their computer screens on videoconferencing platforms to collaboratively complete assessments with their clients.

Before starting their first training cases, several CwWs expressed nervousness about learning IPC didactic material and applying it with their first clients. To mitigate anxiety and increase intervention fidelity, we introduced provider-guided checklists that offer step-by-step instructions on the tasks a provider must complete in each IPC session (e.g., offer psychoeducation), along with some example dialogues (e.g., "depression is treatable"), and time allocation guidelines for each task (e.g., spend around 10 minutes on psychoeducation). These checklists also provide instructions on triaging and IPC assessment tools and concepts

CwWs should review prior to each session. Preliminary feedback from CwWs has suggested that these checklists have been beneficial in helping them navigate the delivery of IPC. CwWs have also shared that they typically study and bring printouts of the checklists to sessions they offer and check off IPC tasks as they progress through them.

IPC CREDENTIALING PROCESS: IMPLEMENTATION CHALLENGES

We have faced several challenges in the IPC credentialing process. First, identifying IPC training clients within agencies instead of research laboratories requires proper planning. To add, clients with comorbidities and suicidality are common in real-world settings, but they are not suitable as training clients. To facilitate the case selection process, we created a working group with IPC supervisors and developed a detailed IPC agency guide for ENGAGE. This guide clearly documented the criteria for training clients (e.g., Patient Health Questionnaire-9 [PHQ-9] scores) and other important features of implementation (e.g., IPC credentialing requirements). After circulating this guide to agencies for feedback, IPC supervisors also met with agency clinical supervisors to support the case selection process.

Client engagement was another initial challenge that required attention. Several training clients did not show up, attended sessions sporadically, canceled scheduled appointments, and eventually dropped out after expressing a lack of interest in participating in IPC. To address these challenges, we worked with agencies to generate a script with sample language CwWs can use during initial outreach to potential clients that could boost interest in IPC. We have also modified processes such that CwWs can contact 2 potential clients at once to ensure a supply of IPC training clients. Last, to ensure that CwWs make steady progress toward becoming credentialed, we worked with agencies to develop guidelines for client attendance (i.e., reminder calls) and IPC termination. If a client does not follow up with 3 consecutive IPC sessions, they are referred for other services, which then allows the CwW to start working with a new training client.

Another challenge of the IPC credentialing process has been technical issues associated with telehealth. CwWs expressed that some of their clients prefer to engage with IPC remotely, as doing so allows for increased flexibility in their daily schedules. Yet, technical difficulties with telehealth within agencies and clients' limited knowledge of or access to remote communication platforms hampered the implementation of IPC. Working closely with the agency leadership teams has helped problem-solve some of these technical challenges.

Finally, the novelty of ENGAGE, which simultaneously assesses and addresses common mental health concerns, hazardous alcohol and substance use, suicide risk, and SDoH, is an important implementation challenge for any agency and its providers, including CwWs, their supervisors, and administrators. Training in each of the ENGAGE evidence-based interventions (e.g., motivational interviewing for hazardous alcohol and substance use, safety planning intervention for suicide risk, and financial wellness for SDoH) is offered separately, and the integration of these interventions within an agency requires thoughtful planning specific to the agency's established procedures. This is because agencies must ensure that these interventions do not disrupt their current services and are offered in a safe and rigorous manner. To support ENGAGE and IPC's integration within agencies' services, we completed site visits to each organization to better understand its internal processes and co-develop ways to integrate our model into existing systems. We also reviewed and discussed with agency leadership teams during weekly meetings and CwWs during subsequent trainings how we can weave ENGAGE into their services. Adjustments and clarifications on how significant elements (e.g., completing IPC case notes in the context of an already demanding workload and clarifying the role difference between IPC supervisors and agency clinical supervisors) fit with agency processes have been included in the IPC agency guide for ENGAGE.

IPC CREDENTIALING PROCESS: IMPLEMENTATION FACILITATORS

The Mental Wellness Equity Center, the 2 community-based organizations' leadership teams, CwWs, and New York States' policymakers share ENGAGE's vision of improving access to mental health services by using a task-sharing approach to offer effective and time-limited interventions. Our common goal facilitates the IPC training and credentialing process by encouraging open communication, active problem-solving, co-development of approaches to implementation, and close collaboration in resolving challenges as they arise.

Additional facilitators of the IPC credentialing process have included small group sizes for weekly supervision that help foster productive group dynamics. IPC supervisors' support and warmth during supervision also encourage CwWs to freely discuss their reactions to and challenges with training clients. Moreover, CwWs have been enthusiastic and proactive, reflected in their active participation, consistent attendance, and preparedness to present their training cases during weekly supervision.

In addition to CwWs' engagement during weekly supervision, a few took the initiative to develop material to support the delivery of IPC. For instance, one CwW created a spreadsheet template that helps graph clients' PHQ-9 and mood rating scores across weekly sessions. This digital template was later circulated to other CwWs and has been beneficial in visually illustrating to clients their symptoms and mood progress throughout IPC. One CwW also translated IPC dialogues in the session checklists into Spanish. This translation effort spurred discussion about the best ways to provide IPC in Spanish, and Spanish-speaking CwWs and staff from the Mental Wellness Equity Center collaborated to tailor existing Spanish IPC material for the ENGAGE context. Last, 1 CwW shared that during an IPC termination session, they documented their client's key takeaways (e.g., IPC skills learned) in writing for them to take home. This prompted the development of a termination pamphlet clients can take home after completing IPC.

Six months after the initial 3-day training in September 2022, we offered a half-day IPC advanced booster workshop for the first cohort of CwWs. This 4-hour, in-person session was facilitated by Kathleen Clougherty, MSW, who also led the initial 3-day training. During the workshop, which was structured as an interactive seminar with guiding prompts, CwWs asked questions, demonstrated how they performed various IPC skills, exchanged reflections, and discussed barriers experienced in completing IPC with their clients. For example, several CwWs shared that it was challenging to get their clients to engage in role play during IPC telehealth sessions. When this topic was raised, the IPC trainer and other CwWs provided useful suggestions on how to resolve challenges with navigating this IPC technique (e.g., ask the client to look into a mirror during role-play activities). CwWs also asked for additional help on how to conduct the communication analysis. CwWs discussed how much they had learned, celebrated how far they have progressed since the initial training, and encouraged each other in completing the remaining training clients required for IPC credentialing.

CASE EXAMPLE

E. M. was a 32-year-old Dominican woman living alone with her young child in Washington Heights. She was placed on a wait list at one of our partner agencies and was contacted by the CwW to offer IPC. E. M. presented with anhedonia, insomnia, feelings of hopelessness, a lack of motivation, and anxiety. The CwW conducted weekly IPC sessions with E. M. in Spanish, and they met through a mix of in-person and phone telehealth appointments.

In the first IPC session, E. M. scored an 11 on the PHQ-9, indicating moderate depression. Through administering the timeline, the CwW learned that E. M.'s husband left their marriage and 2 children 1 year ago without an explanation or notice. Since her husband's departure, E. M. had been depressed, isolated, and unable to enjoy activities she used to like. E. M. struggled with anxiety related to adjusting as a single parent and wished to know why her husband left their marriage. In the second session, the CwW and E. M. jointly decided on "life change," resulting from a shift in her marital status and the ensuing loneliness, as the relevant problem area.

Throughout the working phase, the CwW followed the strategies for life change, which included helping E. M. mourn her broken marriage and look ahead for opportunities. The CwW also assigned E. M. work at home to re-engage in activities she enjoyed before becoming depressed, which included running, socializing at work, and spending time with her younger child. After resuming these activities and exploring what she had lost, E. M.'s mood improved, and she reported feeling less isolated. The CwW helped link E. M.'s mood to events.

During the working phase, the CwW also used IPC techniques of role play and decision analysis to help E. M. gauge whether she wanted to reconnect with her husband or proceed with a formal separation. In the third session, E. M. shared that she had come to terms with the fact that her husband will not return to their marriage and become more involved with their younger child. The CwW and E. M. explored her fears about being a single parent and how E. M. could find support in this new role. E. M. decided that she would talk to her older child, who is attending college away from home, about her worries. This initial conversation went smoothly, and E. M.'s depression symptoms continued to improve. During IPC termination, E. M. scored a 4 on the PHQ-9. She expressed that she was *eternamente agradecida* ("eternally grateful") to have participated in IPC with the CwW.

FUTURE DIRECTIONS

Important elements of ENGAGE's long-term plan include establishing sustainability of the Community Wellness Workforce overtime; maintaining the rigor of training, credentialing, supervision, and clinical services; increasing capacity building of new trainers; and informing policy changes.

The Mental Wellness Equity Center is also developing a versatile digitized training and services platform that guides CwWs and their agency systems in delivering high-quality, high-fidelity, evidence-based assessment, and measurement-based interventions, including IPC. This scalable digital platform, which will be capable of tracking intervention fidelity and quality, clinical outcomes, and other indicators of impact, will interface with electronic health records and is simple to use in diverse clinical and community settings. This platform will also use an open source that can be securely accessed across multiple types of devices (e.g., cell phones, tablets, laptops, and computers) and different users (e.g., clients, providers, and supervisors) to address care-related issues. De-identified data from this platform can also be made available to administrators, researchers, and government actors following Health Insurance Portablity and Accountability Act (HIPAA) protection guidelines. Last, this platform will be built in a modular and standards-based approach, which will make adding new evidence-based interventions as modules to the platform accessible. ENGAGE has already begun incorporating IPC for adolescent populations as the next intervention it will implement.

Currently, we are also working with the 2 partner agencies to identify and train a pipeline of supervisors to provide clinical oversight for IPC within each organization, including recruitment and training of second-year master's students from 3 local social work schools as part of the NYS-OMH Schools of Social Work Project for Evidence-Based Practice in Mental Health. In this project, students will complete their second-year practica in our partner agencies with field supervision provided by ENGAGE. The goal for trainees is to learn to deliver ENGAGE interventions and prepare to serve as future licensed supervisors on graduation.

Additionally, we are working with NYS-OMH to explore reimbursement mechanisms for the delivery of brief interventions offered by nonlicensed lay providers in both a traditional Medicaid or fee-for-service context and more advanced payment models such as Certified Community Behavioral Health Clinics and Federally Qualified Health Centers (FQHCs).

Finally, we are exploring potential opportunities to expand the ENGAGE model to other clinical sites and nontraditional community-based settings (e.g., churches). In addition, we will use the implementation pilot described here to inform the tailoring of a provider-guided IPC application for scale-up in New York State. Piloting IPC under ENGAGE has yielded fruitful learnings. Our first cohort of CwWs continue to increase their IPC knowledge and be empowered by ENGAGE's mission to transform care and improve mental health equity in New York State and the nation.

REFERENCES

1. Centers for Disease Control and Prevention. Mental health: data and publications. 2018. Accessed April 4, 2023. https://www.cdc.gov/mentalhealth/data_publications/index.htm

2. National Institutes of Mental Health. Statistics. 2018. Accessed October 12, 2023. https://www.nimh.nih.gov/health/statistics/mental-illness

3. Murphy AA, Karyczak S, Dolce JN, et al. Challenges experienced by behavioral health organizations in New York resulting from COVID-19: a qualitative analysis. *Community Ment Health J.* 2021;57(1):111–120.

4. Cook BL, Trinh NH, Li Z, Hou SS, Progovac AM. Trends in racial-ethnic disparities in access to mental health care, 2004–2012. *Psychiatr Serv.* 2017;68(1):9–16. https://doi.org/10.1176/appi.ps.201500453

5. American Hospital Association. Statement of the American Hospital Association to the Committee on Ways and Means of the United States House of Representatives "America's Mental Health Crisis." 2022. Accessed February 22, 2023. https://www.aha.org/2022-02-03-aha-house-statement-americas-mental-health-crisis-february-2-2022?utm_source=newsletter&utm_medium=email&utm_campaign=aha-today2022

6. Hankerson SH, Moise N, Wilson D, et al. The intergenerational impact of structural racism and cumulative trauma on depression. *Am J Psychiatry.* 2022;179(6):434.

7. Coombs A, Joshua A, Flowers M, et al. Mental health perspectives among Black Americans receiving services from a church-affiliated mental health clinic. *Psychiatr Serv (Washington, DC).* 2022;73(1):77–82.

8. Ozawa S, Sripad P. How do you measure trust in the health system? A systematic review of the literature. *Soc SciMed.* 2013;91:10–14.

9. Thota AB, Sipe TA, Byard GJ, et al. Collaborative care to improve the management of depressive disorders: a community guide systematic review and meta-analysis. *Am J Prev Med.* 2012;42(5):525–538.

10. Arean PA, Ayalon L, Hunkeler E, et al. Improving depression care for older, minority patients in primary care. *Med Care.* 2005;43(4):381–390.

11. Arean PA, Gum AM, Tang L, Unutzer J. Service use and outcomes among elderly persons with low incomes being treated for depression. *Psychiatr Serv.* 2007;58(8):1057–1064.

12. Archer J, Bower P, Gilbody S, et al. Collaborative care for depression and anxiety problems. *Cochrane Database Syst Rev.* 2012;(10)..

13. Moise N, Shah RN, Essock S, et al. Sustainability of collaborative care management for depression in primary care settings with academic affiliations across New York State. *Implement Sci.* 2018;13(1):128.

14. Hoeft TJ, Fortney JC, Patel V, Unützer J. Task-sharing approaches to improve mental health care in rural and other low-resource settings: a systematic review. *J Rural Health.* 2018;34(1):48–62.

15. Giusto A, Johnson SL, Lovero KL, et al. Building community-based helping practices by training peer-father counselors: a novel intervention to reduce drinking and depressive symptoms among fathers through an expanded masculinity lens. *Int J Drug Policy.* 2021;95:103291.

16. National Academies of Sciences, Engineering, and Medicine; Health and Medicine Division; Board on Population Health and Public Health Practice; Committee on Community-Based Solutions to Promote Health Equity in the United States. In Baciu A, Negussie Y, Geller A, Weinstein JN, eds. *Communities in Action: Pathways to Health Equity.* National Academies Press (US); 2017.

17. Wainberg ML, Lovero KL, Duarte CS, et al. Partnerships in Research to Implement and Disseminate Sustainable and Scalable Evidence-Based Practices (PRIDE) in Mozambique. *Psychiatr Serv.* 2021;72(7):802–811.

18. Wainberg ML, Gouveia ML, Stockton MA, et al. Technology and implementation science to forge the future of evidence-based psychotherapies: the PRIDE scale-up study. *Evid Based Ment Health.* 2021;24(1):19–24.

19. Lovero KL, Basaraba C, Khan S, et al. Brief screening tool for stepped-care management of mental and substance use disorders. *Psychiatr Serv.* 2021;72(8):891–897.

20. Murray LK, Dorsey S, Bolton P, et al. Building capacity in mental health interventions in low resource countries: an apprenticeship model for training local providers. *Int J Ment Health Syst.* 2011;5(1):30.

21. Weissman MM, Hankerson SH, Scorza P, et al. Interpersonal counseling (IPC) for depression in primary care. *Am J Psychother.* 2014;68(4):359–383.

22. Appleton R, Williams J, Vera San Juan N, et al. Implementation, adoption, and perceptions of telemental health during the COVID-19 pandemic: systematic review. *J Med Internet Res.* 2021;23(12):e31746.

PART XI

Reflection and the Future

Reflection

Before we predict the future, let's reflect on this unexpected book journey. We began thinking that our request to learn about interpersonal psychotherapy (IPT) from others around the world would have modest returns. We had little idea of the number of countries where IPT was being used. We were overwhelmed in the enthusiasm, the extent, and quantity of response and the quality of information. Our book doubled, then tripled in size and could have kept going. It was about halfway through writing the book that we realized this enthusiasm should be met with full book access. We explored changing our contract with Oxford University Press, who agreed that both a bound book as well as open access should become available.

Many of the chapters are by clinicians, not researchers, and their ideas may not have been captured in print elsewhere. We believe this information will enrich both the clinical implementation and the research. While we were involved in the clinical trial of IPT in Uganda around 2003, we had little idea of IPT's independent clinical extension in many different parts of Africa: Ethiopia, Zambia, Senegal, Kenya, and more. China had not shown an interest in psychotherapy as a treatment in the past, so the change and massive IPT training there and in Hong Kong were a surprise, as was the use of IPT in Malaysia and Nepal.

We were grateful for the contribution from countries, where, at the time, communication was not easy. We expected to see dissemination efforts progress in the European countries as they were the early users of evidence-based psychotherapy and anticipated the problem of reimbursement for psychotherapy from countries without a generous national health plan, especially in the United States. New Zealand was one of the early users of IPT and the groundwork for the international organization. We welcomed their continued development despite their own countries' natural disaster, a massive earthquake.

The reader will note there is no chapter for the United States except on training. The US work is subsumed inadvertently in the chapters on IPT among diverse populations. Since the early developers of IPT were in the United States they were by now working on specialized adaptations with populations of different ages, life situations, diagnoses, and races/ethnicities. There were some possible generation

Reflection In: *Interpersonal Psychotherapy.* Edited by: Myrna M. Weissman and Jennifer J. Mootz, Oxford University Press.
© Oxford University Press 2024. DOI: 10.1093/oso/9780197652084.003.0058

differences noted within a country. The Netherlands indicated that IPT was popular mostly among the older generation and not so in the younger and questioned
its future. At the same time, a new group in the Netherlands enthusiastically reported on a new IPT delivery that combined face-to-face and online sessions for
major depression. The reader will need to determine common messages across
the globe. We start with a few core concepts.

Most authors described IPT and the interpersonal problem area conceptualization as culturally syntonic, especially in countries where relationships are pivotal to
understanding of well-being. In China, for example, Confucianism centralizes the
concept of interdependence through interpersonal relationships. In Iran, we were
told that people first understand themselves in relation to others before they see
themselves as individuals. IPT's premise that distress is grounded in interpersonal
disruptions is congruent with cultures where community plays an intricate role in
daily lives (Ethiopia). There are settings in Africa that have long harnessed community and the wisdom of interconnectedness to improve the lives of individuals
through collective savings groups, extended kinship networks, church organizations, and other community structures (Kenya). While high-income countries
might traditionally have tended to uphold individualism more than other global
settings, these cultures are far from monolithic. Many populations within high-
income countries likewise centralize the value of relational connectedness. Patel
et al. in Chapter 48 explained, for instance, that Latin(x) people in the United
States have long relied on strong family networks to support well-being, a concept
known as *familismo*.

Many contributions that highlighted IPT's congruence with cultural values of
relational interdependence also described considerations needed to account for
the sophistication of social networks, intricate hierarchies, and varied social roles
that people play. In China, providers spent more time exploring problem areas
and formulating the problem to account for the complexity of relationships and
social roles. Strategies for resolving disputes respected and leveraged hierarchies
within networks and tailored communication to fit with social norms and role
expectations. In some settings, elders were an important part of the therapy and
helped resolve disputes or carry the message of resolution. This was especially
true in African countries, indigenous populations in Australia and New Zealand,
and Iran. In Ethiopia, for example, a well-established community-based approach
called *shemegelena* has involved respected community members in the conflict
resolution process. In Japan, parents were routinely part of the treatment as many
children lived at home into young adulthood, and parents were important figures
in their daily lives. Several authors noted that communication involving direct
confrontation was culturally unacceptable. Dissolution as the resolution of an interpersonal dispute with a family member was a limited option in several places
(e.g., Hong Kong and Iran). The potential outcomes of a dispute were resolution
or an intent to live with a role transition rather than dissolution.

For the problem area of grief, authors tailored IPT to align with cultural expressions of mourning and honoring the deceased. In Mozambique,
nonspecialized providers are trained to follow clients' lead about mourning the

deceased given the numerous ethnic groups and cultural variations for rituals associated with death. There were several settings where expressing affect was incongruent with cultural expectations. These authors tailored the delivery in different ways to include techniques that could help. In a Senegalese predominantly Muslim population, crying is understood to hurt the deceased. Other activities, such as prayer and bringing in objects that remind the person of the loved one, are preferable in Senegal. Forced migration was noted in Malaysia to complicate experiences of grief due to the traumatic nature of deaths and inability to be present for mourning rituals.

The problem area of role transition had a broad application. Authors working in various contexts found it useful to encompass integral and unique life experiences that included developmental milestones (Dietz, Chapter 43; Mufson et al., Chapter 44; and Reynolds, Chapter 46); sexual and gender identity development (Kidd et al., Chapter 53); living with HIV (Heckman et al., Chapter 54); the perinatal period (Swartz et al., Chapter 49); incarceration in the United States (Johnson, Chapter 55); and migration and acculturation stressors (Patel et al., Chapter 48; Pereira and Verghis, Chapter 25). Developmentally, for example, Dietz and Mufson et al. explained how children's and adolescents' lives are full of transition both physically and environmentally (schools, friends, family structure, individuation from parents) and helping them build interpersonal skills to navigate these transitions with use of concrete and visual tools was essential. Older age is also a time when people are susceptible to physical changes and social role transitions (Reynolds). When working with perinatal women, Swartz and colleagues have considered life events, such as complicated pregnancy, as a subtype of role transition.

Role transitions also were relevant for migration experiences and minority identity development. Patel et al. surmised that role transition was useful to account for acculturation among Latin(x) people in the United States, and that acculturation differences among children and parents were often connected to disputes. Reay (Australia; Chapter 39) and Kidd et al. (United States) likewise explained that role transition could encompass disclosure of a sexual or gender minority identity among LGBTQ individuals. Sexual identity disclosures, which Kidd et al. pointed out are continuous and recurring, could be met with disapproval from others and serve as a central reason for disrupted relationships. Because of the interconnectedness of problem areas, some authors have recommended developing interpersonal formulations that acknowledge the interconnectedness.

Those who worked with marginalized populations highlighted structural inequities and the harmful effects of racism, discrimination, heterosexism, colonization, and forced migration. They were careful to root distress outside of individual pathology. Brave Heart et al. (Chapter 47), for example, integrated the concept of historical trauma, the psychological suffering across generations, into their facilitation of IPT among American Indians. They linked experiences of historical trauma to mood and normalized mental health problems as a part of the historical trauma response rather than a person's "fault" or deficit. In working with Indigenous Australians, Reay extended the biopsychosocial explanatory model for mental illness to include historical and structural factors, such as experiences of institutionalized oppression, homophobia, heterosexism, and sexism. Host country recognition of refugee status impacted mental health of refugees in Malaysia, where refugees lived with the persistent threat of arrest and deportation and were unable to work to provide for their families (Pereira et al.). In adapting IPT to work with Black/African American adolescents to reduce loss-of -control eating, Burke et al. (Chapter 45) incorporated a framework that connected loss of control eating to structurally induced pain of exposure to racism and discrimination as opposed to the dominant White framework that eating habits and dieting reflect merit through strength of individual will. In the Netherlands, Peeters et al. (Chapter 31) documented much higher attrition rates among those with an ethnic minority status and have tailored IPT to be more acceptable for diverse populations.

Many authors expanded conceptualization of wellness and connection to be more holistic, extend beyond human attachment, and fit better with local conceptions. For Indigenous populations in both Australia (Reay) and New Zealand (Luty & Nolan), connection to family and community expanded to include connection to land and sea (Australia and New Zealand) and spiritual connection with ancestors or spirits (New Zealand). Luty and Nolan (Chapter 40) provided a tangible example of how IPT could include bringing in or naming objects representative of the earth and sea, describing connection to these elements, and considering how this connection can support relationships with family and community. The authors from different countries reminded us that religions in some communities were an important part of communal activity, for example, shared prayer and adding God to the Interpersonal Inventory among refugees in Malaysia and using the church as a resource in parts of Kenya. In Israel, IPT helped ultra-Orthodox young men function in a secular college.

The title "sick role" was almost universally disliked and thought to be stigmatizing. There was no dispute about the concept behind the sick role, in essence take time and care to recover and get help while symptomatic, but alternative titles were offered. One we liked was "the recovery role," especially as described in the Veterans Administration, where the idea of the veteran having an impairing medical condition did not go over well (Clougherty et al., Chapter 15). Brave Heart et al. and Kidd et al. stressed that given pathologized experiences of underrepresented groups, language like the sick role may be particularly unwelcome. Brave Heart et al. recommended to contextualize distress as part of the historical trauma response. Kidd and colleagues noted that minority stress theory can be applied to externalize distress while supporting agency. Patel et al. gave a practical example of how the cultural formulation interview, which inquires about cultural conceptions of the problem and cultural factors that influence help seeking, could be used to incorporate use of the client's language and meaning within the interpersonal formulation.

The other disliked term was "interpersonal deficits." We had already changed the name of this problem area to "loneliness and social isolation." There is no claim about cause and that this problem area is due to a person's deficits. The problem area is for situations that leave the person with minimal, if any, social contacts and support. It was helpful for practitioners working with veterans in the United States, for example, to assess whether loneliness was present before deployment or resulting from deployment experiences (Clougherty et al., Chapter 15). Isolation can be long term and due to a specific situation like death, moves, or change in status. Suggestions for changing the language of deficits were "interpersonal gaps" and "interpersonal sensitivities."

IMPLEMENTATION OF IPT

Most countries wanted briefer duration of IPT treatment, especially those in low-resource settings. We agree for many settings making efficient use of available resources is imperative. For patients who must find transportation, childcare, manage costs, and overcome other barriers to participation; the desire for briefer interventions also holds true. However, not all places wanted shorter durations. Nepal felt that they needed more time for patients to define the problem, "tell their story," and develop a plan that could be used. They also call IPT a treatment for "distress," not depression, to reduce the stigma of a mental illness. Others, such as those in Israel and Italy, described needing additional sessions to address comorbidities.

The use of professionals trained in psychological treatment—psychiatrists, psychologists, and social workers—has moved to task-shifted care, delivery of mental health services by nonspecialized providers. There was interest and experience in training community health workers (CHWs) in many parts of the world. CHWs included persons with varying levels of education. Careful selection of the trainees and formal training in IPT produced some very favorable results. Task shifting was also covered by new methods of guided and self-guided IPT and by digital online approaches. While these won't cover all needs, they may fill gaps for those who are mildly or moderately distressed.

There was also interest in more training of primary care and family practice doctors in methods of IPT. These professionals often encounter patients who come for a medical problem, but one which is driven by underlying distress and depression. Case examples, such as those from Mozambique and Iran, offer astute examples of how clients present for medical care before psychiatric care.

We are working on a simple, 1-session IPT. This will be mainly a guide on what to cover in 1 session. It may be used for the clinician in primary care or for patients in distress who seek clarification but do not want to enter regular psychotherapy and want to work things out on their own. It might also be useful for patients in remission who have a breakthrough in symptoms. It is too early to tell. IPT may be used as the language that covers these problems and frames a direction of care when the doctor is told in training to "be supportive." Training rarely includes what to cover and what to say during the supportive meeting.

Training in IPT as part of regular graduate programs in psychotherapy (psychiatrist, psychologist, social workers, counselors) would take care of many training needs. However, we learned that, at least in the United States (Flores et al., Chapter 14), this training remains minimal in graduate residency programs and has changed little over the last decade in the United States, except for a new program in the Veterans Administration. However, this is not the case in some countries, which have increased training (e.g., United Kingdom, Switzerland, France, and Finland). There was a real need expressed for certification, and some countries, such as Turkey, have developed their own. The International Society of Interpersonal Psychotherapy (ISIPT) has begun this, and much more is needed. Hopefully, 1-day training and even certification will be handled mainly in the programs that train the professionals, leaving outside training for CHWs or as refreshers or updates as new methods are developed.

We have also seen continued expansion of IPT for treatment of other disorders. In several countries in Africa, IPT/IPC (interpersonal counseling) is being used to treat more comprehensively all common mental disorders, not just depression. In Italy, IPT has been used to treat borderline personality disorder by extending duration of sessions to 10 months with an additional 8-month maintenance phase and offering IPC for family members. Markowitz (Chapter 53) gave an update on the use and testing of IPT for post-traumatic stress disorder, an approach without an exposure component (i.e., describing the traumatic event in detail), among veterans, those experiencing sexual assault, and other populations. Graham and Fitzpatrick (Chapter 33) outlined how IPT has been used across Scotland to treat veterans and teach them about connecting both to people and spaces. They incorporated motivational enhancement to improve engagement and trained veteran peer support workers to deliver the intervention, as these workers carried more credibility with veterans. Given high suicide rates among the veteran population, the specialized veteran program in Scotland adapted IPT to respond to acute self-harm or suicidal crisis (IPT-Acute Crisis) by leveraging social networks, connecting to resources, and engaging in problem-solving. Other settings, such as in Israel, have also adapted IPT for adolescents to address acute and suicidal crises and other comorbidities.

The use of telephones and video for delivery of IPT accelerated during the global pandemic and has been found to be effective and acceptable. While some barriers may be uniquely present for telephone delivery (e.g., lacking privacy or patients needing to multitask for childcare), this mode of therapy can reduce logistical barriers to access. Telehealth may be a permanent feature of delivery. In Germany, Mozambique, and the Netherlands, advances toward digitizing delivery of IPC/IPT have occurred through websites and apps. Some countries added devices to facilitate in-person treatment. For example, China added games and WeChat. StrongMinds in Uganda developed a chatbot (texting communication tool) to provide psychoeducation about depression and help connect people to care. Several settings brought in phones for group members to show pictures while discussing problem areas. Some countries, such as Nepal, used pictures to show how inner feelings might differ from outer expression.

THE FUTURE

We cannot predict the future, but of course will try. With this caveat, we surmise that the move toward continued expansion of the use of lay health workers will increase access to services. While the increase may be partially due to the new onsets of previously treated persons, it will largely come from new and long-needed efforts to treat the underserved not only in the United States and other high-income countries, but also countries where services never before existed.

In many societies, technology has become an integral medium for interpersonal connection and communication. Surely these developments will permeate the training of practitioners, the delivery of treatment, and assessment of outcomes, for both the participant and the provider. In-person office visits, the predominant access mode of training, and treatment will be increasingly administered remotely using cloud-based applications across many different platforms and operating systems with devices, including computers and smartphones to wearable devices and other virtual reality approaches for assessment of outcome. How these deliveries will be assessed for safety and accuracy in many cases will be standard evaluations like clinical trials, and in others, situations will present clear challenges (see Reference 1 for the most recent discussion). What is clear as this book goes to press is that the number of technology-based interventions of psychiatric disorders at the training, treatment, or assessment level are increasing. The scope and possibilities provided by technology are dazzling. However, it is critical to recall that technology is a vehicle to ease the delivery and assessment of content. When used for IPT, the basic contents remain the same, only altered in the extent or detail to meet the particular situation.

COVID-19 has partially helped us to realize that we are globally interconnected and has accelerated efforts to make treatments more accessible. Quarantine and our need to communicate virtually and not in person, facilitated by the increasingly available electronic methods, has brought the world closer in recognition of the importance of attachments. The latter is firmly backed up by research. In 1938, researchers at Harvard set out to learn what makes a person thrive. They recruited 700 participants, including Harvard students and boys from low-income families, following them up with in-depth interviews, surveys, brain scans, and DNA samples every 2 years and in later years. As years went on, they expanded to 3 generations and 1300 descendants of the original group. Reported recently in the *New York Times* "Welcome to the 7-Day Happiness Challenge," Jancee Dunn noted 1 very clear finding emerged for this study. Strong social relationships are what make a happy life more than wealth, IQ, or social class. The strength of our bonds determines whether we feel fulfilled.[2]

Efforts to understand susceptibility are a very different line of psychiatric research. These efforts have moved from success in defining the risks, symptoms, onset, and clinical course of psychiatric disorders, that is its epidemiology, to tackling the mechanism of the disorders through sophisticated research in neuroscience and the available tools of magnetic resonance imaging and electroencephalography. The recent efforts to increase global genetic studies will include more than the US and European populations. In 2023, both the World Psychiatric Association and the Psychiatric Genetic Consortium have accelerated genetic sample collection in Africa. Similar efforts augmented by the electronic communication success of COVID-19 have begun elsewhere. At the same time, "Big Data" has become a new scientific name. Large diverse data sets, with both clinical and biological assessments, are being collected and have become available to scientists all over the world. IPT and other psychotherapies are part of the globalization, as illustrated in this book.

The need for therapist certification through formal institutions, such as the international IPT organization (ISIPT) or several other formats, will increase. It is hoped, the training in IPT will become part of educational programs offering undergraduate and/or graduate counseling degrees. This will ease the need for stand-alone training and should standardize the content and quality of training.

A consistent concern across contributions was the cost of training and supervision. Along with the need for trainers and supervisors fluent in local languages, cost is likely the biggest impediment to scaling up and providing access to care. Johnson highlighted that training and supervision consumed 72% of total implementation costs in prison settings. Law (Chapter 27) described that a barrier to scale-up of IPC-A in Finland was having experienced and knowledgeable supervisors. Settings such as Hong Kong and Japan noted difficulties of having international, often English-speaking, experts leading training and supervision efforts. France and Mozambique provided examples of how building a cadre of national trainers and supervisors could promote scale-up.

Future work must examine scalable, cost-effective solutions that use implementation science methods to better understand and harness organizational processes. From a research perspective, part of this work may explore the minimum effective dose of sessions needed for a reduction in symptoms and maintenance of reduction, given the numerous preferences for briefer versions of IPT. Regarding opportunities for improving policy, cost-effectiveness also needs to consider access to care. Reimbursement for IPT and healthcare coverage emerged as a barrier or facilitator, depending on the context and national level policy. Wesemann and Judge-Ellis in Chapter 51 pointed out how reimbursement for medical treatment is higher than reimbursement for psychotherapy and financial reality affects how nurse practitioners are trained and the treatments they offer (e.g., emphasizing prescription of medications).

While communication has increased, there is little evidence that the rates of distress and suffering from common psychiatric disorders has diminished. Rather, efforts to reach underserved populations have hastened. The need has increased. A recently released report from data collected in 2021 by the Centers for Disease Control in the United States showed that 57% of adolescent girls felt persistently sad or hopeless, 30% had seriously considered attempting suicide, and 18% experienced sexual violence in the past year, all alarming increases from previous surveys.[3] There still will be a need to handle the disabling symptoms of disorders brought on by common situations of stress, grief, disputes, life changes, and loneliness, and great opportunities remain for expansion of care in settings outside of traditional therapeutic ones. For example, some authors have begun implementing IPT in school settings. We should be able to make the simplified and improved evidence-based methods available to the large masses of underserved people globally and consider how the IPT model could be used preventively as standard education teaching the foundational tenets of well-being.

The contributions also highlighted persistent stigma about mental health problems and the need to combat it. More public health efforts and campaigns are needed to provide awareness to populations of mental health problems and how to seek help. These messages could be integrated into other public health programming, such as HIV, maternal/child health, and more. Authors working with special populations, such as those living with HIV, noted additional layers of stigma for medical problems or discriminated against sexual and gender minority statuses. Some settings (e.g., Ethiopia, Kenya, Scotland) gave examples of rolling out educational antistigma messages and recovery videos as a part of the dissemination of IPT. As scale-up and dissemination of IPT continues to happen, incorporating antistigma information that provides facts and normalizes mental health challenges will be critical.

There is so much new in IPT in the expansion into new countries and populations and new adaptations. This book has captured an exciting point in time but not the endpoint, and the good news is that it will be outdated by the time it is published. IPT is at least one, among many other methods, to repair human fractures in attachments. We are hopeful that the realization of our common humanity and need for attachments in many forms will continue to grow.

REFERENCES

1. Harvey PD, Depp CA, Rizzo AA, et al. Technology and mental health: state of the art for assessment and treatment. *Am J Psychiatry*. 2022;179(12):897–914.
2. Waldinger R, Schulz M. *The Good Life: Lessons From the World's Longest Study on Happiness*. Ebury Publishing; 2023.
3. Centers for Disease Control and Prevention. US teen girls experiencing increased sadness and violence. February 23, 2023. Accessed February 26, 2023. https://www.cdc.gov/nchhstp/newsroom/2023/increased-sadness-and-violence-press-release.html

For the benefit of digital users, indexed terms that span two pages (e.g., 52–53) may, on occasion, appear on only one of those pages.

Tables and figures are indicated by *t* and *f* following the page number